IAP Specialty Series on
Rational Antimicrobial Practice in Pediatrics

IAP Specialty Series on
Rational Antimicrobial Practice in Pediatrics

Third Edition

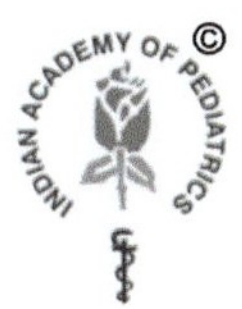

Editor-in-Chief

Tanu Singhal MD MSc Dip LSHTM
Consultant Pediatrics and Infectious Diseases
Kokilaben Dhirubhai Ambani Hospital and Medical Research Institute
Mumbai, Maharashtra, India

Founder Editor

Nitin Shah

Editors

Nitin Shah MD DCH
Section Coordinator
Department of Pediatrics
PD Hinduja National Hospital and Research Centre
Honorary Hematologist Medical Oncologist
BJ Wadia Hospital for Children
Mumbai, Maharashtra, India

Suhas Prabhu MD DCH MNAMS
Consultant Pediatrician
PD Hinduja National Hospital and Medical Research Centre
Mumbai, Maharashtra, India

Vijay Yewale MD DCH FIAP
Head
Department of Pediatrics Institute of Child Health
Apollo Hospitals and Dr Yewale Multispecialty Hospital for Children
Navi Mumbai, Maharashtra, India

Forewords

Digant D Shastri
Santosh T Soans

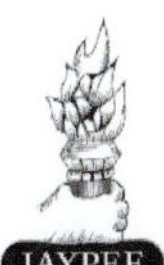

JAYPEE BROTHERS MEDICAL PUBLISHERS
The Health Sciences Publisher
New Delhi | London

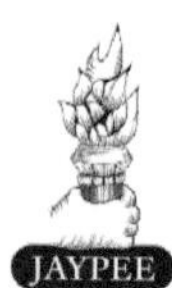

Jaypee Brothers Medical Publishers (P) Ltd

Headquarters
EMCA House
23/23-B, Ansari Road, Daryaganj
New Delhi 110 002, India
Landline: +91-11-23272143,
+91-11-23272703
+91-11-23282021, +91-11-23245672
E-mail: jaypee@jaypeebrothers.com

Corporate Office
Jaypee Brothers Medical Publishers (P) Ltd.
4838/24, Ansari Road, Daryaganj
New Delhi 110 002, India
Phone: +91-11-43574357
Fax: +91-11-43574314
E-mail: jaypee@jaypeebrothers.com

Overseas Offices
J.P. Medical Ltd
83 Victoria Street, London
SW1H 0HW (UK)
Phone: +44 20 3170 8910
Email: info@jpmedpub.com

EU GPSR Authorised Representative
Logos Europe, 9 rue Nicolas Poussin
17000, La Rochelle, France
Phone: +33 (0) 6 67 93 73 78
E-mail: Contact@logoseurope.eu

Website: www.jaypeebrothers.com
Website: www.jaypeedigital.com

IAP Specialty Series on Rational Antimicrobial Practice in Pediatrics

First Edition: 2006

Second Edition: 2013

Third Edition: 2019, Reprint: 2025, **2026**

ISBN 978-93-5270-706-5

Printed in India

Dedicated to

Our families who have patiently borne
Our devotion to and time away from them for this project
and
To all children, whose healthy smiles make it all worthwhile

Contributors

Abhay Shah MD D Ped FIAP
Senior Consultant Pediatrician
Children Hospital
Ahmedabad, Gujarat, India

Ambreen A Pandrowala DNB Fellowship in Infectious Diseases and Immunology (RCPCH)
Consultant
Department of Infectious Diseases and Immunology
SRCC Children's Hospital Managed by Narayana Health
Mumbai, Maharashtra, India

Anjali Shetty MRCP FRCPATH
Consultant Microbiologist
PD Hinduja National Hospital and Medical Research Centre
Mumbai, Maharashtra, India

Ashok Kapse MD
Consultant Pediatrician
Kapse Children Hospital
Surat, Gujarat, India

Atul Kulkarni MD
Assistant Professor
Department of Pediatrics
Ashwini Medical College
Solapur, Maharashtra, India

Ayesha J Sunavala DNB FNB
Consultant Infectious Diseases
PD Hinduja National Hospital and Medical Research Centre
Mumbai, Maharashtra, India

Baldev S Prajapati MD D Ped FIAP MNAMS FICMCH
Head and Professor
Department of Pediatrics
GCS Medical College, Hospital and Research Centre
Ahmedabad, Gujarat, India

Camilla Rodrigues MD
Consultant Microbiologist
PD Hinduja National Hospital and Medical Research Centre
Mumbai, Maharashtra, India

Deepak Karpe MD DNB
Consultant Pediatrician
Siddhivinayak Hospital
Ahmednagar, Maharashtra, India

Dhanya Dharmapalan MD PG Dip PID (Oxford)
Consultant Pediatric Infectious Diseases
Institute of Child Health
Kolkata, West Bengal, India
Apollo Hospitals
Navi Mumbai, Maharashtra, India

Digant Shastri MD PGDHHM
Consultant Senior Pediatrician
Killol Children Hospital
Surat, Gujarat, India

Faria H Farooqi MD
Department of Microbiology
Maulana Azad Medical College
New Delhi, India

Gaurav Patwardhan MD DNB
Consultant Neonatologist
KEM Hospital
Pune, Maharashtra, India

Indu Khosla MD
Consultant Pediatrician and Pulmonologist
Cloudnine Hospital
Mumbai, Maharashtra, India

Ira Shah MD DNB FCPS DCH DPID (UK)
Professor (Addl) Pediatrics and Head
Pediatric Infectious Diseases and Head
Pediatric GI, Hepatology
In-charge
Pediatric HIV, TB, Liver Clinics
BJ Wadia Hospital for Children
Consultant
Pediatric Infectious Diseases (PID) and Hepatology
Nanavati Hospital
Mumbai, Maharashtra, India

Jaideep A Gogtay MD
Global Medical Officer
Cipla Limited
Mumbai, Maharashtra, India

Jaydeep Choudhury DNB MNAMS FIAP
Associate Professor
Department of Pediatrics
Institute of Child Health
Kolkata, West Bengal, India

Jeeson Unni MD DCH FIAP
Consultant Pediatrician
Aster Medcity Hospital
Kochi, Kerala, India

Ketan Kumar MD
Senior Resident
Department of Pediatrics
All India Institute of Medical Sciences
New Delhi, India

Krishnendu Mondal MBBS
Senior Resident
Department of Pediatrics
Institute of Child Health
Kolkata, West Bengal, India

Madhumita Panda DCH
Director
Medical Affairs
Cipla Limited
Mumbai, Maharashtra, India

Mahesh S Kore MD
Consultant Pediatrician
Shree Hospital
Belgaum, Karnataka, India

MR Lokeshwar MD DCH
Consultant Pediatrician and Pediatric
Hematologist Oncologist
Lilavati Hospital, Mumbai
Former Head
Division of Pediatric Hematology
Oncology and
Outdoor Thalassemia Transfusion Center
LTM Medical College and LTMG
General Hospital
Mumbai, Maharashtra, India

Neha Gupta MD FNB
Consultant
Department of Infectious Diseases
Medanta—The Medicity
Gurugram, Haryana, India

Nigam Prakash Narain MD DCH PhD
MRCP (UK) FRCPCH (UK) FIAP FNNF
Professor and Head (Retd)
Department of Pediatrics
Patna Medical College and Hospital
Patna, Bihar, India

Niranjan Shendurnikar MD
Consultant Pediatrician
Ankur Maternity Hospital
Vadodara, Gujarat, India

Nitin Shah MD DCH
Section Coordinator
Department of Pediatrics
PD Hinduja National Hospital and Medical
Research Centre
Honorary Hematologist, Oncologist
BJ Wadia Hospital for Children
Mumbai, Maharashtra, India

Nupur Ganguly DCH DNB FIAP
Associate Professor
Department of Pediatrics
Institute of Child Health
Kolkata, West Bengal, India

Pallavi Bhargava MD
Senior Staff
Infectious Diseases Division
Henry Ford Health System
Detroit, MI, USA

Pankaj Deshpande MD DCH FCPS MRCP (UK)
Consultant Pediatric Nephrologist
PD Hinduja National Hospital and Medical Research
Centre, Mumbai
Institute of Child Health, Kolkata, West Bengal
Apollo Hospitals
Navi Mumbai, Maharashtra, India

Pramod Kulkarni MD MRCPCH Dip PID
Consultant Pediatric Infectious Diseases
KEM Hospital
Pune, Maharashtra, India

Pratima Shah MD DPed
Consultant Pediatrician
Ankur Institute of Child Health
Ahmedabad, Gujarat, India

Prawin Kumar MD
Associate Professor
Department of Pediatrics
All India Institute of Medical Sciences
Jodhpur, Rajasthan, India

Rajal B Prajapati MD D Ped
Professor
Department of Pediatrics
Sheth VS General Hospital
AMC MET Medical College
Ahmedabad, Gujarat, India

Rajeev Soman MD FIDSA
Consultant
Department of Internal Medicine and Infectious Diseases
Jupiter Hospital, Pune
PD Hinduja Hospital and Medical Research Centre
Mumbai, Maharashtra, India
Bharti Vidyapeeth Hospital, Pune
Dinanath Mangeshkar Hospital
Pune, Maharashtra, India

Raju C Shah MD D Ped FIAP FRCPCH (UK)
Consultant Pediatrician
Ankur Institute of Child Health
Ahmedabad, Gujarat, India

Rakesh Lodha MD
Professor
Department of Pediatrics
All India Institute of Medical Sciences
New Delhi, India

Ranjit Sah MD
Fellow
Department of Infectious Diseases
Medanta—The Medicity
Gurugram, Haryana, India

Ritabrata Kundu MD
Professor
Department of Pediatrics
Institute of Child Health
Kolkata, West Bengal, India

S Balasubramaniam MD DCH MNAMS FIAP FRCPCH (UK)
Senior Consultant Pediatrician
Kanchi Kamakoti CHILD Trust Hospital
Chennai, Tamil Nadu, India

Shilpa Kalane MD DNB
Consultant Neonatologist
Deenanath Mangeshkar Hospital
Pune, Maharashtra, India

Shinjini Bhatnagar MD PhD
Dean
Department of Clinical Research
Translational Health Science and Technology Institute
Faridabad, Haryana, India

Simantini Jog MD FRCPATH
Consultant Microbiologist
Queen Elizabeth Hospital Birmingham
Birmingham, UK

Soni Chawla B Tech Dip (Clinical Research)
Clinical Research Coordinator
Medanta—The Medicity
Gurugram, Haryana, India

Soonu Udani MD DAB (Peds) DAB (Neonatology)
Medical Director and Head
Department of Critical Care and Emergency Services
SRCC Children's Hospital Managed by Narayana Health
Mumbai, Maharashtra, India

Suchi Acharya MD
Senior Resident
Department of Pediatrics
Institute of Child Health
Kolkata, West Bengal, India

Sudhir Sane MD DCH
Director
Department of Pediatrics
Jupiter Hospital
Thane, Maharashtra, India

Suhas Prabhu MD DCH MNAMS
Consultant Pediatrician
PD Hinduja National Hospital and Medical Research Centre
Mumbai, Maharashtra, India

Sujata Rege DNB Fellowship (Infectious Disease)
Fellow
Department of Infectious Diseases
Jupiter Hospital
Pune, Maharashtra, India

Sumanth Amperayani DCH DNB
Senior Registrar Pediatrics
Kanchi Kamakoti CHILD Trust Hospital
Chennai, Tamil Nadu, India

Sushil Kabra MD
Professor
Department of Pediatrics
All India Institute of Medical Sciences
New Delhi, India

Tanu Singhal MD MSc Dip LSHTM
Consultant Pediatrics and Infectious Diseases
Kokilaben Dhirubhai Ambani Hospital and Medical Research Institute
Mumbai, Maharashtra, India

Tanushri Mukherjee DNB DCH Fellowship (Neonatology)
Consultant Pediatrician and Neonatologist
Cloudnine Hospital
Mumbai, Maharashtra, India

Umesh Vaidya MD DNB
Chief Neonatologist
KEM Hospital, Pune
Regional Medical Director
Cloudnine Hospital
Pune, Maharashtra, India

Varinder Singh MD
Director Professor
Department of Pediatrics
Lady Hardinge Medical College and
Associated Kalawati Saran Children's Hospital
New Delhi, India

Vijaya Kumar MD
Senior Resident
Department of Pediatrics
All India Institute of Medical Sciences
New Delhi, India

Vijay Yewale MD DCH FIAP
Head, Department of Pediatrics
Institute of Child Health
Apollo Hospitals and
Dr Yewale Multispecialty Hospital for Children
Navi Mumbai, Maharashtra, India

Vikas Manchanda MD MBA
Head, Department of Microbiology
Maulana Azad Medical College
New Delhi, India

Vishrutha Karkera MD
Fellow, Department of Pediatrics
BJ Wadia Hospital for Children
Mumbai, Maharashtra, India

Vivek Kak MD FACP
Clinical Assistant Professor
Department of Medicine
Program Director
Internal Medicine Program
Henry Ford Allegiance Health
Detroit, MI, USA

Vrajesh Udani MD DAB
Consultant Pediatric Neurologist
Department of Child Neurology and Clinical Neurophysiology
PD Hinduja National Hospital and
Medical Research Institute
Mumbai, Maharashtra, India

Winsley Rose MD MSc Fellowship PID
Consultant
Department of Pediatric Infectious Diseases
Christian Medical College
Vellore, Tamil Nadu, India

YK Amdekar MD DCH
Former Professor of Pediatrics
Grant Medical College
Honorary Pediatrician JJ Hospital
Mumbai, Maharashtra, India

Foreword

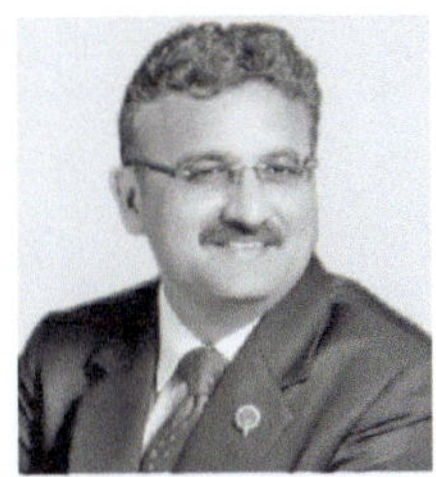

It is a proud privilege for me to write the foreword for the third edition of *IAP Specialty Series on Rational Antimicrobial Practice in Pediatrics*.

Antibiotics are one of the most significant therapeutic reserves of the medical history. Proper selection of antibiotics is a multifaceted process that requires careful clinical judgment, but unfortunately, selection and the use of antibiotics is made lightly without regard to the therapeutic features of the drug and to the infecting microorganisms. The wide use of antibiotics has been associated with increasing antimicrobial resistance, both in the community and hospital settings. Patient care is threatened by treatment failures arising from infection of organisms leading to morbidity and potential mortality. The treatment of these infections is hampered by the lack of efficacious antibiotics, especially for multiresistant gram negative organisms like *Acinetobacter* and *Pseudomonas aeruginosa*. Furthermore, widespread abuse and overuse of antibiotics result in potential drug toxicities leading to increased complications as well as increased healthcare costs.

Looking to the magnitude of problem of irrational antibiotic therapy by doctors, the 1st edition of *IAP Specialty Series on Rational Antimicrobial Practice in Pediatrics* was published in 2006 and within a short span it has become popular amongst readers. Hence, the need for the revised edition arose. Considering this, IAP has come out with the 3rd edition of this book.

In the current publication, all important aspects of rational antibiotic therapy for various pediatric infections are being addressed very diligently through four core sections with section one having details of various antimicrobial agents and chapters on Antimicrobial Resistance and Basics of microbiologic diagnosis, second section having rational management of various infections, while the third section deals with illustrative cases depicting rational antimicrobial therapy and last section having an antimicrobial formulary.

My sincere compliments and congratulations to all the authors who as a part of their sincere efforts to disseminate the knowledge, have contributed chapters for this prestigious publication. I congratulate the entire editorial board Dr Tanu Singhal, Dr Nitin Shah, Dr Vijay Yewale and Dr Suhas Prabhu for their untiring efforts in bringing out the 3rd edition.

I am sure that this new edition of textbook will be as popular as the previous editions amongst the postgraduate students, teaching faculties as well as practicing pediatricians. I wish this landmark publication great success and wish it will contribute in the minimizing menace of misuse/abuse of antimicrobials.

Digant D Shastri
President
Indian Academy of Pediatrics—2019

Foreword

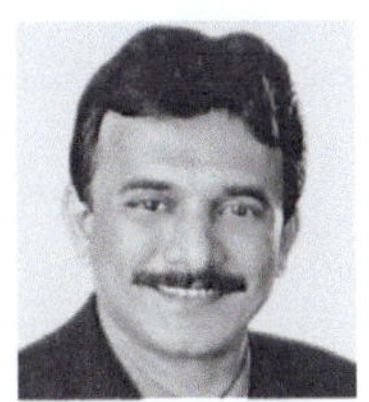

I am delighted to know that *IAP Specialty Series on Rational Antimicrobial Practice in Pediatrics* have been compiled under the editorial stewardship of Dr Tanu Singhal with four different sections and an astonishing 40 chapters contributed by many eminent pediatricians and infectious disease specialists. This is a remarkable and commendable achievement. I am astonished that they have brought out this edition in record time. I wish to congratulate all colleagues involved in this monumental effort.

Rational antibiotic use requires accurate diagnosis and appropriate antibiotic use. Antibiotics have radically improved the prognosis of infectious diseases. Infections that were almost invariably fatal are now almost always curable if treatment is started early. Antibiotics are among our most valuable resources, but their use is threatened by the emergence of resistant strains of bacteria. Physicians need to use antibiotics wisely and responsibly. This means that when deciding which antibiotic to use, we need to consider the likelihood that an antibiotic will induce resistance, as well as traditional evidence-based comparisons of efficacy.

The new edition includes new chapters on antimicrobial resistance, basics of antimicrobial therapy, including escalation and de-escalation, new drugs in the pipeline, intra-abdominal infections and infective endocarditis. All chapters have been written and revised by well-known academicians and an effort has been made to include relevant latest information and guidelines. It is hoped that this book will be a useful resource for postgraduates and practicing pediatricians alike.

I wish the reader an enlightening academic experience. I am sure this book is going to be valued by IAPians and hope to see the next edition in due course.

Santosh T Soans
President
Indian Academy of Pediatrics—2018

Preface

Infections are an important cause of pediatric morbidity and mortality and antimicrobial therapy is an integral part of their treatment. If practiced incorrectly, it can lead to treatment failure, adverse effects as well as antimicrobial resistance. Though several textbooks on the same subject are available, a need was felt to bring out a compendium that discusses these issues in the context of Indian epidemiology.

The previous editions released in 2006 and 2013 were well received. However, antimicrobial therapy is a dynamic subject. There is evolution of antimicrobial resistance; at the same time new drugs are approved and marketed. Several such events have occurred in the past few years. Possibly the most dramatic are increase in penicillin and cephalosporin resistance in meningeal isolates of *S. pneumoniae* as well spiraling carbapenem resistance in gram-negative bacteria. Similarly, certain infections of clinical importance, including intra-abdominal infections, infective endocarditis, brucellosis and rickettsial disease were missing from earlier editions. There was also a need felt to discuss in greater detail the practice of rational antimicrobial therapy. To address all these issues, it was considered necessary to bring out a revised edition.

It gives us great pleasure in presenting the 3rd edition of this book. New chapters have been added and all the previous chapters have been revised and have some change or the other. We hope that this book is useful to practicing pediatricians and postgraduates not only in India but also in South Asia. If this book helps even a little bit in stemming the rise of the antimicrobial resistance monster and improves clinical outcomes in children with infections, the efforts of the contributors and editors will be considered worthwhile.

Tanu Singhal
Nitin Shah
Suhas Prabhu
Vijay Yewale

Contents

SECTION I: BASICS OF MICROBIOLOGY AND PHARMACOLOGY

Rational Antimicrobial Therapy: Need of the Hour

1 Chapter

Tanu Singhal

INTRODUCTION

Rational antimicrobial practice or antimicrobial stewardship implies the use of antimicrobials only when indicated and choosing the right agent in the right dose through the right route for the right duration. Rational antimicrobial choices need to be exercised for both empirical and definitive therapy, the former being more challenging. The hazards of irrational antimicrobial therapy cannot be understated and include:

- Poor clinical outcomes: There is enough evidence supporting the use of the right antimicrobial for a particular infection/pathogen. The supposedly higher antimicrobial may not always be the best one. A salient example is inferior outcomes with vancomycin for methicillin sensitive *Staphylococcus aureus* (MSSA) infections as compared to cloxacillin/first-generation cephalosporins. Choosing the wrong empiric therapy for a serious multidrug-resistant healthcare-associated infection (HAI) is associated with increased morbidity and mortality.
- Increased cost of therapy/drug adverse effects. Using antibiotics when not indicated, multiple antibiotics, broad-spectrum antibiotics for longer than necessary can greatly increase cost of therapy especially in today's era where antimicrobials are highly priced. With this there is also an increased risk of serious adverse events some of which include allergy, nephrotoxicity/hepatoxicity and *Clostridium difficile* infection.
- Increase in antimicrobial resistance. Irrational use of antimicrobials is the biggest driver for antimicrobial resistance owing to selection of resistance strains. This compromises future antimicrobial options for the individual and the community. Antimicrobial resistance which is estimated to cause 700,000 annual deaths presently is projected to cause 10 million annual deaths in 2050.

EXAMPLES OF IRRATIONAL THERAPY

- Prescribing antimicrobials when not indicated. For example, using antibiotics to treat viral upper respiratory tract infections/viral gastroenteritis or treating colonization in critically sick patients.
- Prescribing multiple antimicrobials at the same time using irrational combinations, changing antimicrobials frequently and in case of nonresponse adding rather than substituting drugs.
- Using carbapenems routinely to treat community acquired infections and using drugs for MRSA, such as vancomycin when not indicated.
- Failure to de-escalate to lower antimicrobials after receiving culture reports.

- Using inappropriate empiric therapy for certain serious health care and community acquired infections which are likely multidrug resistant. Here using incorrect empiric therapy is associated with poor outcomes and increased morbidity and mortality.
- Using fewer drugs than indicated for diseases, such as tuberculosis, HIV, falciparum malaria, and serious carbapenem-resistant gram-negative infections.

REASONS FOR IRRATIONAL THERAPY

- Practitioner errors owing to inadequate knowledge about microbial etiology and resistance patterns. Other reasons are fear of missing a diagnosis in order to circumvent investigations and sometimes due to pressure from parents/patients. The belief that newer drugs and multiple drugs are better also drives practitioners to overuse antimicrobials.
- Self-medication by parents and as per pharmacist's recommendations.
- Aggressive and incorrect marketing of antimicrobials by representatives of pharmaceutical companies.
- Ready availability of antimicrobials over-the-counter and licensing of irrational fixed drug combinations.

SOLUTIONS TO PROMOTE RATIONAL ANTIMICROBIAL THERAPY

This involves all stakeholders including the government, pharmaceutical industry, healthcare professionals, and the public and includes:

- Education of medical practitioners about rational antimicrobial practices right from the undergraduate level through postgraduation and practicing doctors.
- Development of evidence-based guidelines to treat common infections and ensuring that they are implemented.
- Educating the public and parents about the hazards of overuse of antibiotics.
- Preventing overuse of antimicrobials in the veterinary industry.
- Legislation to prevent over-the-counter availability of antimicrobials and banning irrational fixed drug combinations.
- Establishing antimicrobial stewardship programs in hospitals.

CONCLUSION

We are facing an "antimicrobial resistance" crises. We are running out of treatment options and not many new drugs are in the pipeline. If we do not use our existing antimicrobials wisely we are destined to return to the preantibiotic era of untreatable infections.

RECOMMENDED READING

1. Ghafur A, Mathai D, Muruganathan A, et al. The Chennai Declaration: a roadmap to tackle the challenge of antimicrobial resistance. Indian J Cancer. 2013;50:71-81.

Basics of Microbiologic Diagnosis

2
Chapter

Anjali Shetty, Simantini Jog, Camilla Rodrigues

INTRODUCTION

Microbiogic diagnosis of infectious disease rests on four basic pillars, viz. smear examination, serology, cultures, and molecular methods.

SMEAR

This is the fastest method to diagnose infection particularly in a sample from a sterile site, e.g. cerebrospinal fluid (CSF), pus, tissue, etc. Salient examples include acid fast bacilli in sputum in tuberculosis, malarial parasite on blood smears, lanceolate gram-positive diplococci suggestive of *Pneumococcus* in sputum/CSF samples, and broad and aseptate right-angle branching hyphae on fluorescent microscopy using calcofluor stain suggestive of Mucorales.

SEROLOGY

These methods include detection of antibodies and antigen. Various methods are available but the common ones are immunochromatographic rapid assays, latex agglutination tests, and enzyme-linked immunosorbent assay (ELISA). Detection of antigen is more reliable than detection of antibody. Common antigen detection tests used in clinical practice include dengue NS1 antigen, malarial antigen, cryptococcal antigen in serum and CSF, latex agglutination test for pneumococcus, hemophilus influenzae, *Meningococcus* in CSF, rotavirus antigen in stool, p24 antigen of human immunodeficiency virus (HIV), surface antigen of hepatitis B virus, filarial antigen, clostridium difficile glutamate dehydrogenase (GDH) and toxin test in stool, and beta-D-glucan/galactomannan in serum/urine histoplasma antigen for diagnosis of invasive fungal infections. Detection of antibodies is limited by poor sensitivity due to the lag time in production and poor specificity owing to past infection or cross reactivity with other pathogens. Commonly used antibody tests in clinical practice include the Widal test/Typhidot immunoglobulin M (IgM) for enteric fever (with its attendant problems), dengue IgG and IgM, leptospira IgM, IgM for scrub typhus and spotted fever, mycoplasma IgM, IgM antibodies for various viral illnesses; including measles, mumps, rubella, varicella, Epstein-Barr virus-viral capsid antigen (EBV–VCA) IgM, parvovirus, hepatitis viruses (hepatitis A, B, C, and E), HIV, *Brucella*, kala-azar, hydatid disease, and *Entamoeba histolytica* liver abscess among others. Toxoplasmosis, rubella, cytomegalovirus, and herpes simplex (TORCH) serology is a commonly performed test, but difficult to interpret and can often be misleading. Serologic tests of no value include the slide Widal, Weil-Felix test, and tuberculosis (TB) IgG and IgM.

MOLECULAR TESTS

These tests have revolutionized microbiology. They are rapid and can be used to detect almost any pathogen. In the past these tests required specialized labs with highly trained staff. Conventionally, molecular tests have been used to diagnose viral infections including HIV, hepatitis B virus (HBV), hepatitis C virus (HCV), *Cytomegalovirus* (CMV) including quantitative estimation, HSV, and influenza. The current tests which are cartridge-based nucleic acid amplification tests (CBNAAT), such as GeneXpert [TB, clostridium difficile, Methicillin-resistant *Staphylococcus Aureus* (MRSA), influenza, etc.] are so simple and require no skill and can be used as point of care tests. We are moving towards the era of syndromic diagnosis with multiplex polymerase chain reaction (PCR) kits like the FILMARRAY® that integrates sample preparation, amplification, detection, and analysis. It requires just a few minutes of hands-on-time and its turnaround time is just about an hour, giving faster results which may lead to better patient care. This syndromic diagnosis is available for respiratory, central nervous system (CNS) and gastrointestinal infections, sepsis, and even tropical fevers (dengue, leptospira, chikungunya). Advanced molecular techniques including deoxyribonucleic acid (DNA) sequencing, ribonucleic acid (RNA)-based sequencing also allow for direct detection of pathogens from specimens when other tests have proved nonrewarding. Molecular tests are also indispensable for diagnosis of emerging pathogens (Zika, Nipah, etc.).

CULTURE

This is the gold standard test in microbiology. However it is time consuming taking up to 6 weeks for mycobacteria and 4 weeks for fungi. Sensitivity is compromised if antimicrobials have been given before cultures and if the organism is fastidious (mycoplasma, lepra bacillus, etc. many viruses). The rest of the chapter discusses cultures, identification of pathogens and susceptibility testing in detail.

Types of Culture

Blood Culture

Automated methods from BD (BACTEC) and Biomerieux (BACT/Alert) have replaced conventional methods in most centers. The advantages of these systems is better recovery since the quality of the media is good and faster diagnosis. These systems depend on automated detection of CO_2 produced by bacterial growth. So if the culture flags positive, a smear can be made from the bottle which will show the pathogen. These can then be further processed. These systems offer aerobic, anaerobic, fungal, mycobacterial, and for patients on antibiotics even resin/charcoal laden bottles. One set of culture includes one aerobic and one anaerobic bottle. For optimum sensitivity adequate amount of blood should be cultured. The sensitivity of one set is 66%, two sets is 85%, and three sets is more than 95%. Preferably two and at least one set should be collected for culture. Sending more sets also helps in differentiating contamination from true infection since in contamination all bottles will not grow the pathogen.

The ideal volume of blood for culture in adults and adolescents is around 30–40 mL (10 mL in each of four bottles containing 40 mL of media), but in younger children it is 1% of circulating blood volume. So a 10 kg child who has blood volume of 800 mL (80 mL/kg) should have 8 mL drawn on culture. Each pediatric culture bottle has 20 mL of media so 4 mL can be inoculated in two bottles. The blood media ratio should be 1:5. Inoculating more blood in one bottle leads to under recovery because of inhibitory substances present in blood. The logic of putting in an anaerobic bottle is not so much for anaerobic organisms, but for better growth of streptococci and enterobacteriaceae which are facultative anaerobes. In newborns due to high levels of bacteremia even 0.5–1 mL of blood is enough. If a patient has a central line then cultures from both the central line (all lumens) and the peripheral venipuncture should be collected at the same time. If the central line culture flags earlier than 120 minutes as compared to the peripheral line, central line may be the focus of infection. While collecting the blood specimen the skin should be cleaned three times with 2% alcoholic chlorhexidine to reduce risk of contamination. The needle need not be changed while inoculating the blood in the bottle to reduce the risk of needle stick injury. If fungal or mycobacterial infection is suspected then special bottles should be used (e.g. Myco/F Lytic). If patient is on antibiotics then media containing resin/charcoal may be used to increase recovery (BACTEC-resin). If the bottle cannot be transported to the lab it should be kept at room temperature or better still at 37°C. It should never be refrigerated. Other sterile site samples including pus and CSF can also be inoculated in blood culture bottles to enhance recovery.

Urine Culture

Contamination of urine by commensal flora adjacent to the urethra is common and unfortunately these organisms are also responsible for true infection. Scrupulous care whilst collecting the sample is important. Patients and staff should be clearly instructed on the procedure for urine collection and the importance of sterile containers should be stressed. In older children it can be a midstream specimen obtained after cleaning the genital area with saline/soap and water and then discarding the first few drops. In smaller children it can be a clean catch sample. If the same is not possible and there is an urgency to start antibiotics then it can be through suprapubic aspiration or one time catheterization. Urine should be cultured with minimal delay, ideally within an hour of collection. Refrigeration at 4°C is required where there is a delay in transport. When collecting urine from catheters it is important to collect from the port and not the bag.

The reports should be interpreted carefully. Multiple organisms usually indicate contamination. A significant colony count is at least 105 organisms/mL of a mid-stream sample, 104 for a sample obtained from a catheter, and any organism from suprapubic puncture. Even if the colony count is significant but there is no pyuria, it may not be a urinary tract infection (UTI) but asymptomatic bacteruria.

Pus/Tissue/Cerebrospinal Fluid/Sterile Body Fluids

Pus or tissue is preferable to a swab. Such samples should be discussed with the microbiologist prior to sending so that the appropriate tests may be requested, adequate volumes of sample may be sent and maximum attention is given to the specimen. Such a discussion will help the microbiologist interpret the culture result appropriately. Samples should be transported in sterile containers at room temperature.

Other Nonsterile Site Cultures

These include tracheal, sputum, wound swab, stool, central line tip, and drain cultures. Nonsterile site samples should be sent only if there is a clinical indication and not as surveillance cultures and if sterile site samples cannot be obtained. Positive results should be interpreted with caution since they may indicate only colonization.

IDENTIFICATION OF PATHOGENS

This can be done manually by biochemical tests. Some of these are rapid giving instantaneous results (e.g. catalase and oxidase) while others need overnight incubation (e.g. esculin hydrolysis). Automated instruments, such as BD Phoenix and Vitek 2 will identify these organisms to species level by using biochemical tests. This usually takes 8–10 hours. Matrix-assisted laser desorption and ionization-time of flight (MALDI-TOF) is a mass spectrometer that identifies organisms (bacteria and fungi) with minutes. Molecular methods are also now used to quickly identify pathogens from cultures and are commonly used for classification of nontuberculous mycobacteria and common gram-positive/gram-negative and fungal pathogens from blood cultures [FILMARRAY® blood culture identification (BCID) panel].

Salmonella and *Staphylococcus* are the easiest to grow while *Hemophilus influenzae* type b (Hib) and *Pneumococcus* are the most fastidious. Hib and *Pneumococcus* are unlikely to grow if the patient is on antibiotics or if sheep's blood has not been used for conventional media preparation, or if the sample has not been incubated appropriately. This is primarily the reason for under diagnosis of invasive Hib and pneumococcal disease. Certain organisms, such as coagulase-negative staphylococcus and diphtheroids are skin commensals and their isolation usually indicates contamination during blood collection. Though isolation of gram-negative bacteria is almost always a true infection, there have been cases of pseudobacteremia due to contamination with the antiseptic (*Pseudomonas* and *Burkholderia cepacia*) or during lab processing. Hence a culture should always be viewed in light of the clinical condition of the patient. Similarly positive central line cultures with negative peripheral cultures may indicate only colonization of the catheter and not true infection.

ANTIMICROBIAL SUSCEPTIBILITY TESTING

One of the principal functions of a clinical microbiology laboratory is to carry out antimicrobial sensitivity testing (AST) which helps to guide the clinician in management of various infectious diseases. With the worldwide development and spread of antimicrobial resistance, treatment options are increasingly limited to newer expensive antimicrobial agents. Hence, the laboratory must give high priority to well standardized in vitro antimicrobial susceptibility tests which generate reliable data. The main objectives of susceptibility testing are:

- To perform susceptibility testing for pathogens for which well standardized methods are available.
- To guide the clinician in the selection of the most appropriate antimicrobial agent for that particular clinical situation. The report should also provide the clinician with alternative agents to which the organism is susceptible.
- To perform quantitative measurement of the sensitivity of pathogens with direct therapeutic relevance, e.g. penicillin minimum inhibitory concentrations (MICs) for *Streptococcus pneumoniae*, MIC's of beta-lactamase inhibitor combinations and carbapenems for gram-negative pathogens.
- Various determining factors need to be kept in mind when performing AST on bacterial isolates. For example, in case normal flora is isolated, sensitivity should not be done as it only leads to further discrepancies between in vitro testing and clinical outcome. Also, when organisms have a predictable susceptibility, e.g. *Streptococcus pyogenes*, additional susceptibility testing need not be done.

Interpretation Results of Susceptibility Testing

Susceptible

There is a high probability that the patient will respond to treatment with the appropriate dosage of that antimicrobial agent.

Resistant

Treatment with the antimicrobial agent is likely to fail.

Intermediate

With the agents that can be safely administered at higher doses, this category implies that higher doses may be required to ensure efficacy or that the agent may prove efficacious if it is normally concentrated in an infected body fluid, e.g. urine. For body compartments where drug penetration is restricted even in the presence of inflammation, e.g. CSF, it suggests that extreme caution should be taken in the use of the agent. Thus, this category represents a "buffer" zone that prevents strains with borderline susceptibility from being incorrectly categorized as resistant.

Evaluation of Susceptibility Tests

The following convention is used to evaluate susceptibility tests:

- *Very major error*: Characterization of a resistant isolate as susceptible.
- *Major error*: Characterization of a susceptible isolate as resistant.
- *Minor error*: Characterization of a susceptible or resistant isolate as intermediate or characterization of an intermediate isolate as susceptible or resistant.

Antimicrobial Susceptibility Testing Methods

- Disk diffusion
- Automated instrument methods
- Antibiotic gradient methods
- Dilution methods (agar and broth dilution and macrobroth and microbroth dilution).

The laboratories worldwide adhere to standardized protocols in order to achieve reproducible results. Clinical and Lab Standards Institute (CLSI) [formerly National Committee for Clinical Laboratory Standards (NCCLS)] is one such organization in USA that publishes standards for susceptibility testing on a continuing basis. European Committee on Antimicrobial Susceptibility Testing (EUCAST) is a similar organization in Europe. It is also important that revised procedures and current recommendations be promptly followed by all clinical laboratories. These standards provide clinical breakpoints to interpret susceptibility tests. Breakpoints are discriminatory antimicrobial concentrations used in the interpretation of results of susceptibility testing to define isolates as susceptible, intermediate or resistant. There are two breakpoints; susceptibility (S) breakpoint and resistance (R) breakpoint. Clinical, pharmacological, microbiological, and pharmacodynamic considerations are important in setting breakpoints. An isolate with MIC/disk diffusion diameter below or equal to the susceptibility breakpoint is termed susceptible while that with an MIC/disk diffusion diameter equal or above the resistance breakpoint is considered resistant. Values in between the S and R breakpoints are classified as intermediate.

There is sometimes discordance between CLSI and EUCAST for breakpoints for certain drugs. For example, by CLSI for Enterobacteriaceae and piperacillin/tazobactam S breakpoint is 16 and R breakpoint is 128, whereas the EUCAST breakpoints are 8 and 16, respectively. This means an isolate with MIC of 16 will be pronounced susceptible by CLSI and R by EUCAST.

Another concept is the MIC:S breakpoint ratio. The drug with the lowest MIC:S breakpoint ratio should be chosen for therapy among all the drugs to which the isolate is susceptible.

Selection of Antimicrobial Agents for Antimicrobial Sensitivity Testing

The choice of antimicrobial agents for AST depends on the organism isolated, the site of infection, the clinical practice setting in which the laboratory functions, the patterns of antibiotic usage and bacterial resistance in the community. Those agents that are prescribed by the physicians on a daily basis should be tested. CLSI publishes tables listing the antimicrobials appropriate for testing various groups of aerobic and fastidious bacteria. These guidelines indicate drugs that are most appropriate for testing each organism group and for treatment based on the specimen source, e.g. CSF, blood, urine or feces. It also includes a few agents that may be tested as surrogates for other agents due to the greater ability of a particular agent to detect resistance to closely related drugs, e.g. the use of cefoxitin to predict overall beta-lactam resistance in staphylococci.

Disk Diffusion Susceptibility Tests

Principle and Method

This is the most commonly used method in laboratories across the country. Commercially prepared filter paper disks impregnated with a specified single concentration of an antimicrobial agent are applied to the surface of an agar medium inoculated with the test organism. When the disk comes into contact with the moist agar surface, water is absorbed into the filter paper and the antibiotic starts diffusing into the surrounding medium. As the distance from the disk increases, the concentration of the antimicrobial agent decreases logarithmically, creating a gradient in the agar medium surrounding each disk (Fig. 1). Simultaneous growth of bacteria occurs on the agar surface when a critical cell mass of bacteria is reached and the inhibitory activity of the antibiotic is overcome. The points at which the critical cell mass is reached appear as a sharply marginated circle of bacterial growth with the middle of the disk forming the center of the circle. The concentration of the antibiotic at this interface of growing and inhibited bacteria is known as the critical concentration and approximates the MIC of the dilution tests. Criteria for the maximum number of disks for plate size should be followed to avoid overlapping of the zones. After incubation for 16–18 hours, the zone diameters of complete inhibition including the disk diameter are measured to the nearest whole millimeter with calipers or a ruler. The measuring device is held at the back of the inverted petridish which is illuminated with reflected light located a few inches above a black and nonreflecting background. The zone diameters are measured around each disk and are interpreted on the basis of CLSI guidelines and the organisms reported as susceptible, intermediate or resistant to the antimicrobial agent tested. Larger zones do not indicate that the antimicrobial is more susceptible. Susceptibility tests have to be interpreted as per the CLSI criteria as susceptible, intermediate and resistant.

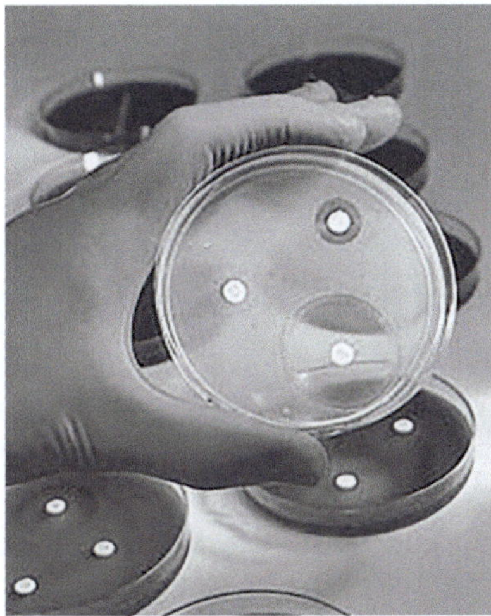

Fig. 1: Disk diffusion method.

Advantages

This include technically simple to perform, reproducible, relatively inexpensive reagents, no special equipment required, and susceptibility results provided are easily understood by the clinicians and flexible as regards to the antimicrobial agents selected for testing.

Disadvantages

This method is standardized for only a limited number of organisms. It is inadequate for the detection of vancomycin-intermediate *S. aureus,* cefoxitin-heteroresistant staphylococci, low level (VanB-type) vancomycin-resistant enterococci, and resistance in nonlactose fermenting gram-negative pathogens. It provides a qualitative and not a quantitative result and does not give an estimate of the MIC.

Automated Instrument Methods

These are being increasingly used in laboratories across the country. These automated MIC systems utilize a tray or other types of panels containing varying concentrations of several antimicrobial agents. Following inoculation, the panels are incubated in the instrument and MIC endpoints are read automatically. Sophisticated software enables MIC to be interpreted and reports are printed automatically.

Examples of automated systems:

- Vitek 2 system (Biomerieux)
- MicroScan system (Dade MicroScan)
- Phoenix system (BD).

Advantages: They are fast, well standardized, and relatively operator independent. They also give an estimate of the MIC of the organism to allow the clinician to make therapeutic decisions.

Disadvantages: These systems are not reliable for susceptibility testing for some nonfermenting gram-negative pathogens including *Elizabethkingia meningoseptica, Chryseobacterium indologenes,* etc. Also recent data indicates that automated systems are not reliable for susceptibility testing for drugs, such as colistin, tigecycline, and fosfomycin. They also do not give the exact MIC. For example, the carbapenem MIC is reported as more than or equal to 16 but the system does not indicate whether it is 32, 64, 128, and so on. This information is sometimes needed to decide whether the infection can be treated with higher than normal doses of the antibiotic.

Gradient Diffusion Method [E test (AB Biodisk, Solna, Sweden)]

This is a method for quantitative AST. A preformed antimicrobial gradient diffuses from a plastic coated strip into an agar medium inoculated with the test organism. The MIC is directly read from a scale on the plastic strip at a point where the ellipse of the organism growth intercepts the strip (Fig. 2).

Advantages: These are very simple and flexible like the disk diffusion test. They can be used to test fastidious and anaerobic bacteria. They can also be used to reconfirm the results of automated susceptibility methods and give exact MIC's.

Disadvantages: These are expensive at a cost of INR 100–150 per drug and are not available for all the drugs.

Dilution Methods

These methods are often used for determination of the MIC of the organism.

Agar Dilution Susceptibility Test

A standardized suspension of bacteria is inoculated onto a series of agar plates, each containing a different concentration of antibiotic. Organisms sensitive to the concentration of the antibiotic contained in the given agar plate do not produce a circle of growth at the inoculum site, whereas if resistant appear as circular colonies. For example, a series of agar plates containing 1, 4, 8, 16, and 32 µg/mL of antibiotic are used to determine the susceptibility of the organism being tested. If the organism grows on the first three plates but not in the plate with 16 µg/mL of the antibiotic, the MIC value is16 µg/mL. It is a well tested reference method for AST.

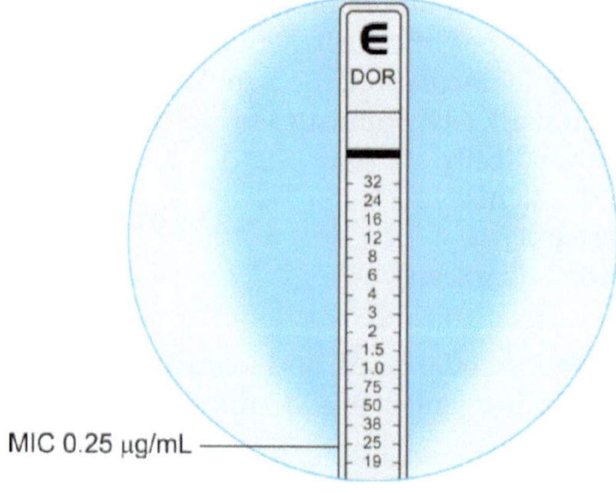

Fig. 2: E-strip for estimation of minimum inhibitory concentration (MIC).

Macrodilution Broth Susceptibility Test

Serial dilutions of the antimicrobial agent are made in the broth after which a standard suspension of bacteria is added. A tube free of antibiotic serves as a growth control. The tubes are then incubated at 35°C for 16–20 hours. Cloudiness indicates bacterial growth that has not been inhibited by the concentration of the antibiotic contained in the medium. The MIC is determined as the lowest concentration of the antibiotic in μg/mL that prevents in vitro growth of bacteria. In this method, the broth volume for each antimicrobial concentration is more than 1.0 mL (usually 2 mL). It is also a reference method and well standardized technique though time consuming and laborious.

Microdilution Broth Susceptibility Test

The principle is the same as macrodilution broth method except that the test is done in a series of microtube wells that are molded into a plastic plate. Each plate may contain 80, 96 or more wells depending on the number and concentration of antibiotics to be included in the susceptibility test panel. The volume of the antimicrobial dilution is most often 0.1 μL. Growth is determined by comparison with the growth control well and is generally indicated by turbidity throughout the well or by buttons in the well buttons. This is a reliable standardized reference method allowing convenient simultaneous testing of several antimicrobial agents against individual isolates. It is now the method of choice for determination of polymyxin/colistin susceptibility.

Breakpoint Susceptibility Tests

These are methods by which antimicrobial agents are tested only at the specific concentrations necessary for differentiating between categories of susceptible, intermediate and resistant rather than in the range of doubling dilutions used to determine the MIC. When two drug concentrations adjacent to the breakpoints defining the intermediate and resistant categories are selected, growth at both the concentrations indicates resistance, growth at the lower concentration only signifies an intermediate result, and no growth at either concentration is interpreted as susceptible. The advantages include the fact that greater number and variety of antimicrobial agents can be incorporated into a broth microdilution panel setup for breakpoint testing rather than full range dilution testing. However, the exact MIC of the isolate is not available.

Indications for use of Dilution Methods and Determination of Minimum Inhibitory Concentration

Minimum inhibitory concentration determination is not required for routine clinical practice. Specific indications for determining MIC include:

- Testing isolates from patients with endocarditis (viridans group of streptococci and penicillin)
- For research purposes, in order to evaluate the relative degrees of susceptibility of bacteria to various antimicrobial agents
- Some species for which MIC is needed to guide selection of therapy and appropriate dosing—penicillin and cephalosporin resistant *S. pneumoniae,* vancomycin for *Staphylococcus* species, and colistin for gram-negative bacilli.

Molecular Methods for Susceptibility Testing

These include CBNAAT and line probe assays for detection of resistance in TB, detection of resistance in HIV/CMV, detection of *mecA* gene in *S. aureus*, and carbapenemase producing genes in gram-negative bacteria.

Choice of Method for Antimicrobial Susceptibility Testing

The advantage of microdilution or agar gradient diffusion methods is the generation of a quantitative result in the form of MIC rather than a category result. These methods can also be used to test anaerobic or fastidious organisms that cannot be tested by disk diffusion method. The Kirby-Bauer disk diffusion method is however the most common method used worldwide. The two major advantages of this method are its low cost and flexibility in drug selection. There is also a direct relationship between the size of the zone of inhibition and the MIC. Both dilution and disk diffusion methods have similar inter- and intralaboratory reproducibility. Hence, the disk diffusion method is sufficient for the vast majority of common rapidly growing bacteria. There are only a limited number of specific clinical indications for determining MIC to assist in patient management and these have been discussed earlier. The automated systems generate results much faster than the manual methods; however, a major challenge posed by such systems is the inflexibility of the standard panels of antimicrobial agents that can be tested. In any case, accuracy should not be sacrificed in an effort to generate a rapid susceptibility testing result. The choice of method for antimicrobial sensitivity testing also depends largely on the local needs and resources.

Caveat of Antimicrobial Susceptibility Testing

There are various reasons why antibiotics may not work despite correct susceptibility and they include:

- *In vivo versus in vitro susceptibility*: Susceptibility tests are based on rapidly growing aerobic organisms determined to be sensitive by established breakpoints in achievable serum concentrations using clinically achievable doses. Susceptibility tests have been designed for monomicrobial infections, but in a polymicrobial infection when one tests the individual pathogens it is difficult to truly ascertain its value in vivo. The presence or absence and the level of expression of virulence factors are determinants which are not considered in in vitro susceptibility tests. The organism may harbor a resistance gene which is inducible and may not be expressed in vitro, e.g. AmpC positive *Enterobacter* species that appears susceptible to third-generation cephalosporins. Another reason for discordance can be poor intracellular penetration of the antibiotic. For example, aminoglycosides do not work for *Salmonella* due to poor penetration in the macrophages. Conversely azithromycin may work for enteric fever despite in vitro resistance due to several fold intracellular concentration of the antibiotic.
- *Inadequate blood/tissue levels*: The breakpoints are based on achievable serum concentrations. The levels of antimicrobials in other sites, such as CSF, prostate, bile, and bone are lower than the serum levels and hence therapy may fail despite susceptibility. To circumvent this very problem, the breakpoints for penicillin in *S. pneumoniae* are much lower for meningeal infections (S breakpoint $\leq$0.06 and R breakpoint of $\geq$0.12) versus nonmeningeal infections (S breakpoint of $\leq$2 and R breakpoint of $\geq$8). Conversely, it is possible to treat UTIs successfully with beta-lactam antibiotics, such as ampicillin/cephalosporins despite in vitro resistance

owing to concentration of the antibiotic in the urine several fold (levels of ampicillin with standard doses is 2.5 μg/mL in serum versus 600 μg/mL in urine).

- *Antibiotic tissue penetration problems*: Most antibiotics penetrate well-defined abscesses poorly, if at all. Surgical drainage remains the cornerstone of the therapeutic approach in the patient with abscesses. Infections involving foreign implant material usually have a glycocalyx around the foreign body which form a biofilm and these cannot be eliminated by antimicrobial therapy. Such infections almost always required removal of the prosthetic device.
- *Colonization versus infection*: The mere recovery of an organism does not implicate its etiological role in the underlying infectious disease process. Certain organisms are almost always associated with colonization and only rarely cause invasive disease, e.g. *Citrobacter* species. Organisms as *Enterobacter* species cause disease in a narrow range of clinical circumstances, e.g. intravenous (IV) line infections, catheter-associated bacteriuria, etc. The recovery of *Pseudomonas aeruginosa* from an endotracheal specimen in an intubated patient in an intensive care unit likewise may represent colonization. Treating colonization not only wastes vital resources, but is almost always unsuccessful.
- *Patient related factors*: Recovery from an infection requires host defenses in addition to antimicrobials. Hence, therapy may fail in a severely immunocompromised or neutropenic patient despite using drugs to which the organism is susceptible.

CONCLUSION

It is crucial to make all efforts to establish the microbiologic etiology of an infection in today's era. The choice of method depends on the clinical setting, cost, and local availability. The results of the diagnostic tests should always be interpreted in the clinical context.

RECOMMENDED READING

1. Caliendo AM, Gilbert DN, Ginocchio CC, et al. Better tests, better care: improved diagnostics for infectious diseases. Clin Infect Dis. 2013;57(S3):S139-70.
2. Cormican M, Whyte T, Hanahoe B. Antimicrobial Susceptibility Testing in Ireland: An introduction to the methods of the National Committee for Clinical Laboratory Standards (NCCLS). Ireland: National University of Ireland Galway; 2001.
3. Jorgensen JH, Turnidge JD. Antibacterial susceptibility tests: dilution and disk diffusion methods. In: Murray PR, Baron EJ, Jorgensen JH, Pfaller MA, Yolker RH. Manual of Clinical Microbiology, 9th edition. Washington DC: ASM Press; 2007. pp. 1152-72.
4. Jorgensen JH. Laboratory issues in the detection and reporting of antibacterial resistance. Inf Dis Clin North Am. 1997;11:785-802.
5. Koneman EW, Allen SD, Janda WM, et al. Colour Atlas and Textbook of Diagnostic Microbiology, 5th edition. Philadelphia, New York: Lippincott; 1997. pp. 785-856.
6. Livermore DM, Winstanley TG, Shannon KP. Interpretative reading: recognizing the unusual and inferring resistance mechanisms from resistance phenotypes. J Antimicrob Chemother. 2001;48 (Suppl 1):87-102.
7. Louie M, Cockerill FR 3rd. Susceptibility testing. Phenotypic and genotypic tests for bacteria and mycobacteria. Inf Dis Clin North Am. 2001;15:1205-26.
8. Turnidge JD, Ferraro MJ, Jorgensen JH. Susceptibility test methods: General considerations. In: Murray PR, Baron EJ, Jorgensen JH, Pfaller MA, Yolker RH (Eds). Manual of Clinical Microbiology, 9th edition. Washington DC: ASM Press; 2003. pp, 1102-7.

Antimicrobial Resistance: Current Scenario

3
Chapter

Vikas Manchanda, Faria H Farooqi

INTRODUCTION

Antimicrobial resistance (AMR) is a global concern. New resistance mechanisms are emerging and spreading globally. When the microorganisms become resistant to most antimicrobials, they are often referred to as "superbugs". Limited ability to manage resistant infections results in prolonged morbidity, disability, and increased mortality. AMR is a natural phenomenon. However, it is accelerated by the inappropriate use of antimicrobials, e.g. using antibiotics for viral infections, such as cold or flu. Low-quality medicines, wrong prescriptions, and poor infection prevention and control also encourage the development and spread of drug resistance. Lack of government commitment to address these issues, inadequate surveillance, limited availability, and use of diagnostic tests available additionally hinders the control of antimicrobial drug resistance.

EMERGENCE AND IMPACT OF ANTIMICROBIAL RESISTANCE

Emergence of resistance among the clinically significant bacterial pathogens is recognized as a major public health threat globally. AMR threatens the effective prevention and treatment of an ever-increasing range of infections caused by bacteria, parasites, viruses, and fungi. Multidrug-resistant (MDR) organisms are not only limited to the hospital environment but are now frequently identified in community settings suggesting that reservoirs of antibiotic-resistant bacteria are also present outside the hospital. The bacterial response to the antibiotic "attack" is the prime example of bacterial adaptation and evolution. "Survival of the fittest" is a consequence of an immense genetic plasticity of bacterial pathogens that trigger specific responses that result in mutational adaptations, acquisition of genetic material, or alteration of gene expression producing resistance to virtually all antibiotics currently available in clinical practice. Resistance has been detected among clinical isolates to the antimicrobials very near to their introduction in clinical practice (Fig. 1). Without effective antibiotics, the success of major surgery and cancer chemotherapy would be compromised. With lack of effective antimicrobials the treatment of infections, medical procedures, such as organ transplantation, diabetes management, and major surgeries (e.g. cesarean sections, joint replacements, coronary artery bypass graft, etc.) would become very high-risk. The cost of healthcare for patients with resistant infections is higher than care for patients with nonresistant infections due to longer duration of illness, additional tests and use of more expensive drugs.

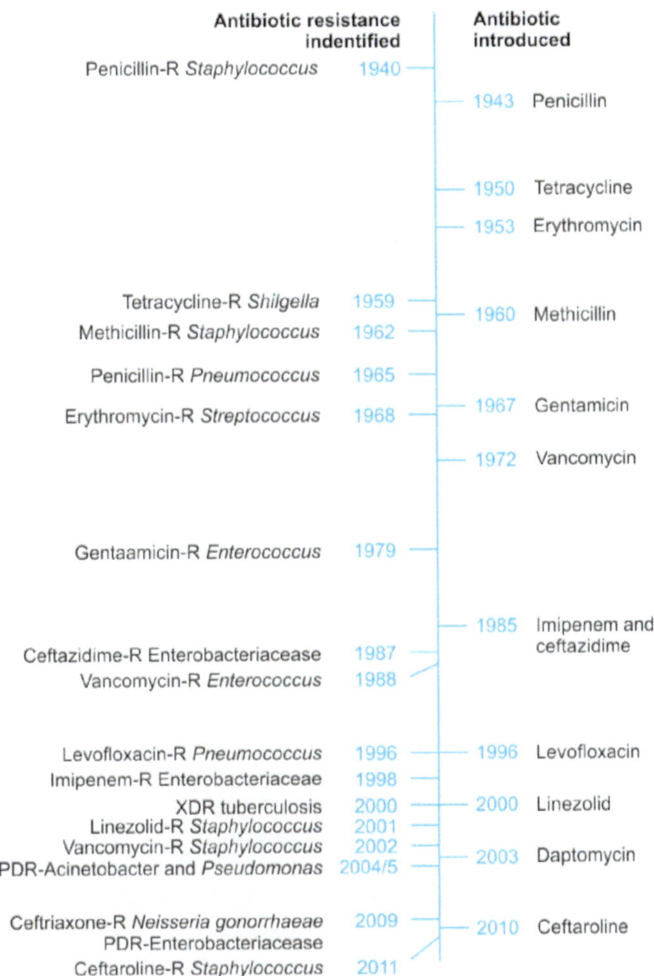

Fig. 1: Timeline for the antimicrobial resistance identified compared to the introduction of an agent in clinical use.

DEFINITIONS OF RESISTANCE

Bacteria are commonly defined as MDR, extensively drug resistant (XDR), pandrug resistant (PDR). The term MDR applies to resistance to at least 1 agent in more than or equal to antimicrobial classes, XDR when there is resistance to all except 1 agent in less than or equal to 2 antimicrobial classes and PDR when the isolate is resistant to all available antimicrobials (Fig. 2).

BASICS OF RESISTANCE MECHANISMS

AMR is an age old phenomenon. Most antimicrobial compounds are naturally produced and coresident bacteria in the environment have evolved mechanisms to overcome their action in order to survive. Thus, these organisms are often considered to be "intrinsically resistant to

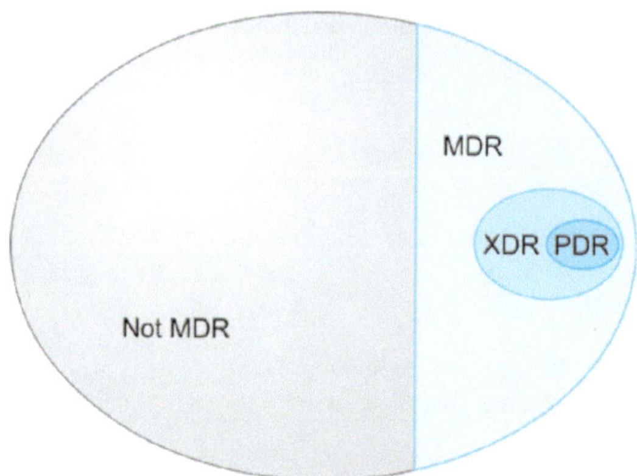

Fig. 2: Relation of MDR, XDR and PDR pathogens.
(MDR: multidrug-resistant; PDR: pandrug-resistant; XDR: extensively drug-resistant)

one or many antimicrobials (Table 1)". In such cases, irrespective of the in vitro susceptibility reported by the microbiology laboratory, these antibiotics should not be used.

It is important to understand that resistance and susceptibility reported in clinical practice are a relative phenomenon. The establishment of clinical susceptibility breakpoints (susceptible, intermediate, and resistant) mainly relies on the in vitro activity of an antibiotic against a sizeable bacterial sample, combined with some pharmacological parameters (e.g. blood and infection site concentrations of the antimicrobial among others). Thus, when treating antibiotic-resistant bacteria, the interpretation of susceptibility patterns may vary according to the clinical scenario and the availability of treatment options. For example, the concentration of gentamicin achieved in the urine may be sufficiently high to treat a lower urinary tract infection caused by an organism reported as gentamicin-resistant. Similarly, different penicillin breakpoints have been established for *Streptococcus pneumoniae* depending if the isolate is causing meningitis versus other types of infections taking into account the levels of the drug that actually reach the cerebrospinal fluid. In addition, the in vivo susceptibility of an organism to a particular antibiotic may vary according to the size of the bacterial inoculum, a situation that has been well documented in *Staphylococcus aureus* infections with some cephalosporins. Indeed, there is evidence to suggest that some cephalosporins (e.g. cefazolin) may fail in the setting of high-inocula deep-seated infections caused by cephalosporin-susceptible *S. aureus*.

GENETIC BASIS OF RESISTANCE

Bacteria have remarkable ability to alter its genetic make-up in response to environmental challenges including exposure to antimicrobial agents. There have been principally two major genetic mechanisms which come into play for the survival, these include—intrinsic genetic mutations without external genetic elements and secondly, through horizontal gene transfer (HGT)—acquisition of external genetic material encoding resistance determinants. The various AMR mechanisms which are obtained by bacteria through genetic mutations include: (1) modifications of the antimicrobial target (decreasing the affinity for the drug), (2) decrease in the drug uptake, (3) activation of efflux mechanisms to pump out the harmful antibiotics, or (4) alterations in important metabolic pathways via modulation of regulatory networks. One of the most important mechanisms is enzyme inactivation of the antimicrobials. Beta-lactamases,

TABLE 1: List of antibiotics to which common clinically relevant bacteria are intrinsically resistant.

Bacteria	*Intrinsic resistance to antibiotics*
Gram-negative bacteria	
Enterobacteriaceae	
Klebsiella pneumoniae	Ampicillin and ticarcillin
Enterobacter aerogenes *Enterobacter cloacae* complex *Citrobacter freundii*	Ampicillin, amoxicillin + clavulanate, ampicillin sulbactam, 1st generation cephalosporins (GC), 2nd GC, and cephamycins
Citrobacter koseri	Ampicillin, ticarcillin, and piperacillin
Proteus species	Ampicillin, 1st GC, 2nd GC, and polymyxins
Morganella morganii	Ampicillin, amoxicillin + clavulanate, 1st GC, 2nd GC, and polymyxins
Providencia species	Ampicillin, amoxicillin + clavulanate, 1st GC and polymyxins; aminoglycosides – gentamicin, netilmicin, and tobramycin
Salmonella and *Shigella*	1st GC, 2nd GC, cephamycins, and aminoglycosides
Nonfermentative gram-negative bacteria	
Acinetobacter species	Ampicillin, amoxicillin + clavulanate, 1st GC, aztreonam, ertapenem, trimethoprim, chloramphenicol, and fosfomycin
Pseudomonas aeruginosa	Ampicillin, amoxicillin + clavulanate, ampicillin + sulbactam, 1st GC, ertapenem, trimethoprim, cotrimoxazole, tetracycline or tigecycline, and chloramphenicol
Burkholderia cepacia	Antipseudomonal penicillins, cefotaxime, ceftriaxone, aztreonam, ertapenem, polymyxins, and fosfomycin
Gram-positive bacteria	
Enterococcus	Fusidic acid, all cephalosporins, erythromycin, clindamycin, quinupristin-dalfopristin, sulfonamides, and aminoglycosides*
Listeria monocytogenes	All cephalosporins

1GC—1st generation cephalosporins (cephalexin and cefazolin)
2GC—2nd generation cephalosporins
Cephamycins (cefoxitin and cefotetan)
*Aminoglycosides resistance is low-level resistance hence should not be used as monotherapy, should always be used in combination with penicillins or glycopeptides.

extended spectrum beta-lactamases (ESBL), and carbapenemases are common among these enzymes. Beta-lactamases hydrolyze beta-lactam rings in natural penicillins. ESBLs hydrolyze all penicillins and most of the cephalosporins including third-generation cephalosporins. Carbapenemases hydrolyze carbapenems.

The common resistance mechanisms for various classes of antimicrobial agents are summarized in Table 2.

ANTIMICROBIAL RESISTANCE IN *STAPHYLOCOCCUS AUREUS*

Overall resistance mechanisms in *S. aureus* include enzymatic inactivation of the antibiotic (penicillinases), alteration of the target with decreased affinity for the antibiotic [notable examples being penicillin-binding protein 2a (PBP2a) of methicillin-resistant *S. aureus* and

TABLE 2: Relative presence of major mechanisms of resistance to different antibiotic classes.

	Enzymatic inactivation	*Decreased permeability*	*Efflux*	*Alteration of target site*	*Protection of target site*	*Over-produce target*	*Bypass of inhibited process*	*Bind up antibiotic*
β-lactam agents	+++	+(Gram-negative)	+	++		–	–	–
Aminoglycoside	+++	+(Gram-negative)	+	++	–	–	–	–
Chloramphenicol	+++	+(Gram-negative)	+	–	–	–	–	–
Macrolide	+(Gram-negative)	++(Gram-negative)	++	+++	–	–	–	–
Sulfonamide	–	–	–	++	–	++	-	-
Tetracycline	–	+(Gram-negative)	+++	+	++	–	–	–
Trimethoprim	–	+(Gram-negative)	–	+++	–	++	+	–
Quinolone	+	+(Gram-negative)	+	+++	+	–	–	–
Glycopeptide	–	++(Gram-negative)	–	+++	–	+	–	++
Lincosamide; Streptogramin	–	+(Gram-negative)	–	+++	–	–	–	–
Rifampin	–	–	–	+++	–	–	–	–

+++, most common mechanism; ++, common; +, less common

D-Ala-D-Lac of peptidoglycan precursors of vancomycin-resistant strains], trapping of the antibiotic (for vancomycin and possibly daptomycin), and efflux pumps (fluoroquinolones and tetracycline). Based on susceptibility to methicillin, all *S. aureus* isolates can be broadly divided into methicillin-susceptible *S. aureus* (MSSA) and methicillin-resistant *S. aureus* (MRSA). This resistance allows cell wall biosynthesis, the target of β-lactams, to continue even in the presence of typically inhibitory concentrations of antibiotic. PBP2a is encoded by the *mec A* gene, which is carried on a distinct mobile genetic element [staphylococcal cassette chromosome (SCC), *mec*]. Due to difficulty with stability of methicillin, susceptibility to oxacillin and cefoxitin is being used as determinant to of identifying MRSA strains. Complex genetic arrays (staphylococcal chromosomal cassette mec elements or the vanA operon) have been acquired by *S. aureus* through HGT, while resistance to other antibiotics, including some of the most recent ones (e.g. fluoroquinolones, linezolid, and daptomycin) have developed through spontaneous mutations and positive selection.

Due to high prevalence (>90%) of staphylococcal strains harboring beta-lactamase enzyme in India, natural penicillins (penicillin G and ampicillin) are no longer used for therapy in treating MSSA infections. The drug of choice for treatment of MSSA infections at all sites is cloxacillin or flucloxacillin. However, there are problems of availability, need for large doses and frequent injections and high cost of the recently marketed formulations. Hence, the first generation cephalosporins cefazolin are being increasingly used with good efficacy for all sites except for central nervous system (CNS). Several retrospective studies have shown equal efficacy of cefazolin in treating bacteremia and endocarditis. Ceftriaxone has also been successfully used for treatment of skin, soft tissue, bone and joint infections, and is useful for outpatient parenteral therapy. It is, however, not recommended for bacteremia or endocarditis. Ceftriaxone may have to be used for CNS MSSA infections, if cloxacillin is not available. Daptomycin is a relatively new drug with equal efficacy for both MSSA and MRSA and may be used, if there is beta-lactam allergy. Glycopeptides are inferior for treating MSSA and should be avoided. With widely disseminated infection or patients with severe toxemia clindamycin is the drug of choice due to its dual effect of bactericidal and toxin neutralizing property.

There is increasing prevalence of MRSA in the Indian setting. Community-acquired MRSA is a resistance mechanism originating in strains circulating in the community and mediated by *mec* A gene. Some of these strains are highly virulent and produce the Panton-Valentine leukocidin toxin (PVL), which leads to rapidly progressive infections with toxemia, necrosis and leukopenia. These strains are commonly associated with pneumonia and skin and soft tissue infections. Paradoxically, they are susceptible to more number of antibiotics as compared to the healthcare-acquired (HA)-MRSA including vancomycin, teicoplanin, linezolid, daptomycin, and often to cotrimoxazole, clindamycin, erythromycin, tetracyclines, and quinolones. Certain studies implicate community-associated (CA)-MRSA as causing 20–40% of community-acquired skin and soft tissue and bone and joint infections bone and joint infections in India.

Conventionally, MRSA strains were first recognized in healthcare-associated infections and these are termed as HA-MRSA. Resistance is mediated through the SCC *mec* gene. These strains are more resistant than the CA-MRSA strains with retained susceptibility to only few drugs including vancomycin, teicoplanin, linezolid, and daptomycin. There is an increase in prevalence of methicillin resistance in nosocomial infections from 30% to 50% in the Indian setting.

However, certain strains of MRSA isolated from healthcare-associated infections have the CA-MRSA phenotype suggesting that there is no clear demarcation between CA-MRSA and HA-MRSA. There is also increase in vancomycin minimum inhibitory concentration's (MIC's) in MRSA. While the susceptibility breakpoint is 2, strains of MRSA with MIC more than 1 show increased incidence of failure with vancomycin. Strains with MIC of 4, 8 are designated as vancomycin-intermediate *S. aureus* (VISA) while those with MIC of 16 and above are designated as Vancomycin-resistant *S. aureus* (VRSA). Options for treating vancomycin-resistant strains include daptomycin and linezolid. Apart from vancomycin resistance strains of *S. aureus* are exhibiting resistance to daptomycin and even linezolid (linezolid resistant *S. aureus*). Several new drugs have been marketed which have anti-MRSA activity including quinolones (delafloxacin), cephalosporins (ceftaroline and ceftobiprole), quinupristin/dalfopristin, and the lipoglycopeptides (telavancin, oritavancin, and dalbavancin).

ANTIMICROBIAL RESISTANCE IN *STREPTOCOCCUS PNEUMONIAE*

The mechanism of resistance to penicillin or other beta-lactams is due to altered penicillin binding proteins (PBPs) in *S. pneumoniae*. The basic mechanisms of resistance to different antibiotics in *S. pneumoniae* are described in Table 3.

Penicillin or cephalosporin resistance in pneumococcal meningitis is emerging in India, however, for nonmeningeal infections there is no resistance. This is because of different drug concentrations available during treatment in different parts of body. Hence, different MIC breakpoints have been described for meningitis and nonmeningitis pneumococcal isolates (Table 4).

TABLE 3: Major antibiotic resistance mechanisms in *Streptococcus pneumoniae.*

Resistance phenotype	*Major resistance mechanism*
β-Lactams	Alteration of target enzymes (PBPs)
Macrolides, lincosamides, streptogramin B	Alteration of ribosomal target sites (methylation of adenine residue in domain V of 23S rRNA-*ermB*); efflux *(mefE)*
Tetracycline	Protection of ribosomal target site *(tetM)*
Trimethoprim and sulfonamides	Alteration of target enzymes (dihydrofolate reductase–trimethoprim; dihydropteroate synthase—*sul1, sul2* in sulfonamines)
Fluoroquinolones	Alteration of target enzymes (DNA gyrase—*gyrA* mutations; topoisomerase IV— *parC* mutations)

(DNA: deoxyribonucleic acid; IV: intravenous: rRNA: ribosomal ribonucleic acid)

TABLE 4: MIC breakpoints for *Streptococcus pneumoniae.*

	Antimicrobial agents	*Interpretive criteria and MIC breakpoints µg/mL*		
		Sensitive	*Intermediate*	*Resistant*
Penicillins				
	Penicillin parenteral (nonmeningitis)	≤2	4	≥8
	Penicillin parenteral (meningitis)	≤0.06	–	≥0.12
	Penicillin (oral penicillin V)	≤0.06	0.12–1	≥2
	Amoxicillin (nonmeningitis) Amoxicillin-clavulanate (nonmeningitis)	≤2 ≤2/1	4 4/2	≥8 ≥8/4
Cephems (parenteral)				
	Cefepime (meningitis)	≤0.5	1	≥2
	Cefepime (nonmeningitis)	≤1	2	≥4
	Cefotaxime (meningitis)	≤1	2	≥4
	Ceftriaxone (meningitis)	≤1	2	≥4
Glycopeptides				
	Vancomycin	≤1	–	–

In a systematic review by Singh et al. which included seven studies published from 2009–2016 in children below 5 years in India, the incidence of penicillin resistance was 10% and cefotaxime resistance was 4%. In the study Alliance for Surveillance of Invasive Pneumococcal Serotypes (ASIP), in children below 5 years which included 361 isolates, penicillin resistance was 8% and no cephalosporin resistance was reported. In yet another study from New Delhi in 1,305 under 5 years' children with suspected acute bacterial meningitis, it was observed that penicillin resistance was 38% using meningitis breakpoint (unpublished data). Among these children, except one isolate all other 28 isolates were susceptible to ceftriaxone. One of the largest retrospective studies till date is from Christian Medical College (CMC), Vellore, which included 861 invasive isolates from both adults and children between 2008 to 2016. Among the 663 nonmeningeal isolates only one was fully resistant to penicillin and three showed intermediate resistance. Of the 148 meningeal isolates, the overall penicillin resistance was

43.7% (increased from 9.5% in 2008 to 42.8% in 2016) while the overall cephalosporin resistance was 14.8% (increased from 4.7% in 2008 to 28.5% in 2016). This data indicates that standard dose penicillins and cephalosporins can be used to manage nonmeningeal infections while for meningeal infections the time has come to move from ceftriaxone monotherapy to ceftriaxone with vancomycin. In fact if the MIC to ceftriaxone exceeds 4, rifampicin should also be added.

Resistance in *S. pneumoniae* to cotrimoxazole in the current era exceeds 50% and that to macrolides ranges from 30% to 40% obviating the use of these antibiotics for pneumococcal infections.

ANTIMICROBIAL RESISTANCE IN *ENTEROCOCCUS* SPECIES

The major resistance mechanisms in *Enterococcus* species are listed in Table 5. It must be remembered that these bacteria are intrinsically resistant to cephalosporins due to presence of low affinity PBP5. Hence, treatment with cephalosporins was not recommended in the past. However, there is emerging data on the synergy of combining ceftriaxone or cefotaxime or ertapenem with ampicillin or daptomycin or vancomycin for the treatment of enterococcal infections. This is due to saturation of PBP2 and 3 by ceftriaxone while PBP4 and 5 are saturated by ampicillin or amoxicillin.

Enterococci intrinsically have low level of resistance to aminoglycosides. Laboratories should routinely check for high level aminoglycoside resistance to gentamicin and streptomycin, if absent aminoglycosides can be used in combination with other antimicrobials to treat enterococcal infections especially bacteremia, endocarditis, CNS infections, and infections in neutropenic hosts. In the presence of HLAR or if there is coexistent nephrotoxicity, ceftriaxone may be used in place of gentamicin for satisfactory results.

In a study from a North Indian Hospital, of 283 isolates of enterococci from various clinical sites (of which half were from urine), *Enterococcus faecalis* was the predominant isolate (82%) and the incidence of high-level gentamicin resistance was 50% and vancomycin resistance was 6%.

TABLE 5: Major antimicrobial resistance mechanisms in Enterococcus species.

Resistance phenotype	*Major resistance mechanism*	*Intrinsic resistance*
β-Lactams (ampicillin)	Alteration of target enzymes (PBP5 in *Enterococcus faecium*); enzymatic inhibition–rare (penicillinase in *E. faecalis*)	Cephalosporins
Aminoglycosides	Altered ribosomal target site mutations, enzymatic inhibition (high-level resistance: aminoglycoside-modifying enzymes)	Low-level resistance
Vancomycin (VRE)	Alteration of cell wall precursor targets (high-level resistance: VanA, B, D phenotypes; low-level resistance—VanC, E, and G phenotypes)	*E. gallinarum* and *E. casseliflavus* intrinsically resistant to vancomycin
Linezolid	Alteration of ribosomal target sites (G2576U mutation in domain V of 23S rRNA)	

ANTIMICROBIAL RESISTANCE IN ENTERIC GRAM-NEGATIVE BACTERIA

Mechanism

Gram-negative bacteria can become resistant by a variety of mechanisms including impaired penetration in the cell, increased efflux, target modification, etc. But the most dramatic of all mechanisms is production of inactivating enzymes chiefly the beta-lactamases. These mechanisms also coexist with each other. The beta-lactamases hydrolyze the beta-lactam ring of penicillins, cephalosporins, monobactams, and carbapenems and will be discussed in detail.

The first-generation beta-lactamases appeared even before penicillin was introduced. These were found in *S. aureus, Moraxella, E. coli* and *Haemophilus influenzae.* The cephalosporins were resistant to these beta-lactamases and hence were widely used for therapy in the 1980's. This efficacy of the cephalosporins was short lived and in 1983 the first ESBL (TEM-3) was described. The number of ESBL's increased phenomenally and now number more than 200. They are plasmid mediated enzymes and are grouped into four major families; TEM, SHV, CTX-M, and OXA. One organism can produce more than one type of ESBL. The ESBLs were first recognized in *E. coli* and *Klebsiella* but are now produced by other gram-negative pathogens as well. The ESBLs hydrolyze all penicillins, cephalosporins, and aztreonam. However, cefoxitin, beta-lactam and beta-lactamase inhibitor combinations and carbapenems are effective against the ESBL's. Even more potent than the ESBLs were the Amp-C beta-lactamases which were chromosomally encoded enzymes produced first by the *Serratia, Pseudomonas,* Indole positive proteus, *Citrobacter,* and *Enterobacter* (SPICE) group of organisms. These are now known to be produced by other gram-negative pathogens too. In the derepressed mutants producing these enzymes, copious quantities are produced such that the beta-lactam and beta-lactamase inhibitor combinations are ineffective and only carbapenems are effective.

Then came the carbapenemases the most potent of all the enzymes that hydrolyze cephalosporins, penicillins, carbapenems but not aztreonam. The conventional beta-lactam and beta-lactamase inhibitor combinations are ineffective against these enzymes. These carbapenemases can further be classified as serine carbapenemases [*Klebsiella pneumoniae* carbapenemases (KPC) and OXA] and the metallo beta-lactamases (NDM, IMP, VIM, etc.). The most common types of carbapenemases seen in India are the NDM and OXA. The only drugs effective against carbapenemases are polymyxins, tigecycline, fosfomycin, and sometimes aminoglycosides, cotrimoxazole, etc. The new beta-lactam and beta-lactamase inhibitor combinations that have recently got regulatory approval but are still not available in India and are effective against KPC-producing organisms include ceftazidime avibactam and meropenem vaborbactam. However, the utility of these drugs in the Indian set up is limited since the main carbapenemase is NDM against which these beta-lactamase inhibitors are ineffective. Aztreonam avibactam a drug still in trial phase is likely to be useful against NDM-producing organisms.

It must be remembered that several different type of beta-lactamases may be coproduced by the same organism, thus making treatment of gram-negative infections even more challenging. Beta-lactamases can be classified in various ways but one classification is the Ambler system, which is based on amino acid homology. Class A includes ESBL's and KPC; Class B includes the metallo beta-lactamases (NDM, IMP, and VIM), Class C includes Amp-C-beta-lactamases, and Class D includes OXA enzymes.

Prevalence of Resistance in Gram-negative Bacteria

Resistance in gram-negative pathogens in community and hospital-associated infections is the most challenging problem facing India today.

Studies in adults indicate 40–50% prevalence of ESBL in *E. coli* causing urinary tract infections in the community. Resistance in *Shigella* to quinolones, cotrimoxazole, and ampicillin is considerable. In *Salmonella*, quinolone resistance rates exceed 90%; while there is return in susceptibility to first-line drugs including ampicillin, chloramphenicol, and cotrimoxazole, there are sporadic reports of ceftriaxone resistance in *Salmonella* due to production of a new type of ESBL.

Prevalence of resistance in healthcare-associated infections is demoralizing. Almost 70–80% of gram-negative healthcare-associated infections are ESBL producing. The rates of carbapenem resistance are increasing and in some tertiary care hospitals in *E. coli* and *Klebsiella* approach 50% while those in *Pseudomonas* and *Acinetobacter* approach 80%. In a recently published study on neonatal sepsis from Delhi, which even included newborns delivered at home and being admitted to a healthcare facility for the first time, the ESBL and carbapenem resistance rates approached 80%. With increase in use of carbapenems, there is excessive use of polymyxins, which has now resulted in emergence of resistance to polymyxins and the prospect of totally drug resistant (TDR) or PDR pathogens.

PREVENTION AND CONTROL OF AMR

The biggest driver of AMR is antimicrobial overuse. In 2010, India was the world's largest consumer of antibiotics for human health at 12.9×10^9 units (10.7 units per person). The next largest consumers were China at 10.0 ×109 units (7.5 units per person) and the US at 6.8 ×109 units (22.0 units per person). Overall, ampicillin and cotrimoxazole use is declining in India, while quinolone consumption is high and increasing in India. Rates of carbapenem use per capita are low compared to other antibiotics in 2,000 but had risen to over 10 million standard units by 2010.

Hence, if we have to stop this gargantuan problem of AMR, we have to first practice rational antimicrobial therapy or antimicrobial stewardship. This concept is revisited several times in this book as we go on. This requires efforts from all stakeholders including patients, physicians, government, and the industry. The second strategy to counter the burden of AMR is to prevent infections by good infection control practices, vaccination, sanitation, and hygiene. No less important is surveillance or tracking of the problem of AMR and development of new antimicrobials and novel treatment strategies for infections including phages, monoclonal antibodies, and the likes.

RECOMMENDED READING

1. Badhan R, Singh DV, Badhan LR, et al. Evaluation of bacteriological profile and antibiotic sensitivity patterns in children with urinary tract infection: A prospective study from a tertiary care center. Indian J Urol 2016;32:50-6.
2. Bennet JE, Dolin R, Blaser MJ. Mandell Douglas and Bennet's Principles and practice of infectious diseases, 8th edition. Philadelphia, PA: Elsevier; 2015. pp. 235-51.

3. Bush K. Bench-to-bedside review: The role of beta-lactamases in antibiotic-resistant gram-negative infections. Crit Care. 2010;14(3):224.
4. CDC. Time line for the antimicrobial resistance identified compared to the introduction of an agent in clinical use. [online] Available from: https://www.cdc.gov/drugresistance/pdf/5-2013-508.pdf [Accessed December, 2018].
5. CDDEP. ResistanceMap Washington DC: Center for Disease Dynamics, Economics & Policy; 2015. [online] Available from: https://cddep.org/partners/resistance-map/ [December, 2018].
6. Clinical and Laboratory Standards Institute. Performance standards for antimicrobial susceptibility testing; 24th informational supplement. Wayne, PA: Clinical and Laboratory Standards Institute; 2014.
7. Clinical and Laboratory Standards Institute. Performance standards for antimicrobial susceptibility testing; 28th informational supplement. Wayne, PA: Clinical and Laboratory Standards Institute; 2018.
8. Datta S, Wattal C, Goel N, et al. A ten year analysis of multi-drug resistant bloodstream infections caused by *Escherichia coli* & *Klebsiella pneumoniae* in a tertiary care hospital. Indian J Med Res. 2012;135(6):907-12.
9. EUCAST. 2018. The European Committee on Antimicrobial Susceptibility Testing – EUCAST.[online] Available from: http://www.eucast.org/ [Accessed December, 2018].
10. Jajoo M, Manchanda V, Chaurasia S, Sankar MJ, Gautam H, Agarwal R et al. Investigators of the Delhi Neonatal Infection Study (DeNIS) collaboration, New Delhi, India. Alarming rates of antimicrobial resistance and fungal sepsis in outborn neonates in North India. PLoS One. 2018 ;13(6):e0180705.
11. Kini AR, Shetty V, Kumar AM, et al. Community-associated, methicillin-susceptible, and methicillin-resistant Staphylococcus aureus bone and joint infections in children: experience from India. J Pediatr Orthop B. 2013;22(2):158-66.
12. Minita JM and Arias CA. Mechanisms of antibiotic resistance. Microbiol Spectr. 2016;4(2):10.
13. Nannini EC, Singh KV, Arias CA, et al. In vivo effect of cefazolin, daptomycin, and nafcillin in experimental endocarditis with a methicillin-susceptible Staphylococcus aureus strain showing an inoculum effect against cefazolin. Antimicrob Agents Chemother. 2013;57(9):4276-81.
14. Pasticci MB, Mencacci A, Moretti A, et al. In vitro antimicrobial activity of ampicillin-ceftriaxone and ampicillin-ertapenem combinations against clinical isolates of enterococcus faecalis with high levels of aminoglycoside resistance. Open Microbiol J. 2008;2:79-84.
15. Roy MP, Gaind R, Aggarwal KC, et al. Pattern of pediatric bacterial infection and antibiotic resistance in New Delhi. Indian Pediatr. 2017;54:153-4.
16. Sachan S, Rawat V, Umesh, et al. Susceptibility pattern of enterococci at Tertiary Care Hospital. J Glob Infect Dis. 2017;9(2):73-5.
17. Singh J, Sundaresan S, Manoharan A, et al. Serotype distribution and antimicrobial susceptibility pattern in children ≤5years with invasive pneumococcal disease in India—a systematic review. Vaccine. 2017;35(35 Pt B):4501-9.
18. Van Boeckel TP, Gandra S, Ashok A, et al. Global antibiotic consumption 2000 to 2010: an analysis of national pharmaceutical sales data. Lancet Infect Dis. 2014;14(8):742-50.
19. Verghese VP, Veeraraghavan B, Jayaraman R, et al. Increasing incidence of penicillin- and cefotaxime-resistant Streptococcus pneumoniae causing meningitis in India: time for revision of treatment guidelines? Indian J Med Microbiol. 2017;35(2):228-36.
20. WHO. Antimicrobial resistance. [online] Available from: http://www.who.int/en/news-room/fact-sheets/detail/antimicrobial-resistance [Accessed December, 2018].
21. WHO. What is antibiotic resistance? [online] Available from: https://www.who.int/features/qa/75/en/ [Accessed December, 2018].

Pharmacokinetics and Pharmacodynamics of Antimicrobials

4
Chapter

Jaideep A Gogtay, Madhumita Panda

INTRODUCTION

Optimizing outcomes for infected patients requires attention to three interconnected factors, namely, patient, pathogen, and drug. While patient and pathogen are uncontrollable factors, the choice of the drug and the way it is administered are modifiable. Against the backdrop of increasing antimicrobial resistance coupled with a poor antimicrobial pipeline, treatment of serious infections has become increasingly challenging. The situation is further aggravated in critically ill patients where resistant organisms are common and in whom pathophysiological change results in alteration of pharmacokinetics (PK) of antimicrobials. This has led to a growing interest in the understanding of PK/pharmacodynamics (PD) parameters and their clinical utility in improving outcomes and minimizing the risk of resistance. This chapter outlines the fundamentals of antimicrobial PK-PD and a few concepts regarding their application in clinical practice, namely, the role of therapeutic drug monitoring (TDM) and prolonged infusion of beta-lactams.

BASICS OF PHARMACODYNAMICS AND PHARMACOKINETICS

Pharmacodynamics describes the effect of the drug on the body and the microorganisms while PK describes the plasma time-concentration course of the drug. It is well known that for a drug to achieve its effect (PD), it has to achieve a certain concentration at the site of the infection via the plasma (PK) (Fig. 1). Looking at the PK-PD together links drug exposure to the antimicrobial and clinical effects after administration of the drug to a patient.

The typical course of a drug after oral administration is illustrated in Figure 2. The drug achieves its maximum concentration (C_{max}) at a particular time point (T_{max}) and is metabolized and finally eliminated from the body depending on its half-life. The "area under the curve (AUC)" represents the total body exposure to the drug. When this is plotted on the same graph as the

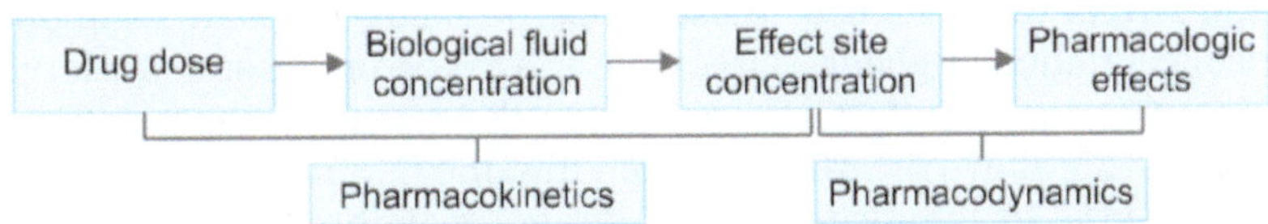

Fig. 1: The relationship between pharmacokinetics-pharmacodynamics (PK-PD) of drugs.

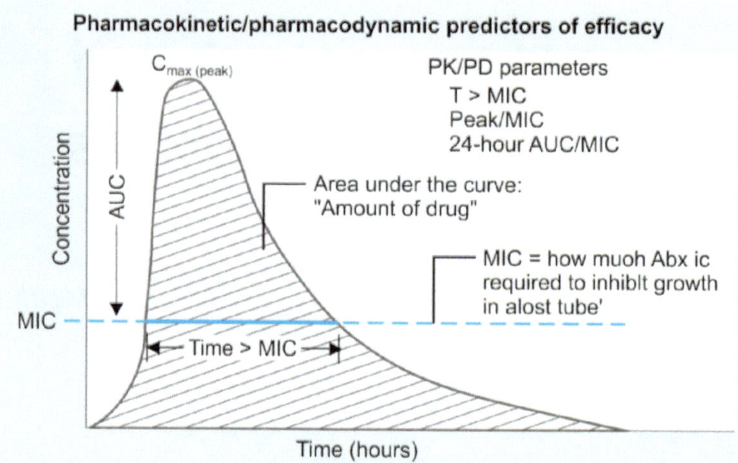

Fig. 2: Plasma time concentration curve of a drug and various pharmacokinetics-pharmacodynamics (PK-PD) parameters.
(AUC: area under the curve; C_{max}: maximum concentration; MIC: minimum inhibitory concentration; T>MIC: time above MIC)

minimal inhibitory concentration (MIC) of the drug against a particular organism, we begin to understand the concept of PK-PD of antibacterial agents.

TYPES OF ANTIBACTERIAL EFFECTS

There are three PD properties of antibiotics that best describe killing activity—these are concentration-dependence, time-dependence, and persistent effects. The rate of killing is determined by either the effect of increasing concentrations (concentration-dependent) or length of time necessary to kill (time-dependent) and persistent suppression of bacterial growth following antibiotic exposure (postantibiotic effect). Using these parameters, antibiotics can be divided into three categories: (1) concentration-dependent killing with moderate-to-persistent bactericidal effects, (2) time-dependent killing with no or minimal persistent bactericidal effects, and (3) time-dependent killing with prolonged persistent effects. PK-PD parameters are interrelated and these are influenced by dose adjustments. Unlike other drugs, it is important to recognize that an organism's MIC strongly influences the likelihood of PK-PD target attainment.

Concentration-dependent Killing with Moderate-to-Persistent Bactericidal Effects

Antibiotics belonging to this group exhibit maximum bactericidal activity at the highest concentration and have a persistent effect in suppressing bacterial growth after the concentration drops below the MIC of the organism. These properties allow a dosing regimen that aims to maximize the concentration by giving a large dose and to keep an extended interval dosing due to the advantage of prolonged effect. Concentration-dependent killing is determined by how much greater is the C_{max} above the MIC and from this, the C_{max} to MIC ratio is calculated. The minimum ratio should be 10; the greater the ratio, the greater is the kill power of the antimicrobial agent. An excellent example of this is the aminoglycoside class of drugs which produce similar or better results when the total dose is given as a once-daily injection versus twice or thrice daily. The other common examples are fluoroquinolones and colistin.

Colistin is increasingly being used to treat multidrug resistant gram-negative infections. With a better understanding of PK-PD of colistin, dosing recommendations have been updated from 1–2 million units (MU) three times a day to initiating treatment with a loading dose. Colistin exhibits concentration-dependent killing and is rapidly bactericidal at concentrations above the MIC. Clinical cure rates of 82% was achieved in adults by using a loading dose of 9 MU followed by 4.5 MU as a maintenance dosage every 12 hours. The loading dose may go up to 12 MU. The logic behind administering the loading dose is because almost two-third of colistin administered as its prodrug colistimethate sodium is excreted unchanged by the kidneys soon after administration. The loading dose should be administered intravenously over 1–2 hours, followed by the first maintenance dose after 12 hours. Recently, a small study in seven children with carbapenem-resistant gram-negative infection aged 46 days–14 years suggests that a loading dose of 150,000 units/kg up to a max of 9 MU followed by a maintenance dose of 75,000 units/kg up–4.5 MU every 12 hours could provide desired plasma concentrations of more than 1 mg/L. However, further studies should be conducted in critically ill children to confirm these results.

Time-dependent Killing with no or Minimal Persistent Bactericidal Effects

On the other hand, some antibiotics demonstrate "time-dependent killing" which means that the efficacy is dependent on how long in the dosing interval the concentration of the drug remains above the MIC levels. For antibiotics in this class, concentrations at four times the MIC are sufficient to kill the organisms and killing is not improved at higher concentrations. Hence, the key PK-PD parameter associated with efficacy is time above MIC (T>MIC) and thus, more frequent administration of antibiotics is often needed. Beta-lactams, such as penicillins, cephalosporins, and carbapenems have this property. Cephalosporins, which have a slow rate of killing require a T>MIC of 60–70% of the dosing interval for maximum efficacy; less time is acceptable for penicillins (50%) and carbapenems (40%), which have faster rates of killing.

Studies have shown that the bacteriological efficacy is greater than 80% in such cases. In children with otitis media, bacteriological cure rates of 80–85% were observed when the serum concentrations exceeded the MIC for 40–50% of the dosing interval and increased to nearly 100% when it was 60–70% of the dosing interval. Table 1 shows the probability of achieving the PK-PD target of piperacillin-tazobactam (P-T) against *Escherichia coli* and *Klebsiella pneumoniae*,

TABLE 1: Probability of attaining pharmacokinetics-pharmacodynamics (PK-PD) targets of piperacillin-tazobactam with different dosing intervals.

Regimen	*Probability of attaining PK-PD target measures*				
	30%	*40%*	*50%*	*60%*	*70%*
Escherichia coli					
3.375 g every 4 hours	0.96	0.92	0.9	0.86	0.77
3.375 g every 6 hours	0.91	0.86	0.73	0.50	0.28
Klebsiella pneumoniae					
3.375 g every 4 hours	0.77	0.72	0.65	0.57	0.48
3.375 g every 6 hours	0.69	0.57	0.43	0.29	0.16

which are extended-spectrum beta-lactamase-producing phenotypes. For example, giving P-T at a dose of 3.375 g every 6 hours had a 73% probability of achieving concentrations greater then MIC against *E. coli* for 50% of the dosing interval. This increased to 90% if the same dose was given every 4 hours. For beta-lactam antibiotics, increasing the dose to increase C_{max} more than four times the MIC does not usually result in achieving greater killing.

Time-dependent Killing with Prolonged Persistent Effects

The time-dependent antimicrobials have additional antibacterial activity after serum concentrations have dropped below the MIC. Efficacy of these antibiotics depends on the total exposure of the organism to the drug and PK-PD parameter associated with efficacy for this category of antibiotics is AUC_{0-24}/MIC ratio. Antimicrobials belonging to this category are macrolides, tetracyclines, clindamycin, linezolid, and vancomycin.

In adults with methicillin-resistant *Staphylococcus aureus* (MRSA) infections being treated with vancomycin, an AUC_{0-24}/MIC of more than 400 has been associated with improved clinical outcomes. However, data in children linking improved outcomes with attainment of an AUC_{0-24}/MIC of more than 400 is lacking. For children with serious or invasive MRSA infections, initiating intravenous (IV) vancomycin 15 mg/kg/dose every 6 hours is recommended as a means of reaching the goal to eradicate isolates with a MIC of less than or equal to 1 mg/mL. It was found in a study that an AUC_{0-24}/MIC of 80–120 and T>MIC of more than 85% of the dosing interval were associated with successful treatment of bacteremia, lower respiratory tract infection, and skin and soft tissue infection in debilitated adult patients. Studies have demonstrated that more frequent doses (every 8 hours) are required for children less than 12 years of age to achieve appropriate exposure.

The other example is azithromycin whose efficacy depends primarily on the total exposure of the organism to the drug and AUC_{0-24}/MIC being more than 100.

Table 2 summarizes the types of killing of antibacterial agents.

TABLE 2: Types of killing for different antibacterial agents.

Pattern of activity	*Antibiotics*	*Goal of therapy*	*PK-PD parameter*
Concentration-dependent killing and prolonged persistent effects	Aminoglycosides Fluoroquinolones Daptomycin Ketolides	Maximize concentrations; increase dose	C_{max}/MIC (should be >10) and AUC_{0-24}/MIC (should be >125)
Time-dependent killing with no or minimal persistent bactericidal effects	Carbapenems Cephalosporins Erythromycin penicillin	Maximize duration of exposure; increase duration of infusion or increase frequency of administration	T>MIC (at least 40% of the dosing interval for carbapenems; 50% for penicillins; and 60–70% for cephalosporins)
Time-dependent killing with moderate-to-prolonged persistent effects	Azithromycin Clindamycin Oxazolidinones Tetracyclines Vancomycin	Maximize amount of exposure; increase dose, frequency of administration or duration of infusion	AUC_{0-24}/MIC (>400 for vancomycin and 80–120 for linezolid)

(C_{max}: maximum concentration; MIC: minimum inhibitory concentration; PK-PD: pharmacokinetics-pharmacodynamics; T>MIC: time above MIC)

AUGMENTED RENAL CLEARANCE IN CRITICALLY ILL PATIENTS

Critically ill patients undergo physiological changes that can alter drug PK. Traditionally, dose adjustments of antimicrobials have been done based on the renal impairment in these patients. However, augmented renal clearance (ARC) has recently begun to be recognized as an alteration in kidney function that can led to accelerated drug elimination and suboptimal drug levels. Around 20–65% of critically ill patients have ARC. Younger age group, polytrauma, and severity of illness have been identified as risk factors.

Augmented renal clearance is a fairly new concept and does not have a standard definition. However, according to broad consensus, ARC is defined as a creatinine clearance (CrCl) of more than 130 mL/minute/1.73m^2. The normal glomerular filtration rate (GFR) in young adults is approximately 125 mL/min/1.73m^2. The mechanism of ARC is not well defined. However, the combination of systemic inflammation coupled with a physiological renal function reserve has been accepted as a possible mechanism for ARC. It has been postulated that systemic inflammatory response syndrome (SIRS), an activation of the immune system could be associated with ARC. The release of inflammatory mediators leads to decrease vascular resistance and increase in cardiac output. This together with intensive fluid therapy and use of inotropic drugs may increase renal blood flow and the GFR. The concept of renal function reserve refers to the capacity of the kidneys to increase GFR in response to certain physiological and pathological stimuli. This would explain the association of ARC and risk factors, such as young age and polytrauma.

It can influence the PK profile of antimicrobial drugs that are renally cleared, such as beta-lactams, vancomycin or aminoglycosides. Enhanced drug clearance leads to shorter half-life, lower C_{max}, and smaller AUC, thereby compromising their efficacy. There are several studies that have shown that the ARC has been significantly and consistently related to subtherapeutic beta-lactam and vancomycin levels. However, the impact of ARC on clinical outcome has not been studied adequately.

An increase in antimicrobial clearance can have negative consequences, but could be overcome with alternative dosing strategies that optimize drug exposure, such as higher daily dose, continuous/extended infusions or loading dose. Further studies are warranted in critically ill patients to explore the dosage adjustment based on the ARC.

CAPSULE SUMMARY

- Augmented renal clearance is defined as a creatinine clearance of (CrCl of >130 mL/minute/1.73 m^2.
- Around 20–65% of critically ill patients have ARC.
- Younger age group, polytrauma, and severity of illness have been identified as risk factors.
- Augmented renal clearance can influence the PK profile of antimicrobial drugs that are renally cleared, such as beta-lactams, vancomycin or aminoglycosides.

THERAPEUTIC DRUG MONITORING

Measurement of the concentration of a specific drug in serum or plasma in a designed interval is known as TDM. This is considered important for antibiotics wherein a strong relationship has been demonstrated between drug concentrations and clinical efficacy and/or toxicity, and more so if the drug shows high PK variability. TDM guides in customizing the optimal dosage of an antibiotic in a particular patient. In other areas where TDM is also useful are drug-drug interactions, compliance, and therapy cessation monitoring. Several methods have been used for measuring serum concentrations of antimicrobial agents, including bioassay, high-performance liquid chromatography (HPLC), and mass spectrometry.

Antimicrobial drugs, such as aminoglycosides, vancomycin, and some azole antifungals (voriconazole and posaconazole) show both significant PK variability and potential toxicity in the patients and in these cases, TDM is a valuable tool for the safe use of these drugs.

Aminoglycosides, such as gentamicin, amikacin, and tobramycin are commonly used antibiotics in children. Irreversible ototoxicity and nephrotoxicity in the form of renal tubular damage are associated with aminoglycosides. These antibiotics are excreted by the kidneys with a lot of interindividual variability. Hence, to prevent this toxicity from happening, TDM is performed at trough level which should be less than 2 mg/mL.

There is a challenge using vancomycin in the neonatal and pediatric patient populations due to the necessity for achieving a high concentration to maintain effective antimicrobial activity and its adverse effects profile. This drug is also renally cleared with significant inter-individual variability. Over the last decade, the recommended pediatric vancomycin dosages have increased as the conventional dosing regimens in children resulted in low initial trough concentrations, thereby leading to treatment failure. The pediatric-specific guidelines from the Infectious Diseases Society of America (IDSA) recommend targeting trough concentration more than 15 mg/mL in critically ill children and more than 10 mg/mL for all pediatric patients. In 2011, the adult guideline by the IDSA was revisited and pediatric-specific guidance was included. However, the authors acknowledged that their recommendation for a target trough concentration of 15–20 mg/mL in critically ill children required additional study and was supported by moderate evidence from respected authorities and expert opinions. In this context, TDM gives clinicians the opportunity to assess whether the drug dose is achieving the expected serum concentration or not. Critically abnormal serum trough concentrations should be followed by an appropriate dosing modification.

Voriconazole is a triazole antifungal administered both orally and intravenously with a high oral bioavailability. It is metabolized in the liver by the cytochrome (CY) P450 system and thus demonstrates significant interindividual variability. It is also susceptible to many drug-drug interactions. In case of voriconazole, concentration-effect, and concentration-toxicity relationships are consistently reported. In a prospective randomized controlled trial, outcomes in patients undergoing TDM (who had plasma concentration maintained between 1.0 mg/L and 5.5 mg/L) were significantly better (81%) than those in the non-TDM group (57%). It is, therefore, recommended to target a trough concentration of more than 1 mg/L for both prophylaxis and treatment of invasive fungal diseases. To reduce the risk of toxicity (visual disturbances, liver dysfunction, skin reactions, and neurotoxicity), the dosage should be adjusted to keep serum concentration less than 5.5 mg/L. The serum trough concentration should be measured within 7 days of initiation of therapy, or following dose adjustment.

In addition, there has been increased interest regarding the application of TDM for drugs used for tuberculosis and for beta-lactam drugs as well. Beta-lactam TDM would be helpful in patients who are critically ill, obese, elderly, cystic fibrosis or infected due to pathogens with high MICs.

CAPSULE SUMMARY

- Therapeutic drug monitoring refers to the measurement of the concentration of a drug in serum or plasma.
- It helps in customizing the dosage of an antibiotic for a patient.
- It is a valuable tool for antimicrobial drugs, such as aminoglycosides, vancomycin and some azole antifungals, all of which have both significant PK variability and potential toxicity.

CONTINUOUS/EXTENDED INFUSION

In clinical practice beta-lactams antibiotics are very commonly used to treat various bacterial infections. Efficacy of these drugs is dependent on how long the concentrations of the drug remain above the MIC levels for the pathogen in the dosing interval (Fig. 3). This can be achieved either by shortening the dosing interval or prolonging the infusion time of the drug. Intermittent dosing regimens are associated with a high peak and low trough. Hence, the serum concentrations falls below the MIC and regrowth of bacteria occurs. So a better strategy is continuous infusion or extended infusion. When the infusion is prolonged for the entire dosing interval, then it is called as continuous infusion whereas when the infusion given for 40–50% of the dosing interval (3–4 hours), then it is known as extended infusion. The total daily milligram per kilogram dose of beta-lactam antibiotics used in continuous or extended infusion dosing is same as used for intermittent infusions. A strategy of administering high dose coupled with prolonged infusion should be adopted for patients infected with organisms having high MICs. However, the first dose should always be given as a bolus to ensure therapeutic levels are achieved quickly.

Evidence of better tissue penetration with continuous infusion into the lungs, subcutaneous tissue, and intra-abdominal tissue has been documented. There were potential clinical benefits associated with prolonged beta-lactam infusion in hospitalized adult patients as per a large meta-analysis comprising 29 studies. Prolonged infusion was associated with a reduction in mortality and improvement in clinical success rates compared with intermittent boluses. Studies have also suggested that giving meropenem as an infusion over 4 hours as against bolus doses reduces the risk of failure; a retrospective Japanese study also showed a significant difference

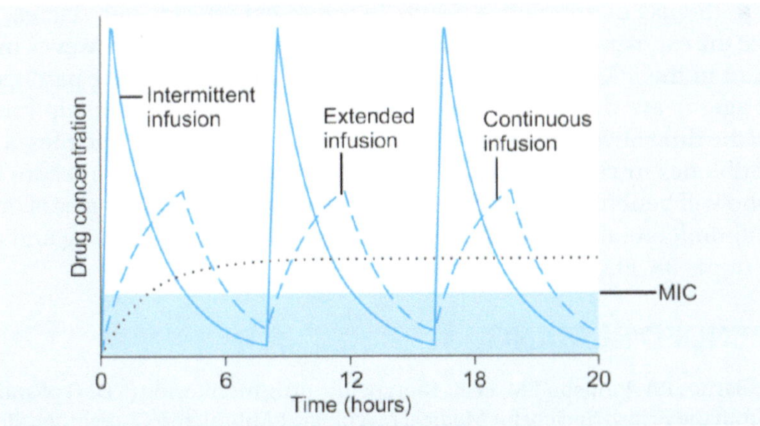

Fig. 3: Time above the minimum inhibitory concentration (MIC) for intermittent, extended and continuous infusion of time-dependent drugs. Extended or continuous infusion of time-dependent drugs can improve the percentage of the dosing interval time above MIC (T>MIC), particularly when treating infections with elevated MICs. Intermittent infusion (solid line), extended infusion (dashed line), and continuous infusion (dotted line) are compared with the time that each dosing regimen is below the MIC, highlighted by the grey area. Curves were generated using the same total daily dose and consistent pharmacokinetic parameters for each regimen.

Source: Downes KJ, Hahn A, Wiles J, et al. Dose optimisation of antibiotics in children: application of pharmacokinetics/pharmacodynamics in paediatrics. Int J Antimicrob Agents. 2014;43(3):223-30.

in mortality. However, in children, there is need for a large, multicenter randomized controlled trial to determine whether there is a clinical benefit of this dosing strategy beyond the PK-PD advantages.

Despite the advantages, practical concerns associated with prolonged infusion should be taken into consideration. Some of these include the limited stability of beta-lactams at room temperature, availability of pump or infusion devices, limited IV access, compatibility issues with other drugs, and patient mobility. Therefore, the use of prolonged infusion should be considered based on patient factors and a clinical setting wherein the benefits outweigh the inconveniences.

Based on available evidence, prolonged infusion dosing of beta-lactam antibiotics in pediatric patients should be considered on a case-by-case basis. Patients who will benefit include those with serious gram-negative infections, such as meningitis, pneumonia, bacteremia, etc. those infected with pathogens with high MIC, and those with repeated exposure to antibiotics. Infants and children have increased clearance of beta-lactams compared to adults and, hence, may benefit from a prolonged infusion strategy.

CAPSULE SUMMARY

- The PK-PD characteristics of beta-lactams make them a suitable candidate for prolonged infusion.
- The infusion can be prolonged for the entire dosing interval (continuous infusion) or it can be extended to 40–50% of the dosing interval (3–4 hours).
- Continuous or extended infusion dosing of beta-lactam antibiotics is the same as the total daily milligram per kilogram dose used for intermittent infusions.

CONCLUSIONS

There are several proof-of-concept studies that have suggested that the application of PK-PD principles to the use of antibiotics results in improved efficacy and decreases the risk of resistance since the exposure to the antimicrobials is not suboptimal. However, one parameter that is important in this PK-PD relationship is the MIC of the offending pathogen. As newer antimicrobial agents are developed, investigating the PK-PD relationship has become an integral part of the drug development process. Knowledge of PK-PD principles is crucial when prescribing antibiotics in children, particularly when treating serious infections. Identifying the patients who will benefit the most from nontraditional dosing strategies is important. The foundation of antimicrobial stewardship is judicious antibiotic prescribing and an important component of this is PK-PD dose optimization.

RECOMMENDED READING

1. Ashbee HR, Barnes RA, Johnson EM, et al. Therapeutic drug monitoring (TDM) of antifungal agents: guidelines from the British Society for Medical Mycology. J Antimicrob Chemother. 2014;69:1162-76.
2. Balch AH, Constance JE, Thorell EA, et al. Pediatric vancomycin dosing: Trends over time and the impact of therapeutic drug monitoring. J Clin Pharmacol. 2015;55(2):212-20.
3. Barker CI, Germovsek E, Hoare RL, et al. Pharmacokinetic/pharmacodynamic modelling approaches in paediatric infectious diseases and immunology. Adv Drug Deliv Rev. 2014;73:127-39.
4. Barker CI, Standing JF, Turner MA, et al. Antibiotic dosing in children in Europe: can we grade the evidence from pharmacokinetic/pharmacodynamic studies—and when is enough data enough? Curr Opin Infect Dis. 2012;25:235-42.

5. Bilbao-Meseguer I, Rodríguez-Gascón A, Barrasa H, et al. Augmented Renal Clearance in Critically Ill Patients: A Systematic Review. Clin Pharmacokinet. 2018; 57(9):1107-21.
6. Cooper TW, Pass SE, Brouse SD, et al. Can pharmacokinetic and pharmacodynamic principles be applied to the treatment of multidrug-resistant Acinetobacter? Ann Pharmacother. 2011;45:229-40.
7. Craig WA, Andes D. Pharmacokinetics and pharmacodynamics of antibiotics in otitis media. Pediatr Inf Dis J. 1995;15:255-9.
8. De Cock PA, Standing JF, Barker CI, et al. Augmented renal clearance implies a need for increased amoxicillin-clavulanic acid dosing in critically ill children. Antimicrob Agents Chemother. 2015;59:7027-35.
9. Downes KJ, Hahn A, Wiles J, et al. Dose optimisation of antibiotics in children: application of pharmacokinetics/pharmacodynamics in paediatrics. Int J Antimicrob Agents. 2014;43(3):223-30.
10. Ebert SC. Application of pharmacokinetics and pharmacodynamics to antibiotic selection. P&T. 2004;29:244-53.
11. Frimodt-Møller N. How predictive is PK/PD for antibacterial agents? Int J Antimicrob Agents. 2002;19:333-9.
12. Huttner A, Harbarth S, Hope WW, et al. Therapeutic drug monitoring of the β-lactam antibiotics: what is the evidence and which patients should we be using it for? J Antimicrob Chemother. 2015;70:3178-83.
13. Itabashi S. Clinical efficacy of prolonged (4 hour) drip infusion of meropenem against severe pneumonia. Jpn J Antibiot. 2007;60:161-70.
14. Jelliff R. Challenges in individualizing drug dosage for intensive care unit patients: Is augmented renal clearance what we really want to know? Some suggested management approaches and clinical software tools. Clin Pharmacokinet. 2016;55:897-905.
15. Karnik ND, Sridharan K, Jadhav SP, et al. Pharmacokinetics of colistin in critically ill patients with multidrug-resistant gram-negative bacilli infection. Eur J Clin Pharmacol. 2013;69:1429-36.
16. Labuschagne Q, Schellack N, Gous A, et al. COLISTIN: adult and paediatric guideline for South Africa, 2016. S Afr J Infect Dis. 2016;31(1):3-7.
17. MacGowan A. Revisiting beta-lactams—PK/PD improves dosing of old antibiotics. Curr Opin Pharmacol. 2011;11:470-6.
18. MacVanea SH, Kutia JL, Nicolaua DP. Prolonging beta-lactam infusion: a review of the rationale and evidence, and guidance for implementation. Int J Antimicrob Agents. 2014;43:105-13.
19. Martinez MN, Papich MG, Drusano GL. Dosing regimen matters: the importance of early intervention and rapid attainment of the pharmacokinetic/pharmacodynamic target. Antimicrob Agents Chemother. 2012;56:2795-805.
20. Pettit RS, Neu N, Cies JJ, et al. Population pharmacokinetics of meropenem administered as a prolonged infusion in children with cystic fibrosis. J Antimicrob Chemother. 2016;71:189-95.
21. Ryback MJ. Pharmacodynamics: Relation to antimicrobial resistance. Am J Infection Control. 2006;34:S38-45.
22. Suchánková H, Lipš M, Urbánek K, et al. Is continuous infusion of imipenem always the best choice? Int J Antimicrob Agents. 2017;49:348-54.
23. Teo J, Liew Y, Lee W, et al. Prolonged infusion versus intermittent boluses of beta-lactam antibiotics for treatment of acute infections: a meta-analysis. Int J Antimicrob Agents. 2014;43:403-11.
24. Yusuf E, Spapen H, Piérard D. Prolonged vs intermittent infusion of piperacillin/tazobactam in critically ill patients: a narrative and systematic review. J Crit Care. 2014;29:1089-95.

Penicillins and Monobactams

5

Chapter

Raju C Shah, Pratima Shah

INTRODUCTION

Beta-lactam (BL) antibiotics are antibiotics possessing a BL ring and include penicillins, cephalosporins, monobactams and carbapenems.

PENICILLINS

Penicillin was the first antibiotic to be used clinically in 1941. It was discovered by Alexender Fleming and originally obtained from the fungus *Penicillium notatum*, but the present source is *Penicillium chrysogenum*. The penicillin nucleus consists of a fused thiazolidine and BL ring to which side chains are attached through an amide linkage. Different side chains can be attached resulting in different semisynthetic penicillins with unique antibacterial activities and different pharmacokinetics. At the carboxyl end of thiazolidine ring, salts may be formed with Na^+ and K^+ which impart stability.

Mechanism of Action

All BL antibiotics interfere with the synthesis of bacterial cell wall. Bacterial cell wall is made of uridine diphosphate N-acetylmuramic acid (UDP NAM) and UDP-N-acetylglucosamine. These peptidoglycan residues are linked together forming long strands. The final step is cleavage of the terminal D-alanine of the peptide chain by transpeptidase, which then facilitates cross-linking of the peptide chains thus providing stability and rigidity to the cell wall. This transpeptidase is inhibited by BL antibiotics hence producing cell wall deficient (CWD) forms, which are prone to lysis. The cell wall of gram-positive bacteria is almost entirely made of peptidoglycan in comparison to gram-negative bacteria, which explains why penicillin is more effective against gram-positive bacteria. Blood, pus, and tissue fluid do not interfere with the antibacterial action of BL antibiotics.

Penicillin G (Benzylpenicillin)

There are four types of natural penicillins designated F, G, X, and K. Out of these, penicillin G (PnG) has a benzyl side chain and has the most desirable properties and is used clinically.

Antibacterial Spectrum

Penicillin G is narrow spectrum antibiotic; activity is limited primarily to gram-positive bacteria and few others. Streptococci (except enterococci) are highly sensitive. Most strains of *Staphylococcus aureus* are resistant. Gonococci and to some extent meningococci have developed partial or high level of resistance. Most of the gram-positive bacilli, gram-positive and gram-negative anaerobes (with the exception of *Bacteroides fragilis*), and *Treponema pallidum* are highly sensitive. Most of the gram-negative bacilli, *Mycobacterium tuberculosis*, rickettsiae, and chlamydia are resistant.

Bacterial Resistance

Two types of bacterial resistance are:

1. *Natural*: This is due to deeper location of penicillin-binding proteins (PBPs) under lipoprotein barrier where PnG is unable to penetrate.
2. *Acquired*: It is mainly by production of penicillinase enzyme which opens the BL ring and inactivates PnG. It is acquired through a plasmid by conjugation or transduction. Second mechanism is that bacteria develop low affinity PBPs which do not bind to penicillin tightly. Third mechanism is either loss or alteration in porin channels in cell wall which transport the antibiotics.

Pharmacokinetics

Penicillin G is acid labile. The oral absorption is poor and infants who have low acidity absorb only one-third of the dose. It reaches most body fluids, but penetration in serous cavities and cerebrospinal fluid (CSF) is poor. It is poorly metabolized and rapidly excreted by kidney, 10% by glomerular filtration (GFR) and rest by tubular secretion. Neonates have imperfect tubular secretion so half-life is longer which reaches adult levels by 3 months of age.

Preparations and Dose

Sodium penicillin G (crystalline PnG) injection: Usual dose 100,000–250,000 units/kg/day q 4–6 hourly intravenous (IV) or intramuscular (IM) (maximum dose 400,000 units/kg/day, 24 million units).

Potassium penicillin G for oral use

Repository PnG injection: Given deep IM and releases PnG slowly

Procaine PnG injection: Levels are sustained for 1–2 days. Usual dose is 50,000 units/kg/day q 24 hourly IM

Benzathine PnG: Levels are sustained for weeks. Dose is 600,000–1,200,000 units IM every 3–4 weeks.

Unfortunately none of the injectable/oral preparations of PnG are easily available in the market.

Therapeutic Uses

- Penicillin G retains its place as the drug of choice for syphilis, anthrax, diphtheria, rat bite fever, erysipeloid, tetanus, trench mouth, actinomycosis, and gas gangrene.
- It remains the drug of choice for treatment of infections caused by sensitive strains of *Streptococcus pneumoniae* particularly pneumonia.

- It is universally effective against group A beta-hemolytic streptococcal infections, such as streptococcal pharyngitis, scarlet fever, and invasive infections. 3 weekly benzathine penicillin is the agent of choice for rheumatic fever prophylaxis. It is also useful for treatment of viridans streptococcal infections, such as endocarditis if the isolate is penicillin sensitive.
- Most anaerobes are sensitive to PnG with exception of *B. fragilis*. It is useful drug for periodontal infections, lung, and brain abscess.
- Penicillin G was till recently the drug of choice for meningococcal infections, but it does not eliminate the carrier state and there are reports of increasing resistance in meningococci.
- Penicillin G is no longer the therapy of choice for gonorrhea, unless it is known that gonococcal isolates of a particular geographical area are susceptible.
- It is also effective against Lyme disease, but amoxicillin is the drug of choice.

Adverse Effects

- *Local irritancy and direct toxicity*: Pain at IM injection site, nausea on oral intake, and thrombophlebitis of injected vein are dose-related expression of irritancy. Large accidental IV injection can cause central nervous system (CNS) sign/symptoms.
- *Hypersensitivity*: An incidence of 1–10% is reported. Frequent manifestations are rashes, itching, urticaria, and fever; anaphylaxis rare (1 to 4/10,000). Allergy is more after following parenteral rather than oral route. Allergy is higher with procaine penicillin and the course of allergy is unpredictable. There is partial cross-sensitivity between different types of penicillins. An intradermal test using benzylpenicilloyl polylysine is done to rule out immediate type of hypersensitivity.
- *Superinfections*: Rare due to narrow spectrum.
- *Jarisch–Herxheimer reaction*: It occurs in syphilitic patients. It last for 12–72 hours, does not recur, and does not need interruption of therapy.

Semisynthetic Penicillins

The aim of producing semisynthetic penicillins has been to overcome the shortcomings of PnG, which are:

- Poor oral efficacy
- Susceptibility to penicillinase
- Narrow spectrum of activity.

Classification

- *Acid-resistant alternatives to PnG*: Phenoxymethylpenicillin (penicillin V)
- *Penicillinase-resistant penicillins:* Methicillin, oxacillin, cloxacillin, nafcillin
- *Extended-spectrum penicillins:*
  - Aminopenicillins: Ampicillin, amoxicillin, and bacampicillin
  - Carboxypenicillins: Carbenicillin and ticarcillin
  - Ureidopenicillins: Mezlocillin and piperacillin
  - Mecillinam
- Combinations of penicillins with beta-lactamase inhibitors (BLIs), such as clavulanic acid, sulbactam, and tazobactam (amoxicillin clavulanic acid, ampicillin sulbactam, ticarcillin clavulanic acid, and piperacillin-tazobactam).

Phenoxymethylpenicillin (Penicillin V)

It is acid stable and hence oral bioavailability is better. The antibacterial spectrum of penicillin V is identical to PnG, but it is about one-fifth the potency of PnG against *Neisseria*, other gram-negative bacteria and anaerobes. It is commonly prescribed for treatment of streptococcal pharyngitis (children 250 mg twice daily and adults 500 mg twice daily for 10 days) and for antibacterial prophylaxis in patients with asplenia and hyposplenia (<5 years 125 mg twice daily and >5 years 250 mg twice daily).

Penicillinase-resistant Penicillins

These agents, in general, are less effective against organisms susceptible to PnG and are not useful against gram-negative organisms. Their use should be restricted to the treatment of infections that are known or suspected to be caused by methicillin-sensitive *Staphylococcus aureus* (MSSA). Owing to their narrow spectrum of action they are the drugs of first choice for MSSA. They are more efficacious than the first-generation cephalosporins (cefazolin) in this respect and are not susceptible to the inoculum effect. However erratic availability in the market, higher cost, need for more frequent administration, and phlebitis are disadvantages as compared to cefazolin. Recently published retrospective analysis has shown cefazolin to be non inferior to cloxacillin for MSSA infections. A randomized clinical trial comparing the two is in the offing. However for CNS MSSA infections, cloxacillin is the drug of choice since cefazolin penetrates the blood brain barrier poorly.

Methicillin

It is highly penicillinase resistant but not acid resistant. Hematuria, albuminuria, and reversible interstitial nephritis are unique adverse effects and it has largely been replaced by cloxacillin.

Cloxacillin and Flucloxacillin

They are highly penicillinase and acid resistant. Oral bioavailability is however variable. It is more active than methicillin against penicillinase producing staphylococci. It is the drug of choice for treating MSSA, such as endocarditis, pneumonia, bone and joint infections, skin and soft-tissue infections, and sepsis. Usual dose is 100 mg/kg/day q 6 hourly IV for skin/soft-tissue and bone/joint infections. After the infection settles, treatment can be switched to oral cloxacillin or first-generation cephalosporins. For serious infections, such as endocarditis and meningitis dose can be increased to 200 mg/kg/day given 4 hourly (maximum dose 12 g/day).

Nafcillin

It is penicillinase resistant and only partially acid resistant. Hepatitis and neutropenia are occasional side effects. It is not commercially available in India.

Aminopenicillins

Ampicillin

It is active against all organisms sensitive to PnG; additionally many gram-negative bacilli, e.g. *Haemophilus influenzae, Escherichia coli, Proteus, Salmonella,* and *Shigella* are inhibited.

Anaerobic activity is lower as compared to PnG. It is not penicillinase resistant. There is increasing prevalence of resistance to ampicillin in *Shigella, H. influenzae, Moraxella catarrhalis,* and *S. pneumoniae. Klebsiella* is inherently resistant to ampicillin. Oral absorption is adequate. Diarrhea is frequent and it alters intestinal flora owing to its broad spectrum. It produces high incidence of rashes (10%), especially in patients with infectious mononucleosis. Probenecid retards normal excretion of ampicillin. Usual childhood dose is 100–200 mg/kg/day q 6 hourly IV/IM. For meningitis the dose is 200–400 mg/kg/day q 4–6 hourly IV (maximum dose 12 g/day). Oral dose is 50–100 mg/kg/day.

A fixed dose combination of ampicillin and cloxacillin is available and used frequently. This combination is not synergistic since cloxacillin is not active against gram-negative organisms and ampicillin is not active against staphylococci. Thus, for any given infection one of the components is useless and adds to cost and adverse effects.

Bacampicillin

It is a prodrug of ampicillin. Tissue penetration is better and incidence of diarrhea is claimed to be lower. It is not commercially available.

Amoxicillin

It is close congener of ampicillin similar to it in all respects except that oral absorption is better, incidence of diarrhea is less, and it is less active against *Shigella.* Usual childhood dose is 25–50 mg/kg/day q 8 hourly oral. For penicillin intermediate/resistant nonmeningeal pneumococcal infections [now defined as those organisms with a penicillin minimum inhibitory concentration (MIC) of >2] a higher dose of 80–90 mg/kg/day is recommended.

Therapeutic Indications for Aminopenicillins

- *Pediatric respiratory infections*: They are first-line drugs for management of otitis media, bacterial sinusitis, streptococcal pharyngitis, and community-acquired pneumonia. However, since they are not penicillinase resistant they do not cover beta-lactamase producing organisms, such as *H. influenzae* and *M. catarrhalis.* Since the prevalence of penicillin resistance in nonmeningeal *S. pneumoniae* infections is still low, ampicillin/amoxicillin in standard doses is effective.
- *Pediatric urinary tract infections*: Rising incidence of beta-lactamase production in *E. coli* has reduced the utility of these drugs for this indication.
- *Enteric fever*: With return of sensitivity in *S. typhi/paratyphi,* ampicillin in doses of 100 mg/kg may be considered for outpatient therapy. However, tolerability to high doses is a problem.
- Ampicillin is the drug of choice for susceptible enterococcal infections. For most isolates, the MIC of ampicillin is two- to fourfold lower than that of penicillin. Combination therapy with an aminoglycoside (e.g. gentamicin and streptomycin) is recommended for enterococcal endocarditis and enterococcal infections in the immunocompromised. Dose is 200 mg/kg/day given 4–6 hourly (maximum dose 12 g/day).
- Prophylaxis of infective endocarditis.
- Drug of choice for Listeria and group B streptococcal disease.
- The use of aminopenicillins in therapy of serious community-acquired infections, such as meningitis, neonatal sepsis, urinary tract infections, severe pneumonia, and intra-abdominal sepsis has been largely replaced by third-generation cephalosporins.

Carboxypenicillins and Ureidopenicillins

Carbenicillin

It is neither penicillinase resistant nor acid resistant. It is however very active against *Pseudomonas aeruginosa* and indole-positive Proteus. High doses are associated with bleeding due to platelet dysfunction. Dose is 400–600 mg/kg/day q 4–6 hourly IV or IM. It is not commercially available.

Ticarcillin

It is more potent than carbenicillin against pseudomonas. Like carbenicillin it is susceptible to penicillinase, has a high sodium load, and also interferes with platelet aggregation. Usual dose is 200–400 mg/kg/day q 4–6 hourly IV. In cystic fibrosis, higher doses of 400–600 mg/kg/day have been used.

Piperacillin

Its antipseudomonal activity is eight times more than carbenicillin. Usual dose is 200–300 mg/kg/day q 4–6 hourly IV (maximum dose is 24 g/day).

Therapeutic Indications of Antipseudomonal Penicillins

These agents are indicated for the treatment of patients with serious infections caused by gram-negative bacteria, such as *Pseudomonas,* indole-positive *Proteus,* and *Enterobacter*. They are relatively less effective against *E. coli* and *Klebsiella* as compared to third-generation cephalosporins. These mainly include nosocomial infections, infections in burns patients, and in the immunocompromised. However, with the increasing prevalence of extended-spectrum beta-lactamases and Amp-C beta-lactamases they have lost most of their utility unless combined with BLIs.

BETA-LACTAM ANTIBIOTICS/BETA-LACTAMASE INHIBITOR COMBINATIONS

The efficacy of BL antibiotics has been seriously hampered with the emergence of bacteria producing beta-lactamase. Hence, the combination of BL antibiotics with BLI drugs has proved to be an easy and efficient way of tackling bacterial resistance and improving clinical efficacy. Three BLIs are currently available, i.e. clavulanic acid, sulbactam, and tazobactam. BLIs act by binding and inactivating the beta-lactamase, hence protecting the BL antibiotic from hydrolysis. They also potentiate the activity of the BL antibiotics by binding directly to the penicillin-binding proteins. Some like sulbactam also have moderate intrinsic antibacterial activity against *Acinetobacter*. The BLIs also vary in their potential to inhibit the different type of beta-lactamases. Clavulanic acid mainly inhibits the first-generation beta-lactamases which are usually present in *H. influenzae* and *S. aureus, Moraxella* and certain *E. coli* and *Klebsiella* while tazobactam/sulbactam inhibit the extended-spectrum beta-lactamases as well. In this chapter we discuss the penicillin based BL-BLI combinations that are usually employed to treat community-acquired infections including amoxicillin clavulanic acid, ampicillin sulbactam, and ticarcillin clavulanic acid. The other BL-BLI combinations are discussed in Chapter 6 and 8.

Amoxicillin/Clavulanic Acid

Amoxicillin/clavulanate is a broad spectrum antibacterial combination that has been used widely for over 2 decades for treatment of respiratory tract infections.

Antibacterial Spectrum

Gram-positive spectrum includes streptococci species, beta-lactamase producing strains of *S. aureus* and *Enterococcus* species, and many gram-positive and gram-negative anaerobes. Gram-negative spectrum includes the first-generation beta-lactamase producing strains of *E. coli*, Proteus species, *H. influenzae, M. catarrhalis,* and *Neisseria gonorrhoeae.*

Pharmacokinetics

The combination ratio varies from 4:1 to 7:1 (amoxicillin:clavulanic acid). Liquid preparations are usually in ratio of 100 mg of amoxicillin to 14.25 mg of clavulanic acid. Available formulations are 200 + 28.5 mg and 400 + 57 mg. Amoxicillin and clavulanic acid are both well absorbed from the gastrointestinal tract, reaching peak serum levels 60–90 and 40–120 minutes, respectively after separate oral administration. Combining the two drugs does not affect their pharmacokinetics. IV co-amoxiclav is available in India and is available as injections of 300 mg, 600 mg, and 1.2 g with ratio of amoxicillin to clavulanic acid being 5:1.

Amoxicillin demonstrates linear pharmacokinetics. Its penetration into respiratory tract secretions is greater than those of ampicillin at peak serum concentrations of each. Also the levels of clavulanic acid in the respiratory tract secretions are comparable to those of amoxicillin despite the obvious dose difference. The elimination half-lives of amoxicillin and clavulanic acid are also similar. Amoxicillin is excreted in the urine mostly unmetabolized whereas clavulanic acid is excreted via feces, urine, and lungs.

Therapeutic Uses

- It is a very effective drug for severe upper respiratory tract infections including otitis media and sinusitis. It is preferred over amoxicillin in treatment of severe infections, infections that do not respond to amoxicillin or infections in children exposed to antibiotics in the previous 3 months where chances of drug resistance are higher. It is recommended for streptococcal pharyngitis where there are frequent recurrences. This is owing to its ability to destroy beta-lactamase in the throat produced by organisms other than *S. pyogenes* which may then destroy amoxicillin. The drug is also useful for management of community-acquired pneumonia especially in children below 5 years where beta-lactamase producing *Moraxella* and *H. Influenzae* are a concern. It is also useful in managing exacerbations of chronic bronchitis and bronchiectasis.
- It is useful for empiric and definitive treatment of urinary tract infections.
- Skin and soft-tissue infections. Here the first-generation cephalosporins are preferred owing to their narrower spectrum.
- Oral, dental infections, and infections following animal bites. Here it is the drug of choice.
- It can also be used for the treatment of melioidosis when there is allergy to cotrimoxazole.

Dosage

- *Oral*: 20–40 mg/kg/day of the amoxicillin component in two-three divided doses (maximum 3 g daily). Thrice daily dose has better efficacy, but poorer compliance. Twice daily dosing can be safely used for *Streptococcus pyogenes* where the MICs are very low.
- *Intravenous*: 50–100 mg/kg of the amoxicillin component daily in divided doses 6–8 hourly.

Adverse Effects

Gastrointestinal side effects include nausea, vomiting, diarrhea; rarely pseudomembranous colitis. Clavulanic acid increases the risk of diarrhea and preparations with lesser amount of clavulanic acid are now available. Other side effects include rashes, hypersensitivity reactions, cholestatic jaundice, and changes in liver function tests.

Ticarcillin-Clavulanate

Ticarcillin-clavulanic acid was one of the first BL, BLI combination made available for parenteral use.

Antibacterial Spectrum

Gram-positive spectrum includes *S. aureus* (methicillin sensitive), *S. epidermidis*, and *Streptococcus* species. Gram-negative spectrum includes beta-lactamase producing *H. influenzae, M. catarrhalis, B. fragilis, N. gonorrhoeae,* and some extended-spectrum beta-lactamase producing pathogens. It has unique activity against *Stenotrophomonas maltophilia.*

Pharmacodynamics/Pharmacokinetics

Concomitant administration of both substances has little effect on the kinetics of either agent alone. It is used in a ratio of 15–30:1. The mean serum half-lives are 1 hour for both drugs. The dose of ticarcillin needs adjustment if creatinine clearance is less than 60 mL/min as it is mainly excreted by the kidneys. But increasing the dosing interval in patients with end-stage renal disease may lead to periods of insufficient clavulanic acid to protect ticarcillin from beta-lactamase degradation. Both drugs achieve adequate levels in body fluids, such as blister fluid, bone, bile, and joint fluid.

Therapeutic Uses

The drug has been largely supplanted by newer BL-BLI combinations, such as piperacillin-tazobactam and cefoperazone-sulbactam due to their superior activity against nosocomial pathogens including *Pseudomonas*. It may be used for infections with *S. maltophilia.*

Dosage

Intravenous 80 mg/kg of ticarcillin every 6–8 hours (every 12 hours in neonates).

Adverse Effects

Rash, allergic reactions, and eosinophilia. Painful if given intramuscularly. Each gram provides 5–6 mEq of sodium and can produce sodium overload. Interferes with platelet aggregation and can cause elevation of liver enzymes and hemorrhagic cystitis (more frequent in children).

Ampicillin-sulbactam

Another combination of sulbactam which has been in use for a while is with ampicillin.

Antibacterial Spectrum

Effective against gram-positive bacteria with the exception of MRSA. It is active against most anaerobes. Gram-negative spectrum includes extended-spectrum beta-lactamase producing *Enterobacteriaceae* mainly *E. coli* and *Klebsiella*. No antipseudomonas activity. The sulbactam component is effective against multidrug-resistant *Acinetobacter baumannii* infections.

Pharmacokinetics

Ampicillin-sulbactam is used in a ratio of 1.5–2:1. Protein binding is 28% for ampicillin and 38% for sulbactam. These drugs are eliminated primarily by the kidney and their elimination may be decreased in neonates as a consequence of underdeveloped renal function. For the same reason dose modification is required in renal failure. Pharmacokinetic studies have demonstrated high drug concentrations at a variety of infection sites, including CSF, peritoneal fluid, and bone.

Dosage

100–200 mg/kg/day of ampicillin in 6 hourly doses; total dose of sulbactam should not exceed 4 g/day.

Indications

May be used for empirically treating serious community-acquired polymicrobial infections, such as intra-abdominal, soft-tissue, and pelvic infections. The drug is commonly used in USA instead of injectable amoxicillin clavulanic acid since the latter is not available. It is indicated in management of enterococcal infections due to strains producing beta-lactamase. This drug is not appropriate as empirical therapy for nosocomial and infections in immunocompromised where *Pseudomonas* is a possibility. It can be used once culture and sensitivity results are available, especially when the culprit is *Acinetobacter*.

MONOBACTAMS

Aztreonam

Monobactams are BLs whose structure differs from that of other BLs because they contain a monocyclic nucleus. Monobactams were first isolated from *Chromobacterium violaceum* and modified thereafter to yield aztreonam, the only currently available monobactam.

Mechanism of Action

Aztreonam has a high affinity for the protein-binding protein 3 (PBP-3) of aerobic gram-negative bacteria. Most of these organisms are inhibited and killed at low concentrations of the drug. Aztreonam binds poorly to PBP sites of the aerobic gram-positive and anaerobic bacteria and consequently has relatively poor inhibitory effects against these bacteria.

Antibacterial Spectrum

Its synthetic structure determines specific areas of activity including enhanced activity against *Pseudomonas* species, exceptional activity against gram-negative bacteria, stability to first-generation beta-lactamases, and lack of activity against gram-positive bacteria. It is not stable against extended-spectrum beta-lactamase producing *Enterobacteriaceae.* It is however stable against the metallo-beta-lactamases/carbapenemases enzymes chiefly New Delhi metallo-beta-lactamase.

Pharmacokinetics

Aztreonam is widely distributed in the body tissues and fluids, and the average elimination half-life is 1.7 hours. IM dosing results in peak serum levels in approximately 1 hour, while IV dosing results in peak levels within 5 minutes. Concentrations above the MIC90 for most gram-negative bacteria are also present within bone, prostate, and CSF. Between 60% and 70% of the drug is excreted unchanged in the urine. Serum clearance of aztreonam is directly proportional to creatinine clearance. Dosage adjustment must, therefore, be made in the presence of reduced clearance.

Therapeutic Uses

The main use of aztreonam was as a substitute to penicillins/cephalosporins in management of serious gram-negative infections when there is history of serious allergy/hypersensitivity to these agents. These indications include community-acquired infections of the urinary tract, sepsis, intra-abdominal and gynecologic infections, nosocomial infections, febrile neutropenia, enteric fever, gonorrhea, and surgical prophylaxis. However, except for enteric fever and gonorrhea, the rising prevalence of extended-spectrum beta-lactamase production in gram-negative infections limits the use of aztreonam for the other indications mentioned above. The other disadvantage is no activity against gram-positive and anaerobic pathogens, and hence other antimicrobial agents including metronidazole/vancomycin may be needed in treatment of suspected polymicrobial infections in seriously sick patients. Though aztreonam is stable against metallo-beta-lactamase producing organisms, it cannot be used since these pathogens produce other beta-lactamases including extended-spectrum beta-lactamase and AmpC which destroy aztreonam. The drug aztreonam-avibactam combination is currently in phase 2 trials for treatment of carbapenem-resistant infections. There may also be a role of combining ceftazidime-avibactam (which will soon be available) with aztreonam in treating refractory carbapenem-resistant gram-negative infections in India (See chapter 8).

Dosage

30–50 mg/kg every 6–8 hours; maximum 6–8 g daily.

Adverse Effects

Gastrointestinal disturbances, nausea, vomiting, diarrhea, abdominal cramps, mouth ulcers, altered taste, gastrointestinal bleeding, and very rarely antibiotic-associated colitis. Occasionally thrombocytopenia, neutropenia, and hepatitis injection-site reactions, skin rash, and eosinophilia may be seen.

RECOMMENDED READING

1. Bush LM, Johnson CC. Ureidopenicillins and beta-lactam/beta-lactamase inhibitor combinations. Infect Dis Clin North Am. 2000;14:409-33.
2. Hardman JG, Limbird LE, Gilman AG. Antimicrobial agents: Penicillin, cephalosporins and other beta-lactam antibiotics. Goodman & Gilman's The Pharmacological Basis of Therapeutics, 10th edition. New York: McGraw Hill; 2001. pp. 1189-218.
3. Lee N, Yuen KY, Kumana CR. Clinical role of beta-lactam/beta-lactamase inhibitor combinations. Drugs. 2003;63:1511-24.
4. Paterson DL, Bonomo RA. Extended-spectrum beta-lactamases: a clinical update. Clin Microbiol Rev. 2005;18:657-86.
5. Rittenbury MS. How and why aztreonam works. Surg Gynecol Obstet. 1990;171S:19-23.
6. Rodríguez-Baño J, Gutiérrez-Gutiérrez B, Machuca I, et al. Treatment of infections caused by extended-spectrum-beta-lactamase-, ampC-, and carbapenemase-producing enterobacteriaceae. Clin Microbiol Rev. 2018;31(2):e00079-17.

Cephalosporins

6 Chapter

Baldev S Prajapati, Rajal B Prajapati

INTRODUCTION

Giuseppe Brotzu observed the good health of recreational bathers on heavily polluted beaches of Gulf of Cagliari on the Southern Coast of Sardinia. He studied the microbial flora of seawater near a sewage outfall and isolated a strain of *Cephalosporium acremonium*. This strain secreted material with activity against a number of gram-positive and gram-negative bacteria. A series of experiments by him and Professor Howard Florey of Sir William Dunn School of Pathology, Oxford lead to production of the antibiotic in 1951. It was active only against certain gram-positive bacteria. Hence, it was called cephalosporin P. Meanwhile, another molecule was found and it was named as cephalosporin N as it was active against gram-negative bacteria. Its name was changed to penicillin N when it was found to have a structure similar to penicillin. The efforts were going on to isolate penicillin N from impurities, another substance was detected and it was named cephalosporin C. The nucleus of cephalosporin C was isolated in 1960 and it opened the doors for future research.

RELEVANT CHEMICAL ASPECTS

All cephalosporins consist of a four-membered beta-lactam ring bound to a six-membered dihydrothiazine ring. It is called cephalosporin or cephem nucleus (Fig. 1). It includes a carbon double bond between positions 3 and 4. Variations on the 7-acylamino side chain and substitutions on the cephem ring have yielded a variety of cephalosporin compounds with different activity profiles. For example, the presence of an amino methoxy group at this position as found in cefuroxime, cefotaxime and ceftriaxone confers increased beta-lactamase stability with some loss of activity against gram-positive organisms. The presence of propyl carboxy group as in a case of ceftazidime at this location produces superior antipseudomonal activity. Substitutions at position 3 of the dihydrothiazine ring play a major role in pharmacokinetics.

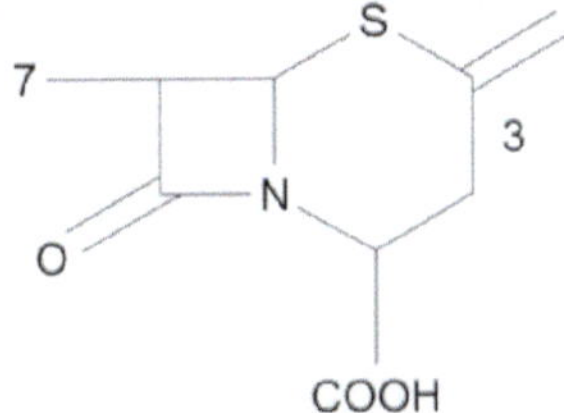

Fig. 1: Cephalosporin (cephem) nucleus.

CLASSIFICATION

The explosive growth of cephalosporins makes a system of classification most desirable. Cephalosporins may be classified by their chemical structure, clinical pharmacology, resistance to beta-lactamase or antimicrobial spectrum, but the well-accepted system of classification by "Generations" is very useful. Classification by generations is based on general features of antimicrobial activity; it also follows the sequence of their discovery.

MECHANISM OF ACTION

Like penicillins, cephalosporins act by binding to penicillin-binding proteins (PBPs) and inhibiting bacterial cell wall synthesis. The highly stressed amide group of the beta-lactam ring is conformationally similar to D-alanyl-D-alanine bond of the peptidoglycan pentapeptide. Consequently, the bacterial enzymes mistake cephalosporins for their normal substrates and react with them to yield stable covalent esters which lack catalytic activity. This in turn interferes with normal synthesis of the peptidoglycan cover.

The fifth-generation cephalosporins exert their antibacterial activity by binding to important PBPs and inhibiting their transpeptidase activity which is essential for the synthesis of bacterial cell wall. The inhibition of transpeptidation leads to inhibition of formation of bacterial cell wall resulting in cell lysis and death.

SPECTRUM OF ACTIVITY

Cephalosporins can be considered as true broad-spectrum antibiotics given their wide spectrum of activity. The first-generation cephalosporins have good activity against gram-positive bacteria and relatively modest activity against gram-negative organisms. The second-generation cephalosporins retain gram-positive activity and have increased activity against certain gram-negative pathogens. The third-generation agents are somewhat less active against gram-positive cocci, but much more active against enteric gram-negative organisms. The fourth-generation cephalosporins have greater beta-lactamase stability and an extended spectrum of activity against both gram-positive as well as gram-negative organisms including *Pseudomonas*. The fifth-generation cephalosporins have broad-spectrum activity against gram-positive and gram-negative organisms. None of the currently available cephalosporins have good activity against *Enterococcus, Mycoplasma, Campylobacter, Listeria* and *Clostridium difficile.*

MECHANISM OF RESISTANCE

Bacterial resistance to cephalosporins is achieved by distinct mechanisms.

- Inability of the drug to reach the site of action, e.g. decreased permeability through the outer membrane of gram-negative organisms.
- *Alterations in PBPs:* Alterations take place in antibiotic-binding proteins and as a result the interaction does not take place, e.g. cephalosporin-resistant pneumococci.
- *Beta-lactamase enzymes:* This is the most common mechanism. These enzymes hydrolyze the beta-lactam ring. Cephalosporins are variably susceptible to beta-lactamases; a good example is the relative resistance of second- and third-generation agents to hydrolysis by beta-lactamases produced by gram-negative organisms compared to first-generation agents. However, the exception is the extended-spectrum beta-lactamases (ESBLs) that hydrolyze the oxyimino side chain of cefotaxime, ceftriaxone, ceftazidime. This plasmid-mediated trait is most often associated with *Klebsiella pneumoniae* and *Escherichia coli* but can be transferred to other enteric bacilli. The AmpC group of beta-lactamases classically produced

by *Enterobacter, Citrobacter, Serratia* and *Pseudomonas* hydrolyze all cephalosporins with the exception of cefepime and are not inhibited by the beta-lactamase inhibitors either.

CLINICAL PHARMACOKINETICS

Cephalosporins formulated for oral administration have excellent bioavailability (>80%) with the possible exception of cefpodoxime proxetil.

The third-generation cephalosporins have exquisite antimicrobial activity and achieve sufficient concentrations for use in central nervous system (CNS) infections. These agents include cefotaxime, ceftriaxone, ceftazidime and ceftizoxime. Cephalosporins also cross the placenta. They are found in high concentrations in synovial and pericardial fluids. Penetration into the aqueous humor of the eye is relatively good after systemic administration of third-generation cephalosporins.

Cephalosporins are primarily excreted by the kidney, so dosage should be altered in patients with renal insufficiency. Third-generation cephalosporins specifically cefoperazone and ceftriaxone have significant biliary excretion. They are useful in the treatment of hepatobiliary infections. Biliary sludge formation by precipitated drug, especially with ceftriaxone is quite common. They may increase alteration of gut flora. Cefotaxime, cephalothin and cephapirin share the property of hepatic biotransformation to potentially active desacetylated compounds. These metabolites have less antimicrobial activity than their parent compounds. Only desacetyl cefotaxime contributes significantly to the microbial action of its parent compound, cefotaxime. None of the other cephalosporins appear to undergo appreciable metabolism in this way.

ADVERSE REACTIONS

The cephalosporins are remarkably free from major adverse reactions. Still any cephalosporins can cause anaphylactic reaction, especially in patients with a previous history of immediate hypersensitivity reaction to cephalosporin or penicillin. Other hypersensitivity reactions include acute interstitial nephritis, autoimmune thrombocytopenia, pulmonary eosinophilia, serum sickness-like reaction, rash and drug fever. Antibiotic-associated diarrhea and *C. difficile*-related pseudomembranous colitis can also occur. Reversible biliary pseudolithiasis seen in children receiving large doses of ceftriaxone is due to precipitation of calcium salts of the drug and can cause transient pain but is not an indication for cholecystectomy. Ceftriaxone has been associated with rapidly fatal immune-mediated hemolytic anemia in patients with underlying sickle cell and myelocytic leukemia in those who had received multiple previous courses of ceftriaxone therapy.

The local side effects of cephalosporins are known in form of pain following intramuscular (IM) injection and thrombophlebitis following intravenous (IV) infusion. For many of the cephalosporins, IM administration using lidocaine as a solvent is recommended by the manufacturer. Thrombophlebitis following IV infusion of cephalosporins can be minimized by increasing the dilution of the drug, slowing infusion rate and introducing a filter into the infusion system.

DRUG INTERACTIONS

Cephalosporins containing the tetrazole thio methyl side chain (cefoperazone, moxalactam, cefotetan) have warfarin like activity, antiplatelet effects and disulfiram-like reactions.

Cephalosporins increase the risk of nephrotoxicity of other agents, such as aminoglycosides, vancomycin, etc. Absorption of cefpodoxime is reduced by H_2 antagonist like famotidine and other agents increasing gastric pH.

FIRST-GENERATION CEPHALOSPORINS

They are active against most gram-positive cocci including penicillinase-producing and non-penicillinase-producing *Staphylococcus aureus, S. epidermidis*, streptococci and pneumococci. These agents have limited activity against some gram-negative bacteria including *E.coli, K. pneumoniae* and *Proteus mirabilis* but not *Haemophilus influenzae.* They have limited activity against anaerobes.

Oral First-generation Cephalosporins

The first-generation cephalosporins for oral use include cephalexin, cefadroxil and cephradine. Cephalexin and cefadroxil are available in India. These agents have a similar antibacterial spectrum (detailed earlier). Cephalexin is well absorbed but due to its short half-life requires four times daily dosing. Cefadroxil has a longer half-life that allows for twice daily administration. These agents are used in the treatment of skin and soft tissue infections and streptococcal pharyngitis. As they have some activity against *E.coli, K.pneumoniae* and *P.mirabilis*, these agents can be used to treat urinary tract infections caused by susceptible strains of these organisms.

Parental First-generation Cephalosporins

The parental first-generation cephalosporins (mainly cefazolin) are the drugs of choice for perioperative prophylaxis. Additionally due to good antistaphylococcal activity, cefazolin is a suitable alternative to cloxacillin for treatment of serious soft tissue, bone and joint, bloodstream infections caused by methicillin-sensitive *S. aureus* (MSSA). Some studies have also reported cefazolin as a possible alternative to cloxacillin in infective endocarditis. However, owing to its poor penetration in the brain, it cannot be used for CNS infections due to MSSA. The dose of cefazolin is 100-150 mg/kg/day in three divided doses.

SECOND-GENERATION CEPHALOSPORINS

The second-generation cephalosporins have spectrum of activity of the first-generation cephalosporins with added activity against gram-negative organisms, such as *H. influenzae, Neisseria meningitidis* and *Moraxella catarrhalis.*

Cefuroxime Axetil

It is available in a pediatric suspension with twice daily dosing schedule. This compound is an ester prodrug to facilitate its absorption, but this characteristic causes an unpleasant metallic after taste. Food enhances the absorption of drug in stomach. Indications include pharyngitis, otitis media, sinusitis, lower respiratory tract infections, soft-tissue and urinary tract infections. This compound is useful for switch on therapy after the patient responds to initial parenteral cefuroxime/ceftriaxone therapy. Its safety and effectiveness for use in infants younger than 3 months is not established. It is a relatively expensive drug. The dose is 20 mg/kg/day in two divided doses.

Cefprozil

Cefprozil has a similar spectrum to that of cefuroxime axetil, but more palatable. Its safety and effectiveness has not been established in children below 6 months of age.

Cefaclor

It has a spectrum of activity similar to other second-generation cephalosporins, except for its somewhat limited activity against *H. influenzae, S. aureus* and penicillin non-susceptible pneumococci. Cefaclor has been associated with an unusual serum sickness-like reaction that appears to be due to an inherited defect in the handling of metabolic products of the drug. This adverse effect, the requirement of thrice daily dosing and the limited spectrum of activity make cefaclor a poor choice for treatment of most pediatric infections.

Cefuroxime Sodium

Among the parenteral second-generation cephalosporins, cefuroxime remains an attractive drug for the inpatient treatment of community-acquired pneumonia in children and severe sinusitis due to its efficacy against beta-lactamase-producing *H. influenzae, M. catarrhalis,* pneumococci and MSSA. It can also be used for skin and soft-tissue infections. Similar to cefazolin, it is also a recommended drug for surgical prophylaxis. The dose is 75 mg/kg/day in two divided doses. Cefuroxime has demonstrable CNS penetration, but its use for treatment of bacterial meningitis is associated with delayed sterilization of cerebrospinal fluid (CSF) and therefore it is not recommended for empiric treatment of bacterial meningitis in children.

THIRD-GENERATION CEPHALOSPORINS

Third-generation cephalosporins have greatly enhanced the armamentarium against serious and life-threatening neonatal and childhood infections. Third-generation cephalosporins were introduced in 1980. The most widely used parenteral third-generation cephalosporins are cefotaxime, ceftriaxone and ceftazidime. They are less active than first-generation against gram-positive cocci. Ceftriaxone and cefotaxime owing to their pharmacodynamics are the only cephalosporins suitable against penicillin-resistant pneumococci. They exhibit increased antibacterial activity against many gram-negative organisms, such as enteric bacilli, *H. influenzae, N. meningitidis, Neisseria gonorrhoeae* and *M. catarrhalis.* They are the mainstay of therapy for inpatient management of many pediatric infections. Among the third-generation cephalosporins, ceftazidime and cefoperazone are active against *Pseudomonas aeruginosa.* However, the usefulness of third-generation cephalosporins in nosocomial infections has become seriously compromised in current day practice due to widespread prevalence of ESBLs and AmpC enzymes.

Oral Third-general Cephalosporins

These drugs are being increasingly prescribed for outpatient therapy of pediatric infections. However, with the risk of promoting drug resistance especially ESBLs, they must be used with great discretion and only when lesser and narrow-spectrum antimicrobials will not work.

Cefixime

Cefixime was the first oral third-generation cephalosporin to become available. Perhaps, it is the reason for its rampant use in the practice. It has poor activity against *Streptococcus pneumoniae*, *S. aureus* and *Pseudomonas*. It is useful in the treatment of urinary tract infections, bacillary dysentery and enteric fever. Cefixime does not work in respiratory tract infections. Broadly speaking, cefixime may be used in the infections developing below the diaphragm and not above the diaphragm. Its half-life is long and therefore can be administered in dose of 8–10 mg/kg/day once a day. For enteric fever, however, the recommended dose is 20 mg/kg/day in two divided doses for 14 days. Combination of cefixime with clavulanic acid is available, but its efficacy in management of ESBL-producing gram-negative infections especially of the urinary tract has not been established.

Cefpodoxime Proxetil

It is the only active ester producing third-generation cephalosporin cefpodoxime. It causes an unpleasant metallic after taste. Unlike cefixime, it has good activity against pneumococci, streptococci and methicillin-susceptible *S. aureus*. It is highly active against Enterobacteriaceae. It is used mainly for respiratory tract infections. However, it does not offer any advantage over amoxicillin-clavulanic acid for this indication and may be associated with treatment failures due to poor tissue levels. There is no sufficient data supporting the use of this drug in enteric fever. The addition of clavulanic acid to cefpodoxime is of no benefit since cefpodoxime is stable to the first-generation beta-lactamases produced by *H. influenzae* and *Moraxella* unlike amoxicillin.

Ceftibuten

It is a once a day oral cephalosporin with good activity against gram-negative organisms, but not against *S. aureus*. Its use is limited by poor clinical efficacy against pneumococci.

Cefdinir

It has a broad-spectrum antimicrobial activity against several organisms including *S. pneumoniae* and *S. aureus*. It has clinical utility is in acute otitis media, streptococcal pharyngitis, skin and soft-tissue infections and uncomplicated urinary tract infections but offers no advantage over cefuroxime or amoxicillin-clavulanic acid.

Cefprozil

It is another oral third-generation cephalosporin which has antimicrobial activity almost similar to cefdinir. It has been found effective in otitis media, respiratory tract infections and skin and soft-tissue infections.

Parenteral Third-generation Cephalosporins

Cefotaxime

Cefotaxime was the first of third-generation parenteral cephalosporins to become available. The drug has good activity against many gram-positive and gram-negative aerobic bacteria. Indications for cefotaxime include community-acquired pneumonia, meningitis, mastoiditis, pyelonephritis, gonorrhea and enteric fever. Its activity against *S. aureus* is poor and it should not be used for serious infections when this pathogen is likely. Cefotaxime is preferred to other cephalosporins in neonates because it has been used more extensively and does not compete with bilirubin for protein binding. Dose of cefotaxime for common infections is 100–150 mg/kg/day, 12 hourly or 8 hourly, but in bacterial meningitis and enteric fever, it should be used in dose of 200 mg/kg/day, 6 hourly.

Ceftriaxone

The distinguishing features of this cephalosporin are its longer duration of action and effectiveness in a wide range of serious infections including bacterial meningitis. It has excellent CSF penetration. CSF sterilization is more rapid with ceftriaxone compared to other cephalosporins. Ceftriaxone is the empirical treatment of choice in bacterial meningitis in children above the age of 2 months. Other indications are community-acquired pneumonia, severe sinusitis/otitis media, complicated urinary tract infections, abdominal sepsis. It is the drug of choice for inpatient management of enteric fever. Initially, its response was obtained in 2–3 days in a case of enteric fever, but now it may take longer time, 5–7 days. It has reasonable activity against *S. aureus* and can be used for treatment of bone and joint infections due to *S. aureus*. It is also the preferred agent for empiric therapy of infective endocarditis due to viridans group streptococci with/without gentamicin. The dose of ceftriaxone is 50–100 mg/kg/day in single or two divided doses by IV or IM route. In a case of bacterial meningitis, ceftriaxone should be used in 100 mg/kg/day in two divided doses by IV route only. For bacterial meningitis single dose and IM route is not recommended. Ceftriaxone for IV route should not be administered as the bolus dose. The calculated amount of reconstituted ceftriaxone should be taken in 50 cc or 100 cc normal saline and it should be infused over 30–45 minutes. It may cause biliary sludging and reversible pseudolithiasis. This side effect is more common in children. The patients of enteric fever on ceftriaxone therapy on ultrasonographic (USG) study of abdomen may be interpreted having gallstone due to biliary sludging and pseudolithiasis. They should be followed up with repeat USG study at appropriate time before labeling them having gallstone. Its affinity to bind albumin can cause displacement of bilirubin. Due to this reason, its use is restricted in neonates as it may cause or aggravate hyperbilirubinemia. Drug fever and skin rashes are also known. Anaphylaxis is very rare but it has been reported. Transient rise in liver enzymes is also seen in the practice. Hemolytic anemia, thrombocytopenia and leukopenia may occur due to ceftriaxone. Concomitant use of aminoglycosides and furosemide may increase the chances of nephrotoxicity, secondary candidiasis is also seen.

Ceftazidime

The most prominent feature of this molecule is its high activity against *Pseudomonas*. Ceftazidime has been found more active in vitro against *Pseudomonas* than cefoperazone or piperacillin. However, ceftazidime is significantly less active than either cefotaxime or ceftriaxone against pneumococci limiting its use in treatment of pneumonia. It has excellent CNS penetration. It is the drug of choice of initial management of melioidosis and respiratory infections in cystic fibrosis. However, the efficacy of ceftazidime in nosocomial infections and febrile neutropenia has been compromised due to rising resistance rates. Hence here, it should not be used as empiric therapy but only when culture results show susceptibility to this drug. However, there are isolates of *Pseudomonas* than can exhibit carbapenem resistance but remain susceptible to ceftazidime.

Cefoperazone

Like ceftazidime it differs from other third-generation cephalosporins in having strong activity against *Pseudomonas*. It is also good for *Salmonella typhi* and *Bacteroides fragilis*. It has poor CSF penetration and should not be used for meningitis. It is concentrated in bile and does not need dose modification for renal dysfunction. It has been found effective in multidrug-resistant enteric fever. It can cause bleeding due to hypoprothrombinemia which can be reversed by administration of vitamin K. Its use in nosocomial infections has been compromised due to organisms producing ESBL and AmpC. A combination of cefoperazone with sulbactam is available for treatment of ESBL infections which will be discussed in Chapter 8.

Ceftizoxime

It has both good gram-positive activity (anti-*Pneumococcus*) and antipseudomonal activity. It has good CNS penetration. However, it does not have a niche indication and is usually supplanted by cefotaxime/ceftriaxone or ceftazidime.

FOURTH-GENERATION CEPHALOSPORINS

These include cefepime and cefpirome. Both are dipolar ionic compounds that diffuse more rapidly in gram-negative bacteria and are poor inducers and substrates for beta-lactamases.

Cefepime

Cefepime has gram-positive coverage similar to cefotaxime and ceftriaxone and excellent gram-negative activity. Its antipseudomonal activity is comparable to ceftazidime. It is relatively more stable as compared to the third-generation cephalosporins against ESBL producing *E. coli* and *Klebsiella* and AmpC producing organisms. There is a disagreement between the European Committee on Antimicrobial Susceptibility Testing (EUCAST) and the Clinical Laboratory Standards Institute (CLSI) for breakpoints for cefepime in enterobacteriaceae. While EUCAST's susceptibility breakpoint is 1 and resistance breakpoint is 2, CLSI classifies isolates with minimum inhibitory concentration (MIC) of 2 and 4 as susceptibility dose dependent and 8 or more as resistant. Cefepime also exhibits an inoculum effect, i.e. the MIC to cefepime rises with rising bacterial load. Retrospective studies have shown higher mortality with cefepime as compared to beta-lactam/beta-lactamase inhibitor (BL-BLI) combinations/carbapenems in treatment of ESBL infections. Hence cefepime should be used with caution in management of resistant gram-negative infections and only when the MIC is 1 or less. While it has good CNS penetration, cefepime has no any added advantage over cefotaxime or ceftriaxone in bacterial meningitis. The dose of cefepime is 50 mg/kg 12 hourly and 50 mg/kg 8 hourly in severe infections. It has been approved in patients older than 2 months. It may cause phlebitis, headache, blurred vision, rash, urticaria, fever and gastrointestinal (GI) tract disturbances. Transient elevation of hepatic enzymes is known. There is recent data about increased risk of seizures in patients treated with cefepime especially with higher doses. Cefepime is also available in India in combination with tazobactam which will be discussed further in Chapter 8.

Cefpirome

Cefpirome is another fourth-generation cephalosporin. It is a potentially useful agent for therapy of childhood bacterial meningitis because of enhanced activity against pneumococci

TABLE 1: Dosage of third- and fourth-generation cephalosporins.

Molecule	*Dose (mg/kg/day)*	*Route of administration*	*Interval*
Cefixime	8	Oral	Single dose
	For enteric fever: 20	Oral	12 hourly
Cefpodoxime proxetil	10	Oral	12 hourly
Cefdinir	14	Oral	12 hourly
Ceftibuten	9	Oral	Single dose
Cefprozil	15–20	Oral	12 hourly
Cefotaxime	100–150	IV/IM	8 hourly
	Bacterial meningitis: 200	IV only	6 hourly
Ceftriaxone	50–100	IV/IM	Single dose or 12 hourly
	Bacterial meningitis and typhoid:100	IV only	12 hourly
Ceftizoxime	50–200	IV/IM	6–8 hourly
Cefoperazone	50–100	IV/IM	8–12 hourly
Ceftazidime	Newborn: 100 Children: 150–200	IV/IM	6–8 hourly
Cefepime	100	IV/IM	12 hourly
Cefpirome	50–100	IV/IM	12 hourly

and good penetration into the CSF but has not shown any significant benefit over the traditional ceftriaxone/cefotaxime.

In view of the almost similar efficacy of third-generation cephalosporins and fourth-generation cephalosporins for most severe community-acquired infections and limitations of the fourth-generation cephalosporins for severe nosocomial infections (due to inoculum effect), the fourth-generation cephalosporins have not really broken any new ground in treatment of resistant bacterial infections. Dosage of third and fourth generation cehalosporins is summarized in Table 1.

FIFTH-GENERATION CEPHALOSPORINS

Fifth-generation cephalosporins mainly include two drugs, ceftobiprole and ceftaroline. Whether these two agents should be considered as fifth-generation cephalosporins or unclassified is not certain. Currently ceftaroline and ceftobiprole are on an unnamed subclass of cephalosporins by CLSI.

Ceftaroline

Ceftaroline is modified from cefozopran, a fourth-generation cephalosporin. The prodrug, ceftaroline fosamil, which contains a phosphono group to increase water solubility, is rapidly converted in plasma into the bioactive agent, ceftaroline. The 1,3-thiazole ring attached to the 3-postion of cephalosporin nucleus and the oxime group in C7 acyl moiety are responsible for the enhanced anti-MRSA activity observed with ceftaroline. Ceftaroline is a broad-spectrum cephalosporin. Ceftaroline has the ability to bind PBP2a, an MRSA-specific PBP that has low affinity for most other beta-lactam antibacterials. The high-binding affinity of ceftaroline to PBP2a (median inhibitory concentration 0.90 μg/mL) correlates well with its low MIC for MRSA.

Ceftaroline is active in vitro against gram-positive cocci including MRSA, methicillin-resistant *S. epidermidis*, penicillin-resistant *S. pneumoniae* and vancomycin-resistant *Enterococcus faecalis* (not *Enterococcus faecium*). It is active against many gram-negative pathogens but not ESBL/Amp C producing organisms. Ceftaroline has limited activity against anaerobes, such as *B. fragilis* and non-fragilis *Bacteroides* spp.

The dose of ceftaroline fosamil is 600 mg IV every 12 hours over 1 hour in adults, more than 18 years of age. Dosage adjustment is necessary in patients with moderate to severe renal impairment. The drug has been evaluated in randomized controlled trials for treatment of complicated skin and soft-tissue infections where it has been found to be noninferior to vancomycin with/without aztreonam. It is currently approved for management of skin and soft-tissue infections and community-acquired pneumonia in adults. It has also been used successfully in management of MRSA bacteremia but not approved for the same. The drug has not been evaluated in children and is not available in India at present.

Ceftobiprole

Ceftobiprole a new anti-MRSA cephalosporin has spectrum of activity similar to ceftaroline. Among the gram-positive pathogens, it has shown good activity against MRSA strains with reduced susceptibility to linezolid, daptomycin or vancomycin. Ceftobiprole has also displayed potent activity against *S. pneumoniae* (including penicillin-sensitive, penicillin-resistant and ceftriaxone-resistant) and *E. faecalis*, but not against *E. faecium*. It is active against many gram-negative pathogens but not against ESBL/AmpC-producing pathogens. The drug has been approved for management of community and healthcare-associated pneumonia. It is not been evaluated in children and not available in India at present.

The new anti-MRSA cephalosporins are of uncertain clinical value in the Indian context where the major problem is resistant gram-negative pathogens against which these agents are inactive.

RECOMMENDED READING

1. Abraham EP. Cephalosporins 1945-1986. Drugs. 1987;34 Suppl 2:1-14.
2. Biek D, Critchley IA, Riccobene TA, et al. Ceftaroline fosamil: a novel broad-spectrum cephalosporin with expanded anti-gram-positive activity. J Antimicrob Chemother. 2010;65 Suppl 4;iv9-16.
3. Bowlware KL, Stull T. Antimicrobial agents in pediatrics. Infect Dis Clin N Am. 2004;18:513-31.
4. Chuang YY, Hung IJ, Yang CP, et al. Cefepime versus ceftazidime as empiric monotherapy for fever and neutropenia in children with cancer. Pediatr Infect Dis J. 2000;21:203-9.
5. Goldberg DM. The cephalosporins. Med Clin North Am. 1987;71:1113-33.
6. Gulati S, Marwaha RK, Singhi S, et al. Third-generation cephalosporins in multi-drug resistant typhoid fever. Indian Pediatr. 1992;29:513-6.
7. Gupta AK, Wadhwa A, Anand NK. Ceftriaxone. Indian Pediatr. 1990;27:381-3.
8. Hathi GS. Cephalosporins today. In: Gupte S (Ed). Recent Advances in Pediatrics. New Delhi: Jaypee Brothers Medical Publishers (P) Ltd.; 1994. pp. 357-82.
9. Heim-Duthoy KL, Caperton EM, Pollock R, et al. Apparent biliary pseudolithiasis during ceftriaxone therapy. Antimicrob Agents Chemother. 1990;34:1146-9.
10. John S, Jason S. Antimicrobial agents. In: Long SS, Pickering LK, Prober CG (Eds). Principles and Practice of Pediatric Infectious Diseases, 3rd edition. Philadelphia, PA: Elsevier, Churchill Livingstone; 2008. pp. 1420-60.
11. Kurchavov VA, Beloborodeva NV, Biriukov AV, et al. The comparative activity of cefepime and other current antibiotics against microorganisms isolated from patients in pediatric intensive therapy units. Antibiot Khimifer. 1999;44:23-30.

12. LeBel MH, Hoyt MJ, McCracken GH Jr. Comparative efficacy of ceftriaxone and cefuroxime for treatment of bacterial meningitis. J Pediatr. 1994;114:1049-54.
13. Mandell GL, Sande MA. The cephalosporins. In: Gilman AG, Rall TW, Nies AS, Taylor P (Eds). The Pharmacological and Basis of Therapeutics, 8th edition. New York: Pergamon Press; 1991. pp. 1085-92.
14. Mishra S, Niranjan S, Kumar H, et al. Ceftriaxone: use in multidrug resistant typhoid fever. Indian Pediatr. 1993;30:67-70.
15. Nisha AR, Vanishree H, Mahesh DM. Fifth-generation cephalosporins: drugs to overcome antibiotic resistance. IJSRSET. 2017;3:228-32.
16. Norrby SR. Side effects of cephalosporins. Drugs. 1987:34 Suppl 2:105-20.
17. Rizvi MW, Shujatullah F, Malik A, et al. Ceftobiprole: a novel cephalosporin to combat MRSA. East J Med. 2011;16:1-8.
18. Saez-Llorens X, O'Ryan M. Cefepime in the empiric treatment of meningitis in children. Pediatr Infect Dis J. 2001;20:356-61.
19. Schaad UB, Wedgewood-Krucko J, Tschaeppeler H. Reversible ceftriaxone-associated biliary pseudolithiasis in children. Lancet. 1988;2:1411-3.
20. Singhal T. Irrational fixed dose antibiotic combinations. In: Shivananda, Yewale V, Prajapati B, Kundu R (Eds). Rational Antimicrobial Therapy: Desktop Reference Manual. Mumbai: IAP Infectious Disease Chapter Publication. 2009. p. 57.
21. Tripathi KD. Essentials of Medical Pharmacology, 5th edition. Jaypee Brothers Medical Publishers (P) Ltd.; 2003. pp. 662-7.
22. Update on cephalosporins in pediatrics. In Clinical Updates in Pediatric Infectious Disease. Bethesda, MD: National Foundation for Infectious Diseases, Vol. IV, Issue 1, Nov. 2001.
23. Vidaillac C, Rybak MJ. Ceftobiprole: first cephalosporin with activity against methicillin-resistant Staphylococcus aureus. Pharmacotherapy. 2009;29:511-25.
24. Wakiguchi H, Fujieda M, Maeda A, et al. Clinical efficacy of cefpirome against various infectious diseases in children. Jpn J Antibiot. 1991;44:241-5.
25. Zhanel GG, Sniezek G, Schweizer F, et al. Ceftaroline: a novel broad-spectrum cephalosporin with activity against methicillin-resistant Staphylococcus aureus. Drugs. 2009;69:809-31.

Carbapenems

7
Chapter

Vijaya N Kumar, Rakesh Lodha

INTRODUCTION

Serious bacterial infections in children cause significant morbidity and mortality and need effective antimicrobial agents to combat them. With widespread use of third-generation cephalosporins, there has been the emergence of strains of bacteria that produce extended-spectrum beta-lactamases (ESBLs) which are capable of hydrolyzing third-generation cephalosporins, penicillins, and aztreonam. They are most often associated with *Klebsiella pneumoniae* and *Escherichia coli*, but can be produced by other gram-negative bacilli as well. Data from AIIMS, New Delhi, shows an increasing prevalence (66.8–71.5%) of infections due to ESBL-producing bacteria. In addition to the ESBLs, certain gram-negative bacteria (GNB) such as *Pseudomonas, Serratia, Citrobacter*, and *Enterobacter* produce chromosomally mediated AmpC β-lactamases. These hydrolyze cephalosporins and penicillins and are not inhibited by beta-lactamase inhibitors. In addition, plasmid-mediated AmpC β-lactamases, first reported in 1988, which differ from the chromosomal AmpC in being non-inducible have further complicated management of gram-negative infections.

Carbapenems are the most potent class of β-lactams, with stability against ESBL and AmpC chromosomal β-lactamases. They have a relatively broad spectrum of activity against gram-negative and gram-positive organisms, including anaerobes. They are mainly used for serious infections in hospitalized patients where the organism is unknown or is suspected or proven to be resistant. The commonly used members of this class of antibiotics include imipenem, meropenem, and ertapenem. Other carbapenems are doripenem, razupenem, tebipenem, tomopenam, biapenem, panipenem, faropenem, and sanfetrinem.

CHEMISTRY

Carbapenems are derivatives of *thienamycin*, a compound produced by the soil organism, *Streptomyces cattleya*, which was first discovered in 1976. Like other beta-lactams, carbapenems contain a four-member lactam ring fused to a five-member thiazolidinic secondary ring through the nitrogen and adjacent tetrahedral carbon atom. The basic structure differs from that of penicillins only by the substitution of sulfur for a carbon at position 1 and an unsaturated bond between C2 and C3 in the five-member ring. It is the side chains attached to this basic two-ring structure that differentiates the carbapenems from each other. The trans 1-hydroxyethyl present on the beta-lactam ring prevents the drug from hydrolysis by beta lactamase.

MECHANISM OF ACTION

Carbapenems, like other β-lactams, exhibit their bactericidal activity by binding to critical penicillin-binding proteins (PBP). This inhibits growth and also results in damage to the cell wall, thus causing cell lysis and death. This interaction occurs near the cell surface in gram-positive bacteria. However, in GNB, carbapenems first gain entry into the periplasmic space between the cell wall and surrounding membrane by passing through channels in the membrane that normally function to provide access for essential nutrients (porin channels). After traversing this membrane the carbapenems permanently acylate the PBPs inhibiting the peptidase domain of it, thereby preventing the peptide cross linking. Cell wall synthesis is a three-dimensional process where formation and autolysis occur simultaneously. Due to the inhibition of PBPs formation of cell wall gets affected and autolysis continues ultimately leads to cell burst due to osmotic pressure. The ability to pass through these channels, along with a high affinity for critical PBPs and resistance to a broad range of β-lactamases, is thought to account for the broader spectrum of activity of carbapenems versus most other antibiotics. Different members of the carbapenem class exhibit a varying affinity for different PBPs, like, imipenem binds preferentially to PBP2, followed by PBP1a and 1b, and has weak affinity for PBP3, while meropenem preferentially binds to PBPs 2, 3, and 4.

SPECTRUM OF ACTIVITY

The carbapenems possess broad spectrum in vitro activity against gram-positive and gram-negative aerobic and anaerobic bacteria. However, none of the carbapenems demonstrate clinically useful activity against *Enterococcus faecium*, methicillin-resistant *Staphylococcus aureus* (MRSA), *Stenotrophomonas maltophilia,* and other non-fermenters, such as *Elizabethkingia meningoseptica/Chryseobacterium indologenes,* Rickettsia, Chlamydia, and Mycoplasma.

Based on their affinity for various PBPs, there can be differences in the activity of individual carbapenems and can be broadly grouped into three. There are subtle differences between drugs within a group also. Group 1 includes ertapenem which inactive against *Pseudomonas* and *Acinetobacter* but suitable for community acquired infections caused by ESBL/AmpC-producing bacteria including *E. coli* and *Klebsiella*. Group 2 has imipenem, meropenem, biapenem, and doripenem with activity against *Pseudomonas, Acinetobacter* apart from other gram-negative aerobes and hence better suited for nosocomial infections. Within the group, imipenem has better activity against gram-positive cocci while meropenem is better against GNB. In vitro, meropenem is more potent than imipenem-cilastatin against *Enterobacteriaceae, Pseudomonas aeruginosa,* and *Acinetobacter*. Group 3 has investigational carbapenems with activity against MRSA as well.

DRUG RESISTANCE

To combat infections by multidrug resistant bacteria, carbapenems are among the last resort especially in intensive care units (ICUs) and high risk wards. Resistance to them, is however increasing rapidly. In a study from AIIMS, which looked into the prevalence of carbapenem resistance among ESBL positive GNB isolates, it was found that 22% isolates were resistant to meropenem and 17% to imipenem. Resistance in *Pseudomonas* species was even higher. Other centers in India are now reporting almost 50% resistance in nosocomial bloodstream infections due to *E. coli* and *Klebsiella* and up to 80% resistance in ventilator associated pneumonia due to *Pseudomonas* and *Acinetobacter*. Mortality in carbapenem resistant pathogens approaches 50%. Resistance may be mediated by the following mechanisms:

- Production of carbapenemases
- Downregulation of porin channels/impermeable porin channel
- Active efflux of the drug from the cell by a multidrug efflux pump
- Alteration of critical PBPs (carbapenem insensitive transpeptidase).

Carbapenem resistance in gram-positive cocci is mainly due to alteration PBPs, while rest of the mechanisms either alone or in combination are responsible for resistance in gram-negative organisms.

Production of carbapenemases: These are either chromosomally encoded or plasmid-mediated metallo/serine periplasmic enzymes that hydrolyze the β-lactam ring of virtually all β-lactams, including carbapenems and prevent them from reaching the PBPs. There are four types of carbapenemases Ambler class A, B, C, and D. Class B uses zinc, while the rest of them use serine as a nucleophile to hydrolyze β-lactam bond. Class B carbapenemases are clinically threatening. In 2009, an increasing number of carbapenem-resistant Enterobacteriaceae strains were identified in UK hospital patients, many of whom were recently hospitalized in India and Pakistan. A new type of MBL was isolated from these patients and was designated as NDM-1 (New Delhi Metallo-1), a class B MBL. The Indian subcontinent became a reservoir of blaNDM-1 gene. An environmental study from New Delhi showed that NDM-1 can be environmental, as well as hospital or community acquired. It was initially mapped in *K. pneumoniae* and *E. coli*, later other Enterobacteriaceae, *Acinetobacter*, and *Pseudomonas* were also found to express it. The major concern is NDM-1 MBLs producing organisms are resistant to almost all class of antibiotics including fluoroquinolones and aminoglycosides. Besides, the carbapenem minimal inhibitory concentrations (MICs) are exceedingly high (usually more than 16 µg/mL). They are sensitive only to colistin and tigecycline and variably to fosfomycin. The other class B metallo-β-lactamases not commonly reported from India include IMP (described in Enterobacteriaceae, *Pseudomonas*, and *Acinetobacter*) and VIM (mainly *Pseudomonas*). The most common carbapenemase in the USA and Europe is the class A *K. pneumoniae* carbapenemase (KPC); however, the carbapenem MICs associated with KPC are usually lower than the NDM. The class D carbapenemase OXA initially described in Acinetobacter but now in other gram-negatives as well is increasing in prevalence all over the world including India (OXA-48).

Downregulation of porin channels/impermeable porin channel: Porin channels are water filled channels extending across the cell membrane of GNB that help in uptake of nutrients. Porin loss or alteration in the channels can cause reduced drug entry of carbapenems resulting in resistance to them. Though a single mutation that reduces porin channels (OprD mutants) can confer resistance to imipenem, resistance to meropenem requires two independent mutations, a mutation to reduce porin channels (OprD mutation), as well as a mutation to upregulate cellular efflux mechanisms (nalB mutation at the mexR locus). Consequently, the rate of selection of resistance to meropenem in vitro is lower than that for imipenem. In *K. pneumoniae* resistance to imipenem is with loss of outer membrane porins (OMPs) such as Opr K-35/36. Carbapenem resistance in *Acinetobacter* is associated with CarO, Omp33-36, and OprD homologue.

Active efflux of the drug from the cell by a multidrug efflux pump: Efflux pumps are grouped into superfamilies, small multidrug resistant (SMR), the resistance nodulation division (RND), the major facilitator superfamily (MFS), the ATP-binding cassette (ABC), and the multidrug and toxic compound extrusion (MATE) superfamily. In *Pseudomonas*, OprM, and OprJ are involved in resistance against carbapenems. AdeABC efflux pump of RND superfamily confers resistance to carbapenems in *Acinetobacter baumannii*.

Alteration of critical PBPs: This mechanism usually operates in gram-positive cocci for acquiring resistance against carbapenems. Mutation in PBPs or acquisition of novel PBPs result in carbapenem resistance in *Haemophilus influenzae, Bacteriodes fragilis, S. aureus, E. faecium, Proteus mirabilis, Listeria monocytogenes, Streptococcus pneumoniae.*

PHARMACOKINETICS

All the currently available carbapenems (except tebipenem and faropenem, oral drugs) are formulated as parenteral agents as they are not absorbed from the intestinal tract. Imipenem-cilastatin and ertapenem can be given intramuscularly and rest by intravenous route. Imipenem lacks 1-β-methyl group so it undergoes hydrolysis by the enzyme dehydropeptidase-1 (DHP-1) in the brush border of proximal renal tubular cells and hence it is always administered with an inhibitor of DHP-1, cilastatin, in a ratio of 1:1 to achieve an appropriate in vivo half-life and prevent potential nephrotoxicity. Half-life of imipenem is 1 hour which is prolonged in renal impairment where dose modification is required. Protein binding of imipenem and cilastatin are 20% and 40% respectively. In the presence of cilastatin, 60–70% of imipenem is excreted unchanged in urine. Intravenous infusion of imipenem-cilastatin results in penetration of the drug into almost all tissues (lung, bone, skin, fascia, endometrium, and myometrium) and body fluids (aqueous and vitreous humor, pleural and peritoneal fluid, bile).

Meropenem is dimethyl carbamoyl pyrrolidinyl derivative of thienamycin demonstrate increased stability to DHP-1 due to the presence of 1-β-methyl group which also improves anti *H. influenzae* activity and is administered without a DHP-1 inhibitor. Approximately 70% of meropenem is excreted by kidneys as the parent compound. Meropenem has good tissue penetration and penetration studies in cerebrospinal fluid (CSF) show that at doses of 40 mg/kg, its CSF concentration is much higher than the reported MIC_{90} for most bacterial pathogens associated with meningitis. However, as with other β-lactams, its penetration into CSF is effective only in the presence of inflamed meninges.

The plasma half-life of both meropenem and imipenem approximately 1 hour and peak plasma levels attained after intravenous dose decline to less than 1 μg/mL after 4–6 hours. The usual dosing interval is 6 hours for imipenem and 8 hours for meropenem in patients with normal renal function. Ertapenem is long-acting carbapenem with half-life of 4 hours and 94% protein bound. It is administered once daily and eliminated mainly through glomerular filtration and secretory process. As kidneys are the primary route of elimination of carbapenems, different levels of renal impairment require dosage and/or dosage interval changes. The pharmacokinetics of carbapenems show age-associated changes. Their elimination half-life is the longest in preterm neonates and it decreases with advancing age. The volume of distribution of meropenem is greater in infants than in children in view of their reduced renal functional capacity and increased extracellular fluid volume. Similar studies with imipenem-cilastatin in preterm neonates show linear elimination pharmacokinetics with peak plasma concentrations showing a linear increase with increase in doses.

Imipenem and meropenem are available as dry powder in vials, which should be stored below 25°C before reconstitution. After reconstitution, they may be kept at room temperature for up to 2 hours and under refrigeration (4°C) for up to 24 hours. The detailed pharmacokinetic data and dosing for these compounds in children is shown in Table 1. Doses less than or equal to 500 mg should be given by intravenous infusion over 15–30 minutes and those more than 500 mg over 40–60 minutes. Studies show that administering the carbapenem over 3–4 hours as infusion may help in treatment of infections with organisms with relatively higher MIC.

PHARMACODYNAMICS

The activity of carbapenems is dependent on the time for which the drug levels remain above the MIC for the organism (T > MIC). A T > MIC of ~ 20% achieves bacteriostatic effects and T > MIC of ~ 40% results in bactericidal effects. Unlike other β-lactams, carbapenems also exhibit a post-antibiotic effect (PAE) against both gram-positive and gram-negative. So their effect may last even longer than that predicted by their half-life and on evaluating the PAE of imipenem against *E. coli* at varying drug concentrations and times of exposure, the area under the concentration-time curve (AUC) is a better predictor of the PAE than concentration or time alone.

Carbapenems provide a significant advantage in treating ESBL +ve strains since they do not exhibit the "inoculum effect". Cefepime can theoretically be used for the treatment of ESBL +ve strains and can demonstrate effective levels above the MIC values (1 mg/L) for a colony count of 10^5 CFU/mL. However at higher bacterial loads, like 10^7 CFU/mL, the MIC for cefepime increases dramatically (64 mg/L). This reduced efficacy in relation to the size of the inoculum has been called the "inoculum effect". In addition to this effect, use of cefepime has also been associated with selection of ESBL +ve strains and outbreaks of infection and with higher mortality as compared to carbapenems. Hence cefepime may not be effective for treatment of severe bacterial infections with ESBL +ve strains. Similarly the BL-BLI combinations may also exhibit an inoculum effect where in the presence of high organism burden with excess β-lactamase production, the efficacy is low. In contrast, the MIC data of meropenem does not show the inoculum effect. Its MIC for a bacterial load of 10^7 CFU/mL is not very high as compared to that for 10^5 CFU/mL. Clinical studies show that the plasma trough concentrations (8.5 ± 1 mg/L) on an 8-hour dosing schedule remain persistently above the MIC values for most infecting organisms.

CLINICAL USE

Carbapenems have broad-spectrum antibacterial activity and are therefore useful agents for a wide variety of infections. To prevent the development of resistance, the use of carbapenems must be judicious. If carbapenems have been started, therapy should be de-escalated if possible once cultures are available. Of the available carbapenems, imipenem-cilastatin, meropenem, and ertapenem are approved by the FDA for use in children. Imipenem was the first carbapenem approved for clinical use in 1985. Meropenem was approved in 1996.

Meropenem/imipenem are primarily indicated as empiric/definitive therapy of serious healthcare-associated infections including bloodstream infections, pneumonia, urinary tract infections (UTIs), surgical site infections, nosocomial meningitis as there is a high probability of these infections being due to ESBL-producing organisms. Here there is a choice to be made between BL-BLI combinations and carbapenems. In the beginning, trials showed superiority of carbapenems as compared to BL-BLI in management of ESBL infections and they were the preferred drugs. Over time, several retrospective, observational studies and meta-analysis showed noninferiority of BL-BLI in managing ESBL infections. Recently, the MERINO trial showed superiority of carbapenems over piperacillin tazobactam in treating serious ESBL infections. So the jury is still out. Therefore in seriously sick patients with suspected ESBL infections carbapenems are drugs of choice. However in less sick patients where adequate source control has been done and where the BL-BLI MICs are low, BL-BLIs should be used to spare carbapenems and reduce the selection pressure. Ertapenem should not be used for empiric therapy since it does not work against the non-fermenters (Pseudomonas/Acinetobacter). It can be used for de-escalation once the patient is stable and cultures show susceptibility.

The other important indication for meropenem/imipenem is in treatment of febrile neutropenia. With the increasing prevalence of ESBL production and AmpC production in gram-negative organisms causing febrile neutropenia empiric therapy with carbapenems with/without aminoglycosides is front-line therapy for febrile neutropenia in many units (alternative option being BL-BLI combinations with/without aminoglycosides). In areas where prevalence of carbapenem-resistant strains is high, combination of carbapenems with polymyxins may also have to be considered.

Neonatal sepsis is another area where empiric therapy with carbapenems may have to be initiated in critically sick babies or those with hospital acquired sepsis. Imipenem is approved for use in neonates but cannot be given in the setting of meningitis due to risk of seizures (discussed later). Meropenem is an excellent drug for neonatal sepsis and meningitis but is not approved for infants less than 3 months. However, there is a significant off-label use in newborn and infant patients younger than 3 months of age. In neonates with sepsis due to multidrug-resistant gram-negative organisms, meropenem showed excellent results (100% cure rates for sepsis and 87.5% for nosocomial pneumonia) with almost no side effects in this age group.

There is a limited indication for use of carbapenems in critically sick children with community acquired infections due to ESBL-producing organisms such as those of the urinary tract or intra-abdominal sepsis. However, the use of carbapenems for other community acquired infections such as meningitis, pneumonia, skin and soft tissue infections in previously healthy children should be discouraged since ESBL-producing pathogens are not a concern in this setting.

Meropenem/imipenem with clavulanic acid have been used as salvage therapy for MDR/XDR tuberculosis. The other less common indications for carbapenems is for melioidosis (meropenem instead of ceftazidime), infections due to rapidly growing mycobacteria (imipenem), and nocardia (imipenem/meropenem).

The role of carbapenems as combination therapy with polymyxins for treatment of carbapenem-resistant infections is controversial. It was earlier proposed that this combination is synergistic with the polymyxin destroying the cell membrane and allowing penetration of the carbapenem. However, this is true when carbapenem MICs are in the range of 2–8 μg/mL. In India, where carbapenem resistance is mediated by NDM, the usual MICs are more than 16 μg/mL. The additive benefit of using carbapenems in this setting is of limited utility.

DOSAGE (TABLES 1 AND 2)

Dosing of carbapenems and dose modification of imipenem and meropenem in renal insufficiency have been given in Tables 1 and 2.

SIDE EFFECTS

Carbapenems are contraindicated in patients with known hypersensitivity to any component. In those with history of serious penicillin/β-lactam hypersensitivity reactions, carbapenems should be used with great caution. Before initiating therapy, an enquiry should be made regarding history of previous anaphylactic reactions and history of allergy to multiple allergens.

TABLE 1: Dosing of carbapenems.

Characteristic	*Imipenem-cilastatin*	*Meropenem*	*Ertapenem*
FDA status	Approved 1985	Approved 1996	Approved 2001
Dose and Dosing interval	*Age:* • <1week: 25 mg/kg q12h • 1–4 weeks: 25 mg/kg q8h • 4 weeks to-3 months: 25 mg/kg q6h • 3 months to 12 years: 15–25 mg/kg q6h • Maximum daily dose: 3 g • Adults: 0.5–1 g q6–8 h	• >3 months: 20 mg/kg q8h • Meningitis: 40 mg/kg (maximum 2 g) q8h • Respiratory infection in cystic fibrosis: 40 mg/kg (maximum 2 g) q8h • Adults and children >50 kg: 1–2 g q8h	• 3 months to 12 years: 15 mg/kg q12h • Adults: 1 g q24h

TABLE 2: Dose modification of imipenem and meropenem in renal insufficiency.

Creatinine clearance (mL/min/1.73 m^2)	*Imipenem-cilastatin*		*Meropenem*		*Ertapenem*	
	% individual dose	Dose interval	% individual dose	Dose interval	% individual dose	Dose interval
30–50 (mild insufficiency)	50%	q8h	100%	q12h	100%	q24h
10–30 (moderate insufficiency)	50%	q12h	50%	q12h	50%	q24h
<10 (severe insufficiency)	50%	q24h	50%	q24h	50%	q24h

Imipenem-cilastatin is generally well tolerated and serious side effects requiring cessation of therapy are rare. Side effects include local reactions in the form of erythema, induration and thrombophlebitis; nausea, vomiting, diarrhea, oliguria/anuria and renal failure. In addition, a harmless discoloration of urine has been seen in children. Laboratory abnormalities include transient thrombocytosis, liver enzyme elevations, eosinophilia, and neutropenia. The overall incidence of seizures is about 2%, with a slightly higher incidence noted in children with cancer (3.6%). A study of imipenem-cilastatin use in children with suspected bacterial meningitis was in fact terminated when 33% of children with meningitis developed seizures after imipenem administration. The pathogenesis of its neurotoxicity is by virtue of its interaction with $GABA_A$ receptor and this interaction depends upon the side chain of the second carbon atom in the carbapenem nucleus. The more basic the side chain is, the better is the binding to the $GABA_A$ receptor, and this results in higher convulsant activity. Imipenem and panipenem have basic C-2 side chains whereas meropenem's side chain is not. Hence imipenem should not be used in treatment of CNS infections in children and should also be avoided in children with risk factors for seizures, such as prior seizure episode, metabolic derangement, anoxia, and renal impairment.

Norrby et al. reviewed the safety profile of meropenem in 5,000 patients from 46 trials. The review included 758 pediatric patient episodes of treatment with meropenem out of which 246 children had meningitis. The review included the studies comparing meropenem to cephalosporin-based therapies. The doses of meropenem administered were 10 mg/kg, 20 mg/kg, and 40 mg/kg. There were no major differences in clinical profile of the participants in meropenem and comparator groups. Around 16% of meropenem-treated and 11% of cephalosporin-treated patients developed drug-related adverse events. Diarrhea (4.1%), rash (2.2%), nausea/vomiting and injection site inflammation were the most common adverse events in the meropenem group. Even when taking into account non-drug-related adverse events, no specific event was reported in more than 5% of meropenem treatment exposures, reflecting a low frequency for individual adverse events. Thrombocytosis and increase in liver enzymes were common laboratory adverse effects which occurred in small proportion of participants.

The common side effects of ertapenem are diarrhea, nausea, vomiting, thrombophlebitis, vaginitis, elevated aminotransferases, and seizures.

DRUG INTERACTIONS

There are reports of occurrence of seizures on concurrent administration of imipenem-cilastatin with ganciclovir and their concomitant use is not recommended unless the benefit outweighs the risk. Concomitant administration of imipenem with cyclosporin is also known to cause central nervous system effects in the form of confusion, agitation and tremor. Concomitant administration with probenecid results in minimal increase in plasma levels and half-life of imipenem but the levels of cilastatin are almost doubled. The urinary recovery of imipenem is reduced to 60% of the administered dose and hence its concomitant administration is not recommended. Probenecid could also increase the plasma levels of meropenem, doripenem, and faropenem by decreasing their excretion. Carbapenems (meropenem, imipenem, and ertapenem) can decrease the drug levels of sodium valproate when coadministered and hence increase the seizure potential; maximum reduction is by meropenem.

OTHER CARBAPENEMS

Doripenem

It was first developed in Japan and then marketed worldwide. Doripenem has similar structure to meropenem except the presence of sulfamoxil-aminomethyl chain instead of dimethyl-carboxyl chain. It is not approved for pediatric use. Doripenem like other carbapenem binds with PBPs and inactivates them leading to death of the organisms. It binds with PBPs 3, 4, and also 2. Its antibacterial spectrum is similar to other carbapenems but has superior activity against *P. aeruginosa*. However superior clinical efficacy has not been demonstrated. Its half-life is 1 hour and protein binding is around 8%. Excretion of doripenem depends on creatinine clearance and it is metabolized by DHP-1. However coformulation with cilastatin is not needed. The drug is more stable in reconstituted solution as compared to other carbapenems hence more suitable for prolonged infusion as compared to other carbapenems. Meta-analysis on doripenem showed that it was safe, effective and noninferior to comparators. The adult dose is 500 mg thrice daily. Clinical experience with use of doripenem is less as compared to the other group 2 carbapenems.

Faropenem

It is a member of the unique penem class of β-lactams but actually not a carbapenem. Penems are hybrid of penam (penicillin) and cepham (cephalosporin) nuclei. The microbiological properties of faropenem are different when compared with carbapenems. Faropenem acts by binding to PBPs and it binds more with high molecular weight PBPs (1, 2, and 3) than low molecular weight PBPs. It demonstrates broad-spectrum in vitro antimicrobial activity against many gram-positive and gram-negative aerobes and anaerobes, and is resistant to hydrolysis by TEM, SHV, CTX-M type ESBLs. The half-life of faropenem is 1–1.5 hour and it is 80–90% protein bound, excreted by kidneys. Faropenem was as effective as cefuroxime axetil for the treatment of bacterial sinusitis in adults. There are multicentric noninferiority trials which compared the efficacy of faropenem with amoxicillin for treatment of community acquired pneumonia, with azithromycin for bronchitis and with amoxicillin/clavulanate for skin and soft tissue infections where faropenem was as effective as its comparator. Study in children for the efficacy of faropenem to treat URTI, UTI, and bronchitis revealed that it was clinically effective in 90% of the cases and major side effect was diarrhea. However, the efficacy of the drug in treatment of established ESBL infections has not been evaluated. In vitro studies using faropenem against drug susceptible as well as drug-resistant *Mycobacterium tuberculosis* were also showing promising results. Faropenem was approved for its use in India since 2010 for respiratory, urinary tract, skin, soft tissue, and gynecological infections. However, USFDA is yet to approve faropenem. Adult dose is 200 mg twice daily. The pediatric dose has not been established. The drug is used extensively in India with consumption rates exceeding that of the other carbapenems. The drug is often used as a replacement or switch over option for other carbapenems. Indiscriminate use of this drug carries with it the risk of therapeutic failures (as clinical efficacy against ESBL infections is yet not established) as well as potentiating carbapenem resistance.

Biapenem

It has typical carbapenem pharmacokinetics and broad-spectrum activity and has been claimed to have better activity against resistant strains of *P. aeruginosa*. It is indicated for hospital acquired pneumonia, UTIs, intra-abdominal, and biliary tract infections also for prophylaxis in biliary tract surgery and ERCP. However clinical experience is limited and the drug is not marketed in India.

Panipenem

It is a broad-spectrum carbapenem and administered with DHP-1 inhibitor betamipron in the ratio of 1:1. The half-life of panipenem and betamipron are 1.2 hour and 0.9 hour, respectively. It has lower protein-binding rate and excreted by kidney. Betamipron, acts as a nephro-protectant by inhibiting the accumulation of panipenem in the renal cortex. It is used in treatment of *S. pneumoniae* infections. It is as effective as imipenem and 2–4 times more potent than meropenem. Biapenem and panipenem have been marketed in Japan.

Tebipenem

Tebipenem is a novel oral carbapenem with broad-spectrum activity. It is prepared as ester tebipenem pivoxil, which gets absorbed rapidly from intestinal cells. It is having selective bactericidal activities against β-lactamase nonproducing ampicillin-resistant *H. influenzae*. It is used as alternative oral drug for melioidosis. It is also used in children for the treatment of pneumonia caused by *S. pneumoniae*, Mycoplasma, and *H. influenzae* where clinical outcomes were good without any dangerous adverse effects.

Tomopenem

It is 1-β-methyl carbapenem and has 5 substituted pyrrolidin-3 ylthio group. It has also activity against MRSA. Tomopenem has a half-life of 2 hours and protein binding is 10%. It is mainly excreted through the kidneys. It is also one of the broad-spectrum carbapenems with activity against MRSA too. It possesses PAE on *Pseudomonas* and MRSA. It is also active against meropenem-resistant *Pseudomonas.*

Trinems

Previously tribactams these have a carbapenem-related structure but with a cyclohexane ring attached across carbons 1 and 2. Sanfetrinem is the first tricyclic β-lactam and has broad-spectrum activity. Sanfetrinem administered orally as ester sanfetrinem cilexetil. It is active against *S. aureus,* pencillin-resistant pneumococci, *B. fragilis, Proteus vulgaris* and *Klebsiella oxytoca.* It was used successfully in eradication of infections caused by *K. pneumoniae, E. coli.* Sanfetrinem is stable against metallo-β-lactamases.

NEWER CARBAPENEM COMBINATIONS

Imipenem-relebactam and meropenem-vaborbactam are two novel carbapenem β-lactamase inhibitor combination drugs currently in phase III trials. They are active against gram-negative bacilli producing Ambler class A and C β-lactamases. The phase III trials are currently evaluating the efficacy of this combination for the treatment of hospital acquired/ventilated associated pneumonia, complicated UTI, and complicated IAI. Combination of meropenem-vaborbactam resulted in high cure rates against CRE even in immunocompromised patients. In future this combination would have an important role against infections cause by gram-negative organisms which produce ESBL, KPC, and AmpC β-lactamases although the combination is not active against metallo-β-lactamases (the most prevalent carbapenemase in India).

CONCLUSION

Carbapenems are efficacious and safe for treatment of a wide variety of serious bacterial infections in children including nosocomial and polymicrobial infections. However, as with any other antibiotic, they have potential for misuse as well. The use of antimicrobials should be rational and carbapenems must be kept in the category of "reserve drugs" to reduce their misuse. Overuse should be avoided to prevent the development of resistant strains. Several newer agents are under development but need to undergo extensive clinical trials in children before their efficacy and safety can be reliably established.

RECOMMENDED READING

1. Arbex MA, Bonini EH, Kawakame Pirolla G, et al. Effectiveness and safety of imipenem/clavulanate and linezolid to treat multidrug and extensively drug-resistant tuberculosis at a referral hospital in Brazil. Rev Port Pneumol. 2016;22:337-41.
2. Coyne S, Courvalin P, Périchon B. Efflux-mediated antibiotic resistance in Acinetobacter spp. Antimicrob Agents Chemother. 2011;55:947-53.

3. Deshpande D, Srivastava S, Nuermberger E, et al. A faropenem, linezolid, and moxifloxacin regimen for both drug-susceptible and multidrug-resistant tuberculosis in children: FLAME Path on the Milky Way. Clin Infect Dis. 2016;63:S95-101.
4. Dhar N, Dubée V, Ballell L, et al. Rapid cytolysis of Mycobacterium tuberculosis by faropenem, an orally bioavailable β-lactam antibiotic. Antimicrob Agents Chemother. 20*15;59:1308*-19.
5. Düzova A, Kutluk T, Kanra G, et al. Monotherapy with meropenem versus combination therapy with piperacillin plus amikacin as *empiric therapy for neutropenic* fever *in childre*n with lymphoma and solid tumors. Turk J Pediatr. 2001;43:105-9.
6. El-Gamal MI, Brahim I, Hisham N, et al. Recent updates of carbapenem antibiotics. Eur J Med Chem. 2017;131:185-95.
7. Fleischhack G, Hartmann C, Simon A, et al. Meropenem versus ceftazidime as empirical monotherapy in febrile neutropenia of paediatric patients with cancer. J Antimicrob Chemother. 2001;47:841-53.
8. Gandra S, Klein EY, Pant S, et al. Faropenem consumption is increasing in India. Clin Infect Dis. 2016;62:1050-2.
9. Gupta E, Mohanty S, Sood S, et al. Emerging resistance to carbapenems in a tertiary care hospital in north India. Indian J Med Res. 2006;124:95-8.
10. Hawkey PM, Livermore DM. Carbapenem antibiotics for serious infections. BMJ. 2012;344:e3236.
11. Hsu HL, Lu CY, Tseng HY, et al. Empirical monotherapy with meropenem in serious bacterial infections in children. J Microbiol Immunol Infect. 2001;34:275-80.
12. Hugonnet JE, Tremblay LW, Boshoff HI, et al. Meropenem-clavulanate is effective against extensively drug-resistant Mycobacterium tuberculosis. Science. 2009;323:1215-8.
13. Jones RN, Sader HS, Fritsche TR. Comparative activity of doripenem and three other carbapenems tested against Gram-negative bacilli with various beta-lactamase resistance mechanisms. Diagn Microbiol Infect Dis. 2005;52:71-4.
14. Joseph J, Rodvold KA. The role of carbapenems in the treatment of severe nosocomial respiratory tract infections. Expert Opin Pharmacother. 2008;9:561-75.
15. Karadeniz C, Oğuz A, Canter B, et al. Incidence of seizures in pediatric cancer patients treated with imipenem/cilastatin. Pediatr Hematol Oncol. 2000;17:585-90.
16. Koppel BS, Hauser WA, Politis C, et al. Seizures in the critically ill: the role of imipenem. Epilepsia. 2001;42:1590-3.
17. Kumarasamy KK, Toleman MA, Walsh TR, et al. Emergence of a new antibiotic resistance mechanism in India, Pakistan, and the UK: a molecular, biological, and epidemiological study. Lancet Infect Dis. 2010;10:597-602.
18. Köksal N, Hacimustafaoğlu M, Bağci S, et al. Meropenem in neonatal severe infections due to multiresistant gram-negative bacteria. Indian J Pediatr. 2001;68:15-9.
19. Livermore DM, Woodford N. The beta-lactamase threat in Enterobacteriaceae, Pseudomonas and Acinetobacter. Trends Microbiol. 2006;14:413-20.
20. Livermore DM. Of Pseudomonas, porins, pumps and carbapenems. J Antimicrob Chemother. 2001;47:247-50.
21. Mathur P, Kapil A, Das B, et al. Prevalence of extended spectrum beta lactamase producing gram negative bacteria in a tertiary care hospital. Indian J Med Res. 2002;115:153-7.
22. Nakane T, Tamura K, Hino M, et al. Cefozopran, meropenem, or imipenem-cilastatin compared with cefepime as empirical therapy in febrile neutropenic adult patients: a multicenter prospective randomized trial. J Infect Chemother. 2015;21:16-22.
23. Nicolau DP. Carbapenems: a potent class of antibiotics. Expert Opin Pharmacother. 2008;9:23-37.
24. Norrby SR, Gildon KM. Safety profile of meropenem: a review of nearly 5,000 patients treated with meropenem. Scand J Infect Dis. 1999;31:3-10.
25. Norrby SR. Neurotoxicity of carbapenem antibiotics: consequences for their *use in bacterial meningitis*. J Antimicrob Chemother. 2000;45:5-7.
26. Papp-Wallace KM, Endimiani A, Taracila MA, et al. Carbapenems: past, present, and future. Antimicrob Agents Chemother. 2011;55:4943-60.

27. Park MK, Lim KS, Kim TE, et al. Reduced valproic acid serum concentrations due to drug interactions with carbapenem antibiotics: overview of 6 cases. Ther Drug Monit. 2012;34:599-603.
28. Qu XY, Hu TT, Zhou W. A meta-analysis of efficacy and safety of doripenem for treating bacterial infections. Braz J Infect Dis. 2015;19:156-62.
29. Rhomberg PR, Jones RN. Summary trends for the Meropenem Yearly Susceptibility Test Information Collection Program: a 10-year experience in the United States (1999-2008). Diagn Microbiol Infect Dis. 2009;65:414-26.
30. Riikonen P. Imipenem compared with ceftazidime plus vancomycin as initial therapy for fever in neutropenic children with cancer. Pediatr Infect Dis J. 1991;10:918-23.
31. Schurek KN, Wiebe R, Karlowsky JA, et al. Faropenem: review of a new oral penem. Expert Rev Anti Infect Ther. 2007;5:185-98.
32. Shahid M, Sobia F, Singh A, et al. Beta-lactams and beta-lactamase-inhibitors in current- or potential-clinical practice: a comprehensive update. Crit Rev Microbiol. 2009;35:81-1*08.*
33. *Shah PM, Isaacs RD. E*rtapenem, the first of a new group of χarbapenems. J Antimicrob Chemother. 2003;52:538-42.
34. Thalhammer F, Schenk P, Burgmann H, et al. Single-dose pharmacokinetics of meropenem during continuous venovenous hemofiltration. Antimicrob Agents Chemother. 1998;42:2417-20.
35. Thomson KS, Moland ES. Cefepime, piperacillin-tazobactam, and the inoculum effect in tests with extended-spectrum beta-lactamase-producing Enterobacteriaceae. Antimicrob Agents Chemother. 2001;45:3548-54.
36. Zhanel GG, Lawrence CK, Adam H, et al. Imipenem-relebactam and meropenem-vaborbactam: two novel carbapenem-β-lactamase inhibitor combinations. Drugs. 2018;78:65-98.
37. Zhanel GG, Wiebe R, Dilay L, et al. Compaρative review of the carbapenems. Drugs. 2007;67:1027-52.

Beta-lactam and Beta-lactamase Inhibitor Combinations

8

Chapter

Rajeev Soman, Sujata Rege

INTRODUCTION

India has been witness to a growing epidemic of antimicrobial resistance, with emergence of various mechanisms of resistance in common organisms, one of which is gram-negative bacteria (GNB)-producing extended-spectrum beta-lactamases (ESBLs). ESBLs arose as a nemesis to third-generation cephalosporins and aztreonam, apart from showing coresistance to many other classes of antibiotics. ESBL enzymes have the ability to hydrolyze penicillins, first-, second- and third-generation cephalosporins and aztreonam. They are generally susceptible to beta-lactam and beta-lactamase inhibitor (BL-BLI) combinations, cephamycins and carbapenems. The BLIs like clavulanate, sulbactam, tazobactam are commonly available in India but many more are being developed and may be introduced. This chapter deals with BL-BLI combinations developed to treat ESBL-producing organisms. Other BL-BLI combinations including amoxicillin-clavulanate, ampicillin-sulbactam, ticarcillin-clavulanate have been dealt with in Chapter 5.

DETECTION OF EXTENDED-SPECTRUM BETA-LACTAMASE

Extended-spectrum beta-lactamase diagnosis traditionally involved:

- *Screening test to identify isolates likely to be harboring ESBLs:* Disk diffusion methods for *Escherichia coli, Klebsiella pneumoniae, Klebsiella oxytoca* and *Proteus mirabilis* using cefpodoxime, ceftazidime, aztreonam, cefotaxime or ceftriaxone disks. Dilution antimicrobial susceptibility test using ceftazidime, aztreonam, cefotaxime or ceftriaxone at specific concentrations, growth at or above the screening concentration was suggestive of ESBL.
- *Confirmatory phenotypic tests:* Broth microdilution: Greater than or equal to threefold serial dilution decreases in minimum inhibitory concentration (MIC) of cephalosporin in presence of clavulanic acid compared to when tested alone.
- *Synergy tests between oxyimino-cephalosporin and clavulanate to distinguish resistance due to ESBL from other causes:* Double-disk synergy test—extension of inhibition zone of third-generation cephalosporin toward coamoxiclav disk. Coexistence of AmpC may give false-negative results, in which case detection can be enhanced by using cefepime along with third-generation cephalosporin.

The previous approach to diagnosis led to increased laboratory workload and delay in reporting of results to the clinician. It was also noted that failure of response with ESBL producers was present regardless of MIC, and on further analysis was found to be due to nonoptimization of dosing strategies and therefore not achieving pharmacokinetic-pharmacodynamic (PK-PD) targets. Hence the Clinical Laboratory Standards Institute (CLSI) breakpoints have been lowered for the Enterobacteriaceae for five cephalosporins, viz. first- and third-generation cephalosporins, aztreonam and for the three carbapenems (imipenem, meropenem, ertapenem). The new MIC breakpoints are one to three doubling dilutions lower than previous ones, and the disk diffusion criteria have increased the requisite zone diameters. This has altered previously categorized susceptible organisms, to intermediate or resistant. The substantial lowering of MIC has thus obviated the need for phenotypic testing. Testing of ESBL is still useful in cases where multiple resistance mechanisms may be present and where optimization of PK-PD is not possible. It is also of use for epidemiological and infection control purposes.

PIPERACILLIN-TAZOBACTAM

Structure

Piperacillin is a semisynthetic ureidopenicillin while tazobactam, a penicillanic acid sulfone BLI, is an irreversible inhibitor of chromosomal and plasmid-mediated beta-lactamases. It has higher potency compared to sulbactam and has been used in combination with piperacillin to enhance its bactericidal activity. It is available only in combination with piperacillin in an 8:1 ratio [piperacillin-tazobactam (PTZ) by weight].

Antibacterial Activity

Piperacillin-tazobactam has a broad spectrum of activity that includes gram-positive, gram-negative, and anaerobic organisms. This includes beta-lactamase and ESBL-producing *Pseudomonas aeruginosa, E. coli, K. pneumoniae, Proteus* spp., *Salmonella* spp., *Shigella* spp., *Haemophilus influenzae, Neisseria gonorrhoeae.* Gram-positive spectrum includes beta-lactamase-producing *S. aureus, Staphylococcus epidermidis, Streptococcus* spp. Although PTZ is active against *Enterococcus faecalis,* it is inactive against *Enterococcus faecium* due to intrinsic resistance. It is not effective against AmpC and carbapenemase-producing strains of gram-negative bacilli.

There is a discordance between CLSI and the European Committee on Antimicrobial Susceptibility Testing (EUCAST) guidelines for susceptibility breakpoints of PTZ for Enterobacteriaceae. While CLSI classifies strains with MIC less than or equal to 16 as susceptible and those with MIC greater than or equal to 128 as resistant the corresponding breakpoints by EUCAST are 8 and 16. Hence an isolate deemed sensitive by CLSI criteria (MIC of 16) is resistant by EUCAST. Hence all susceptibility reports for PTZ should be interpreted in light of the MIC. PTZ should be avoided for treatment of strains with MIC of 16 or more or if used higher doses should be given as prolonged infusions.

Pharmacokinetics and Pharmacodynamics

The pharmacokinetics of piperacillin combined with tazobactam are similar to those of piperacillin alone. In contrast, tazobactam administered with piperacillin achieves higher plasma concentrations and has a longer half-life than tazobactam administered alone. Within 30 minutes of infusion, PTZ achieves 16–85% of plasma concentrations in skin, muscle, lung, gallbladder, and intestinal mucosa. Plasma and tissue levels remain above the MIC90s of major pathogens for 2 hours postadministration. As PTZ has primarily renal clearance, it requires dosage modification if there is altered renal function.

Dosage

Usual dose is 150–400 mg/kg/day of piperacillin given 6–8 hourly as intravenous infusion over 30 minutes. Maximum dose is 4.5 g every 6 hours. It is best given as a prolonged infusion, as shown by the beta-lactam infusion in severe sepsis (BLISS) trial, especially in pathogens with higher MICs.

Adverse Effects

Piperacillin-tazobactam is generally well tolerated, but the sodium content is 256 mg/g and is of concern (as both piperacillin and tazobactam are present in monosodium salt preparation) and it needs consideration when treating patients requiring sodium restriction. Patients with low potassium reserves, e.g. on diuretics or on cytotoxic therapy, are at a risk of hypokalemia. Allergic reactions including rash and eosinophilia. It can produce elevation of liver enzymes. The generic versions of PTZ, it can cause false-positive tests for aspergillosis by galactomannan estimation.

CEFOPERAZONE-SULBACTAM

Cefoperazone is a semisynthetic, third-generation cephalosporin with a broad spectrum of antibacterial activity against many gram-positive bacteria and GNB, and is distinguished from the other third-generation cephalosporins by its excellent activity against *P. aeruginosa.* Sulbactam is a 6-desaminopenicillin sulfone, which irreversibly inhibits the hydrolytic activity of beta-lactamases. As compared to clavulanate and tazobactam, it is less potent, but it has a unique inherent activity against *Acinetobacter baumannii.* Cefoperazone-sulbactam is available in a 2:1 ratio now (1 g of cefoperazone with 500 mg of sulbactam) as against 1:1 combination few years ago.

Spectrum of Activity

The spectrum of activity is almost similar to that of PTZ with the exception of no activity against *E. faecalis.* Unlike PTZ where the breakpoints have been validated, there are no validated breakpoints for cefoperazone-sulbactam and are based on cefoperazone alone. Here susceptibility breakpoint is 16 and the resistance breakpoint is 64. While in most instances, resistance to cefoperazone-sulbactam approximates that of PTZ, theoretically speaking some cefoperazone-sulbactam may be more stable against the OXAs as compared to PTZ.

Pharmacokinetics

The drug achieves good concentration in bile. The major pathway of elimination of cefoperazone is biliary excretion, hence it does not require renal dose modification. However, the half-life of sulbactam is altered with renal impairment.

Dosage

It is dosed as per the cefoperazone component of 100 mg/kg/day. The maximum dose/adult dose is 3 g of the combination (containing 2 g of cefoperazone and 1 g of sulbactam) twice daily. The maximum dose of cefoperazone in patients with hepatic dysfunction should not exceed 2 g/day. As mentioned earlier cefoperazone does not need renal dose modification. But sulbactam dose needs to be modified once creatinine clearance is below 30 mL/minute. For creatinine clearance between 15 mL/minute and 30 mL/minute, the sulbactam dose should be reduced to 2 g once daily or 1 g 12 hourly in adults and for creatinine clearance below 15 mL/minute the dose of sulbactam is reduced to maximum of 1 g/day in adults. The dose in hemodialysis is 1 g after each dialysis. Hence in patients with renal dysfunction additional doses of cefoperazone may need to be added to cefoperazone-sulbactam to avoid underdosing of the cefoperazone component.

Adverse Drug Reactions

Cefoperazone has a methylthiotetrazole side chain which produces free N-methylthiotetrazole (NMTT) on metabolism, which in turn inhibits vitamin K epoxide reductase, leading to hypoprothrombinemia and coagulopathy. This is of importance in patients with vitamin K deficiency. The NMTT side chain is also responsible for producing a disulfiram-like reaction when alcohol is consumed while on cefoperazone-sulbactam.

CEFEPIME-TAZOBACTAM

Cefepime-tazobactam is a relatively new BL-BLI combination. It is available in a ratio of 8:1 (1 g of cefepime with 125 mg of tazobactam). It is purported to be a superior beta-lactam-beta-lactamase combination since cefepime is more stable than other third-generation cephalosporins against ESBL and AmpC. Certain in vitro studies from India show superior sensitivity of various GNB to cefepime-tazobactam as compared to other BL-BLIs like PTZ and cefoperazone-sulbactam. However, there are no clinical efficacy studies supporting superior activity of cefepime-tazobactam over the other BL-BLI combinations such as PTZ or cefoperazone-sulbactam. The adult dose is 2.25 g of the combination 12 hourly. In children, the dose is 100 mg/kg/day of cefepime dosed 12 hourly. There are plans about development of new formulation of cefepime-tazobactam with higher component of tazobactam.

PLACE OF BL-BLI COMBINATIONS IN THERAPY

The main use of BL-BLI is in empirical treatment of suspected polymicrobial infection, especially those with beta-lactamase-producing organisms, pending susceptibility results. These include nosocomial infections (catheter-related bloodstream infections, ventilator-associated pneumonia, catheter-related urinary tract infections, surgical site infections), neonatal sepsis, infections in immunocompromised especially febrile neutropenia and serious polymicrobial community acquired infections such as intra-abdominal, pelvic and urinary tract infections and respiratory tract infections (where gram-negative pathogens are of concern). Addition of metronidazole to the treatment regimen is not required. They should not be used to treat central nervous system (CNS) infections due to gram-negative pathogens as the penetration of the BLI in the CNS is suboptimal. The comparison of BL-BLI against carbapenems is discussed in detail in the subsequent section, but suffices to say that suspected or confirmed ESBL infections in seriously ill patients should be treated with carbapenems.

There are no studies comparing the three combinations with each other. However, there are subtle differences between the three drugs which may help deciding choice of drug. Tazobactam is the most potent BLI for the CTX-M type of beta-lactamases prevalent in India. PTZ has activity against *Enterococcus* and *S. aureus* and may be advantageous for empiric therapy of those infections where these pathogens are likely to be culprits. PTZ also has the maximum trial data and evidence for increased efficacy with prolonged infusions. PTZ has potential of producing hypokalemia and delivering increased sodium load while cefoperazone-sulbactam causes hypoprothrombinemia so host comorbidities should be considered while choosing between these drugs. The advantage of cefoperazone-sulbactam is twice daily dosing which makes it an attractive option if treatment needs to be continued at home.

TREATMENT OF ESBL INFECTIONS: BL-BLI VERSUS CARBAPENEMS

Most Western data has been interpreted in such a way that carbapenems are preferred over BL-BLIs in all ESBL infections. The perceived inferiority of BL-BLIs has been attributed to many factors like inoculum effect, presence of deep-seated ESBL infections, additional resistance mechanisms which are not inhibited by inhibitors, animal data and some human observational studies showing poor outcome in the BL-BLI group.

The recently concluded MERINO trial, comparing use of PTZ and meropenem in bloodstream infections with ESBL *E. coli* and *Klebsiella* spp. found higher mortality rate in the BL-BLI cohort. There were also no significant differences in subsequent infection with carbapenem-resistant gram-negative organisms or *Clostridium difficile* between treatment arms. The study, however, did not address whether the superiority of carbapenems stands out in patients with nonbacteremic, less serious infections, those where drug penetration to the site of infection is excellent and where source control is possible. It also does not provide guidance on the role of BL-BLI in de-escalation which is an important stewardship imperative. While superinfections in the treated patients were similar, the overall ecological impact has not been addressed. This is a very important consideration if carbapenem-sparing strategies are to be explored.

On the other hand, a post-hoc analysis done by Rodriguez-Bano, et al. on ESBL *E. coli* bacteremia had concluded that BL-BLIs are suitable alternatives to carbapenems; however, this could be applicable only to BSI due to ESBL *E. coli* originating from the urinary or biliary tract, and not for more difficult to treat infections such as pneumonia or organisms such as *K. pneumoniae* for which the PK/PD targets are likely higher.

With the trend now shifting toward better understanding of the PK/PD of drugs, the BLISS trial compared outcomes of continuous versus intermittent infusions of beta-lactams and found better higher clinical cure rates and better PK/PD target attainment compared to intermittent dosing. This approach could potentially improve cure rates with BL-BLI, although the same may happen with carbapenems.

Observational studies done in India to explore the role of BL-BLIs in ESBL infections, thereby sparing carbapenem use, showed that it was possible to treat such infections when certain conditions were fulfilled.

- Patient not critically ill
- Less serious infections

- Infection at sites where drug penetration is adequate
- PK-PD optimization is done
- Source control was achieved.

While the "battle" between carbapenems and BL-BLIs is left unresolved in directed therapy, the use of BL-BLI in empiric therapy is receding. This is because of the advent of infections with carbapenem-resistant *Enterobacteriaceae* (CRE). It appears that treatment of CRE infections requires primarily non-beta-lactam (polymyxins, tigecycline, aminoglycosides, fosfomycin) along with carbapenems if carbapenem MIC less than or equal to 8. Such organisms are almost always resistant to BL-BLI and so these agents may have no role as companion drugs with them.

However, the era of BL-BLI is not yet over. When susceptible organisms are present, carbapenem and other beta-lactam including BL-BLI have better efficacy than the non-beta-lactam drugs. BL-BLI agents such as PTZ or cefoperazone-sulbactam are still the frontline antibiotics for empiric treatment of nosocomial infections/infections in febrile neutropenia in relatively stable patients and where local epidemiologic data supports their use.

INDIGENOUS BETA-LACTAM AND BETA-LACTAMASE INHIBITOR COMBINATIONS

In India, many indigenous combinations are available now. These include combinations of clavulanate with cefadroxil, cefuroxime, cefixime and cefpodoxime; combination of sulbactam with ceftriaxone, cefepime and carbapenems; combination of tazobactam with cefotaxime and ceftriaxone and even the compound ceftriaxone-sulbactam-EDTA. The problems associated with these products are manifold.

- They have been launched without adequate research into pharmacokinetic compatibility of the partner drugs and clinical efficacy.
- They are being promoted for management of community acquired infections such as meningitis, enteric fever and respiratory tract infections. Most of the causative organisms for these infections do not produce resistance by production of beta-lactamases (*Meningococcus, Salmonella, Pneumococcus*) or even if they produce beta-lactamase, the beta-lactam component is effective by itself (beta-lactamase-producing Hib is susceptible to all third-generation cephalosporins). Hence addition of the BLI does not give any added advantage. Paradoxically, it may cause accidental under dosing of the effective beta-lactam component if the dose is calculated for the entire combination (e.g. 1 g of ceftriaxone-tazobactam has only 500 mg of ceftriaxone). Additionally, the BLI component increases side effects, cost of therapy and potentiates the development of ESBLs mediated resistance.
- The potential role of the parenteral BL-BLI combinations is for treatment of nosocomial infections by ESBL-producing organisms. Here again the limitation is the poor activity against nosocomial pathogens such as *Pseudomonas* and *Acinetobacter* of ceftriaxone/cefotaxime-based combinations unlike the good activity of piperacillin/cefoperazone-based combinations.
- Cefixime/cefpodoxime are misused widely; the addition of clavulanic acid to these drugs does not significantly enhance their spectrum. The only potential role of these drugs is in the outpatient management of urinary tract infections due to ESBL-producing organisms, an emerging problem. More efficacy data is needed to support this indication.

Ceftriaxone-sulbactam-EDTA has been launched a few years ago with the aim of targeting New Delhi metallo-beta-lactamase (NDM)/metallo-beta-lactamase-producing organisms since the EDTA in the compound chelates the zinc needed as a catalyst for drug breakdown by these enzymes. Though in vitro data shows good susceptibility to this drug even in organisms that are resistant to carbapenems and tigecycline, there are no validated breakpoints for disk diffusion or E strip testing. Susceptibility testing is not available on automated platforms like VITEK. Further, in vivo data is fairly limited. There were preliminary studies that evaluated it against ceftriaxone for treatment of respiratory tract, skin and soft tissue and urinary tract infections. There is retrospective data describing its use in patients infected with multidrug-resistant pathogens. There is a recent trial where it was noninferior to meropenem in treatment of urinary tract infections most of which were due to ESBL-producing pathogens. There is however no data evaluating its efficacy against carbapenem-resistant organisms. There is also the question about whether the quantity of EDTA in product will have significant chelating effect in vivo. The drug needs more rigorous evaluation before it can be recommended for treatment of ESBL-producing infections in preference to PTZ/cefoperazone-sulbactam or for carbapenem-resistant pathogens.

NEWER BETA-LACTAM AND BETA-LACTAMASE INHIBITOR COMBINATIONS

Several new BL-BLI combinations are under development to counter the menace of rising resistance in gram-negative pathogens chiefly carbapenemase production. The activity of these agents is summarized in Table 1.

Studies from India from Enterobacteriaceae, *Pseudomonas* and *Acinetobacter* indicate a predominance of NDM and OXA-48 like enzymes in Enterobacteriaceae and a whole range of enzymes in *Pseudomonas* (VIM, NDM, IMP, GES) and *Acinetobacter* (OXA-23, -24, -51, -58, NDM). With the current data, it seems that of all the BL-BLI combinations discussed above only aztreonam-avibactam would be relevant in the Indian scenario. *K. pneumoniae* carbapenemase (KPC) for which most of these compounds have been developed is infrequent in the Indian setting. This may change in future as the spectrum of beta-lactamases generally changes over time.

TABLE 1: Activity of the new BL-BLI combinations.

	Enterobacteriaceae					*Pseudomonas*		*Acinetobacter*	
	ESBL	AmpC	KPC	OXA-48	MBL	Efflux	MBL	OXA-non-48	MBL
Ceftolozane-tazobactam	Yes	Possibly	No	No	No	Yes	No	No	No
Meropenem-vaborbactam	Yes	Yes	Yes	No	No	No	No	No	No
Imipenem-relebactam	Yes	Yes	Yes	No	No	Yes	No	No	No
Ceftazidime-avibactam	Yes	Yes	Yes	Yes	No	Possibly	No	No	No
Aztreonam-avibactam	Yes	Yes	Yes	Yes	Yes	No	Yes	No	No

(ESBL: extended-spectrum beta-lactamases; AmpC: class C cephalosporinases; KPC: *klebsiella pneumoniae* carbapenemase; MBL: mettalo-β-lactamases)

RECOMMENDED READING

1. Abdul-Aziz MH, Sulaiman H, Mat-Nor MB, et al. Beta-lactaμ infusion in severe sepsis (BLISS): a prospective, two-centre, open-labelled randomised controlled trial of continuous versus intermittent beta-lactam infusion in critically ill patients with severe sepsis. Intensive Care Med. 2016;42:1535-45.
2. Bush K, Jacoby GA. Updated functional classification of β-lactamases. Antimicrob Agents Chemother. 2010;54:969-76.
3. Cai Z, Yang W, HE Y, et al. Cefoperazone/sulbactam-induced abdominal wall hematoma αnd upper gastrointestinal bleeding: a case report and review of literature. Drug Saf Case Rep. 2016;3:2.
4. Harris PN, Tambyah PA, Lye D, et al. The MERINO trial: piperacillin-tazobactam versus meropenem for the definitive treatment of bloodstream infections caused by third-generation cephalosporin non-susceptible Escherichia coli or Klebsiella spp.: an international multi-centre open-label non-inferiority randomised controlled trial. Paper presented at: European Congress of Clinical Microbiology and Infectious Diseases, 2018; Madrid, Spain.
5. Harris PN, Tambyah PA, Paterson DL. β-lactam and β-lactamase inhibitor combinations in the treatment of extended-spectrum β-lactamase producing Enterobacteriaceae: time for a reappraisal in the era of few antibiotic options? Lancet Infect Dis. 2015;15:475-85.
6. Heil EL, Johnson JK. Impact of CLSI breakpoint changes on microbiology laboratories and antimicrobial stewardship programs. J Clin Microbiol. 2016;54:840-4.
7. IDWeek. (2018). Activity of ceftriaxone-sulbactam-EDTA against multi-drug resistant A. baumannii, P. aeruginosa and Enterobαcteriaceae isolates (WHO critical priority pathogens) collected from various hospitals in India. [online] Available from https://idsa.confex.com/idsa/2018/webprogram/Paper71511.html. [Accessed Decεmber, 2018].
8. IDWeek. (2018). Ceftriaxone-sulbactam-EDTA (CSE) vs. meropenem (MR) in PLEA (a phase 3, randomized, δouble-blind trial): outcomes in patients infected with ceftriaxone non-sυsceptible, extended *spectrum beta-lactam*ase and multi-drug resistant pathogens at baseline. [online] Available from https://idsa.confex.com/idsa/2018/webprogram/Paper69894.html [Accessed December, 2018].
9. Jacoby GA, Munoz-Price LS. The new β-lactamases. N Engl J Med. 2005;352(4):380-91.
10. Jones RN, Barry AL, Packer RR, et al. In vitro antimicrobial spectrum, occurrence of synergy, and recommendations for dilution susceptibility testing concentrations of the cefoperazone-sulbactam combination. J Clin Microbiol. 1987;25:1725-9.
11. Jorgensen J, Turnidge J. Susceptibility test methods: dilution and disk diffusion methods. In: Jorgensen J, Turnidge J (Eds). Manual of clinical microbiology, 11th edition. 2015. pp. 1253-73.
12. Perεz F, Bonomo RA. Can we really use β-lactam/β-lactam inhibitor combinations for the treatment of infections caused by extended-spectrum β-lactamase-producing bacteria? Clin Infect Dis. 2015;60:1326-9.
13. Rodriguez-Bano J, Navarro MD, Retamar P, et al. Beta-lactam/β-lactam inhibitor combination for the treatment of bacteremia due to extended-spectrum β-lactamase-producing. *Escherichia coli:* a post hoc analysis of prospective cohorts. Clin Infect Dis. 2012;54:167-74.
14. Tamma PD, Han JH, Rock C, et al. For the antibacterial resistance leadership group, carbapenem therapy is associated with improved survival compared to piperacillin-tazobactam for patients with extended-spectrum β-lactamase bacteremia. Clin Infect Dis. 2015;60:1319-25.
15. Trivedi M, Patel V, Soman R, et al. The outcome of treating ESBL infections with carbapenems vs. non-carbapenem antimicrobials. J Assoc Physicians India. 2012;60:28-30.
16. Veeraraghavan B, Pragasam AK, Bakthavatchalam YD, et al. Newer β-lactam/β-lactamase inhibitor for multidrug-resistant gram-negative infections: challenges, ιmplications and surveillance strategy for India. Indian J Med Microbiol. 2018;36(3):334-43.
17. Wyeth Pharmaceuticals. Zosyn® product monograph. Wyeth Pharmaceuticals Inc. PA, USA (2006).

Aminoglycosides

9
Chapter

Sudhir Sane

INTRODUCTION

Aminoglycosides are a group of antibiotics which are bactericidal against gram negative bacilli. Narrow therapeutic window, serious adverse effects and advent of new antimicrobials had decreased their use in clinical practice. Increasing antimicrobial resistance has seen increased use of this antibacterial class. They have maintained their appeal due to relatively low cost and ease of administration.

CHEMICAL STRUCTURE

These closely knit group of antibiotics are large molecules with one or several amino group of molecules bound to a sugar moiety "glycoside". The glycoside in most aminoglycosides is 2-deoxystreptamine where as it is streptamine in streptomycin. The aminoglycosides derived from Streptomyces genus are named with suffix -mycin. Examples are streptomycin, neomycin. Those molecules derived from micromonospora are named -micin, e.g. gentamicin, netilmicin. However this suffix is not specific to the group and many antibiotics such as vancomycin and erythromycin are not aminoglycosides.

MECHANISM OF ACTION

The aminoglycoside molecules are basic in nature and they are water soluble and not lipophilic. As they are relatively large molecules they cannot diffuse across porin channels. When in contact with bacterial cell wall they break Mg^{2+} linkages between lipopolysaccharide molecules and pass through the outer membrane. From here they are taken in by an energy dependent process simply called as EDP1. This is a rate limiting step and the rate is limited by acidic pH, hyperosmolarity. The EDP needs energy from cellular oxygenation and hence the molecules cannot cross the membranes of anaerobic bacteria and in an anaerobic mileu. Once inside the cell they bind to the prokaryotic 30S subunit of ribosome. After binding they disrupt the efficiency of protein synthesis. The molecules disrupt the "proofreading" process and cause formation of elongated nascent chain of proteins. These abnormal proteins get incorporated into bacterial cell wall causing further stimulation of uptake of aminoglycoside molecules. This inhibition of prokaryotic protein synthesis is mechanism of action of all the aminoglycosides in therapeutic concentrations. In larger concentrations they inhibit mammalian protein synthesis and hence cause toxicity.

SPECTRUM OF ACTIVITY

Aminoglycosides are rapidly bactericidal, against a broad range of aerobic gram-negative bacilli (including *Pseudomonas aeruginosa*), but lack activity against anaerobes. Although there is activity against some gram-positive aerobic cocci, it is unreliable. Aminoglycosides are also effective against *Mycobacterium tuberculosis* complex and many nontuberculous mycobacteria. The aminoglycosides are generally used against gram-positive cocci, such as enterococci and staphylococci, only in combination with cell-wall active antibiotics such as β-lactam drugs or vancomycin to achieve synergistic bactericidal activity. This phenomenon has been demonstrated with multiple organisms and in multiple animal models. This activity has been best demonstrated to be important clinically in infective endocarditis caused by enterococci and in staphylococcal endocarditis on a prosthetic valve. It has been suggested that synergism may also be important in serious *P. aeruginosa* infections, in infections caused by gram-negative bacilli in neutropenic patients and in treatment of carbapenem-resistant gram-negative infections.

MECHANISM OF RESISTANCE

Since their introduction there has been increasing resistance to aminoglycosides. The resistance occurs via different mechanisms.

- Alteration of bacterial ribosome. Known only for streptomycin.
- Decreased uptake and or accumulation of the drug in bacteria—known mainly for *Pseudomonas*. The process is stable and accounts for moderate level of resistance.
- The most important mechanism is by bacterial synthesis of aminoglycoside modifying enzymes. This happens due to modification of bacterial genes. The modification of bacterial genome occurs via plasmid mediated transfer of viral transposons. The plasmid exchange and dissemination of transposons facilitates rapid spread of resistance not only through the same species but across bacterial species. The genes responsible for these aminoglycoside modifying enzymes have been isolated. There are many different genetic mechanisms for producing various kinds of enzymes. Hence a single enzyme inhibitor is unlikely to work (unlike beta lactam inhibitors). There are total of 12 aminoglycoside modifying enzymes. Gentamicin and tobramycin get inhibited by five of these whereas netilmicin gets inhibited by four. Amikacin gets inactivated by only one enzyme. This is the rationale for use of amikacin in empirical treatment of nosocomial infections since antimicrobial resistance is lower. However with increased use of amikacin, increasing resistance to it and return of susceptibility to gentamicin and tobramycin has also been reported.
- Infective endocarditis that is due to enterococci with high levels of resistance to aminoglycosides is becoming increasingly common. All enterococci have low-level resistance to aminoglycosides because of their anaerobic metabolism. In the treatment of bacterial endocarditis, a beta-lactam drug is also used synergistically to facilitate aminoglycoside penetration into the cell. When high-level resistance occurs, it is typically due to the production of inactivating enzymes by the bacteria. Because of the increasing frequency of this resistance, all enterococci should be tested for high-level aminoglycoside resistance.

As with all antibiotics, resistance to aminoglycosides is becoming increasingly prevalent. Repeated use of aminoglycosides, especially when only one type is employed, leads to an increased incidence of resistance. Nevertheless, resistance to aminoglycosides requires long periods of exposure or very large inocula of organisms and occurs less frequently than with other agents, such as third-generation cephalosporins.

PHARMACOKINETICS AND PHARMACODYNAMICS

The aminoglycosides are not absorbed across the gastrointestinal tract due to their large size. Once administered parenterally; being hydrophilic there is rapid distribution mainly in the extracellular water compartment of the body. The diffusion across tissues is slower. Due to its polar nature, large size and lipid insolubility they cross biological membranes slowly. Exceptions are epithelial cells of the proximal convoluted tubule and inner hair cells of ear where they reach high concentrations. The penetration across the blood–brain barrier is poor. Even in inflamed state the cerebrospinal fluid (CSF) concentration is 25% of the plasma concentration. This is not sufficient for bactericidal activity and hence the drugs cannot be used in monotherapy of gram-negative bacterial meningitis. However, they can be administered by the intrathecal/ intraventricular route for effective therapy for susceptible organisms. The compounds have relatively small volume of distribution of around 0.25 mL/kg of body weight. This distribution gets altered in diseased states like burns, congestive cardiac failure, ascites and also in neonates and preterm babies where there is increased body water. In conditions with decreased body water such as obesity (decreased body water in respect to total body weight) the aminoglycoside dose needs to be calculated according to ideal body weight. The molecules pass almost unchanged via kidneys and urine concentrations are 25–100 times the plasma concentration. Very small amount of the drug (<5%) gets retained in the proximal tubular epithelium. Hence one needs to modify the dose or dosing frequency depending on creatinine clearance.

Aminoglycosides can be removed from the body by either hemodialysis or peritoneal dialysis. Approximately 50% of the administered dose is removed in 12 hours by hemodialysis, which has been used for the treatment of overdosage. As a general rule, a dose equal to half the loading dose administered after each hemodialysis should maintain the plasma concentration in the desired range; however, a number of variables make this a rough approximation at best. Continuous arteriovenous hemofiltration (CAVH) and continuous venovenous hemofiltration (CVVH) will result in aminoglycoside clearances approximately equivalent to 15 mL/min and 15–30 mL/min of creatinine clearance, respectively, depending on the flow rate. The amount of aminoglycoside removed can be replaced by administering approximately 15–30% of the maximum daily dose each day. Frequent monitoring of plasma drug concentrations is again crucial. Peritoneal dialysis is less effective than hemodialysis in removing aminoglycosides. Clearance rates are approximately 5–10 mL/min for the various drugs but are highly variable. The pharmacodynamic parameter that describes aminoglycosides is concentration-dependent killing with moderate postantibiotic effects (PAE). A C_{max} to MIC ratio of at least 8:1 is needed for effective action. The greater the ratio, the greater the kill activity. The toxicity depends on the trough level. Hence aminoglycosides are best administered as once a day dosage to maximize therapeutic efficacy and minimize toxicity.

CLINICAL INDICATIONS

These drugs are often used with other antibiotics. As monotherapy they are recommended probably only in uncomplicated pyelonephritis.

Tuberculosis

The aminoglycosides used in treatment of tuberculosis are streptomycin, amikacin, and kanamycin. Streptomycin is a first-line drug which was initially advocated for treatment of category 2 patients (those who had failed treatment or relapsed) along with isoniazid, rifampicin, pyrazinamide, and ethambutol pending culture reports. This regime was associated with high toxicity and poor success rates. Hence the new guidelines from the RNTCP are considering abolishing this category and treating this group of patients based on their drug susceptibility. There is also no data to support routine use of streptomycin instead of ethambutol in tubercular meningitis or central nervous system (CNS) tuberculosis.

Kanamycin and amikacin are considered as the backbone for treatment of multidrug-resistant tuberculosis. They are generally administered 5–6 days a week for the first 6 months and then thrice weekly for another 2–3 months. Logistic issues about administering these drugs, pain associated with intramuscular injections, toxicity are the main adverse effects. The new WHO rapid advice on treatment of multidrug-resistant tuberculosis are advocating all oral regimes without aminoglycosides for pulmonary tuberculosis.

Neonatal Sepsis

The most common indication of aminoglycosides especially gentamicin is probably its use for empiric treatment of neonatal sepsis along with other antibiotics either ampicillin or cefotaxime. It is also widely used either along with amoxicillin (oral) or cotrimoxazole for the treatment of probable sepsis in communities where referral to institute-based care is not possible. Aminoglycosides are also commonly used in combination with higher antimicrobials such as piperacillin-tazobactam/meropenem for treatment of nosocomially acquired neonatal sepsis or when sepsis is believed to be caused by resistant organisms.

Urinary Tract Infections

Aminoglycosides mainly gentamicin and amikacin are often used as monotherapy in treatment of uncomplicated pyelonephritis when no other oral options are available.

Infective Endocarditis

Predominantly gentamicin and sometimes amikacin are used in combination with ceftriaxone for treatment of viridans group endocarditis, in combination with ampicillin/vancomycin for enterococcal endocarditis and in combination with either cloxacillin/vancomycin for staphylococcal endocarditis of the prosthetic valve. The use of gentamicin routinely for native valve staphylococcal endocarditis has been given up. New trials have also demonstrated ampicillin and ceftriaxone to be as efficacious as ampicillin and gentamicin for enterococcal endocarditis.

Topical/Local Therapy

Aminoglycosides are widely used as topical therapy for ear and eye infections and surface infections. They can also be used for local therapy including antibiotic lock therapy for catheter infections where the catheter cannot be removed as a mixture with beads/cement for orthopedic infections (prosthetic joint/bone implant associated infections), intraperitoneally for continuous ambulatory peritoneal dialysis (CAPD) associated infections and intraventricularly/intrathecally for nosocomial meningitis (dose of gentamicin is 1–8 mg/amikacin 5–50 mg).

TABLE 1: Usual doses of aminoglycosides.

Drug	*Route*	*Total dose mg/kg/day*	*Peak level*	*Trough level*
Gentamicin	IV/IM	3–5	4–6	1–2
Tobramycin	IV/IM	3–5	4–6	1–2
Netilmicin	IV/IM	3–5	4–6	1–2
Amikacin	IV/IM	15	20–30	5–10
Streptomycin	IM	15	20–30	<5
Kanamycin	IM	15		

(IV: intravenous; IM: intramuscular)

DOSAGE

The doses of aminoglycosides have been given in Table 1.

THERAPEUTIC DRUG MONITORING

Aminoglycosides are potentially toxic compounds with narrow therapeutic window. Besides cumulative dose, the efficacy and ototoxicity is determined mainly by peak drug level where as nephrotoxicity by trough level. The peak levels of the drug are achieved after 30–60 minutes of parenteral administration whereas trough levels are measured prior to next dose. Typically after first dose of the antibiotic the levels are obtained after 6–8 hours and the dosing schedule is determined by availability of nomograms. Unfortunately, the nomograms are not validated for use in children and toxicity has been reported in spite of therapeutic range of drug levels. Not all pediatric patients who receive aminoglycosides require therapeutic drug monitoring. Cost and availability is also a problem with therapeutic drug monitoring (TDM). Indications for measuring aminoglycoside concentrations are:

- Treatment course more than 5 days
- Patients with decreased or changing renal function
- Infants less than 3 months of age
- Signs of ototoxicity or nephrotoxicity
- Patients on hemodialysis or chronic ambulatory peritoneal dialysis
- Clinical need for higher doses or longer intervals (cystic fibrosis, major burns, endocarditis, febrile granulocytopenia)
- Concomitant use of other nephrotoxic agents.

EXTENDED INTERVAL DOSING/ONCE DAILY DOSING OF AMINOGLYCOSIDES

Basis

The pharmacodynamic characteristics of aminoglycosides that allow the use of once-daily dosing are: (i) concentration-dependent killing; (ii) PAE and postantibiotic leukocyte enhancement (PALE); and (iii) adaptive resistance.

Concentration-dependent killing: Bacterial killing by aminoglycosides is *concentration-dependent*. In vitro studies have shown increases in the rate of bacterial killing as aminoglycoside concentrations increase. A strong relationship between peak aminoglycoside concentrations and response to therapy has been described in a cohort of patients with serious gram-negative bacillary infections treated with thrice-daily dosing of gentamicin or tobramycin. This suggests that concentration-dependent killing is clinically important. It might be expected that bolus dosing of aminoglycoside antibiotics, with resultant higher peak levels, would result in improved clinical efficacy.

Postantibiotic effect: The use of once-daily dosing regimens in aminoglycoside therapy results in intervals during which drug concentrations are below the minimum inhibitory concentration (MIC). This might foster concern that target pathogens would proliferate once concentrations of drug fall below the MIC; however, aminoglycoside antibiotics have a potent PAE; that is, suppression of bacterial growth persists despite concentrations of antibiotic below the MIC. An aminoglycoside PAE has been demonstrated with both staphylococci and with gram-negative bacilli. The measured duration of PAE tends to be longer in vivo than in vitro, even in neutropenic animals, suggesting that this difference is not only due to the presence of host neutrophils. The PAE in vivo following aminoglycoside administration is prolonged and lasts from 1 hour to 13 hours in animal models of gram-negative bacterial infection. The PAE is extended by higher doses of aminoglycosides and concurrent administration of a cell-wall active antibiotic. Enhanced phagocytosis of aminoglycoside-exposed bacteria by host leukocytes has also been observed in vitro. This has been referred to as PALE.

Adaptive resistance: The term *adaptive resistance* refers to the reduction in rate of bacterial killing by an antibiotic following pre-exposure to that drug. Adaptive resistance to aminoglycoside agents has been observed principally in *P. aeruginosa* but also in other gram-negative bacilli. Adaptive resistance to aminoglycosides appears to be transient and reversible. The mechanism of adaptive resistance may be a decrease in drug uptake by aminoglycoside-exposed organisms caused by downregulation of enzymes that control accelerated energy-dependent uptake of aminoglycoside antibiotics. Adaptive resistance peaks between 6 hours and 16 hours after drug administration, although it may last longer following higher doses of drug. Once-daily dosing may circumvent the possibility of adaptive resistance through the provision of a drug-free interval. The transient nature of adaptive resistance means that organisms exposed to once-daily doses of aminoglycosides can revert to the sensitive phenotype during the interval when antibiotic concentrations are low.

Clinical Efficacy of Once-daily Dosing

The possibility of increased efficacy with once-daily aminoglycoside dosing has been evaluated in a multitude of randomized clinical trials. The interpretation of these studies has been complicated by the fact that individual trials have had insufficient power to determine whether observed differences in efficacy between once-daily and multiple-daily dosage regimens are due to chance alone. Meta-analysis has been used in an attempt to synthesize the data contained in these multiple studies. The performance of these meta-analyses has been complicated by heterogeneity in the patient populations, disease states, and drug regimens studied, and the different definitions of drug efficacy used. Most meta-analyses have shown an improvement in the clinical efficacy of once-daily aminoglycoside dosing; for example, the meta-analyses by Ali and Goetz and Bailey et al. found once-daily dosing to be associated with a 4 to 5% decrease in risk of clinical failure.

The heterogeneity of the studies evaluated has led some authors to perform subgroup analyses, with exclusion of some study types. Investigators have found that estimates of efficacy do not change when analyses are restricted to intravenous (as opposed to intramuscular) dosing, infections with microbiologically documented cure, or infections in neutropenic individuals. Despite methodologic flaws in the available literature, current evidence would suggest that when single and multiple daily dosing regimens are compared there is no difference in efficacy, and there is a trend toward reduced toxicity with the single regimens.

Several studies have evaluated the use of once-daily dosing of aminoglycosides in pediatric populations. These studies have included children younger than 6 months and children with neutropenia and sepsis. Pharmacokinetic analyses have suggested that children have a higher volume of distribution than adults and that higher antibiotic dose per unit of body mass may be warranted in children. Once-daily dosing appears to be safe and effective in children.

Dosing of Once-daily Aminoglycosides

It has been suggested that once-daily doses should be based upon maximum daily doses of aminoglycoside antibiotics (5 mg/kg/day for gentamicin and tobramycin, 6.5 mg/kg/day for netilmicin, and 15 mg/kg/day for amikacin).

Monitoring of Levels with Once-daily Aminoglycosides

Traditional multiple-daily dosing of aminoglycoside antibiotics requires the determination of both peak and trough serum levels; measurement of peak concentrations is not necessary with once-daily full dosage aminoglycoside administration, as serum concentrations will be predictably high. Some authors have suggested that monitoring trough concentrations only, with dose adjustments for troughs greater than 2 mg/L, should prove adequate in individuals on decreased dose once-daily dosing regimens. This monitoring scheme, however, does not allow clinicians to appreciate under dosage of drug and will delay adjustment of the dosing regimen. Another proposed approach to monitoring of once-daily dosage, which overcomes these limitations, is monitoring with a drug level taken 8 hours after infusion. Netilmicin levels between 1.5 and 6 mg/L 8 hours after infusion appear to be safe and effective, and this approach permits adjustment of drug dosage before the next dose is given.

Once-daily Dosing in Selected Disease States

Individuals with altered volume of distribution: Individuals with a variety of pathologic states, including ascites, septic shock, severe burns, pancreatitis as well as pregnant and postpartum women have increased volumes of distribution for aminoglycoside antibiotics. It is unclear whether existing data on once-daily dosage can be safely extrapolated to these populations, and it may be prudent to avoid the use of once-daily dosage in these groups until further data are available.

Infections in individuals with neutropenia: Postantibiotic leukocyte enhancement of bacterial killing is expected to be impaired in individuals with neutropenia, and some animal experiments have demonstrated once-daily dosing of aminoglycoside antibiotics to be less effective in neutropenic animals than in non-neutropenic animals. Because of this, concern has been raised that once-daily aminoglycoside dosage is inappropriate in neutropenic individuals. Randomized trials comparing once-daily to multiple-daily dosing of netilmicin, tobramycin, and amikacin in combination with beta-lactam antibiotics have been performed. These studies have included individuals with neutropenia and fever without a documented focus as well as individuals with a septic focus or bacteremia. All studies included individuals with granulocyte count less than 100 cells/mm^3, and in one trial, prolonged (>7 days) neutropenia was present in more than half the study subjects. No significant difference was seen between once-daily and multiple-daily dosing of aminoglycosides, either within individual trials or when these trials were subjected to a meta-analysis. Presently available data suggest that once-daily and multiple-daily dosing of aminoglycosides in combination with beta-lactam antibiotics are equally effective for individuals with neutropenia and fever.

Gram-positive coccal endocarditis: Aminoglycosides are commonly used to provide antibacterial synergy against infecting organisms in bacterial endocarditis caused by gram-positive organisms (including viridans streptococci, enterococci, and staphylococci). Traditionally, the synergistic doses of aminoglycosides used in the treatment of endocarditis have been lower than those used for serious gram-negative infections (target serum peak levels 3–4 mg/L). The use of once-daily dosing of aminoglycosides in enterococcal endocarditis has been assessed in vitro and in animal models. Multiple-daily dosing regimens are superior to once-daily regimens in the treatment of experimental enterococcal endocarditis. Once-daily gentamicin dosing for streptococcal endocarditis has been assessed in a randomized clinical trial, comparing 4 weeks of ceftriaxone (2 g/d) to 2 weeks of ceftriaxone combined with gentamicin. This study showed cure rates of 96% in both treatment groups. The use of once-daily dosing of aminoglycoside therapy in the treatment of staphylococcal endocarditis has not been assessed. At present, the use of once-daily dosing of aminoglycosides for the treatment of gram-positive coccal endocarditis remains controversial, and further data are needed before such regimens can be recommended.

Cost

A comparison of the costs of single daily dosing and traditional multiple dosing should include not only the cost of the antibiotic but also the costs of labor, laboratory monitoring and drug toxicity. A pharmacoeconomic comparison of single daily dosing versus traditional dosing of gentamicin found a 54% reduction in drug supply and labor costs with single daily dosing. The same study showed a 62% reduction in monitoring costs with single daily dosing. Since single daily dosing is often at least equally effective (and may be less toxic and more cost-effective), it may be the preferred method of administration in most clinical situations. It is especially useful for Nocardia, *Mycobacterium avium intracellulare*, and some rapidly growing atypical mycobacteria. It is currently the preferred injectable agent for management of drug resistant tuberculosis.

INDIVIDUAL AMINOGLYCOSIDES

Amikacin: It is mainly used in empirical treatment of serious bacterial infections where gentamicin resistance is anticipated. Amikacin is active against a vast majority of gram-negative bacilli including most strains of Proteus, *P. aeruginosa* and Serratia. It is also active against nearly all strains of *Klebsiella, Escherichia coli*, and Enterobacter that are resistant to gentamicin and tobramycin. Unusual pathogens like *Acinetobacter*, *Providencia*, and *Flavobacter* and strains of *Pseudomonas* other than *P. aeruginosa* show resistance to amikacin. It is especially useful for *Nocardia*, *Mycobacterium avium* intracellulare, and some rapidly growing atypical mycobacteria. It is currently the preferred injectable agent for management of drug resistant tuberculosis. Amikacin is less active than gentamicin against enterococci and must not be used for this indication.

Gentamicin: Used mainly for empirical treatment of gram-negative infections in areas where there is low aminoglycoside resistance. It is also used as monotherapy in tularemia. Gentamicin is used in combination with doxycycline and rifampin in the initial phase of brucellosis and is the aminoglycoside of choice for gram-positive endocarditis. In the multiple-daily dosing regimen, gentamicin sulfate is given in a loading dose of 2 mg/kg followed by 3–5 mg/kg in three divided doses intramuscular or intravenous. The once-daily dose of gentamicin sulfate is 5 mg/kg given over 30–60 minutes for patients with normal renal function. In newborns the dose is 3 mg/kg once daily for preterm infants less than 35 weeks gestation and 4 mg/kg once daily for newborns more than 35 weeks gestation.

Tobramycin: Its indications and clinical usages are similar to gentamicin. Its role mainly is now in nebulized form in treatment of chronic bronchiectasis as seen in patients with cystic fibrosis and sometimes ventilator associated tracheobronchitis.

Netilmicin: Similar spectrum of activity as gentamicin but apparently less ototoxic. Less active against *P. aeruginosa*.
Neonates (<6 weeks): 4.0–6.5 mg/kg/day given as 2.0–3.25 mg/kg every 12 hours.
Infants and children (6 weeks through 12 years): 5.5–8.0 mg/kg/day given either as 1.8–2.7 mg/kg every 8 hours, or as 2.7–4.0 mg/kg every 12 hours.

Streptomycin: It is mainly used in treatment of tuberculosis in a dose of 15–20 mg/kg/day. Streptomycin is the drug of choice for the treatment of tularemia. The recommended dose is 15–25 mg/kg/day for 7–10 days. It is also indicated in plague 30 mg/kg/day divided every 8–12 hours till patient is afebrile for at least 3 days. It is also used with doxycycline and rifampin in therapy of brucellosis (alternative being gentamicin).

Neomycin: It is too toxic for systemic use and is used mainly as local gastrointestinal decontaminant. Here also even miniscule of the drug that gets absorbed can worsen the nephrotoxicity in patients with renal disease. It is often used as topical therapy in combination with other drugs for cuts, wounds.

TOXICITY

The three main side effects of aminoglycoside drugs are ototoxicity (often largely irreversible), nephrotoxicity (usually reversible) and neuromuscular blockade.

The antibiotics have curare like effect and can cause reversible neuroparalysis. This action gets potentiated by use of anesthetic drugs and in presence of hypomagnesemia in neonates. Very rare instances of allergic reactions, anaphylaxis or drug fever are reported. The drugs are not irritant to the tissues on parental administration hence incidences of thrombophlebitis or injection site pain are unusual.

Ototoxicity

This is one of the most feared side effects of aminoglycoside therapy and occurs in up to 10% of patients. It is reported even after instillation of ear drops especially in presence of ear drum perforation or tympanostomy tubes. The ototoxicity is of two types some drugs are classically cochleotoxic (amikacin, kanamycin) some are more vestibulotoxic (streptomycin, gentamicin). The ototoxicity is associated with prolonged use and with high drug levels. With therapy of some duration the drug damages outer hair cells of cochlea. This causes loss in high tone hearing capabilities. Humans typically have most of the speech at 0.3–3 kHz whereas they have ability to hear sounds up to 20 kHz. So the initial loss of hearing in high frequencies is not clinically apparent. Only when the loss reaches to 4–8 kHz then there is diminished ability to hear in noisy surroundings (Background noise interference). The hearing loss is irreversible and can come after a latency of even up to 6 months after therapy. Serial audiograms should be requested in patients on prolonged therapy.

Nephrotoxicity

Nephrotoxicity is characterized by non-oliguric renal failure. There is slow rise in creatinine and diminished capacity of renal concentration. This effect is largely reversible and happens due to damage to the endothelium of the proximal renal tubules. The nephrotoxicity of aminoglycoside is potentiated by coadministration of other drugs notably nonsteroidal anti-inflammatory drugs (NSAIDs). The third-generation cephalosporins also potentiate the renal toxicity of aminoglycosides. The nephrotoxicity is related to trough levels. Box 1 lists the risk factors for aminoglycoside-induced nephrotoxicity. Serial monitoring of urine output, blood urea nitrogen, serum creatinine, and urine analysis should be done for all patients on aminoglycosides.

How to Minimize Aminoglycoside Toxicity?

- Aminoglycosides should be used only when their unique antibiotic potency is needed, such as treatment of infection in critically ill patients, and in nosocomial infections or infections with organisms resistant to less toxic therapies.
- The clinician should change to a potentially less toxic antibiotic as soon as the infecting organism and its antibiotic sensitivities have been determined.
- Potential risk factors that predispose to nephrotoxicity should be identified and, when possible, corrected (Box 1).

DURATION OF TREATMENT

It is desirable to limit the duration of treatment with aminoglycosides to short-term whenever feasible. The usual duration of treatment of all patients is 7–14 days. In complicated infections,

BOX 1: Risk factors predisposing to aminoglycoside nephrotoxicity.

Potentially alterable factors
- Use of diuretics*
- Effective circulating volume depletion
- Use of other nephrotoxic medications
- Concomitant use of amphotericin
- Use of ACE (angiotensin converting enzyme) inhibitors†
- Use of nonsteroidal anti-inflammatory agents†
- Radiographic contrast exposure
- Use of cisplatin

Unalterable factors
- Age
- Pre-existing renal disease

*May cause effective circulating volume depletion.
†May cause prerenal acute renal failure in the setting of volume depletion.

a longer course of therapy may be necessary. Although prolonged courses of aminoglycosides have been well tolerated, it is particularly important that patients treated for longer than the usual period be carefully monitored for changes in renal, auditory, and vestibular functions. Dosage should be adjusted if clinically indicated.

CONCLUSION

In spite of narrow therapeutic window and availability of newer antibiotics, aminoglycoside antibiotics have a place in therapy especially in empirical therapy of serious gram-negative infections including early onset neonatal sepsis. They are also important components of certain drug regimens against *M. tuberculosis*. Therapeutic drug monitoring and extended interval dosing are two important tools to use these antibiotics more safely and effectively.

RECOMMENDED READING

1. Ali MZ, Goetz M. A meta-analysis of the relative efficacy and toxicity of single daily dosing versus multiple daily dosing of aminoglycosides. Clin Infect Dis. 1997;24:796-809.
2. Bailey T, Little J, Littenberg B, et al. A meta-analysis of extended interval dosing versus multiple daily dosing of aminoglycosides. Clin Infect Dis. 1997;24:786-95.
3. Barclay ML, Begg MJ, Chambers ST. Adaptive resistance following single doses of gentamicin in a dynamic in vitro model. Antimicrob Agents Chemother. 1992;36:1951-7.
4. Barza M, Ioannidis J, Cappelleri J, et al. Single or multiple daily doses of aminoglycosides: a meta-analysis. BMJ. 1996;312:338-44.
5. Chambers HF, Sande MA. The Aminoglycosides. In: Hardman JG, Limbird LE, (Eds). Goodman and Gilman's The Pharmacological Basis of Therapeutics. New York: McGraw-Hill; 1996. pp. 1103-21.
6. Choudhury D, Ahmed Z. Drug-induced nephrotoxicity. Med Clin North Am. 1997;81:705-17.
7. Craig WA, Gundmundson S. Postantibiotic effect. In: Lorian V, (Ed). Antibiotics in laboratory medicine. Baltimore: Williams and Wilkins; 1991. pp. 403-31.
8. Dager W. Aminoglycoside pharmacokinetics: Volume of distribution in specific adult patient subgroups. Ann Pharmacother. 1994;28:944-51.
9. Edson RS, Terrell CL. The Aminoglyosides. Mayo Clin Proc. 1999;74:519-28.
10. Elhanan K, Siplovich L, Raz R. Gentamicin once-daily versus thrice-daily in children. J Antimicrob Chemother. 1995;35:327-32.
11. Germovsek E, Barker CI, Sharland M. What do I need to know about aminoglycoside antibiotics? Arch Dis Child Educ Pract Ed. 2017;102:89-93.
12. Gilbert DN. Aminoglycosides. In: Mand ll GL, Bennett JE, Dolin R, (Eds). Douglas and Bennett's Principles and Practice of Infectious Diseases. New York: Churchill Livingstone; 1995. pp. 279-301.
13. Hatala R, Dinh TT, Cook DJ. Single daily dosing of aminoglycosides in immunocompromised adults: A systematic review. Clin Infect Dis. 1997;24:810-5.
14. Hock R, Anderson RJ. Prevention of drug-induced nephrotoxicity in the intensive care unit. J Crit Care. 1995;10:33-43.
15. Karlowsky JA, Zelenitsky SA, Zhanel GG. Aminoglycoside adaptive resistance Pharmacotherapy. 1997;17:549-55.
16. Kothari U, Krilov LR. Aminoglycosides. Pediatr Rev. 2012;33(11):531-3.
17. Livornese LL, Slavin D, Gilbert B, et al. Use of antibacterial agents in renal failure. Infect Dis Clin North Am. 2004;18:551-79.
18. Lortholary O, Tod M, Cohen Y, et al. Aminoglycosides. Med Clin North Am. 1995;79:761-87.
19. Marangos MN, Nicolau DP, Quintiliani R, et al. Influence of gentamicin dosing interval on the efficacy of penicillin-containing regimens in experimental Enterococcus faecalis endocarditis. J Antimicrob Chemother. 1997;39:519-22.

20. Marik P, Havlik I, Monteagudo F, et al. The pharmacokinetics of amikacin in critically ill adult and paediatric patients: comparison of once-daily and twice-daily dosing regimens. J Antimicrob Chemother. 1991;27 Suppl C: 81-9.
21. Montie T, Patamasucon P. Aminoglycosides: the complex problem of antibiotic mechanisms and clinical applications. Eur J Clin Microbiol Infect Dis. 1995; 14:85-87.
22. Salehifar E, Rafati M. Extended-interval dosing of aminoglycosides in pediatrics: a narrative review. J Pediatr Rev. 2015;3(2):e2652.
23. Sexton DJ, Tenenbaum MJ, Wilson WR, et al. Ceftriaxone once daily for four weeks compared with ceftriaxone plus gentamicin once daily for two weeks for treatment of endocarditis due to penicillin-susceptible streptococci. Endocarditis Treatment Consortium Group. Clin Infect Dis. 1998;27:1470-4.
24. Swatrz MN. Use of antimicrobial agents and drug resistance. N Engl J Med. 1997;337:491-2.
25. Tunkel AR, Hasbun R, Bhimraj A, et al. Infectious Diseases Society of America's Clinical Practice Guidelines for Healthcare-Associated Ventriculitis and Meningitis. Clin Infect Dis. 2017;14. doi: 10.1093/cid/ciw861.
26. WHO. (2018). Rapid communication: key changes to treatment of multidrug- and rifampicin-resistant tuberculosis (MDR/RR-TB). License: CC BY-NC-SA 3.0 IGO. [online] Available from http://www.who.int/tb/publications/2018/WHO_RapidCommunicationMDRTB.pdf [Accessed December, 2018].

Macrolides and Azalides

10

Chapter

Abhay Shah, Niranjan Shendurnikar

INTRODUCTION

Macrolides have been known for more than 5 decades, and, since the introduction of erythromycin into therapy, a number of these molecules have been developed for clinical use. For years, these antibiotics have represented a major alternative to penicillins and cephalosporins for the treatment of infections due to gram-positive microorganisms. The first macrolide "erythromycin" is a prototype of all the macrolides. It is a metabolic product of a naturally occurring strain of *Streptomyces erythreus* isolated in 1952 from Philippines. Since then it was extensively used in penicillin allergic patients. However it was associated with many limitations including erratic bioavailability, frequent gastrointestinal (GI) intolerance, short serum half-life, drug-drug interactions and toxicity. Hence new macrolides were developed.

Azithromycin and clarithromycin are the prototypes of advanced, synthetic macrolides approved by US FDA in 1991-1992. These synthetic compounds are prepared by modifying the erythromycin base by structural modification and alteration in chemical ring and thereby resulting in compounds with extended spectrum of activity, better pharmacodynamics, infrequent dosing, and good tolerability. Since their introduction, these advanced macrolides have been used extensively for the treatment of respiratory tract infections, sexually transmitted diseases, and infections caused by susceptible gram-positive organisms.

CHEMICAL STRUCTURE

The macrolides are hydrophobic molecules with a central 14- to 16-membered-ring lactone with few or no double bonds and no nitrogen atom. Several amino or neutral sugars may be attached to the lactone nucleus. Commercially available macrolides usually have a 14-membered ring (clarithromycin, dirithromycin, erythromycin, and roxithromycin). Those with 16-membered ring (josamycin, midecamycin, miocamycin, rokitamyin, and spiramycin) are available in certain countries or used in veterinary practice. The azalides which have a 15-membered ring such as azithromycin or tulathromycin are technically not included in macrolides as they have an endolactone nitrogen atom and will be referred as such in the course of the chapter. Nevertheless, they are semisynthetic derivatives of erythromycin A and due to their antibacterial spectrum, belong to the macrolide family. Ketolides were derived from erythromycin by substituting the cladinose sugar with a keto-group and attaching a cyclic carbamate group in the lactone ring. These modifications give ketolides much broader spectrum than other macrolides. Telithromycin was the ketolide that received marketing approval but is no longer widely used due to severe adverse effects including reversible visual disturbance, syncope, exacerbation of myasthenia gravis and hepatic failure and is not available in India. It will not be discussed further.

MECHANISM OF ACTION

Macrolides are bacteriostatic and their mechanism of action includes suppression of RNA-dependent protein synthesis by reversibly binding to 50s subunit of 23s bacterial ribosome. This interaction inhibits RNA-dependent protein synthesis by preventing transpeptidation and translocation reactions.

SPECTRUM OF ACTIVITY

The macrolides have activity against susceptible strains of *Streptococcus pneumoniae, Staphylococcus aureus,* and *Streptococcus pyogenes.* They are generally inactive against methicillin-resistant *S. aureus* (MRSA). Staphylococci and streptococci that are resistant to erythromycin are also resistant to azithromycin and clarithromycin. The other gram-positive bacteria inhibited by macrolides include *Listeria* spp., *Erysipelothrix insidiosa, Corynebacterium* spp., *Lactobacilli* spp., *Leuconostoc* spp., and *Pediococcus* spp. They inhibit gram-negative cocci including meningococci and gonococci along with some fastidious gram-negative bacilli (e.g. *Pasteurella* spp. and *Bordetella* spp.). Some anaerobic bacteria, rickettsia, atypical bacteria such as mycoplasma/chlamydia and legionella and some but not all susceptible strains of gram-negative bacilli causing respiratory infections *(Haemophilus influenzae* and *Moraxella catarrhalis),* and are also susceptible to the macrolides. Some atypical mycobacteria, spirochetes, bacteria responsible for GI infections (*Vibrio cholerae* and other *Vibrio* spp., *Campylobacter* spp. and *Helicobacter pylori*), remain susceptible to macrolides. They also display activity against *Leptospira, Borrelia,* and *Bartonella* spp. However, these molecules are weakly active against enterococci and only have moderate activity against the viridans group of streptococci.

The structural modifications in the newer macrolides broaden the spectrum of activity. Clarithromycin has superior gram-positive activity and azithromycin has superior gram-negative activity when compared to erythromycin. Both newer macrolides have significantly improved effectiveness against *H. influenzae* and *M. catarrhalis,* although clarithromycin's activity is significant only when combined with its synergistic 14-hydroxy metabolite. Azithromycin is even more active against *H. influenza/M. catarrhalis* with a minimal inhibitory concentration (MIC) fourfold to eightfold lower than erythromycin. The advanced macrolides also demonstrate enhanced activity against atypical respiratory pathogens as compared to erythromycin. Clarithromycin seems more active than azithromycin and erythromycin against *Legionella pneumophila* and *Chlamydia pneumoniae,* whereas azithromycin demonstrates better in vitro activity against *Mycoplasma pneumoniae.*

Azithromycin and clarithromycin have similar or increased in vitro activity against genital pathogens compared with erythromycin. *Neisseria gonorrhoeae, Haemophilus ducreyi,* and *Ureaplasma urealyticum* are susceptible to both antibiotics with azithromycin demonstrating better activity as evidenced by a lower MIC. Clarithromycin is approximately 10-fold more active than erythromycin against *Chlamydia trachomatis,* whereas azithromycin activity is similar to that of erythromycin.

Azithromycin has the best gram-negative activity of the group. Azithromycin has activity against enteric pathogens including *Escherichia coli, Salmonella* spp., *Yersinia enterocolitica,* and *Shigella* spp. Clarithromycin has no in vitro activity against these gram-negative organisms.

Azithromycin is more active against *Campylobacter jejuni* than erythromycin or clarithromycin, whereas clarithromycin has greater activity against *H. pylori*. Azithromycin also has activity against organisms contracted via animal bites, such as *Pasteurella multocida*, and human mouth bites, such as *Eikenella corrodens*.

Clarithromycin is the most active macrolide against nontuberculous mycobacteria, notably, *Mycobacterium avium-intracellulare* complex (MAC), at concentrations that are achievable in lung tissue. *Treponema pallidum* is susceptible to both newer macrolides. Azithromycin has activity equivalent to erythromycin against *Toxoplasma gondii*. It must be remembered that in vitro MIC measurements do not take into account properties of an antimicrobial like tissue penetration, intracellular half-life or postantibiotic effect and thus may not predict its relative efficacy at the site of infection. Azithromycin also shows some activity against plasmodia. However currently, there is no evidence for the superiority or equivalence of azithromycin monotherapy or combination therapy for the treatment of *Plasmodium falciparum* or *Plasmodium vivax* compared with other antimalarials or with the current first-line antimalarial combinations.

Although it is known that macrolides possess immunomodulatory properties, it is difficult to independently assess the immunomodulatory and antimicrobial effects. Administration of macrolides has been shown to be beneficial in patients with chronic pulmonary inflammatory diseases, including diffuse pan bronchiolitis, cystic fibrosis and asthma. Whether macrolides also exert favorable immunomodulatory effects during acute pulmonary infection is less clear. Moreover, even the exact mechanism of the beneficial effect of macrolides is a matter of debate. In vitro effects of macrolides show that these drugs can moderate the inflammatory response independent of antibacterial activity.

MECHANISM OF RESISTANCE

Bacteria resist macrolide antibiotics in three ways: (1) through target-site modification by methylation or mutation that prevents the binding of the antibiotic to its ribosomal target, (2) through efflux of the antibiotic, and (3) by drug inactivation. Modification of the ribosomal target confers broad-spectrum resistance to macrolides, whereas efflux and inactivation affect only some of these molecules.

Altered binding, caused by methylation of the ribosomal target of the antibiotics, confers high-level resistance (MICs ≥ 64 mg/L) to all macrolide, azalide, lincosamide (clindamycin), and streptogramin type B compounds, a phenotype that is known as "MLSB resistance". Resistance to erythromycin implies cross-resistance to clarithromycin and azithromycin. The mLSB phenotype is encoded by a variety of *erm* (erythromycin ribosome methylase) genes and is reported in a large number of microorganisms. Nearly 40 *erm* genes have been reported so far. Expression of MLSB resistance can be constitutive or inducible. In inducible resistance, the bacteria produce inactive mRNA that is unable to encode. The presence of an inducer leads to rearrangements of mRNA, which allow ribosomes to translate the methylase coding sequence. The strains harboring an inducible erm gene are resistant to the inducers but remain susceptible to non-inducer macrolides and lincosamides (clindamycin). By contrast, constitutive production of a methylase generally confers a characteristic phenotype with high-level cross-resistance to the MLSB drugs. Drug efflux, the second important mechanism of macrolide resistance, is mediated by the macrolide efflux (mef) genes and is specific for 14- and 15-membered macrolides. Macrolide resistance is usually low-level (MICs 1–32 mg/L) and in vitro susceptibility to ketolides, lincosamides, and streptogramins is maintained. Similar to penicillin resistance, macrolide resistance in vitro may not result in treatment failures for levels of resistance that can be exceeded by tissue levels of certain macrolides chiefly azithromycin. A third mechanism of macrolide resistance, drug inactivation, is believed to be of minor clinical importance.

INCIDENCE OF MACROLIDE RESISTANCE

Macrolide resistance in *S. pneumoniae* is most commonly caused by either ribosomal methylation (ermA, ermB) resulting in inducible cross-resistance to lincomycins and streptogramins (mLS$_B$ phenotype) or to efflux pumps (mefA, mefE) resulting in variable-level resistance to macrolides alone (M phenotype). The clinical implications of M-type resistance for use of newer macrolides and azalides remains controversial. Huge geographic differences, from 3%–74%, are observed in the resistance frequencies against pneumococci reported for individual countries. In addition, considerable variations can be seen within a country, depending on the source of the strains (teaching/nonteaching hospital, or community), patient age, sample origin, seasonal factors, and pneumococcal serotype. For this reason, local statistics are of crucial value for empiric therapy. Similar to the case of penicillin resistance, higher prevalence of macrolide resistance is generally seen among children and for pneumococci from middle ear fluids. In general, the higher the rate of penicillin resistance, the higher the rate of macrolide resistance. In a large study that involved hospitals from 21 countries around the world, macrolide resistance was detected in 12.8% of penicillin-susceptible pneumococci versus 55.7% of penicillin-resistant strains. No substantial difference was observed between percentages of resistance to azithromycin, clarithromycin, and erythromycin, which confirms cross-resistance between the 3 antimicrobials. By contrast, in several countries, the incidence of clindamycin resistance may be much lower than that of erythromycin resistance. The incidence of macrolide resistance in *S. pneumoniae* in India is 30%.

In the vast majority of *S. pyogenes* strains, erythromycin resistance is caused by the presence of the efflux gene *mef*(A) or the methylase genes *erm*(TR) [*erm*(A)] and *erm*(B). The *mef*(A) and *erm*(TR) genes are frequently predominant. The incidence of macrolide resistance in *S. pyogenes* in India is around 30%.

Similarly for treatment of community-acquired MRSA infections, clindamycin is often effective, but should be restricted to erythromycin-susceptible isolates. This is because macrolide resistance is a surrogate marker of MLSB mechanism which may indicate inducible resistance to clindamycin.

PHARMACOKINETICS AND PHARMACODYNAMICS

Erythromycin base and its various oral salts (estolate, stearate, and ethylsuccinate) are absorbed well from the fasting GI tract. Food reduces absorption of all but the estolate form. As erythromycin is degraded in an acidic environment, oral bioavailability is variable and depends on the preparation studied. Enteric-coating of erythromycin base overcomes acid lability but can delay therapeutic blood levels (unpredictably) and does not decrease the incidence of common erythromycin GI adverse effects. Enteric-coated erythromycin can be taken with food. Erythromycin stearate is converted to base in vivo and produces serum levels that are identical to that of uncoated base. The ethylsuccinate salt is used frequently when an oral suspension is needed, because only the estolate and ethylsuccinate salts are available in this dosage formulation. Erythromycin is excreted primarily in bile (bile concentrations exceed

10 times those in plasma); only 2–5% is excreted in urine. Erythromycin diffuses readily into most tissues except brain and cerebrospinal fluid, crosses the placenta, and is present in breast milk. The structural alterations of the erythromycin base used to synthesize the advanced macrolides result in improved pharmacokinetic properties. Table 1 shows a comparison of these properties (clarithromycin and azithromycin are more acid-stable and have greater oral bioavailability (55% and 37%, respectively). The oral bioavailability of the suspension formulation of clarithromycin is similar to the equivalent tablet doses. The extended-release formulations of clarithromycin should be administered with food, whereas the immediate-release tablets can be taken with or without food. Clarithromycin is biotransformed rapidly to its active, 14-hydroxy metabolite, which peaks 3 hours after administration. The absorption of azithromycin is decreased with food and therefore it should be taken 1–2 hours before a meal. Aluminum- and magnesium-containing antacids reduce the peak serum concentrations of azithromycin but not the total absorption. Both clarithromycin and azithromycin may also be given parenterally.

The macrolides are lipophilic and are extensively distributed in body fluids and tissues. Azithromycin is taken up, rapidly and extensively, from the circulation into intracellular compartments, followed by a much slower release. Tissue concentrations do not peak until 48 hours after administration of azithromycin and persist for several days afterward. The elimination of azithromycin is polyexponential. The initial serum half-life is 11–14 hours, followed by a more prolonged half-life of approximately 68 hours as drug is slowly removed from the tissue. Clarithromycin concentrates well in tissues (better than erythromycin) but azithromycin's steady-state tissue or fluid concentrations are substantially higher than serum levels. Mean tissue concentrations of clarithromycin are 2- to 20-fold greater than serum concentrations and those of azithromycin 10- to 100-fold greater than serum concentrations. Both drugs are also concentrated in alveolar macrophages and polymorphonuclear cells. Azithromycin remains in pulmonary macrophages, tonsillar tissue, and genital or pelvic tissue for extended periods of time with a mean tissue half-life of 2–4 days. This feature allows single-dose therapy for STDs and 3- to 5-day regimens for skin, soft tissue, and some respiratory infections. The terminal half-life of azithromycin is long enough to allow once-daily dosing. Twice-daily dosing of the immediate-release formulation of clarithromycin is necessary based on the terminal half-life of 4–5 hours.

Like β-lactams, vancomycin and clindamycin, macrolides demonstrate time-dependent killing (i.e. longer time with the drug concentration above the MIC of the target organism increases bacterial killing). They also have significant postantibiotic effects. The goal of the macrolide dosing regimen is therefore to optimize the amount of drug exposure, with the ratio

TABLE 1: Comparative pharmacokinetics of the macrolide antibiotics.

Parameter	*Erythromycin*	*Azithromycin**	*Clarithromycin**
Bioavailability (%)	25	37	55
C_{max} (mg/L)	0.3–0.9	0.4	2.1–2.4
t_{max} (h)	3–4	2	2
t½ (h)	2–3	40–68	3–5
AUC (mg h/L)	8	3.4	19

*Mean values after a single 500 mg oral dose (azithromycin or clarithromycin)

AUC: Area under plasma concentration time curve; C_{max}: Peak serum concentration; t_{max}: Time to peak serum concentration; t1/2: Serum half-life of AUC (area under the serum-concentration-time curve) to MIC being the major parameter correlating with efficacy. For *S. pneumoniae*, the therapeutic goal is to achieve an AUC to MIC ratio of 25–35.

Clarithromycin is metabolized in the liver by the cytochrome P-450 3A4 (CYP3A4) enzymes to the active 14-hydroxy form and other products. 30–40% of an oral dose of clarithromycin is excreted in the urine either unchanged or as the active 14-hydroxy metabolite. The remainder is excreted into the bile. In patients with moderate-to-severe renal impairment (i.e. creatinine clearance less than 30 mL/min), the dose should be reduced. In patients with moderate-to-severe hepatic impairment and normal renal function, there is less metabolism of clarithromycin to the 14-hydroxy form resulting in decreased peak plasma concentrations of the metabolite and increased renal excretion of unchanged clarithromycin. Dosing modifications do not seem to be necessary for these patients. Azithromycin elimination is primarily in the feces as the unchanged drug and urinary excretion is minimal. Unlike clarithromycin, azithromycin does not interact with the cytochrome P-450 system. In patients with mild or moderate hepatic impairment, dosing modifications do not seem to be necessary.

CLINICAL INDICATIONS

Upper Respiratory Tract Infections

Like erythromycin, clarithromycin, azithromycin seem attractive options for treating acute pharyngitis, otitis media, and sinusitis as they can be administered once or twice daily for shorter duration. However, an area of concern is the increasing macrolide resistance that is being reported with some of the common pathogens, particularly *S. pneumoniae*, group A streptococci, and *H. influenzae*. A longitudinal study conducted in a pediatric population detected the emergence of erythromycin resistance in 50% of pharyngeal isolates of group A streptococci. Azithromycin has been demonstrated to perform no better than placebo in the treatment of acute otitis media caused by penicillin-nonsusceptible bacteria. Owing to increasing resistance, the routine use of macrolides in upper respiratory tract infections should be avoided and limited only to patients with significant penicillin allergy.

Lower Respiratory Tract Infections

Atypical pathogens including *M. pneumoniae, Chlamydophila pneumonia,* and *L. pneumophila,* are common causes of community-acquired pneumonia in older children and adults. These are susceptible to the macrolides which are therefore considered to be components of antimicrobial regimes for community acquired pneumonia. However, these drugs are not recommended alone for empiric therapy of CAP due to rising incidence of macrolide resistance in *S. pneumoniae* and *H. influenzae*, the other common causes of CAP. Also recent meta-analysis have shown non-inferiority of regimes not containing macrolides with those containing macrolides in treatment of CAP in children. Further, Cochrane reviews also report no significant benefits in treatment outcomes of children with *Mycoplasma pneumonia* with use of macrolides. Notwithstanding all these limitations, macrolides should be prescribed in childhood CAP in children above the age of 5 years if there are clinical features to suggest mycoplasma, or if there is nonresponse to β-lactam antibiotics or in children hospitalized with very severe community acquired-pneumonia. Similarly adult guidelines recommend addition of macrolide to β-lactams in outpatient treatment of CAP if there are comorbidities or exposure to antibiotics in past 3 months and all hospitalized patients with CAP. Macrolides are preferred to fluoroquinolones as atypical cover for CAP in India to prevent masking of tuberculosis presenting as CAP and to prevent fluoroquinolone resistance in *M. tuberculosis*.

Pertussis

Macrolides remain the first-line treatment against *Bordetella pertussis*. Traditionally, erythromycin has been the first-line agent in the treatment of pertussis and chlamydia infections in the newborn infant. Its association with an increased risk of hypertrophic pyloric stenosis, however, has prompted some clinicians to use azithromycin instead. A 5-day course of azithromycin or a 7-day course of clarithromycin is better tolerated and is comparable with 14 days of erythromycin when treating pertussis. Early introduction of macrolides in pertussis is associated with better outcomes with reduced transmission.

Sexually Transmitted Diseases

The unique pharmacokinetics of azithromycin, including high tissue concentrations and a prolonged tissue half-life, allows single-dose treatment courses, directly observed therapy, and improved patient compliance. Guidelines published by the US Public Health Service currently recommend either doxycycline, 100 mg twice a day for 7 days, or azithromycin, 1 g as a single dose, for either chlamydial infections or nongonococcal urethritis among adolescents and adults A single 1-g dose of azithromycin is also one of the recommended treatments for genital ulcer disease (chancroid) caused by *H. ducreyi*. Azithromycin is also efficacious in the treatment of uncomplicated gonorrhea. Gastrointestinal side effects, however, occur frequently with single large doses.

Helicobacter Pylori Infections

Numerous studies have documented the efficacy of clarithromycin in the treatment of *H. pylori* infections associated with peptic ulcer disease. Antibiotic therapy for *H. pylori*-associated peptic ulcer disease decreases ulcer recurrence and promotes healing. Regimens include a proton pump inhibitor with clarithromycin, with either amoxicillin or metronidazole; or ranitidine with bismuth citrate with clarithromycin and either amoxicillin, metronidazole, or tetracycline. Treatment courses are for 14 days and all agents are given twice daily.

Nontuberculous Mycobacteria

Both clarithromycin and azithromycin are effective against most nontuberculous mycobacteria and are the back bone of therapy. There is more experience with use of clarithromycin as compared to azithromycin and hence it is preferred. Clarithromycin in combination with rifampicin/rifabutin and ethambutol is the preferred regime for treating MAC in both patients with or without HIV. Daily clarithromycin or weekly azithromycin are recommended in HIV-infected patients with CD4 counts less than 50 to prevent disseminated MAC disease. Clarithromycin/azithromycin in combination with other drugs are used for treating infections with rapidly growing mycobacteria including *Mycobacterium chelonae, Mycobacterium fortuitum,* and *Mycobacterium abscessus.*

Toxoplasmosis

Clarithromycin or azithromycin (or clindamycin) may be used (as an alternative to sulfadiazine) in combination with pyrimethamine in the treatment of toxoplasmosis. The macrolide spiramycin is used to treat primary toxoplasmosis in pregnant women.

Skin and Soft Tissue Infections

Studies have proven the efficacy of erythromycin and the newer macrolides in the treatment of pyoderma, abscesses, infected wounds, ulcers, or erysipelas. However, narrow spectrum antibiotics such as first-generation cephalosporins including cephalexin/cefadroxil are more efficacious, better tolerated and are recommended as first-line in view of increasing macrolide resistance. Macrolides both topical and systemic have been used in acne but resistance in as many as 60% of *Propionibacterium acnes* have compromised their efficacy.

Gastrointestinal Infections

Azithromycin has been proposed as effective treatment for enteric fever. Azithromycin has been demonstrated to be as efficacious as third-generation cephalosporins in treatment of enteric fever with reduced relapse rates. Other advantages include once a day therapy and shorter duration of therapy leading to better compliance. Similarly, trials have demonstrated noninferiority of azithromycin in treating shigellosis as compared to third-generation cephalosporins. Additionally some of the cephalosporin-resistant shigella may be azithromycin susceptible. Single dose azithromycin is also a recommended drug for management of severe cholera in both adults and children.

Gastroesophageal Reflux Disease

Erythromycin evokes striking changes in gastric motor activity by its action as a motilin receptor agonist. It has been used in the treatment of gastroesophageal reflux disease for its prokinetic effects.

Other Uses

Erythromycin has a well-established role as an alternative to penicillin, e.g. in the prophylaxis of rheumatic fever and bacterial endocarditis and in the treatment of anthrax and actinomycosis. The role of erythromycin as an alternative drug to penicillin, particularly in the prevention of bacterial endocarditis in patients who have underlying cardiac conditions recently has been replaced because of erythromycin-associated GI intolerance and unpredictable blood levels with the various erythromycin formulations. The newer macrolides are considered alternatives. Azithromycin has been mentioned as an effective treatment of erythrasma and rosacea as well as in the treatment of donovanosis. It has been used in the treatment of erythema migrans (Lyme disease) but amoxicillin has been found to be superior. Treatment of patients with typical cat-scratch disease with oral azithromycin for 5 days offers significant clinical benefit. Azithromycin and clarithromycin are also effective for treating rickettsial diseases in children. Azithromycin is useful in treating cyclosporine-induced gingival hyperplasia. Oral azithromycin was as effective as ocular tetracycline in treating trachoma and may be more convenient. Erythromycin is the drug of choice for *C. trachomatis* inclusion conjunctivitis. Azithromycin is also used as an alternative to doxycycline for prophylaxis against leptospirosis following flood water exposure.

DOSAGE

For erythromycin, the dose is 30–50 mg/kg/day given orally 4–6 hourly. Equivalent dosage of ethylsuccinate to erythromycin base (and the other erythromycin salts) is 400 mg to 250 mg. Azithromycin may be administered as 30 mg/kg single dose, 10 mg/kg once daily for 3 days, or 10 mg/kg on the first day followed by 5 mg/kg on days 2 through 5. If used for pharyngitis, azithromycin should be given in the dose of 12 mg/kg/day for 5 days. The recommended dose of clarithromycin for streptococcal pharyngitis is 7.5 mg/kg every 12 hours for 10 days. Dosage for treatment of acute maxillary sinusitis is 7.5 mg/kg every 12 hours for 14 days. For management of enteric fever azithromycin is dosed as 10–20 mg/kg/day (max 1 g) for 5–7 days.

ADVERSE DRUG REACTIONS

The most common adverse reactions to erythromycin are GI symptoms, including nausea, vomiting, abdominal cramps, and diarrhea. These side effects are dose-related and result from erythromycin's action on the gastric hormone motilin. Motilin activates duodenal/jejunal receptors to initiate peristalsis. There is a 25% incidence of typical GI symptoms with oral or intravenous administration. Antibiotic-associated colitis should be considered in patients with diarrhea that does not resolve on discontinuation of erythromycin. There is less GI distress with the newer macrolides.

Allergic reactions occur rarely (most often with the estolate salt). Erythromycin estolate can cause cholestatic hepatitis, which manifests with nausea, vomiting, abdominal pain, jaundice, fever, liver function abnormalities, and occasionally eosinophilia. It may be confused with viral hepatitis or acute cholecystitis. It is probably an allergy and recovery is usual. The use of the estolate salt is not recommended. There have also been reports that erythromycin has been associated with cardiac conduction abnormalities, allergic reactions of a mild to severe nature, skin eruptions that range from mild to severe, and reversible hearing loss. Side-effects of topical erythromycin include erythema, scaling, tenderness, burning, itching, irritation, oiliness, and dryness. It is a very weak sensitizer, and only a handful of reports of contact dermatitis to it have been published.

Both azithromycin and clarithromycin are well-tolerated by children. Gastrointestinal intolerance is the primary adverse side effect of these agents, but occurs at a significantly reduced rate when compared with erythromycin. Azithromycin has shorter treatment regimens and improved tolerance which may improve compliance in the treatment of respiratory tract, skin, or soft tissue infections. The most common adverse effects reported with azithromycin were diarrhea (3.6%); nausea (2.6%); abdominal pain (2.5%); and headache or dizziness (1.3%). Laboratory abnormalities were infrequent and minor including transient increases in transaminases in 1.5% of patients. Adverse events related to the intravenous infusion of azithromycin were pain at the injection site (6.5%) and local inflammation (3.1%). A recent large-scale retrospective analysis of azithromycin in adults found that the risk of cardiac death was significantly increased with azithromycin compared with no antibiotics or amoxicillin. Deaths were more likely in patients with pre-existing risk of heart disease. It is worthwhile to be cautious with the use of this drug especially in patients with heart disease. The most common adverse reactions reported with clarithromycin are similar to azithromycin, e.g. nausea (3.8%), diarrhea (3%), abdominal pain (1.9%), and headache (1.7%). There was no difference in the spectrum and frequency of adverse reactions between the extended-release or immediate-release formulations of clarithromycin. Gastrointestinal adverse events with the extended-release formulation, however, tended to be less severe and resulted in fewer discontinuations of the medication. Laboratory abnormalities were also rare and included abnormal liver function tests and decreased white blood cell counts. It can also induce mania, especially when given with steroids. Clarithromycin can also increase the QT interval especially in patients with preexisting cardiac disease and if other drugs that prolong QT interval such as moxifloxacin are administered. ECG monitoring is recommended for both azithromycin and clarithromycin in predisposed individuals.

CONTRAINDICATIONS AND SPECIAL PRECAUTIONS

Hypersensitivity to macrolides occurs rarely. Erythromycin estolate should not be used in patients with liver disease. Appropriate dose reductions, clinical monitoring and therapeutic drug level monitoring are necessary when drugs metabolized by the CYP3A4 enzymes are given concurrently with macrolides.

DRUG INTERACTIONS

Erythromycin and clarithromycin are oxidized by the cytochrome P-450 system, primarily the CYP3A4 subclass of hepatic enzymes. This converts the macrolide to a nitrosalkalane metabolite that forms an inactive metabolite-enzyme complex by binding to the iron of the CYP3A4 enzyme. This interaction inhibits the CYP3A4 enzymes resulting in decreased clearance of other agents given concurrently that are metabolized by the same enzyme system. Interference with the hepatic CYP3A4 enzyme system is responsible for increased blood levels of benzodiazepines (triazolam, midazolam, and alprazolam), carbamazepine, cyclosporine, ergot alkaloids, pimozide, protease inhibitors, "statins", i.e. 3-hydroxy-3-methylglutaryl-coenzyme A reductase inhibitors (atorvastatin, lovastatin, and simvastatin), tacrolimus, theophylline, and warfarin. Clarithromycin is a less potent inhibitor of the CYP3A4 enzymes than erythromycin. Azithromycin interferes poorly with this system and no major interactions have been reported with azithromycin. There are case reports, however, of toxicity related to coadministration of azithromycin and lovastatin, warfarin, cyclosporine, disopyramide, and theophylline.

Erythromycin, troleandomycin, and clarithromycin are the most potent inhibitors of carbamazepine metabolism by CYP3A4 enzymes; some patients have up to four times the normal plasma concentration of carbamazepine, which can cause serious toxicity. Macrolides that have reduced (e.g. roxithromycin) or absent (e.g. azithromycin, spiramycin) potential for such interaction are recommended for the treatment of patients receiving carbamazepine. Oxcarbazepine, tiagabine, and felbamate are not affected by coadministration of erythromycin. Rhabdomyolysis has occurred secondary to a drug interaction between simvastatin and clarithromycin.

The concurrent use of cisapride, pimozide, terfenadine, and astemizole with clarithromycin is contraindicated because of the possible cardiotoxic effects of these agents and the occurrence of torsades de pointes. Class 1A antiarrhythmic agents (quinidine, disopyramide) too should be used cautiously when given with clarithromycin. Both clarithromycin and azithromycin have been associated with digoxin toxicity.

Clarithromycin may reduce the absorption of zidovudine (AZT) by 20%, whereas azithromycin does not. Data suggest that when the two agents are separated by at least 2 hours, no reduction in zidovudine levels is found. Clarithromycin interacts with rifabutin in such a way that coadministration of the two agents can result in a 50% decrease in the AUC of clarithromycin. The current theory points to enzyme induction secondary to rifabutin administration. When coadministered, desloratadine or fexofenadine increase levels of azithromycin.

CONCLUSION

The advanced macrolides (azithromycin and clarithromycin) are structural analogs of erythromycin that have similar mechanisms of action. These antimicrobials have several distinct advantages over erythromycin including improved oral bioavailability, longer half-life allowing once- or twice-daily administration, higher tissue concentrations, enhanced antimicrobial activity, and less GI adverse effects. Between the two, azithromycin is cheaper, allows once a day dosing and shorter therapy and has no drug interactions. This makes this wonderful molecule the most potential candidate for drug resistance. Treatment guidelines have emphasized the roles of azithromycin in the treatment of certain sexually transmitted diseases, enteric fever, shigellosis and clarithromycin for the treatment of *H. pylori*-associated peptic ulcer disease. Azithromycin and clarithromycin have been used successfully for preventing and treating disseminated MAC infections in HIV-infected patients. Due to ever rising resistance macrolides should not be used as a first-line choice for the treatment of bacterial URTI, LRTI (other than mycoplasma), and skin and soft tissue infections. The incidence of resistance is highly variable with regard to the country and, most importantly, the patterns of infections observed among patients. For this reason, local statistics are of crucial value for empiric therapy.

RECOMMENDED READING

1. Black DJ, Ellsworth A. Practical overview of antibiotics for family physicians. Clin Fam Pract. 2004;6:265.
2. Bowlware KL, Stull T. Antibacterial agents in pediatrics. Infect Dis Clin North Am. 2004;18:513-31.
3. Cunha BA. Newer macrolide antibiotics: Advantages and uses. Adv Ther. 1996;13(1):29-37.
4. Daga NR, Klugman KP, Craig WA, et al. Evidence to support the rationale that bacterial eradication in respiratory tract infection is an important aim of antimicrobial therapy. J Antimicrob Chemother. 2001;47:129-40.
5. Dagan R, Leibovitz E. Bacterial eradication in the treatment of otitis media. Lancet Infect Dis. 2002;2:593-604.
6. File TM. Telithromycin new product overview. J Allergy Clin Immunol. 2005;115:S1-13.
7. Hasler WL. Pharmacotherapy for intestinal motor and sensory disorders. Gastroenterol Clin North Am. 2003;32:707-32.
8. Hyde TB, Gay K, Stephens DS, et al. Macrolide resistance among invasive *Streptococcus pneumoniae* isolates. JAMA. 2001;286:1857-62.
9. Kataja J, Huovinen P, Seppala H. Erythromycin resistance genes in group A streptococci of different geographical origins: the Macrolide Resistance Study Group. J Antimicrob Chemother. 2000;46:789-92.
10. Kaye KS, Engemann JJ, Fraimow HS, et al. Pathogens resistant to antimicrobial agents: epidemiology, molecular mechanisms, and clinical management. Inf Dis Clin North Am. 2004;18:467-511.
11. Leclercq R. Mechanisms of resistance to macrolides and lincosamides: nature of the resistance elements and their clinical implications. Clin Infect Dis. 2002;34(4):482-492. [online]. Available from https://doi.org/10.1086/324626 [Accessed December, 2018].

12. Meijvis SC, van de Garde EM, Rijkers GT, et al. Treatment with anti-inflammatory drugs in community acquired pneumonia. J Internal Med. 2012;272:25-35.
13. Patsalos PN, Perucca E. Clinically important drug interactions in epilepsy: interactions between antiepileptic drugs and other drugs. Lancet Neurol. 2003;2:473-81.
14. Roberts MC, Sutcliffe J, Courvalin P, et al. Nomenclature for macrolide and macrolide-lincosamide-streptogramin B resistance determinants. Antimicrob Agents Chemother. 1999;43:2823-30
15. Scheinfeld NS, Tutrone WD, Torres O, et al. Macrolides in dermatology. Dis Mon. 2004;50:350-68.
16. Shah D. Role of azithromycin in enteric fever. Indian Pediatr. 2009;46:51-2.
17. Tait-Kamradt A, Clancy J, Cronan M, et al. mef E is necessary for the erythromycin-resistant M phenotype in Streptococcus pneumonia. Antimicrob Agents Chemother. 1997;41:2251-5.
18. Van Eijk AM, Terlouv DJ. Azithromycin for treating uncomplicated malaria. Cochrane Database Syst Rev. 2011;16(2):CD006688.
19. Whitney CG, Farley MM, Hadle J, et al. Increasing prevalence of multidrug-resistant Streptococcus pneumoniae in the United States. N Engl J Med. 2000;346:1917-24.
20. Zuckerman JM. Macrolides and ketolides: azithromycin, clarithromycin, telithromycin. Infect Dis Clin North Am. 2004;18:621-49.

Quinolones

11

Chapter

Indu Khosla, Tanushri Mukherjee

INTRODUCTION

The era of quinolone antibiotics began with the serendipitous discovery of the prototype quinolone antibiotic, nalidixic acid during the synthesis of the antimalarial agent chloroquine in the early 1960s. In the 90s, fluoroquinolones (quinolones) had become a dominant class of antibiotics in adults because of their excellent tissue penetration and their bactericidal activity. They were, however, not authorized for pediatric use because of the potential for joint toxicity reported from experiments with young animals. Despite the absence of official approval of the Food and Drug Administration (FDA) [except ciprofloxacin for postexposure treatment for inhalation anthrax and complicated urinary tract infection (UTI)] and the Indian drug regulatory authority they are still widely used in pediatrics. In the USA alone, the number of annual ciprofloxacin prescriptions for patients younger than 18 years is estimated at 150,000; 20% for children less than 1 year of age. Newer generation fluoroquinolones have become indispensable for the management of drug resistant tuberculosis in both adults and children both in India and globally. This article describes the pharmaceutical profile of fluoroquinolones with special reference to the clinical applications. Table 1 lists the various generations of fluoroquinolones.

MECHANISM OF ACTION

The quinolones act primarily on a group of enzymes called topoisomerases (type I and type II). Topoisomerases are a class of enzymes that maintain the cellular deoxyribonucleic acid (DNA) molecule in a physicochemically stable and biologically active state as well as play an important role in bacterial DNA replication and safe decatenation of the subsequent daughter chromosome. Type I topoisomerases are active during the replication of single-stranded DNA and type II topoisomerases the double-stranded DNA. The quinolones are strong inhibitors

TABLE 1: Generations of fluoroquinolones.

Generation	*Example*	*Activity*
First	Nalidixic acid	Achieves minimal serum levels
Second	Class 1—norfloxacin Class 2—ciprofloxacin, ofloxacin, and levofloxacin	Class 2 have higher tissue concentrations and some action against atypical pathogens
Third	Sparfloxacin, gatifloxacin, gemifloxacin, and grepafloxacin	Expanded activity against gram-positive bacteria and atypical pathogens
Fourth	Moxifloxacin and trovafloxacin	Added significant activity against anaerobes

of type II topoisomerases (DNA gyrase and topoisomerase IV). Both are large and complex enzymes composed of two pairs of subunits. The subunits of DNA gyrase are GyrA and GyrB. The corresponding subunits of topoisomerase IV are ParC and ParE. The two enzymes work together in the replication, transcription, recombination, and repair of DNA. The enzymes transiently break both strands of double-stranded DNA, pass a second DNA double helix through the break, and seal it. Quinolones block the reaction and trap gyrase or topoisomerase IV as a drug-enzyme-DNA complex, with subsequent release of lethal, double-stranded DNA breaks. DNA gyrase is the primary target of quinolones in gram-negative organisms and topoisomerase IV in the gram-positive organisms. Several aspects of the quinolone structure directly influence antibacterial activity. The addition of a fluorine molecule at position 6 was one of the earliest changes (thus known as fluoroquinolone) to the structure. This single alteration provides a more than 10-fold increase in gyrase inhibition and up to 100-fold improvement in potency.

SPECTRUM OF ACTIVITY

The first- and second-generation quinolones mainly act on aerobic gram-negative rods. The third- and fourth-generation quinolones have been designed to build up range of activity towards the gram-positive organisms and atypical organisms, but no change in gram-negative activity. On the basis of activity, quinolones can be classified into four groups as shown in Table 2.

Newer fluoroquinolones such as levofloxacin, moxifloxacin, gatifloxacin, and gemifloxacin have excellent intrinsic activity against *Streptococcus pneumoniae, Haemophilus influenzae, Moraxella catarrhalis,* and the atypical respiratory pathogens. With respect to penicillin-resistant pneumococci, newer fluoroquinolone minimum inhibitory concentrations (MICs) remain the same in both resistant and susceptible strains. Antipneumococcal activity is present in all newer quinolones with levofloxacin having highest MIC50–MIC90 (1–3.13 µg/mL) and hence relatively lower activity. A recently published study in Canada (1988–1998) has however tracked a decreased susceptibility to fluoroquinolones in *S. pneumoniae* probably due to increased prescriptions. Newer quinolones also have activity against group A and group

TABLE 2: Spectrum of activity of uoroquinolones.

Agents	*Activity*	*Clinical use*
1. Urinary agents (1960–1985) - Nalidixic acid - Norfloxacin	Enterobacteriaceae Short serum half-lives renal elimination	Main use in urinary tract infection (UTI)
2. Gram-negative systemic agents (1985–1995) - Ciprofloxacin - Ofloxacin - Levofloxacin	Gram-negatives including *Pseudomonas aeruginosa*, marginal activity against gram-positive, longer serum half-lives	Widely used against tissue-based and urinary infections
3. Broad spectrum systemic agents (1990–2000) - Temafloxacin - Trovafloxacin	Gram-negative, including *P. aeruginosa*, gram-positive, anaerobe, long serum half-lives	Widely used against a broad range of tissue-based infections
4. Respiratory agents (>1995) - Levofloxacin - Sparfloxacin - Moxifloxacin - Gatifloxacin	Enterobacteriaceae, gram-positive, especially *Streptococcus pneumoniae*, active against atypical bacteria, variable activity against anaerobes, long serum half-life	Respiratory tract infections

B hemolytic streptococci. As far as antipseudomonal activity is concerned ciprofloxacin is the best. All quinolones have moderate activity against *Mycobacterium tuberculosis*, the best being moxifloxacin. Levofloxacin has a wide range of potential uses, but its main focus is respiratory infection. The quinolones have in vitro activity against *Staphylococcus aureus*, but resistance develops rapidly if used as monotherapy. The quinolones do not have any activity against *Nocardia* and *Treponema*. Trovafloxacin is the only quinolone specifically approved for use in the treatment of anaerobic infections; but rarely prescribed because of hepatotoxicity. Gatifloxacin, moxifloxacin, and sparfloxacin have demonstrated in vitro activity, but have not been studied in diseases caused by anaerobes.

RESISTANCE TO QUINOLONES

Resistance to quinolones may occur via three mechanisms; mutations that alter the drug targets, mutations that reduce drug accumulation, and plasmids that protect cells from the lethal effects of quinolones.

- *Target-mediated quinolone resistance:* Quinolone resistance is most often associated with specific mutations in gyrase and/or topoisomerase IV that weaken the quinolone-enzyme interaction. This is most common cause of high level of resistance. Mutation of one type II enzyme confers less than or equal to 10-fold drug resistance whereas mutation of both enzymes causes higher levels of resistance (~10–100-fold).
- *Plasmid-mediated quinolone resistance:* Plasmids carrying quinolone resistance genes cause low-level (≤10-fold) resistance by three mechanisms.
    1. *Klebsiella pneumoniae, Escherichia coli,* and other enteric bacteria may express Qnr proteins which decrease topoisomerase DNA binding and protect enzyme-DNA complex from quinolones.
    2. aac(6')-Ib-cr is an aminoglycoside acetyltransferase that acetylates the free nitrogen on the C7 ring of ciprofloxacin and norfloxacin, decreasing their effectiveness. This mediates low-level resistance to ciprofloxacin, as well as high-level resistance to tobramycin and amikacin. This enzyme variant has been present since at least 1999 and is now widely disseminated in enteric gram-negative bacteria such as *E. coli, Klebsiella* species, and *Enterobacter* species.
    3. Plasmid-encoded efflux pumps decrease the concentration of quinolones in the cell. QepA, which pumps fluoroquinolones such as norfloxacin and ciprofloxacin out of the cell, confers low-level resistance. Isolates encoding the QepA protein have been found in Europe, Japan, China, and North America, but usually only in low frequency. Another plasmid-encoded efflux pump, OqxAB, has been found in *E. coli* isolates from humans and swine.
- *Chromosome-mediated quinolone resistance*: The cellular concentration of quinolones is regulated by the opposing actions of diffusion-mediated drug uptake and pump-mediated efflux. Underexpression of porins in gram-negative species decreases drug uptake and overexpression of chromosome-encoded efflux pumps decreases drug retention in the cell.

Though, plasmid-mediated and chromosome-mediated resistance is low-level resistance, but lowering the cellular concentration of quinolones creates a favorable background for other forms of resistance to develop and propagate leading to high-grade resistance.

PHARMACOKINETICS AND PHARMACODYNAMICS

The pharmacokinetic profile of the commonly used quinolones is given in Table 3. As quinolones have developed larger serum area under the curve (AUC) or peak serum (C_{max}) values are

TABLE 3: Pharmacokinetics and pharmacodynamics of quinolones with standard adult doses in healthy volunteers.

Pharmacokinetic property	*Ciprofloxacin*	*Norfloxacin*	*Ofloxacin*	*Levofloxacin*	*Gatifloxacin*	*Moxifloxacin*
Oral bioavailability	60–80	35–45	85–95	99%	90%	90%
Plasma protein binding	20–35	15	25	40%	20%	50%
C_{max} (mg/mL)	2.5	-	4.4	5.2	3.4	3.1
AUC (mg/h/L)	11.6	-	36.8	47.7	32.4	30.8
Elimination half-life (hours)	3–5	4–6	6	7	7	8–12
Route of administration	Oral/IV	Oral	Oral/IV	Oral/IV	Oral/IV	Oral/IV
Route of elimination	Hepatic, renal	Hepatic, renal	Renal	Renal	Renal	Hepatic

(AUC: area under the curve; IV: intravenous)

consistently seen and oral absorption has markedly improved compared with that of nalidixic acid. Norfloxacin does not achieve good systemic levels and should be used only as a urinary antiseptic. Quinolones achieve high concentrations in kidneys, lung, and gallbladder. Similar concentrations are also achieved in bone. The CSF penetration of the newer fluoroquinolones is better than the older ones with moxifloxacin having the best penetration. They are excreted largely by the kidneys and need renal dose adjustment with the exception of moxifloxacin.

The fluoroquinolone antibiotics are concentration-dependent agents with prolonged postantibiotic effect (PAE). The parameter that correlates most closely with clinical and/or bacteriological success and development of bacterial resistance is the ratio of the area under plasma concentration curve to MIC. A very high free drug peak (C_{max}) and AUC combined with low MIC are having a significant clinical effect and increase the ratios. Schentag et al. have described a relationship between the ratio of AUC and the MIC called area under the inhibitory curve (AUIC). To achieve maximal therapeutic benefit, the peak to MIC ratio should be maintained at more than 8–10 and the AUC/MIC should be more than or equal to 125 for gram-negative organisms and more than or equal to 30 for gram-positive organisms. In addition, to prevent the development of resistance maintenance of peak to MIC ratio at more than or equal to 10 or AUC/MIC more than or equal to 125 for gram-negative organisms and more than or equal to 50 for gram-positive organisms is necessary.

CLINICAL INDICATIONS

The inappropriate use of fluoroquinolones in children and adults is likely to be associated with increasing bacterial resistance and toxicity. The use of a fluoroquinolone in a child or adolescent may be justified in special circumstances after careful assessment of the risks and benefits for the individual patient. According to the American Academy of Pediatrics (AAP), fluoroquinolones should be used in children only in the following circumstances:

- Infection is caused by multidrug-resistant pathogens for which there is no safe and effective alternative exists.
- Parenteral therapy is not feasible and no other effective oral agent is available.

The FDA licensed systemic indications are:

- Complicated UTIs caused by *Pseudomonas aeruginosa* or other multidrug-resistant, gram-negative bacteria, and pyelonephritis attributable to *E. coli* in patients (1–17 years of age). Use of quinolones for prophylaxis though effective, is associated with risk of increased resistance.
- Exposure to inhalational *Bacillus anthracis* and plague.

In 2011, the AAP published an updated clinical report because of the increased ophthalmologic and topical use of fluoroquinolones as well as data on lack of toxicity when used in children. Widely used, but not FDA licensed indications are:

- *Acute otitis media, sinusitis, lower respiratory tract infection, and chronic suppurative otitis media*: Newer fluoroquinolones show enhanced in vitro activity against *S. pneumoniae*, compared with ciprofloxacin. Current otitis media and acute bacterial sinusitis guidelines from the AAP and Pediatric Infectious Diseases Society/Infectious Diseases Society of America guidelines on community-acquired pneumonia in children support the use of levofloxacin as an alternative therapy for those with severe (type I) penicillin allergy and for those infected with suspected multidrug-resistant pneumococcus (i.e. patients in whom amoxicillin and amoxicillin-clavulanate have failed). Levofloxacin being the only fluoroquinolone in which well-defined pharmacokinetic data is available for children 6 months and older. Although pneumococcal resistance to new fluoroquinolones is currently low, there is still concern about the potential for widespread emergence of resistance to these agents if they are indiscriminately used. There is a concern about using fluoroquinolones in lower respiratory infections in India where tuberculosis can sometimes present as a community-acquired pneumonia and use of fluoroquinolones can delay the diagnosis.
- *Tuberculosis*: The antitubercular activity of the newer fluoroquinolones is superior to the older ones. The phase II OFLOTUB trial tested three fluoroquinolones against ethambutol and found that moxifloxacin was slightly better than gatifloxacin in the speed of sputum conversion, and both were better than ofloxacin, which was equivalent to ethambutol. Trials that evaluated utility of moxifloxacin as compared to ethambutol in drug-susceptible tuberculosis did not demonstrate significant efficacy in shortening the duration of therapy to 4 months from 6 months. Hence, use of quinolones in drug-susceptible tuberculosis is at present not recommended unless there is poor tolerance/adverse effects with the first-line drugs. However, quinolones are indispensable for drug-resistant tuberculosis and this is discussed in detail in the chapter on antitubercular therapy.
- In cystic fibrosis bronchopulmonary infections with *P. aeruginosa* and *S. aureus* are a major cause of morbidity and mortality. There is now unanimous support for the treatment of *P. aeruginosa* pulmonary super infections in children with cystic fibrosis with ciprofloxacin, but in higher doses (40–60 mg/kg/day).
- Gastrointestinal tract infection caused by multidrug-resistant *Shigella* species, *Salmonella* species, *Vibrio cholerae*, or *Campylobacter jejuni*. However, studies from various parts of the Indian subcontinent and Southeast Asia show increasing resistance to quinolones. Although ciprofloxacin has been regarded as an effective agent for traveler's diarrhea in the past, resistance in *Campylobacter* species is increasing.
- Chronic or acute osteomyelitis or osteochondritis caused by *P. aeruginosa*. A combination of quinolones and rifampicin is often used to treat chronic osteomyelitis due to methicillin-sensitive *Staphylococcus aureus*/methicillin-resistant *Staphylococcus aureus* (MSSA/MRSA) where the isolate is susceptible to both drugs.
- Ciprofloxacin was in the 1990s drug of choice for enteric fever, but very high resistance rates in the current era preclude its empiric use for this indication. Quinolones are however

the preferred drugs for nontyphoidal salmonella infections including osteomyelitis and meningitis particularly in patients with sickle cell anemia, if the isolate is susceptible.

- Ciprofloxacin is effective in eradicating nasal carriage of *Neisseria meningitidis* (single dose, 500 mg for adults and 20 mg/kg for those older than 1 month).
- Gram-negative bacterial infections in immunocompromised/neutropenic hosts in which oral therapy is desired or resistance to alternative agents is present. Very high resistance rates make this a theoretical indication in the Indian scenario.
- Documented bacterial septicemia or meningitis attributable to organisms with in vitro resistance to approved agents or in immunocompromised infants and children in whom parenteral therapy with other appropriate antimicrobial agents has failed.
- Serious infections attributable to fluoroquinolone-susceptible pathogen(s) in children with life-threatening allergy to alternative agents.
- *Topical indications*: External otitis, tympanostomy tube-associated otorrhea, conjunctivitis, levofloxacin, ofloxacin, moxifloxacin, and ciprofloxacin (FDA approved for children older than 12 months).

DRUG DOSES

Dosages of commonly used quinolones are given in Table 4.

ADVERSE DRUG REACTIONS

The restriction of quinolone use and paucity of prospective studies have limited safety data in children. Most studies seem limited to detailing and retrospectively analyzing incidents reported to the drug monitoring agencies.

Musculoskeletal Side Effects

Quinolone-induced cartilage toxicity in immature animals has been the basis for nonapproval of their use in children. Each quinolone has a different potential to cause cartilage toxicity, but given a sufficiently high exposure, cartilage changes will occur in all animal models with all quinolones. In 2004, the FDA released data about the safety of ciprofloxacin from an analysis of clinical trial 100169, which evaluated ciprofloxacin for the treatment of complicated UTI or pyelonephritis in children 1 through 17 years of age. Arthropathy rates were 9.3% for ciprofloxacin

TABLE 4: Dosages of commonly used quinolones.

Drug	*Route*	*Dose (mg/kg/dose)*	*Frequency*
Ciprofloxacin	Oral IV	10–15 10	Q12 hours Q12 hours
Norfloxacin	Oral	5–7.5	Q12 hours
Ofloxacin	Oral IV	7.5 7.5	Q12 hours Q12 hours
Gatifloxacin	Oral	10	Q24 hours
Levofloxacin	Oral IV	10 10	Q12–24 hours (12 hourly in children below 5)
Moxifloxacin	Oral IV	10 10	Q24 hours

(IV: intravenous)

versus 6% for the comparator group. Levofloxacin safety data were collected on a large cohort of 2,523 children who participated in prospective, randomized, and unblended clinical efficacy trials. All subjects from both treatment arms were followed up for 12 months safety assessments, including musculoskeletal events (tendinopathy, arthritis, arthralgia, and gait abnormality). Results showed a greater rate of musculoskeletal events in levofloxacin-treated group compared to comparator group at 2 months (1.9% vs 0.7%; P = .025) and at 12 months (2.9% vs 1.6%; P = .047). A long-term follow-up study (5 years) in selected subjects from this cohort was published recently showing similar growth characteristics at the 5-year.

Tendinitis and tendon rupture are also adverse effects of quinolones. Tendon rupture has a predilection for the Achilles tendon (and is often bilateral). It happens more in adults with advanced age, antecedent steroid therapy, and underlying diseases, i.e. hypercholesterolemia, gout, rheumatoid arthritis, and end-stage renal disease/dialysis, have been identified as risk factors. Pefloxacin and ciprofloxacin have a high tendency to cause tenotoxicity while ofloxacin and levofloxacin have low potential for causing this effect. The symptoms are joint pain and swelling followed by difficulty in movement. Rupture of the involved tendons has been reported and can cause permanent disability. The symptoms may start within 1–2 days after starting therapy. Tendinitis resolves in a few weeks, but may persist over months.

Nonmusculoskeletal Side Effects

The adverse drug reactions associated with quinolones include gastrointestinal, central nervous system (CNS) side effects, phototoxicity, renal effects, hepatic effects, mutagenicity, and cardiotoxicity.

- *Gastrointestinal*: Most common but well tolerated. Anorexia, nausea, vomiting, and abdominal discomfort are mild. Quinolone use in adults is significantly associated with *Clostridium difficile* infection.
- *Central nervous system*: The effects on the central nervous system are a real risk for children and are probably underestimated (incidence close to 3–6%). Intracranial hypertension is a known side effect of nalidixic acid in young children. Other side effects include dizziness, drowsiness, headaches, and sleep disorders. Hallucination, delirium, and seizures are rare. These side effects occur as a result of direct action on gamma-aminobutyric acid (GABA) and N-methyl-D-aspartate (NMDA) receptors.
- *Cardiovascular system*: The principal cardiac risk associated with quinolones toxicity is an increased QT interval due to inhibition of potassium channels leading to life-threatening arrhythmia and torsades de pointes. Sparfloxacin is most potent followed by grepafloxacin, both of which had been removed from the market. Moxifloxacin, levofloxacin, ofloxacin, and ciprofloxacin have decreasing effects in that order.
- *Rash and allergic reaction*: Occur in 0.4–2.2% patients. Photosensitive reactions caused by quinolones are predominantly phototoxic in nature, but typical photoallergic features can also be demonstrated with certain quinolones such as nalidixic acid, sparfloxacin, and lomefloxacin. The reported incidence of phototoxicity ranges from less than 0.05% (ciprofloxacin) to as high as 19% for a high dose fleroxacin. The methoxy group found at eighth position in moxifloxacin and gatifloxacin reduces the phototoxic potential. Other allergic reactions include drug fever, urticaria, angioedema, vasculitis, serum sickness like illness, anaphylactoid reactions, etc.
- *Liver failure*: Trovafloxacin has been removed from market.

- *Hypoglycemia and hyperglycemia*: Diabetic patients are more commonly affected. Moxifloxacin confers highest risk compared to levofloxacin and ciprofloxacin.
- *Hematologic*: Hemolysis in glucose-6-phosphate dehydrogenase (G6PD)-deficient people can occur. Leukopenia and eosinophilia may happen rarely.
- *Others*: However, more serious effects that infrequently occur seem to be an idiosyncratic reactions, e.g. hemolytic uremic syndrome with temafloxacin.

CLINICALLY SIGNIFICANT DRUG INTERACTIONS AND PRECAUTIONS

The absorption of all quinolones can be altered by the coadministration of divalent or trivalent cation-containing agents. Aluminum, magnesium, and lesser extent calcium containing antacids, sucralfate if coadministered with quinolones form cation-quinolone complex leading to poor bioavailability. Generally H2 blockers and proton pump inhibitors do not affect the absorption. Concurrent administration of ferrous sulfate and zinc containing multivitamin reduce absorption of quinolones. The intravenous formulation of ciprofloxacin precipitates when infused through same intravenous tubing with aminophylline and amoxicillin, so separate infusions are indicated.

Some of the quinolones inhibit the cytochrome P450 1A2 isozyme, responsible for metabolism of methylxanthines derivatives including theophylline and caffeine. Enoxacin, ciprofloxacin, and grepafloxacin have been shown to reduce the total body clearance of theophylline. This may result in increase in serum levels of theophylline by 30–84% and can cause theophylline toxicity, manifested as nausea, vomiting, and seizures. Moxifloxacin, levofloxacin, and ofloxacin have less effects.

Nonsteroidal anti-inflammatory drugs (NSAIDs) and theophylline potentiate the central nervous system stimulant effect of quinolones by displacing GABA from its receptor leading to seizures.

Quinolones prolong QT interval by inhibiting potassium channels. So coadministration of quinolone along with other drugs (class IA antiarrhythmic quinidine, procainamide, and class III amiodarone and sotalol) that prolong QT interval should be avoided. Other drugs that can prolong the QT interval include clarithromycin, clofazimine, and bedaquiline. Caution should also be taken in hypokalemia, hypomagnesemia, and in patients with organic heart disease including congestive cardiac failure. Moxifloxacin and sparfloxacin have a greatest tendency to prolong the QT interval while ciprofloxacin and ofloxacin the least. Quinolones increase the levels of warfarin and other coumarin derivatives, so coadministration should be avoided.

CONTRAINDICATIONS

Quinolones are contraindicated in persons with a history of hypersensitivity to ciprofloxacin or any member of the quinolone class of antimicrobial agents. They are also contraindicated in children with seizure disorders.

DELAFLOXACIN

Several new fluoroquinolones are in various phases of development. Delafloxacin is a new fluoroquinolone that has been recently approved by the US FDA. It differs from the other fluoroquinolones in having an anionic character that allows it to have better intracellular penetration and efficacy in acid environments. It has good activity against MRSA unlike other fluoroquinolones and shares the other antibacterial spectrum of the newer generation quinolones. The drug has been found noninferior to comparator drugs including tigecycline/linezolid and vancomycin with aztreonam in phase 3 trials for treatment of skin and soft-tissue infections and is approved for this indication. More than half the patients in these trials were infected with MRSA. A trial evaluating its efficacy in community-acquired pneumonia is in progress. The drug is not available in India at present.

CONCLUSION

The quinolones are a valuable addition to our armamentarium of antibiotics. The class of drugs would continue to grow with time. Each new addition would bring with it a unique spectrum of activity, safety, and tolerability profile. Clinicians must remain abreast with these particular aspects so that their clinical applications are appropriate. Despite rare, specific problems associated with individual quinolones, this class of antibiotics generally is well-tolerated and effective and the safety data in children seem to be similar to those in adults. A number of controversies, however, exist due to observations of joint toxicity in animals. The increasing use of quinolones in pediatric infections has been associated with good results with no clear demonstration of chondrotoxicity. Quinolones are indispensable in children with cystic fibrosis and multidrug-resistant tuberculosis and recommended in children with complicated UTI, pyelonephritis, shigellosis, nontyphoidal salmonella infections, and enteric fever when the isolate is susceptible. The newer quinolones though excellent for respiratory tract infections, should be used only as second-line drugs owing to fear of drug resistance in both bacterial and mycobacterial infections and as other alternatives are available.

RECOMMENDED READING

1. Alghasham AA, Nahata MC. Clinical use of fluroquinolones in children. Ann Pharmacother. 2000;34:347-59.
2. Andersson MI, MacGowan AP. Development of the quinolones. J Antimicrob Chemothery. 2003;51(Suppl S1):1-11.
3. Blondeau JM. Expanded activity and utility of new fluoroquinolones: a review. Clin Ther. 1999;21:3-40.
4. Bradley JS, Byington CL, Shah SS, et al. The management of community acquired pneumonia in infants and children older than 3 months of age: clinical practice guidelines by the Pediatric Infectious Diseases Society and the Infectious Diseases Society of America. Clin Infect Dis. 2011;53(7):e25-76.
5. Bradley JS, Jackson MA, Committee on Infectious Diseases, et al. The use of systemic and topical fluoroquinolones. Pediatrics. 2011;128(4):e1034-45.
6. Bradley JS, Jackson MA, Committee on Infectious Diseases. The Use of Systemic and Topical Fluoroquinolones. Pediatrics. 2011;118(3):1287-92.
7. Bradley JS, Kauffman RE, Balis DA, et al. Assessment of musculoskeletal toxicity 5 years after therapy with levofloxacin. Pediatrics. 2014;134(1):e146.
8. Chalumeau M, Tonneliere M. Fluoroquinolones safety in pediatric patients: a prospective multicenter cohort study in France. Pediatrics. 2003;111:e714-19.
9. Church DA, Kanga JF, Kuhn RJ, et al Sequential ciprofloxacin therapy in pediatric cystic fibrosis: comparative study versus ceftazidime/tobramycin in the treatment of acute pulmonary exacerbations. Pediatr Infect Dis J. 1997;16:97-105.
10. Dheda K, Chang KC, Guglielmetti L, et al. Clinical management of adults and children with multidrug-resistant and extensively drug-resistant tuberculosis. Clin Microbiol Infect. 2016;23:131-40.
11. Garau J, Xercavins M, Rodriguez-Carballeira M, et.al. Emergence and dissemination of quinolone resistant *E Coli* in the community. Antimicrob Agents Chemother. 1999:43:2736-41.

12. Gendrel D, Chalumeau M, Moulin F, et al. Fluoroquinolones in pediatrics: a risk for the patient or for the community? Lancet Infect Dis. 2003;3:537-45.
13. Harish BN, Menezes GA. Antimicrobial resistance in typhoidal salmonellae. Indian J Med Microbiol. 2011;29(3):223-9.
14. Hooper DC. Fluoroquinolone resistance among Gram-positive cocci. Lancet Infect Dis. 2002;2:530-8.
15. Jackson MA, Schutze GE, Committee on Infectious Diseases. The use of systemic and topical fluoroquinolones. Pediatrics. 2016;138(5):e20162706.
16. Jacoby GA. Mechanisms of resistance to quinolones. Clin Infect Dis. 2005;41:S120-6.
17. Lieberthal AS, Carroll AE, Chonmaitree T, et al. The diagnosis and management of acute otitis media. Pediatrics. 2013;131(3):e964-99.
18. McEwan SR, Davey PG. Ciprofloxacin and tenosynovitis. Lancet. 1988;2:900.
19. Nelson JD, McCracken GH. Fluoroquinolone use in children. Pediatr Infect Dis J. 2002;21:A7-8.
20. Noel GJ, Bradley JS, Kauffman RE, et al. Comparative safety profile of levofloxacin in 2523 children with a focus on four specific musculoskeletal disorders. Pediatr Infect Dis J. 2007;26(10):879-91.
21. O'Donnell JA, Gelone SP. Fluorouinolones. Infect Diseases Clin N Am. 2000;14:489-513.
22. O'Donnell JA, Gelone SP. The newer fluoroquinolones. Infect Diseases Clin N Am. 2004;18:691-716.
23. Parry CM, Hien TT, Dougan G, et al. Typhoid fever. N Engl J Med. 2002;347:1770-82.
24. Patrick CC. Use of fluoroquinolones as prophylaxis in patients with neutropenia. Pediatr Infect Dis J. 1997;16:135-9.
25. Petrilli AS, Dantas LS, Campos MC, et al. Oral ciprofloxacin versus intravenous ceftriaxone administered in outpatient setting for fever and neutropenia in low-risk pediatric oncology patients: a randomized prospective trial. Med Pediatr Oncol. 2000:34:87-91.
26. Polk RE, Johnson CK, McClish D, et al. Predicting hospital rates of fluoroquinolone-resistant *Pseudomonas aeruginosa* from fluoroquinolone use in US hospitals and their surrounding communities. Clin Infect Dis. 2004;39:497.
27. Richard DA, Nousia-Arvanitakis S, Sollich V, et al. Oral ciprofloxacin vs. intravenous ceftazidime plus tobramycin in pediatric cystic fibrosis patients: comparison of anti pseudomonas efficacy and assessment of safety with ultrasonography and magnetic resonance imaging. Cystic Fibrosis Study Group. Pediatr Infect Dis J. 1997;16:572-8.
28. Rustomjee R, Lienhardt C, Kanyok T, et al. A phase II study of the sterilising activities of ofloxacin, gatifloxacin and moxifloxacin in pulmonary tuberculosis. Int J Tuberc Lung Dis. 2008;12:128-38.
29. Saravolatz LD, Stein GE. Delafloxacin: A new anti-MRSA fluoroquinolone. Clin Infect Dis. 2018.
30. Schaad UB, Wedgwood J, Ruedeberg A, et al. Ciprofloxacin as antipseudomonal treatment in patients with cystic fibrosis. Pediatr Infect Dis J. 1997;16:97-105.
31. Sher L, Arguedas A, Husseman M, et al. Randomized, investigator-blinded, multicenter, comparative study of gatifloxacin versus amoxicillin/clavulanate in recurrent otitis media and acute otitis media treatment failure in children. Pediatr Infect Dis J. 2005;24:301-8.
32. Szarfman A, Chen M, Blum MD. More on fluoroquinolones antibiotics and tendon rupture. N Engl J Med. 1995;332:193.
33. Takiff H, Guerrero E. Current prospects for the fluoroquinolones as first-line tuberculosis therapy. Antimicrob Agents Chemother. 2011;55(12):5421-9.
34. US Food and Drug Administration. Division of Special Pathogen and Immunologic Drug Products. Summary of clinical review of studies submitted in a response to a pediatric written request: ciprofloxacin. [online] Available from www. fda.gov/downloads/drugs/developmentapprovalprocess/developmentresources/ucm447421. pdf [Accessed December 2018].
35. Wald ER, Applegate KE, Bordley C, et al. Clinical practice guideline for the diagnosis and management of acute bacterial sinusitis in children aged 1 to 18 years. Pediatrics. 2013;132(1):e262-80..
36. Wright DH, Brown GH, Peterson ML, et al. Application of fluoroquinolone pharmacodynamics. J Antimicrob Chemother. 2000;46(5):669-83.
37. Zabraniecki L, Negrier I, Vergne P, et al. Fluoroquinolone induced tendinopathy: report of 6 cases. J Rheumatol. 1996;23(3):516-20.

Glycopeptides, Lipopeptides, Oxazolidinones, and Glycolipopeptides

12
Chapter

Pallavi Bhargava, Vivek Kak

GLYCOPEPTIDES

Vancomycin

Vancomycin is a large complex glycopeptide that was first isolated in the early 1950s from a sample of soil that contained the organism *Nocardia orientalis*. Its use re-emerged in late 1980s after the widespread emergence of methicillin-resistant *Staphylococcus aureus* (MRSA) as a pathogen. However, the widespread use of this antibiotic has led to emergence of vancomycin resistance among various pathogens including enterococci as well as decreasing susceptibility of MRSA to vancomycin.

Mechanism of Action

The drug exerts its antimicrobial action by restricting cell wall synthesis in susceptible organisms by preventing formation of the peptidoglycans required for the bacterial cell wall. The amino acids in these peptidoglycans terminate in D-alanyl-D-alanine residue and vancomycin binds to these residues and prevents elongation of the peptidoglycan backbone. Vancomycin may also impair ribonucleic acid (RNA) synthesis. The drug exhibits time dependent killing with moderate persistent effects and the 24-hour area under the curve/minimum inhibitory concentration (AUC/MIC) ratio has been described as the optimum pharmacokinetic-pharmacodynamic (PK-PD) parameter.

Spectrum of Activity

Vancomycin is primarily a drug with activity against gram-positive organisms. Except for certain *Neisseria* species (not *gonorrhea* or *meningitides*) and *Elizabethkingia meningosepticum* (formerly known as *Flavobacterium meningosepticum*), it has no gram-negative activity. Vancomycin has no activity against mycobacteria, rickettsiae or chlamydia. The drug is slowly bactericidal against sensitive organisms; however, enterococci are only inhibited and not killed if the drug is used alone with achievable serum concentrations. The combination of vancomycin and an aminoglycoside is bactericidal against enterococci unless high-level aminoglycoside resistance is present.

Its spectrum of activity includes both methicillin-sensitive and resistant strains of *Staphylococcus aureus* and most strains of coagulase-negative staphylococci. These organisms have vancomycin MICs in the range 0.25–4.0 mg/L. There have been case reports of coagulase-negative *Staphylococcus* resistant to vancomycin from the late 1980s, however, these are still fairly rare. Streptococci, including viridans species, anaerobic and microaerophilic strains, and penicillin-sensitive and resistant pneumococci are all susceptible to vancomycin. The clinically achievable levels of vancomycin in serum inhibit most strains of *Listeria monocytogenes*, however therapeutic failures have been reported and this drug is not recommended for Listeria infections, especially of the central nervous system (CNS). The nondiphtheroid corynebacteria including *Corynebacterium jeikeium* are susceptible in vitro to vancomycin. The anaerobic spectrum of vancomycin includes anaerobic and microaerophilic streptococcus, and clostridia species, including both *Clostridium perfringens* and *Clostridium difficile*. The susceptibility of actinomycetes is variable.

The clinician should be aware of gram-positive organisms, which should be considered intrinsically vancomycin resistant unless shown to be otherwise by MICs. These include opportunistic pathogens like *Lactobacillus, Leuconostoc, Pediococcus,* and often *Listeria*.

Drug Resistance

Acquired resistance to vancomycin was unusual until the late 1980s, when reports of enterococci resistant to glycopeptides were reported. Vancomycin-resistant enterococci (VRE) usually are *Enterococcus faecium*, but vancomycin resistance has also been seen in *E. faecalis, E. gallinarum, E. casseliflavus, and E. avium.* The mechanism of resistance in these organisms is usually due to a change in the amino acids at the site of action of vancomycin. Instead of the peptidoglycan ending in D-alanyl-D-alanine bipeptide the drug-resistant organisms bipeptide terminates in D-alanyl-D-lactate. This removes the site for vancomycin to bind and causes the organism to become resistant to the drug.

Beside enterococci, over the last 5 years, this mechanism of resistance has also been recently reported in a few clinical strains of *S. aureus*. These strains, the first isolates of *S. aureus* truly vancomycin resistant have been labeled as vancomycin-resistant *S. aureus* (VRSA) (MIC > 16 μg/mL), were first seen in a patient in USA who was infected with a MRSA isolate and had concomitant isolation of a VRE from wounds and stool. The *VanA* gene complex, which mediated the vancomycin resistance in VRE was transferred to the MRSA isolate leading to *S. aureus* isolate that was both MRSA as well as vancomycin resistant. Prior to this, there had been isolates of *S. aureus* that had reduced susceptibility to vancomycin labeled as vancomycin or glycopeptide-intermediate *S. aureus* (VISA/GISA), MIC of 4–8 μg/mL. These isolates become less susceptible to vancomycin by increasing their cell wall size with increased production of D-alanyl-D-alanine bipeptides in its peptidoglycan cell wall. Vancomycin binds to these dipeptides and is unable to reach in sufficient amount at the level of the cytoplasmic membrane leading to a decreased susceptibility.

It is important to note that the major factor that has driven the rise of both methicillin/oxacillin resistance in *S. aureus* as well as VRSA is the use/overuse of vancomycin in the hospital setting. Thus, it is imperative that the drug be used carefully and if culture results show that therapy can be simplified, it be done as soon as possible.

Pharmacokinetics

The drug is primarily used in IV form. The oral route may be effectively used for treating pseudomembranous colitis, but cannot be used for treating systemic infections, as there is minimal to no absorption of the drug from the gastrointestinal (GI) tract. However, in exceptional circumstances in individuals with both inflammation in the GI tract and renal failure, administration of vancomycin orally may result in potentially high serum concentrations of vancomycin. The drug can be used intraperitoneally for treating continuous ambulatory peritoneal dialysis (CAPD)-associated peritonitis. The intramuscular route of administration causes severe pain and should not be used.

When treating systemic infections in critically sick patients, vancomycin is administered using a loading dose by slow IV therapy to avoid infusion related side effects. The duration of the dose should be longer than 1 hour. The PK distribution of vancomycin is consistent with two or three compartment model, with an initial distribution phase followed by an intermediate half-life of approximately 1 hour. The half-life varies between 3 hours and 11 hours in patients with normal renal function. The drug does have a significant postantibiotic effect, which has been demonstrated both in vitro and in vivo.

At a steady state, drug levels above 75% of serum levels are achievable in synovial, ascitic, and pericardial fluid. Vancomycin also achieves good levels in pleural fluid and in bile. It, however, does not achieve good cerebrospinal fluid (CSF) levels, except in the presence of meningeal inflammation. The degree of vancomycin penetration of the CSF increases in direct proportion to the severity of meningeal inflammation, but higher doses of 15 mg/kg are recommended to treat patients with meningitis. When used intraperitoneally greater than 50% of the drug can be found in the serum suggesting significant systemic absorption. The drug has good bone penetration, enough to treat osteomyelitis however its lung parenchymal penetration is controversial. This low penetration in lungs is suggested as a cause of vancomycin's failure in severe MRSA pneumonia.

The drug is excreted primarily unchanged by the kidneys by glomerular filtration, and as renal function declines, its half-life increases and may exceed 7 days in patients with no renal function.

The recommended trough levels for serious infections and children are 15–20 mg/L while in nonserious skin and soft-tissue infections levels of 5–10 mg/L are generally adequate. While routine monitoring of vancomycin trough drug levels is desirable, it is often not possible due to cost and availability. However, monitoring is recommended in obese patients, presence of renal failure, patients on hemodialysis (HD), and those with rapidly changing renal function and for serious infections. There is no indication to monitor peak levels of the drug.

Indications

Vancomycin is indicated for use for serious infections due to susceptible bacteria. As the above spectrum of activity discussion indicates, these would be infections caused by most gram-positive bacteria with exception of those caused by *Leuconostoc, Lactobacillus, Pediococcus,* and often *Listeria.* The main utility of the drug is to treat infections caused by MRSA, ampicillin-resistant enterococci, and for serious infections caused by penicillin-resistant pneumococci. It is also used to treat gram-positive infections in patients who are unable to tolerate beta-lactam antibiotics due to side effects or allergy. The drug can be used for infections such as endocarditis, bacteremias, brain abscesses, meningitis, ventriculitis, osteomyelitis, septic arthritis, peritonitis, renal infections, and skin and soft-tissue infections such as cellulitis and pyomyositis. The drug is indicated for use in meningitis, but physicians using it should be aware of its poor penetration into CSF and patients should be carefully monitored for any signs of therapeutic failure. However, the drug should be used cautiously in patients with vancomycin MIC of 2 μg/mL; though this MIC is at the susceptibility breakpoint of 2 mcg/ml, data suggests higher risk of therapeutic failure.

The addition of a second drug such as an aminoglycoside or rifampin is often suggested when dealing with persistent bacteremia due to MRSA, however, recent studies suggest an increase in toxicity when using dual therapy especially when using aminoglycosides hence routine use is not recommended. The addition of rifampin is recommended especially when dealing with infections involving prostheses, such as prosthetic joints infections or prosthetic valve endocarditis or treatment of penicillin-resistant *Streptococcus pneumoniae* meningitis with ceftriaxone MIC more than 4 µg/mL or where repeat CSF does not show improvement or where dexamethasone has been used.

Oral vancomycin is used for treatment of pseudomembranous colitis caused by *C. difficile*. The use of IV vancomycin is not effective for this infection because of the lack of excretion/penetration of IV vancomycin into the gut.

Vancomycin is useful for the prevention of bacterial endocarditis in high risk, penicillin-allergic patients undergoing dental procedures. Vancomycin is also used for surgical prophylaxis into patients known or suspected of being colonized with MRSA.

Dosage

In adult patients with normal renal function 15–20 mg/kg every 8–12 hours is the usual dose of vancomycin. For serious infections including meningitis, osteomyelitis the vancomycin troughs should be between 15 mg/L and 20 mg/L. To achieve these levels, it is recommended to follow weight and age-based dosing to avoid underdosing. The maximum single individual dose should not exceed 2 g. In patients who are very sick and with severe infections, a loading dose of 20–30 mg/kg may be given (maximum dose 2 gm); the efficacy of loading dose is uncertain.

Pediatric Dosage

The 2011 guidelines from Infectious Diseases Society of America recommend dosing vancomycin at 15 mg/kg every 6 hours when treating MRSA infections in pediatrics and aiming for a trough of 15–20 g/mL.

Vancomycin doses in premature infants are based on gestational age as follows:

- Less than 27 weeks: 27 mg/kg every 36 hours
- 27–30 weeks: 24 mg/kg every 24 hours
- 31–36 weeks: 18 mg/kg every 24 hours
- More than 37 weeks: 22.5 mg/kg every 12 hours.

Vancomycin is virtually eliminated by the kidney, and since vancomycin elimination correlates directly with creatinine clearance, the dosage can be based on creatinine clearance rather than on a simple determination of serum creatinine level. With decrease in creatinine clearance the duration of the interval between doses can be progressively increased from 12 hours based on the drop in the clearance. The trough of the drug should be monitored on a regular basis to adjust the interval of administration and for achieving therapeutic levels. Patients on HD should be given 500 mg intravenous (IV) every 2 days. Vancomycin dose can be repeated if necessary by monitoring serum vancomycin levels. Patients on CAPD can receive a loading dose of 30 mg/kg intraperitoneally, followed by 1.5 mg/kg in each peritoneal exchange or 7 mg/kg once daily. An option of using continuous vancomycin infusion giving a dose of around 2.5 g a day is used in parts of Europe and has efficacy similar to traditional divided dosing.

The suggested daily dose for intrathecal administration of vancomycin is 5–10 mg every 48 72 hours. Higher initial dose of 5–10 mg/day in infants and 15–20 mg/day in children and adults for treatment of meningitis, ventriculitis, and shunt infection is recommended.

When used orally for treatment of *C. difficile* colitis the dose is generally 125 mg four times a day for 10 days. Higher doses up to 500 mg QID are reserved for severe or fulminant colitis. Pediatric dose is 10 mg/kg four times a day with a maximum of 125 mg QID for nonsevere disease and maximum of 500 mg QID for severe colitis.

The duration of treatment with the drug is dependent entirely on the site and severity of the infection and the infecting organism. 2 weeks therapy is recommended for simple bacteremias, pneumonia, and pyelonephritis. Longer duration of therapy of up to 4–6 weeks is necessary for endocarditis, meningitis, brain abscess, and staphylococcal necrotizing pneumonias.

Side Effects

The initial preparations of vancomycin contained large amounts of impurities, and it was termed "Mississippi Mud" because of its brown discoloration. These impurities also led to significant side effects and thus early reports in the literature list a lot of side effects of the drug. With improvements in the manufacturing process of the drug these side effects have also decreased.

The most common side effect is the so-called "red man syndrome". It is an infusion rate related event and occurs 10–20 minutes after the start of infusion. The patient complains of itching and flushing of skin over the upper part of the body. This reaction occurs due to vancomycin-mediated histamine release and can be minimized and prevented by slowing the infusion rate. The occurrence of this reaction does not constitute vancomycin allergy and does not preclude its use. Vancomycin allergy though rare does occur and usually manifests as hypotension and urticarial rash.

The incidence of nephrotoxicity due to vancomycin was initially reported as high as 25%, but is generally considered a vast overestimation due to confounding factors in those studies. It is estimated that in individuals receiving vancomycin alone, the rate of reversible nephrotoxicity is less than 5%. However, in individuals receiving vancomycin with an aminoglycoside the risk of nephrotoxicity is enhanced and these patients need to have both drugs carefully monitored by drug levels and estimation of renal function. A retrospective review has suggested that vancomycin nephrotoxicity is associated with serum trough more than 15 mg/L.

Vancomycin-associated ototoxicity like tinnitus, vertigo, and hearing loss are usually associated with high serum levels (>40 mg/L) of the drug or concurrent use of ototoxic drugs or conditions such as meningitis that by themselves can cause hearing loss.

Hematological toxicity has been reported with vancomycin including neutropenia and thrombocytopenia. Vancomycin induced neutropenia usually occurs after weeks of therapy and is reversible after stopping the drug. It has no relationship to serum levels.

The drug can also cause phlebitis when infused via a peripheral vein. Other rare side effects reported include diarrhea, nausea, and abnormal liver function tests. It rarely can cause drug fever and two cases of hypotension and cardiac arrest due to the drug have been reported and were probably manifestations of severe allergy to the drug.

Clinically Significant Interactions

The only clinically significant drug interaction of vancomycin is with aminoglycosides when used together. This use may result in increased nephrotoxicity than associated with the use of either drug alone.

Contraindications

The only absolute contraindication to the drug is true vancomycin allergy. The drug should be carefully used and monitored in individuals with renal dysfunction or decreased hearing, however these conditions are not contraindication to its use. Patients with these conditions should have drug levels carefully monitored and a high trough level more than 15 mg/L as well as very high peak levels more than 55 mg/L should be avoided. The use of aminoglycosides and other nephrotoxic agents along with vancomycin should be minimized unless necessary and if used together both aminoglycoside as well as vancomycin levels should be carefully followed along with frequent monitoring of renal function.

Teicoplanin

Teicoplanin was first isolated through fermentation of an *Actinomyces* species from a soil sample from India in 1978. Teicoplanin is a mixture of different glycopeptides that are related to each other. Basic structure has a linear heptapeptide, the carbohydrates D-mannose and D-glucosamine, and an acyl residue that carries fatty acids. It is a large molecule with estimated weight of about 1,900 daltons.

Mechanism of Action

Teicoplanin like vancomycin inhibits bacterial cell wall synthesis and has bactericidal action. It interferes with the process of building new sections of cell wall peptidoglycan by binding to the D-Ala-D-Ala portion subunit. This step prevents growth of the new cell wall units and final cross-binding step.

Spectrum of Activity

Teicoplanin has activity against a wide variety of gram-positive organisms namely staphylococci (*S. aureus* and *S. epidermidis* including methicillin-resistant strains), most streptococci (*S. pneumoniae, S. pyogenes, and S. viridans)* and enterococci. It also has activity against *Corynebacterium* species (including *C. jeikeium*), *L. monocytogenes* and gram-positive anaerobic bacteria namely *Clostridium species, Peptostreptococcus, Actinomycetes,* and *Propionibacterium species. S. aureus* strains susceptible to vancomycin but resistant to teicoplanin have been described. VanA-type VRE strains are resistant to teicoplanin. Certain VanB-type VRE strains are susceptible to teicoplanin.

Pharmacokinetics

Teicoplanin is primarily used intravenously or intramuscularly, as its oral absorption is poor. Teicoplanin at the dose of 6 mg/kg IV achieves mean peak concentration of 111.8 mg/mL and trough levels of 14 mg/mL and the volume of distribution is 800–1600 mL/kg. It has high protein and tissue binding and it has low clearance and long half-life (83–168 hours). Teicoplanin achieves adequate concentrations in heart, pericardium, mediastinal tissues, lung and synovial, pleural, peritoneal and pericardial fluid. The bone concentrations are better than that achieved with vancomycin, as shown in animal studies. Penetration into CSF and vitreous fluid is not adequate. The teicoplanin population PK is highly variable in children, with a wider AUC distribution spread than for adults. Investigators from United Kingdom and Japan have proposed that therapeutic drug monitoring (TDM) should be a routinely carried out to minimize suboptimal concentrations. Children and burn patients clear the drug faster and need higher doses for treatment. Teicoplanin excretion is mainly through the renal route. It is dialyzable in significant quantities.

Indications

Teicoplanin is safe in all age groups ranging from neonates to elderly. Teicoplanin is indicated perioperatively for knee or hip implant related surgeries and prevention of bacterial endocarditis in penicillin-allergic patients. It can also be used perioperatively in patients known or suspected to have MRSA colonization or are at risk for it. Teicoplanin is used frequently in following clinical situations for resistant gram-positive coverage. Intraperitoneal instillation in CAPD-related peritonitis, neutropenic fever, nosocomial lower respiratory tract infections due to MRSA (teicoplanin achieves better levels in the epithelial lining fluid than vancomycin) and complicated skin and soft-tissue infections, and osteoarticular (osteomyelitis, native or prosthetic joint septic arthritis) infections. *C. difficle* colitis responds just as well to teicoplanin as it does to oral vancomycin, but is not commonly used for this purpose. Though teicoplanin has in some trials shown equal efficacy as compared to vancomycin in MRSA bacteremias and endocarditis, it is not recommended as the first-line agent for these indications.

The need for once daily administration, shorter infusion time, lack of infusion related side effects, less nephrotoxicity, and effectiveness by the intramuscular route make it an attractive alternative to vancomycin. However, clinical experience with vancomycin use is much higher than teicoplanin and hence vancomycin is considered the gold standard agent.

Dosage

Dose for normal renal function is 6 mg/kg/day and needs to be given once in 48 hours for creatinine clearance between 10 mL/min and 50 mL/min and once in 72 hours for clearance less than 10 mL/min, in HD and CAPD patients. Higher maintenance dose (12 mg/kg) of teicoplanin is recommended for treatment of septic arthritis. In serious infections caused by MRSA an initial loading dose of 12 mg/kg twice daily for 3 doses followed by 12 mg/kg once daily is recommended. Trough level monitoring is indicated for serious infections with recommended levels more than 20 mg/L (not available routinely). Duration depends on the site and severity of infection and to some extent on the causative pathogen. Please refer to the suggested duration guideline in the vancomycin section above. Intramuscular teicoplanin 400–600 mg/day can be given over several weeks to treat osteomyelitis caused by MRSA.

The recommended dose in children are three loading doses of 10 mg/kg every 12 hours followed by 10 mg/kg/day. These loading doses may be insufficient in children with normal kidney function and hence investigators in UK and Japan have recommended TDM and measurement of trough level to achieve recommended levels (15–30 mg/L) (not routinely available). A higher teicoplanin MIC value (≥2.0 μg/mL) in patients receiving teicoplanin may lead to treatment failure among patients with MRSA pneumonia. Teicoplanin can be administered as a bolus over 3–5 minutes or as a 30-minute infusion. Only the latter is recommended for neonates.

Adverse Effects

The toxicity profile of teicoplanin is much superior than vancomycin. Meta-analysis of the frequency of adverse events occurring in treatment groups shows significantly fewer reports of adverse events in patients receiving teicoplanin (13.9%) than in those receiving vancomycin (21.9%), less nephrotoxicity (4.8% versus 10.7%), and less potentiation of nephrotoxicity of aminoglycosides. Drug fever and rash are its most common side effects. There is some degree of cross-sensitivity between vancomycin and teicoplanin however the red man syndrome described with vancomycin infusion is extremely rare with teicoplanin. Ototoxicity is rare, and thrombocytopenia, leukopenia, and eosinophilia are other less frequent side effects. There was no significant difference found in renal (2.3%) or hepatotoxicity (5.8%) between teicoplanin trough levels of less than 20 μg/mL or more than 20 μg/mL.

Drug Interactions and Contraindications

The combination with rifampicin has been reported as no effect to synergistic to frankly antagonistic in small number of old studies. A more recent study done on biofilm-embedded MRSA isolates did not demonstrate synergy between teicoplanin and rifampin and all surviving isolates of MRSA developed resistance to rifampin. The only contraindication is a serious allergic reaction to teicoplanin.

LIPOPEPTIDES

Daptomycin

Daptomycin is a drug belonging to the lipopeptide class, is effective against many gram-positive organisms including MRSA and VRE and is characterized by very rapid bactericidal activity. The drug received approval for use by the US Food and Drug Administration (FDA) in 2003 for adults and in 2017 for children age 1–17 years. It is not recommended to be used in neonates based upon muscular and nervous system adverse effects observed in neonatal dogs, but has been used off-label in certain cases of recalcitrant MRSA/vancomycin-resistant enterococcal bacteremias.

Chemical Structure and Mechanism of Action

Daptomycin, a fermentation product of *Streptomyces roseosporus* is a 13-member amino acid cyclic lipopeptide with a decanoyl side chain. The proposed mechanism involves insertion of the lipophilic daptomycin tail into the bacterial cell membrane, causing rapid membrane depolarization and a potassium ion efflux. This is followed by arrest of deoxyribonucleic acid (DNA), RNA, and protein synthesis resulting in bacterial cell death. The bactericidal effect of daptomycin is rapid with greater than 99.9% of both MRSA and methicillin-susceptible *S. aureus* (MSSA) bacteria dead in less than 1 hour. This rapid cell death does not result in rapid bacterial cell lysis. The antimicrobial activity of daptomycin like the aminoglycosides and quinolones is concentration dependent and is associated with a prolonged postantibiotic effect. The drug is inactivated by pulmonary surfactant and therefore should not be used for pulmonary infections.

Spectrum of Activity

Daptomycin's spectrum of activity includes MRSA, MSSA, glycopeptide-intermediate *S. aureus* (GISA), methicillin-resistant coagulase-negative *Staphylococcus* species (CONS), and VRE. Daptomycin has also demonstrated potency against vancomycin-resistant *S. aureus* as well as linezolid and quinupristin/dalfopristin-resistant *S. aureus* and *E. faecium*. Furthermore, daptomycin is also effective against a variety of streptococcal groups such as the β-hemolytic streptococci including *S. pyogenes* (Group A) and *S. agalactiae* (Group B) as well as other *Streptococcus* species. Daptomycin is also potent against *C. jeikeium*, and a variety of gram-positive anaerobic species including *Peptostreptococcus* species, *C. perfringens*, *C. difficile*, and *Propionibacterium acnes*. It has no activity against gram-negative and atypical organisms.

Resistance

Daptomycin resistance appears to emerge gradually via multiple steps resulting in a heteroresistant subpopulation with elevated MICs to daptomycin. This is due to altered cell membrane charge, which leads to reduced binding of daptomycin and consequent reduced cell depolarization. The development of resistance has often occurred in patients with prolonged use, underdosing of the drug or uses in indications were the drug did not penetrate the site of infection. Resistance is more also common in those patients treated previously with vancomycin or those with high vancomycin MICs suggesting some cross-resistance with vancomycin.

Pharmacokinetics

The drug has poor oral bioavailability and hence must be dosed parenterally. Following parenteral administration, more than 95% of the drug binds to serum albumin and distributes primarily in the vascular compartment. The penetration into various tissues including bone, lung, and CSF is very low. The drug has a half-life of 8 hours and is primarily excreted unchanged in urine (80%). The developmental differences in children compared to adults such as the presence of increased total body water content lead to changes in the PK parameters of daptomycin in children such as lower peak daptomycin concentrations, increased volume of distribution, and more rapid clearance of the drug.

Therapeutic Uses

The drug has received FDA approval for management of complicated skin and soft-tissue infections and bacteremia with or without right sided endocarditis due to various gram-positive infections including MRSA and VRE. In children it has received approval for treatment of acute bacterial skin and soft-tissue infections.

Randomized controlled trials that evaluated daptomycin in adults from Europe, South Africa, and US patients with complicated skin and soft-tissue infections showed noninferiority of daptomycin against the comparator drug. Another randomized controlled trial that compared daptomycin with a β-lactam and aminoglycoside (given for the first 4 days only) combination therapy in adults with *S. aureus*, bacteremia with or without right sided endocarditis showed noninferiority of daptomycin to the comparator drug. Patients with left-sided endocarditis were excluded from the trial. While in the case of MSSA bacteremia both groups showed equal success rates, in those with MRSA bacteremia, the outcome of the daptomycin group was superior to the comparator. The difference was most pronounced in those with uncomplicated right-sided endocarditis. Excellent outcomes in patients with MSSA bacteremia (unlike with the experience with vancomycin) suggested that daptomycin may be useful empirical therapy in patients with suspected staphylococcal bacteremia where susceptibility results were pending. Several uncontrolled case series and the Cubicin Outcome Registry and Experience (CORE) database have reported successful outcomes with daptomycin in patients with diverse gram-positive infections including bacteremia and left-sided endocarditis with MRSA/VRE. Conversely, there have been case reports that describe treatment failures and emergent drug resistance with use of daptomycin in MRSA and enterococcal infections. Recent data advocates use of combination therapy of daptomycin with cephalosporins, tigecycline, gentamicin, rifampicin, and other drugs for serious infections including endocarditis.

As mentioned earlier, it should not be used to treat pulmonary infections unless these are septic infarcts arising from right-sided endocarditis, CNS, and urinary tract infections.

Pediatric Use

Data on efficacy and safety of daptomycin in children are limited, however in a recent study, data on the retrospective use of daptomycin in 146 pediatric patients was presented. In this study 109 out of the 146 patients had a documented gram-positive infection. The median age of these patients was 12 years and they received a median duration of therapy for 12 days. The most common indication for the use of daptomycin was catheter-related bacteremia. The majority of the patients (107 out of 109) had improvement in their condition and resolution of their infection by discharge.

Dosage

The recommended adult dosage of daptomycin is 4–6 mg/kg/day for skin and soft-tissue infections and 6–8 mg/kg/day for bacteremia/endocarditis dosed once daily. Recent studies have evaluated higher doses up to 12 mg/kg/day for endocarditis and have not noticed increased toxicity. In patients with renal failure and creatinine clearance less than 30 mL/minute, daptomycin should be given once every 48 hours.

However, these doses do not achieve adequate PK parameters in pediatrics and thus pediatric dosages are much higher. The usual dose recommended for children aged:

- 1–2 years is 10 mg/kg daily
- 2–6 years is 9 mg/kg daily
- 7–11 years 7 mg/kg daily
- 2–17 years 5 mg/kg daily.

Higher doses have been recommended in bacteremia and endocarditis. When used in salvage therapy in neonatal bacteremia dosage recommended is 6 mg/kg twice daily.

Adverse Effects

The most common side effects noted in clinical trials are nausea, constipation, and injection site reactions. The most significant side effect with daptomycin is elevation of creatine phosphokinase (CPK), noticed in about 3% of patients treated with daptomycin at dose of 4 mg/kg/day. Occasionally, it can cause rhabdomyolysis. Muscle complications usually present in the first week of starting therapy. CPK should be monitored weekly and daptomycin stopped if levels exceed 10 times normal or if there are symptoms of myopathy and CPK levels exceed 1,000. The symptoms resolve quickly after stopping therapy, but CPK elevation can persist for weeks.

Daptomycin can also cause acute eosinophilic pneumonia. The risk factors for development of this side effect based on unpublished data from the authors include use of high dose (>8 mg/kg) daptomycin and prolonged (>2 weeks) use. Patients typically present with development of fevers, and cough and bilateral infiltrates while on daptomycin. The condition can mimic hospital-acquired pneumonia and can lead to initiation of broader antimicrobial use, while typically discontinuation of daptomycin and initiation of steroids can lead to a rapid resolution of this condition.

Daptomycin can also be associated with development of acute interstitial nephritis (AIP), patients typically present with sudden and rapid development of acute nonoliguric renal failure usually within the first week of use. The condition is reversible with discontinuation of daptomycin and use of steroids. There are case reports of daptomycin-induced transaminase elevation and hence monitoring of liver function besides complete blood count (CBC), renal function tests (RFTs), and CPK is recommended. A rising C-reactive protein (CRP) after initial improvement in both clinical and laboratory parameters including CRP level has often been an early clue to daptomycin-induced toxicity and acute AIP in our experience.

The studies that have studied use of daptomycin in children have reported similar side effects with the caveat that because of limited number of patients in these studies, some of the more unusual side effects have not been reported.

Drug Interactions

Daptomycin is neither inducer nor stimulator of CYP450 system and hence has no significant interactions. Concomitant use of statins should be avoided due to increased risk of muscle complications.

Conclusion

Daptomycin is a welcome addition to the armamentarium of agents for gram-positive infections. Data is limited in children. Use of the drug can be considered in certain instances of severe MRSA and enterococcal (especially VRE) infections such as endocarditis, bacteremia, and infections of the skin and soft-tissue. It is also useful for treating MSSA infections in patients with serious beta lactam allergy. A relative indication is for outpatient parenteral therapy (OPAT) for *S. aureus* bacteremia and endocarditis since it is dosed once daily. The drug should not be used for CNS, bone and joint and lung infections, and when other effective agents are available.

OXAZOLIDINONES

Linezolid

The oxazolidinones belong to a new class of antimicrobials first synthesized in 1970s. They have a unique molecular structure and mechanism of action. Linezolid is the first molecule from this class approved for clinical use in year 2000. It has antibacterial activity against a broad range of gram-positive pathogens and few other types of pathogens.

Mechanism of Action

Oxazolidinones act via inhibition of initiation phase of bacterial protein synthesis. They bind to 50S ribosome and prevent synthesis of the 70S initiation complex. Because of this unique mechanism of action linezolid is not likely to develop cross-resistance with other antibacterial drugs.

Spectrum of Activity

Linezolid has good activity against a variety of clinically important gram-positive organisms including strains resistant to other antimicrobial agents, a few gram-negative organisms, anaerobes, and mycobacteria. Linezolid is bacteriostatic against *S. aureus* (methicillin sensitive and methicillin resistant strains), CONS, *E. faecalis*, and *E. faecium*. It has been shown to have bactericidal activity against *S. pneumoniae* and *S. pyogenes* (Group A streptococcus) and a few anaerobes. There are other gram-positive bacteria against which linezolid has been shown to have activity namely, *Corynebacterium* species, *Gemella, L. monocytogenes, Rhodococcus equi, and Erysipelothrix rhusiopathiae.*

Linezolid has some activity against *Neisseria* species and *Haemophilus influenzae,* but no useful activity against *Enterobacteriaceae*. It does have good activity against all species of *Pasteurella* which is a gram-negative. Linezolid has good in vitro activity against *Mycobacterium tuberculosis* including resistant strains and nontubercular mycobacteria as well as *Nocardia* species.

Resistance to linezolid remains rare with rates lower than 0.1%, mutations conferring resistance have been found on the *23S rRNA* genes. Resistance to linezolid has been reported in strains of MRSA and VRE. Resistance has been associated with prolonged linezolid courses in association with undrained abscesses and indwelling devices and has occurred most frequently in enterococci.

Pharmacokinetics

Linezolid is rapidly and completely absorbed after oral administration achieving bioavailability of 100%. IV dose of 600 mg 12 hourly results in peak concentration of 15 mg/mL. Elimination half-life of linezolid is about 5 hours. Linezolid achieves good levels in bone, lung, pancreas, and skin to inhibit pathogens of concern. It achieves higher lung epithelial lining fluid concentrations in comparison to glycopeptides like vancomycin. Linezolid exhibits several characteristics that promote CNS penetration including low plasma protein binding, neutral charge, low molecular weight, and amphiphilic nature.

Linezolid is metabolized by oxidation, 85% is excreted through renal route and rest fecal, 30–40% is excreted unchanged. Dosage of linezolid need not be adjusted in presence of mild to moderate renal or hepatic insufficiency. In HD patients, linezolid should be given postdialysis as the molecule and its metabolites are removed by dialysis.

Indications

Linezolid was approved in 2000 by US FDA for treatment of infections caused by gram-positive organisms (Table 1). Linezolid has shown great promise for the treatment of multi-resistant gram-positive organisms. Concurrently with the increase in serious infections in children due to resistant gram-positive bacteria, linezolid use in pediatrics has expanded and will likely result in a widening of the current linezolid indications. Linezolid use in children was found to be associated high clinical cure rates (75.0–93.2%).

TABLE 1: Linezolid: US Food and Drug Administration (FDA) approved indications for clinical use.

Condition	*Caused by*
Infections	*Enterococcus faecium* (VRE)
Nosocomial pneumonia	*Staphylococcus aureus* (MRSA and MSSA) *Streptococcus pneumoniae*
Community-acquired pneumonia	*Streptococcus pneumoniae* *Staphylococcus aureus*
Uncomplicated skin and skin structure infections	*Staphylococcus aureus* *Streptococcus pyogenes*
Complicated skin and skin structure infections	*Staphylococcus aureus* *Streptococcus pyogenes* *Streptococcus agalactiae* (Group B *Streptococcus*)

(MRSA: methicillin-resistant *Staphylococcus aureus*; MSSA: methicillin-susceptible *Staphylococcus aureus*; VRE: vancomycin-resistant enterococci)

Methicillin-resistant Staphylococcal Infections (MRSA and MRSE)

In multiple multicenter randomized controlled phase 3 trials, efficacy and safety of linezolid has been found comparable to vancomycin and other standard treatment options for infections caused by gram-positive bacteria. Linezolid has been shown to be as effective as oxacillin and vancomycin for the treatment of skin and soft-tissue infections caused by MSSA and MRSA. MRSA infections of skin and soft-tissue, lung, and urinary tract have been treated with linezolid with success rate comparable to vancomycin. Some evidence suggests that linezolid may be superior to vancomycin for treatment of ventilator-associated pneumonia due to MRSA due to better lung penetration and faster microbiologic clearance. More recent meta-analysis data has failed to show superiority in clinical cure rates. With the rise in incidence of community-acquired MRSA, the need for using linezolid is increasing further. Linezolid can also be used as a protein synthesis inhibitor in patients presenting with toxic shock syndrome due to MRSA. Linezolid is not approved for treatment of catheter associated bloodstream infections since the trial did not demonstrate noninferiority to the comparator drug, but may be considered in patients whose bacteremia rapidly clears and is not related to an endovascular focus. Adults and children have been successfully treated with complicated skin and soft-tissue infections, bone and joint infections, pneumonia and empyema, and postneurosurgical infections caused by MRSA with IV linezolid followed by oral linezolid. Linezolid is not recommended for the treatment of bacterial endocarditis and meningitis caused by *S. aureus.*

Vancomycin-resistant Enterococcal Infections

Bacteremia, osteomyelitis, endocarditis, and even postoperative CNS infections have been successfully treated with linezolid.

Streptococcus Pneumoniae

Community-acquired pneumonia (CAP) caused by penicillin-resistant strains have been successfully treated by linezolid. Linezolid should not be used alone as a first-line drug for treatment of CAP as it has limited activity against other agents causing CAP namely *H. influenzae, Mycoplasma,* and *Chlamydia* species. It has also been used to treat penicillin/cephalosporin-resistant *S. pneumoniae* meningitis in place of vancomycin.

Multidrug-resistance and Extensively Drug-resistant Tuberculosis

A key PD parameter for *M. tuberculosis* has been reported to be the area under the curve over a 24-h dosing interval $(AUC)_{24}$/MIC. This fact along with the slow growth of *M. tuberculosis* and the high concentration achievable in serum and tissues allows daily-half dosage of linezolid to be effective. Some studies have shown effectiveness of even 300 mg daily in treatment. The drug is a very important component in regimes for treating pre-extensively drug-resistant (XDR) and XDR tuberculosis and has been significantly associated with cure in multidrug regimes. However, side effects such as peripheral and optic neuropathy have been reported from its long-term use. Recently, this drug has been upgraded to a category A drug by the WHO for inclusion in an all oral regime to treat multidrug-resistance (MDR) tuberculosis.

Nontuberculous Mycobacteria Infections

Linezolid has shown promising results when used as combined treatment with other drugs against antibiotic-resistant nontuberculous mycobacteria (NTM), especially the rapid growers including *Mycobacterium abscessus.*

Nocardia Infections

Linezolid has been successfully used for the treatment of infections due to *Nocardia asteroides, Nocardia otitidiscaviarum, Nocardia brasiliensis,* and *Nocardia farcinica,* in studies including adult patients. *N. farcinica* is most often associated with antibiotic resistance and more than 50% of cases involve disseminated infection. Linezolid appears to be a good alternative for the treatment of *Nocardia* species infections in cases in which trimethoprim-sulfamethoxazole (TMP-SMX) has failed or its use is contraindicated (allergy or side effects) or where a second agent is indicated, and no other options exist.

Dose, Frequency, and Duration

The recommended dose of linezolid for adults is 600 mg orally or IV twice daily for most infections and 400 mg twice daily for skin and soft-tissue infections. In infants and children 10 mg/kg 8 hourly (maximum 600 mg thrice daily) is recommended. Duration of administration usually depends upon the site and severity of infection and clinical response. Duration as short as 7 days for skin and soft-tissue infections and as long as 6 weeks for bone and joint infections have been used. The maximum approved duration is 28 days.

It is dosed as 300–600 mg once daily in adults and 10 mg/kg once daily for treatment of mycobacterial infections.

Side Effects

Linezolid is a well-tolerated drug. Most commonly reported side effect is GI intolerance. The most frequently reported adverse events are diarrhea (from 3.1% to 16.8%), nausea and or vomiting (from 2.9% to 11.9%), and thrombocytopenia (from 1.9% to 4.7%). Reversible thrombocytopenia has been commonly observed worldwide in patients receiving linezolid for more than 2 weeks. The drug also depresses the white and red cell line with longer use. Serial monitoring of hematologic parameters especially platelet count is recommended. Linezolid must be used cautiously in patients already at risk for bleeding, patients with pre-existing low platelets, and patients on other medications that cause low platelet count.

Cases of peripheral neuropathy, optic neuritis, and vision loss have been described in children and adults. This side effect is most common with linezolid use duration of more than 28 days. Peripheral neuropathy is now being reported increasingly following its use in drug-resistant tuberculosis; it is painful and irreversible.

Serotonin syndrome with selective serotonin reuptake inhibitors (SSRIs) has been described (incidence about 3% with concomitant use). Serotonin syndrome has been reported with the use of linezolid because of its monoamine oxidase (MAO) inhibitory activity. Review of the cases reported in literature suggests that if clinical situation requires use of linezolid in patient on an SSRI, the two can be used together without waiting for a 14-day washout period and careful monitoring of symptoms and signs of serotonin syndrome.

Lactic acidosis (LA) from mitochondrial toxicity has been described with longer duration of linezolid use (6.8% in a retrospective chart review). Some patients can be asymptomatic with early linezolid induced LA, therefore, even if there are no symptoms, it is recommended that serum lactate concentrations are checked regularly especially patients on long-term treatment. Reversible tongue discoloration, superinfection with *Candida* species are some of the other less serious side effects.

Drug Interactions

Owing to its MAO inhibitory activity it should not be combined with adrenergic drugs such as adrenaline, dopamine, noradrenaline, phenylpropanolamine, and ephedrine, as well as with other drugs with MAO inhibitory activity including tricyclic antidepressants and SSRIs. It is suggested that drug-drug interaction (free online tools available) check be done each time linezolid is prescribed.

Contraindications

Linezolid formulations are contraindicated for use in patients who have known hypersensitivity to linezolid or any of the other product components. Linezolid should not be used in patients taking any medicinal product which inhibits MAOs A or B (e.g. phenelzine and isocarboxazid).

Caution

The cost of therapy of oral linezolid turns out to be nearly one-tenth of vancomycin and teicoplanin. However, because of ready availability and relatively low cost in India there exists a big potential for drug misuse and resistance. Widespread and prolonged uses of linezolid, especially amongst patients with device-associated orthopedic infections, have led to emergence of linezolid-resistant *S. aureus* (LRSA) at much higher numbers in India. Linezolid and other agents from this class have excellent activity against mycobacteria both tubercular and NTM and unnecessary use of this drug may lead to development of resistance and loss of a last resort option for drug resistant *M. tuberculosis* and NTM. Resistance in MTB and NTM to linezolid has already been described. Linezolid use in children should be limited, and to avoid unnecessary expansion of resistance its use should be reserved for situations where no other safe and effective options are available.

NEWER ANTIMICROBIAL AGENTS FOR TREATMENT OF GRAM-POSITIVE INFECTIONS (NOT AVAILABLE IN INDIA)

Lipoglycopeptides

The lipoglycopeptides are a relatively new semisynthetic class of antibiotics that have a lipophilic side chain attached to the glycopeptide molecule. The addition of the lipophilic side chain leads to an improvement in the activity of the drug against the bacterial cell membrane. The three lipopeptides that are available in the United States include telavancin (initial FDA approval 2009), oritavancin, and dalbavancin (FDA approved in 2014). These drugs are not available in India and are not yet indicated among children however, the unique PKs of oritavancin and dalbavancin deserve mention. These two drugs have long half-lives, which leads to infrequent dosing of these drugs. In addition, oritavancin is metabolized primarily via the liver which makes it an attractive option in patients with renal failure. The three drugs have indications for the treatment of skin and soft-tissue infections in adults caused by gram-positive organisms, while telavancin also is indicated in adults for the treatment of hospital-acquired pneumonia and ventilator-associated pneumonia caused by susceptible bacteria.

Structure

Telavancin is a synthetic derivative of vancomycin with dual mechanism of action. It inhibits cell wall synthesis and disrupts the bacterial cell membrane as well. Oritavancin is a semisynthetic lipoglycopeptide that has mechanism of action similar to telavancin and it inhibits RNA synthesis in addition. Dalbavancin is a semisynthetic compound that is partly derived from *Nonomuraea* species, an actinomycete with modification and substitution of the sugar moiety. It resembles teicoplanin by having a lipophilic side chain that binds to the bacterial cell membrane and prolongs the interaction of this drug with the bacteria. Dalbavancin acts by restricting cell wall synthesis in susceptible organisms by preventing formation of the peptidoglycans. It binds to the D-alanyl-D-alanine residue of the cell wall and thus disrupting the cross-linking of the cell wall, it also inhibits peptidoglycan synthesis by impairing transglycosylase activity leading to a dual mechanism of activity.

Spectrum of Activity

All three agents have good in vitro activity against *S. aureus* and *S. epidermidis* regardless of whether they are methicillin-resistant or methicillin-sensitive, as well as *Streptococcus* species. Both dalbavancin and telavancin are active against vancomycin-intermediate *S. aureus* (VISA), but not against VRSA. Oritavancin has activity against VISA and VRSA. Dalbavancin, oritavancin, and telavancin exhibit activity against VanB VRE, but have no activity against VanA with exception of oritavancin. The three lipoglycopeptides have activity against streptococci (including multidrug-resistant pneumococci) and clostridia. They have no activity against gram negative bacteria.

Pharmacokinetics/Pharmacodynamics

Dalbavancin is 95% protein bound and has excellent tissue distribution with half-life of 14.5 days. After a single 1,000 mg IV dose, serum and bone levels are above MIC90 for *Staphylococcus* even after 14 days. It has both renal and nonrenal excretion via feces. A single IV dose of the drug often is adequate to treat skin and soft-tissue infections and makes this an attractive option for use in situations where compliance with daily IV therapy may be a problem. Likewise, oritavancin has a prolonged half-life and treatment of soft-tissue infections does not require repeat dosing after the initial dose of 1,200 mg over 3 hours. No dose adjustment is required for renal or hepatic insufficiency.

Dosage

The PKs of dalbavancin have been studied in children suggesting that an age and weight-based dosing regimen may mimic adult parameters:

- *3 months to 6 years*: 15 mg/kg (1,000 mg maximum) on day 1 and 7.5 mg/kg (500 mg maximum) on day 8
- *6–18 years*: 12 mg/kg (1,000 mg maximum) on day 1 and 6 mg/kg (500 mg maximum) on day 8
- *Adults*: 1,500 mg once.

Side Effects

The side effects reported among adults include taste disturbances, risk of nephrotoxicity, and QT interval prolongation (especially in the presence of at-risk comedications) especially with telavancin; and transaminitis with dalbavancin and oritavancin. The drugs oritavancin and telavancin can interfere with coagulation tests results.

Future Role in Pediatrics

These newer agents, especially dalbavancin and oritavancin, may have a future role in treating children especially infections that often require long-term IV therapy such as MRSA bloodstream infections, endocarditis and osteomyelitis and septic arthritis. The advantage of the long half-life can lead to dosing these agents every 2 weeks and finishing treatment within two to three infusions.

Tedizolid

Tedizolid is a novel oxazolidinone prodrug (converted into active form by phosphatases) and like linezolid, it works by binding to the 23S ribosomal RNA of the 50S subunit, thereby preventing the formation of the 70S initiation complex and inhibiting protein synthesis. Its spectrum of activity is similar to linezolid, also covers some linezolid-resistant pathogens. Tedizolid has a longer half-life and good oral bioavailability that allows for once daily dosing and easy conversion to oral from IV. Tedizolid (a weak MAO inhibitor) has not been shown to interact with serotonergic agents in clinical studies. Its once daily dosing of 200 mg daily, shorter course of 6 days compared to 10 days of linezolid (for acute bacterial skin and skin structure infection) amounts to less GI and hematologic side effects. It was approved for clinical use by US FDA in 2014.

RECOMMENDED READING

1. Abdel-Rahman SM, Chandorkar G, Akins RL, et al. Single-dose pharmacokinetics and tolerability of daptomycin 8 to 10 mg/kg in children aged 2 to 6 years with suspected or proved Gram-positive infections. Pediatr Infect Dis J. 2011;30:712-4.
2. Arbeit RD, Maki D, Tally FP, et al. The safety and efficacy of daptomycin for the treatment of complicated skin and skin structure infections. Clin Infect Dis. 2004;38:1673-81.
3. Ardura MI, Mejías A, Katz KS, et al. Daptomycin therapy for invasive Gram-positive bacterial infections in children. Pediatr Infect Dis J. 2007;26(12):1128-32.
4. Burdette SD, Trotman R. Tedizolid: The first once-daily oxazolidinone class antibiotic. Clin Infect Dis. 2015;61:1315-21.
5. Charbonneau P, Hading I, Garaud JJ, et al. Targocid: a well-tolerated and easily administered alternative to vancomycin for gram-positive infections in intensive care patients. Intensive Care Med. 1994;20: S35-42.
6. Chiappini E, Conti C, Galli L, et al. Clinical efficacy and tolerability of linezolid in pediatric patients: a systematic review. Clin Ther. 2010;32(1):66-88.
7. Chow AW, Azar RM. Glycopeptides and Nephrotoxicity. Intensive Care Med. 1994;20:S23-9.
8. Cox H, Ford N. Linezolid for the treatment of complicated drug-resistant tuberculosis: a systematic review and meta-analysis. Int J Tuberc Lung Dis. 2012;16:447-54.
9. Cunha BA. Vancomycin. Med Clin North Am. 1995;79:817-31.
10. Dryden MS, Jones NF, Phillips I. Vancomycin therapy failure in Listeria monocytogenes peritonitis in a patient on continuous ambulatory peritoneal dialysis. J Infect Dis. 1991;164:1239-41.
11. Farber BF, Moellering RC. Retrospective study of the toxicity of preparations of vancomycin from 1974 to 1981. Antimicrob Agents Chemother. 1983;23:138-41.
12. Fowler VG Jr, Boucher HW, Corey GR, et al. Daptomycin versus standard therapy for bacteremia and endocarditis caused by *Staphylococcus aureus*. N Engl J Med. 2006;355:653-65.
13. Goetz MB, Sayers J. Nephrotoxicity of vancomycin and aminoglycoside therapy separately and in combination. J Antimicrob Chemother. 1993;32:325-34.
14. Graziani AL, Lawson LA, Gibson GA. Vancomycin concentrations in infected and noninfected human bone. Antimicrob Agents Chemother. 1988;32:1320-132.

15. Harwick HJ, Kalmanson GM, Guze LB. In vitro activity of ampicillin or vancomycin combined with gentamicin or streptomycin against enterococci. Antimicrob Agents Chemother. 1973;4:383-7.
16. James A, Koren G, Milliken J, et al. Vancomycin pharmacokinetics and dose recommendations for preterm infants. Antimicrob Agents Chemother. 1987;31:52-4.
17. Johnson AP, Uttley AH, Woodford N, et al. Resistance to vancomycin and teicoplanin: an emerging clinical problem. Clin Microbiol Rev. 1990;3:280-91.
18. Karkow DC, Kauer JF, Ernst EJ. Incidence of serotonin syndrome with combined use of linezolid and serotonin reuptake inhibitors compared with linezolid monotherapy. J Clin Psychopharmacol. 2017;37:518-23.
19. Levine DP. Clinical experience with daptomycin in bacteremia and endocarditis. J Antimicrob Chemother. 2008;62 (Suppl 3):iii35-9.
20. Liu C, Bayer A, Cosgrove SE, et al. Clinical practice guidelines by the infectious diseases Society of America for the treatment of methicillin-resistant *Staphylococcus aureus* infections in adults and children. Clin Infect Dis. 2011;52:e18-55.
21. Park IN, Hong SB, Oh YM, et al. Efficacy and tolerability of daily-half dose linezolid in patients with intractable multidrug-resistant tuberculosis. J Antimicrob Chemother. 2006;58(3):701-4.
22. Plouffe JF. Emerging therapies for serious gram-positive bacterial infections: a focus on Linezolid. Clin Infect Dis. 2000;31:S144-9.
23. Polk RE, Healy DP, Schwartz LB, et al. Vancomycin and the red-man syndrome: pharmacodynamics of histamine release. J Infect Dis. 1988;157:502-7.
24. Ramos-Martín V, Neely MN, Padmore K, et al. Tools for the individualized therapy of teicoplanin for neonates and children. Antimicrob Agents Chemother. 2017;61(10): e00707-17.
25. Roberts KD, Sulaiman RM, Rybak MJ. Dalbavancin and oritavancin: an innovative approach to the treatment of gram-positive infections. Pharmacotherapy. 2015;35:935-48.
26. Rose PC, Hallbauer UM, Seddon JA, et al. Linezolid-containing regimens for the treatment of drug-resistant tuberculosis in South African children Int J Tuberc Lung Dis. 2012;16(12):1588-93.
27. Schaison G, Graninger W, Bouza E. Teicoplanin in the treatment of serious infection. J Chemother. 2000;12(Suppl 5):26-33.
28. Spitzer PG, Eliopoulos GM. Systemic absorption of enteral vancomycin in a patient with pseudomembranous colitis. Ann Intern Med. 1984;100:533-4.
29. Steenbergen JN, Alder J, Thorne GM, et al. Daptomycin: a lipopeptide antibiotic for the treatment of serious Gram-positive infections. J Antimicrob Chemother. 2005;55:283-8.
30. Stevens DL, Herr D, Lampiris H, et al. Linezolid versus vancomycin for the treatment of methicillin-resistant *Staphylococcus aureus* infections. Clin Infect Dis. 2002;34:1481-90.
31. Stevens DL, Herr D, Lampiris H, et al. Linezolid versus vancomycin for the treatment of methicillin-resistant Staphylococcus aureus infections. Drugs. 2001;61:525-51.
32. Su E, Crowley K, Carcillo JA, et al. Linezolid and lactic acidosis: a role for lactate monitoring with long-term linezolid use in children. Pediatr Infect Dis J. 2011;30:804-6.
33. Thool VU, Bhoosreddy GL, Wadher BJ. Detection of resistance to linezolid in *Staphylococcus aureus* infecting orthopedic patients. Indian J Pathol Microbiol. 2012;55:361-4.
34. Van Bambeke F. Lipoglycopeptide antibacterial agents in gram-positive infections: a comparative review. Drugs. 2015;75(18):2073-95.
35. Yamada T, Kubota T, Yonezawa M, et al. Evaluation of teicoplanin trough values after the recommended loading dose in children with associated safety analysis. Pediatr Infect Dis J. 2017;36(4):398-400.

Polymyxins, Newer Tetracyclines and Fosfomycin

13
Chapter

Ketan Kumar, Rakesh Lodha

INTRODUCTION

Colistin, polymyxin B, tigecycline, minocycline, and fosfomycin are a significant addition to the armamentarium of drugs against gram-negative infections. They have assumed great importance in the current era with the advent of carbapenem resistance. Herein, colistin or polymyxin B is the backbone of therapy. The other drugs are generally used as companion drugs to improve efficacy and decrease emergence of resistance to colistin. They also have some niche indications as monotherapy. It is of paramount importance that these drugs are used wisely in proper doses since they constitute our current last line of defense against gram-negative infections.

COLISTIN

INTRODUCTION

Antimicrobial resistance among gram-negative bacteria, in particular *Pseudomonas aeruginosa, Acinetobacter baumannii*, and *Klebsiella pneumoniae*, has become a worldwide healthcare crisis with many of these pathogens showing limited or no susceptibility to currently available antimicrobial treatments. This problem is further compounded by the marked decline in the discovery and development of novel antibiotics. The limited therapeutic options have forced infectious disease clinicians and microbiologists to reappraise the clinical value of older antibiotics like polymyxins.

Colistin, or polymyxin E, is a cationic polypeptide antibiotic obtained from *Bacillus polymyxa* subspecies *colistinus*. It was discovered in 1949, and was initially used therapeutically in Japan and in Europe during the 1950s and in the United States in the form of colistimethate sodium (CMS) in 1959. Colistin was one of the first antibiotics with significant activity against gram-negative bacteria, notably *P. aeruginosa*. It exhibits rapid and concentration-dependent bactericidal activity. Colistin was largely replaced by aminoglycosides in the 1970s because of concern about nephrotoxicity and neurotoxicity. In the last 10–15 years, however, colistin has been used as a "salvage" therapy for infections caused by extensively drug resistant (XDR) gram-negative bacteria. These bacteria are usually resistant to carbapenems and only susceptible to two antimicrobial classes.

Because such a large gap exists between the years that colistin was used clinically, available pharmacokinetic and pharmacodynamic data are very limited. Thus, information regarding colistin toxicities and optimum dosing is not well defined, and no universal dosing for the antibiotic exists. In addition, reports have begun to surface of colistin resistance among the organisms that the drug is currently being used to treat. This increased rate of resistance has emphasized the need to provide adequate, effective dosing with minimal toxicity.

CHEMISTRY

Colistin consists of a cationic cyclic decapeptide linked to a fatty acid chain through an amide linkage. Based on the composition of amino acids and fatty acids, at least 30 different components have been isolated from colistin. Two major components are colistin A (polymyxin E1) and colistin B (polymyxin E2). The proportion of colistin A and colistin B in commercial material differs between pharmaceutical suppliers and batches.

Colistin is commercially available in two forms, (1) colistin sulfate and (2) CMS. Colistin sulfate is cationic and stable, whereas CMS is anionic and not stable in vitro or in vivo. Colistin sulfate has greater antimicrobial activity, but is also more toxic, so it is restricted to topical use. CMS is the form that is safer to administer parenterally because of its lower toxicity. CMS by itself has been shown to display little to no antibacterial activity and is considered an inactive prodrug of colistin. On parenteral administration, CMS is readily hydrolyzed to form partially sulfomethylated derivatives, as well as colistin sulfate, the active form of the drug.

MECHANISM OF ACTION

The mechanism behind colistin's bactericidal ability is thought to be indistinguishable from that of polymyxin B, the standard of the polymyxins. The target of antimicrobial activity of colistin is the bacterial cell membrane. Colistin binds with the anionic lipopolysaccharide (LPS) molecules by displacing calcium and magnesium from the outer cell membrane of gram-negative bacteria, leading to permeability changes in the cell envelope. The disruption of the outer membrane leads to leakage of the cell content and subsequently cell lysis and death. Another characteristic of colistin, which is of potential benefit, is its unique antiendotoxin activity, being able to neutralize bacterial LPSs. The significance of this mechanism for in vivo antimicrobial action, namely prevention of induction of shock through the release of cytokines, is not clear. There might be other, as yet unknown mechanisms, by which colistin brings about its bactericidal activity, but they have not been evaluated in clinical practice.

SPECTRUM OF ACTIVITY

Colistin has a narrow antibacterial spectrum of activity, with susceptibility mostly against common gram-negative aerobic bacilli. Most significantly, it displays in vitro activity against multidrug-resistant (MDR) or XDR gram-negative pathogens such as *A. baumannii*, *P. aeruginosa*, *E. coli*, *Enterobacter cloacae*, and *K. pneumoniae*.

Colistin is not active against some gram-negative aerobic bacilli (including *Pseudomonas mallei*, *Burkholderia cepacia*, *Proteus* species, *Providencia* species, *Serratia* species, *Edwardsiella* species, and *Brucella* species), gram-negative and gram-positive aerobic cocci, gram-positive aerobic bacilli, anaerobes, fungi, and parasites.

DRUG RESISTANCE

Resistance to colistin is uncommon and the mechanism of colistin resistance is poorly defined. Studies of colistin-resistant *P. aeruginosa* strains have suggested that alterations of the outer membrane of the bacterial cell are related to the development of resistance. These alterations may be in the form of:

- Reduction in LPS
- Reduced levels of specific outer membrane proteins
- Reduction in cell envelope magnesium and calcium contents
- Lipid alterations.

Resistance is postulated to be induced by a gene (PmrA), which modifies LPS resulting in reduced binding affinity of colistin and possibly related antimicrobial peptides to the outer membrane.

There are no standardized methods for colistin susceptibility testing. Recent data indicates that automated methods such as VITEK should not be used. They are prone to very major error misclassifying resistant isolates as susceptible. The broth microdilution method is preferred for susceptibility testing. The disk diffusion method cannot be used to test for resistance since polymyxins diffuse poorly in agar.

Development of resistance to colistin is a serious concern. As colistin is the last line of defense against virulent pathogens, resistance to this antibiotic may have devastating effects. Moreover, researchers have found that clinically selected colistin-resistant organisms, once emerged, have a potential to persist in the patients and the hospital environment and cause subsequent transmission. With the continued use of colistin for treatment of infection with various MDR gram-negative pathogens, it is likely that we will see an increasing number of instances of both de novo emergence of resistance and nosocomial spread. One of the possible methods to decrease the selection of colistin resistant strains without exposing the patient to toxicity associated with higher dosages might be to use a combination of colistin with other antibiotics.

PHARMACOKINETICS

Colistin sulfate and CMS are not absorbed by the gastrointestinal tract with oral administration. Following parenteral administration, ~ 60% of CMS is excreted in the urine during the first 24 h. The rest is converted by the kidney and the bladder to the active drug colistin. Hence, CMS is a relatively inefficient prodrug of colistin.

After nebulization with CMS, the systemic bioavailability of colistin is low but high levels of colistin have been found in the lungs. Even though meningeal inflammation enhances passage, the penetration across blood-brain barrier is limited, administration via the intraventricular or intrathecal route might be better.

The pharmacokinetics of intravenous CMS in adolescents with cystic fibrosis (CF) with a dose of 5–7 mg/kg/day in three divided doses has demonstrated a half-life of 3.4 h, volume of distribution of 0.09 L/kg, and total body clearance of 0.35 mL/min/kg. In patients on intermittent hemodialysis, repeating the dose after the session is advised. CMS is eliminated predominantly by the kidneys. In renal failure, the renal excretion of CMS is decreased resulting in a greater conversion to colistin. This explains the need to decrease the dose of CMS in renally impaired patients. Colistin is eliminated predominantly by the nonrenal route by means of mechanisms not yet fully understood. No biliary excretion has been reported in humans.

PHARMACODYNAMICS

Most pharmacodynamics data on colistin are from in vitro studies. Colistin displays concentration-dependent killing against susceptible strains of *P. aeruginosa, A. baumannii,* and *K. pneumoniae*, including MDR strains. Colistin concentrations in the vicinity of minimum inhibitory concentrations (MICs) or above result in extremely rapid initial killing, with large decreases in colony forming units per mL occurring as early as 5 min following exposure. For the susceptible strains of *P. aeruginosa*, the MICs of colistin sulfate range from 1 mg/L to 4 mg/L, while the values for CMS are significantly higher and range from 4 mg/L to 16 mg/L. A very modest postantibiotic effect (PAE) is seen only at high concentrations against *P. aeruginosa*. It has been shown in recent studies that colistin demonstrates "inoculum effect", i.e. both the rate and extent of killing by colistin are decreased at high compared to low inocula. Despite the often extensive initial killing observed against colistin-susceptible strains with exposure to colistin alone, regrowth is a common feature both in vitro and in vivo. Though, the exact reason for this regrowth is not known, but it is proposed that the colistin-susceptible strains harbor a subpopulation of colistin-resistant cells, which contribute to regrowth, and emergence of colistin resistance later.

Studies to determine which pharmacokinetic or pharmacodynamic index best predicted the antibacterial activity of colistin found that the overall killing was best correlated with AUC or MIC (the ratio of Area under curve to MIC). The identification of this index will be the key to designing optimal dosage regimens for patients.

CLINICAL USES

The use of colistin should be considered for the treatment of infections caused by gram-negative bacteria resistant to other antimicrobials or when treatment with these agents has been clinically ineffective. In the last decade colistin has been used to treat a wide range of infections [Ventilator-associated *Pneumonia* (VAP), bacteremia, central nervous system (CNS) infections, and urinary tract infection (UTI)] caused by carbapenem resistant gram-negative bacteria, in particular *P. aeruginosa, A. baumannii,* and *K. pneumoniae*, in critically-ill adult and pediatric patients. For antibiotic stewardship reasons colistin should not be employed for therapy, if other alternatives exist. Colistin is also a weaker and less efficacious drug if the isolate is susceptible to other beta-lactams including carbapenems and beta-lactam-beta-lactam inhibitor combinations.

Combination therapy is proposed for treatment of carbapenem-resistant infections. This is because case series describing the use of colistin in patients with carbapenem-resistant Enterobacteriaceae (CRE) have revealed high mortality (as high as that seen in patients receiving inappropriate therapy) in those patients who received monotherapy as compared to those who received dual therapy with carbapenem and colistin or triple drug therapy with carbapenem, colistin, and tigecycline. Combination therapy is also purported to reduce development of resistance as well as to be synergistic (due to enhanced entry of drugs in a cell membrane that has been disrupted with colistin). The cons of combination therapy include cost, adverse effects, and increased ecologic damage. Literature is divided on the role of combination therapy in treatment of carbapenem resistant infections. In a recently conducted randomized controlled trial (RCT) by Michel Paul et al. that compared use of colistin alone with colistin and meropenem in patients with severe carbapenem-resistant infections where most were *A. baumannii*, the latter was not found to be superior. However, most of the study patients had meropenem MIC's more than or equal to 16. A recent meta-analysis by Zusman et al. included data till 2016 from 22 studies, 28 comparisons (3 RCT) with CRE, pseudo, and *Acinetobacter*. The overall results favored combination with odds ratio (OR) of polymyxins versus combination with carbapenems of 1.58 (1.03–2.42) and Poly versus combination with tigecycline, aminoglycosides and fosfomycin

1.57 (1.06–2.32). If subgrouped by type of infection for *Klebsiella* bloodstream infection (BSI) OR was 2.09 (1.21–3.60) and hospital-acquired pneumonia (HAP) or VAP 0.69 (0.39–1.24). The high risk of bias and low quality of studies were limitations of this meta-analysis. The INCREMENT (Effect of appropriate combination therapy on mortality of patients with bloodstream infections due to carbapenemase-producing Enterobacteriaceae) study was a retrospective cohort study of 437 (375 *Klebsiella*) CPE bacteremias from 26 hospitals, 10 countries from 2004 to 2013. The most frequent carbapenamase was *K. pneumoniae* carbapenemase (KPC) (low carbapenem MIC) there was no difference between combination (35%) and monotherapy (41%). However, the combination was better than mono in the group with high mortality score (48% vs 62%). In the low mortality score, there was no difference (24% vs 20%).

Hence, the consensus is to use combination therapy for sick patients while monotherapy can be used to treat localized infections such as urinary tract, bone and joint and skin, and soft tissue. The other drugs used in the regime should be on the basis of susceptibility or local epidemiologic data and prior exposure and include carbapenems (only is MIC is ≤ 8, high doses and prolonged infusions), tigecycline, fosfomycin, aminoglycosides, cotrimoxazole, and sometimes rifampicin. Source control is crucial for carbapenem resistant infections to reduce the burden.

Bloodstream Infections

No specific comparative trials have assessed the effectiveness of colistin in MDR or carbapenem resistant gram-negative bacteremia. However, there are multiple case rep reports and case series in literature, which have demonstrated successful use of colistin in treating BSIs with carbapenem-resistant bacteria with response rates ranging from 60% to 100%. Combination therapy should be used as far as possible.

Pneumonia

The XDR gram-negative bacilli including carbapenem-resistant *Acinetobacter* and *Pseudomonas* have become a major cause of nosocomial pneumonia, especially in critically-ill patients requiring mechanical ventilation. Colistin is indicated for management of VAP caused by carbapenem-resistant organisms in combination with other drugs especially high dose tigecycline.

Inhaled colistin has been used as an adjunctive therapy to intravenous antibiotics for nosocomial pneumonia due to MDR organisms. However, there is minimal evidence of benefit when used in this setting. In a recent study, aerosolized colistin resulted in no extra benefit when given as an adjunct to intravenous colistin to patients with MDR gram-negative VAP. In a separate study, inhaled colistin was compared with inhaled saline in patients with VAP caused by either *A. baumannii* or *P. aeruginosa*. Although patients who used inhaled colistin had increased microbial eradication from the respiratory secretions, they had no difference in clinical outcomes and had an increased rate of bronchospasm compared with patients who used inhaled saline. Also, when used prophylactically, nebulized colistin did not appear to reduce the rates of VAP in intubated patients as compared to normal saline in an RCT involving 168 intubated adult patients. If inhaled colistin is used it should be administered with caution.

Respiratory Infections in Cystic Fibrosis

Pseudomonas aeruginosa frequently colonizes the airway of patients with CF, initially only intermittently, but generally evolving toward a chronic infection, almost impossible to eradicate.

As infection by *P. aeruginosa* has been related to a significant worsening in lung function, a need for aggressive treatment of the initial cases of intermittent colonization is commonly accepted, in order to prevent it from becoming chronic. Inhalation of CMS has been used in CF over the last two decades both for the treatment of initial colonization as well as for the treatment of chronic infections.

- *Treatment of initial colonization:* For the treatment of initial colonization, different treatment regimens have been proposed including inhaled tobramycin (80 mg every 12 h) or colistin (1–3 million IU every 12 h) alone or associated with systemic antibiotics (oral ciprofloxacin or other intravenous antipseudomonal agents) for a total duration of 3 weeks–3 months. Nevertheless, no properly designed studies have proved the superiority of any of these strategies or established their optimal duration.
- *Treatment of chronic infections:* CF patients with chronic *P. aeruginosa* infection are recommended to receive regular nebulized antipseudomonal antibiotic treatment, to avoid the development of acute exacerbations and preserve respiratory function. Nebulized tobramycin or colistin (eventually associated with oral ciprofloxacin) has been proposed, though no clinical differences have been proved so far.
- *Treatment of acute exacerbations:* For treatment of acute exacerbations of CF, a combination of two intravenous antipseudomonal agents is recommended. Antimicrobial treatment in these cases should be tailored by previous isolations and usually includes an antipseudomonal beta-lactam associated with an aminoglycoside. Colistin should be reserved as a second-line treatment in patients infected by XDR-gram-negative bacilli (GNB) or presenting intolerance to aminoglycosides.

CNS Infections

Intravenous treatment with colistin alone is not recommended for CNS infections with carbapenem-resistant GNB because colistin does not consistently cross the blood brain barrier in noninflamed or inflamed meninges. There are several case reports in literature citing successful treatment with intraventricular or intrathecal administration of colistimethate in children and adults with gram-negative meningitis. Literature has reported doses ranging from 3.2–10 mg given once daily for intrathecal administration and 10–20 mg/day for intraventricular administration in adults.

Other Uses

Good outcomes with intravenous colistin therapy have been reported in patients with carbapenem resistant gram-negative infections at other sites including UTIs, surgical site and soft tissue infections, intra-abdominal infections, bone and joint infections, and infective endocarditis.

Topical colistin sulfate has been used for conditions such as otitis externa and eye infections due to *P. aeruginosa*. Oral colistin sulfate has also been used in certain conditions for decontamination and sterilization of the gut especially prior to liver transplant.

Colistin in Febrile Neutropenia

With increasing prevalence of carbapenem resistant pathogens in febrile neutropenics, colistin in combination with other drugs is recommended therapy for febrile neutropenia especially in those who are in septic shock, have failed first-line regimes of beta-lactam–beta-lactam inhibitor or carbapenems or are known to be colonized with carbapenem resistant pathogens. The need to combine colistin with other drugs is especially important in this group of patients due to impaired host defenses.

Colistin Use in Neonates

There is increasing prevalence of carbapenem resistance in neonatal sepsis. A recent study published from New Delhi has reported carbapenem resistant rates of 40–80% in newborns even in neonates who were delivered at home and admitted directly to the study hospital. Studies have reported good outcomes and excellent tolerability with use of colistin.

Colistin Use in Children

In clinical studies, CMS has been safely and successfully administered to the pediatric population (including infants, children, and adolescents). The adverse effects related to colistin in this patient population appear to be no different from that of the adult population. In a recent systematic review of the use of colistin in children without CF, 271 children were evaluated and 86.5% were cured of infection. Nephrotoxicity occurred in 2.8% of children and no neurotoxicity was reported. In a prospective study of 29 critically-ill children, the authors concluded that intravenous colistin was well tolerated and effective for treatment of nosocomially acquired gram-negative organisms. There is also evidence for use of inhaled colistin in addition to intravenous colistin in children as it led to a quicker eradication of bacteria in a retrospective study, although it did not affect the clinical outcomes.

DOSING AND ADMINISTRATION

Systemic administration: Two formulations are commercially available for parenteral use. Both contain CMS powder for reconstitution, but they are formulated differently and have distinct dosing recommendations. The product available in the United States is supplied in vials containing 360 mg of CMS per vial (equivalent to 150 mg colistin base activity). The product available in India and many European countries is provided in vials of 1 and 2 million international units (IU) of CMS (One IU is defined as the amount of colistin that inhibits the growth of *E. coli* 95 I.S.M. in 1 ml broth at pH 7.2).

12,500 IU CMS = 1 mg CMS = 0.42 mg colistin base activity

The doses recommended by the Indian manufacturers are as follows:
- For patients less than 60 kg: 50,000–75,000 units/kg per day, in three divided doses.
- For patients More than 60 kg: 3–6 million units/day in three divided doses.

In patients with renal dysfunction, the systemic dose must be modified (Tables 1 and 2). Inspite of these dosing recommendations by the manufacturers, studies have shown that alternative dosing regimens including dose escalation and use of a loading dose may be more efficacious. As per this regime in adults, a loading dose of 9 million units followed by dosing @ 4.5 million units twice daily. This translates to a loading dose of 10–12 mg/kg of salt and maintenance dose of 5–6 mg/kg twice daily in neonates, infants, and children. Cure rates of more than 80% were achieved in patients with infections due to organisms susceptible only to colistin and reversible

TABLE 1: Dosing and equivalences of colistimethate in patients with normal renal function.

	Dosage recommended	*Equivalence in IU#*	*Equivalent dose of colistin base#*
Colistimethate sodium	12 mg/kg/day (q 8–12 h)	150,000 IU/kg/day (q 8–12 h)	5 mg/kg/day (q 8–12 h)

#1 mg colistin base = 2.4 mg CMS

TABLE 2: Dosing and equivalences of colistimethate in patients with impaired renal function.

Creatinine clearance	*Dose of colistimethate*	*Equivalence in IU#*	*Equivalent dose of colistin base#*
80–50 mL/h	9–12 mg/kg/day (q 12 h)	112,000 IU–150,000 IU/kg/day (q 12 h)	3.8–5 mg/kg/day (q 12 h)
50–10 mL/h	6 mg/kg/day (q 12 h–24 h)	75,000 IU/kg/day (q 12 h–24 h)	2.5 mg/kg/day (q 12 h–24 h)
<10 mL/h (anuria)	4.8 mg/kg/day (q 24 h)	60,000 IU/kg/day (q 24 h)	1.5 mg/kg/day (q 36 h)

#1 mg colistin base = 2.4 mg CMS; 1 mg colistin base = 30.000 IU; 1 mg CMS = 12.500 IU

nephrotoxicity was seen in around 15%. Though, the efficacy and safety of this regime needs to be evaluated further but it should be considered in critically-sick patients. At the same time, in a prospective cohort study that included critically sick adults, colistin administered at a dose of 6 million units per day without any loading, did not confer any mortality benefit on patients with MDR *A baumannii* VAP compared to those with colonization with the same pathogen. There is controversy regarding when to start the maintenance doses after the loading dose and intervals ranging from 12 h to 24 h have been suggested. Attempts have also been made to use a higher dose of colistin and studies using doses as high as 18 million units per day have been reported, however, the clinical outcomes have not been significantly different.

Inhaled administration: Inhalational administration of CMS is not approved by the Food and Drug Administration (FDA), but is common in CF clinics throughout the world. The dosage of CMS commonly used for inhalation in adults with CF is 40–60 mg two or three times a day. If inhaled CMS is used, it should be administered with caution. The drug breakdown products can cause direct damage to lung tissue, leading to potentially serious, and life-threatening side effects. This is particularly true for the premixed, ready to use liquid forms of the products. If colistin is to be used for nebulized inhalation, it must be mixed immediately prior to administration.

ADVERSE REACTIONS

The most important side effect of intravenous colistin is nephrotoxicity; neurotoxicity also occurs, although the frequency and severity are much less. Both renal and neurologic toxicity are dose-dependent and usually reversible after early discontinuation of the drug.

Nephrotoxicity

Colistin has been associated with hematuria, proteinuria, and oliguria and acute renal failure due to acute tubular necrosis. Colistin nephrotoxicity is ascribed to high delivery rates of CMS to kidney and conversion to the active drug. Nephrotoxicity rates of 30–40% have been described in patients on colistin therapy. It may be difficult to determine the relative contribution of colistin to development of acute renal failure since patients who receive colistin typically have complex clinical circumstances and many may be receiving other concomitant nephrotoxins. Nephrotoxicity, if it occurs, usually occurs within the first 4 days of therapy and mainly includes acute tubular necrosis, manifested as decreased CrCl and increased serum urea and creatinine levels. In a prospective cohort of adult patients, who were part of an RCT comparing colistin alone to colistin with rifampicin for XDR *A. baumannii*, one-third to half of the patients developed acute kidney injury (AKI), however, there was no effect on mortality and the therapy did not need to be discontinued. Higher risk was found to be associated with older age and pre-existing renal impairment. While using colistin, frequent monitoring of renal function is advised. Use of other nephrotoxic drugs should be avoided whenever possible.

Neurotoxicity

Neurological symptoms, which have been associated with the use of colistin, include dizziness, weakness, facial and peripheral paresthesia, vertigo, visual disturbances, confusion, ataxia, and neuromuscular blockade, which can lead to respiratory failure or apnea. The incidence of colistin-associated neurotoxicity reported in initial studies was about 7%; paresthesias were the main neurotoxic adverse event.

Other Adverse Effects

Hypersensitivity reactions (including rash, pruritus, urticaria, and fever) have been reported in 2% of patients. Other rare complications related to colistin administration are ototoxicity, drug fever, and gastrointestinal disturbances. Complications related to administration of aerosolized colistin are sore throat, cough, bronchoconstriction, and chest tightness. Bronchodilation prior to administration may be beneficial.

DRUG INTERACTIONS

Other antibiotics, which interfere with the nerve transmission at the neuromuscular junction (like aminoglycosides) should not be given concomitantly with colistin. Curare-like muscle relaxants (e.g. tubocurarine) and other drugs, including ether, succinylcholine, gallamine, and decamethonium potentiate the neuromuscular blocking effect. Concomitant administration of other nephrotoxic agents (gentamycin, amikacin, streptomycin, vancomycin, etc.) should be avoided, if possible. However, there may be instances when in the absence of other effective agents combination of aminoglycosides and colistin may be indicated for serious carbapenem resistant infections.

POLYMYXIN B

INTRODUCTION

Polymyxin B is one of the two polymyxin antibiotics, who have regained popularity in recent years in view of the burgeoning problem of antibiotic resistance, especially among gram-negative organisms, the other being colistin or polymyxin E. Interest in polymyxin B followed colistin due to some inherent disadvantages with colistin that will be discussed later. Data about polymyxin B is less as compared to colistin but is likely to increase with time.

CHEMISTRY

Polymyxins are composed of a fatty acid chain linked to a cyclical peptide ring via a tripeptide side chain. Single amino acid chain of D-leucine in polymyxin E or colistin is replaced by D-phenylalanine in polymyxin B. Commercially, polymyxin B is available as a sulfate salt. There can be variation among different batches of the antibiotic as it is a mixture of compounds having different molecular formula because of the polypeptide component, namely polymyxin B1, B2, B3, and B1-I. However, batch-to-batch variation of polymyxin B is less as compared to colistin.

MECHANISM OF ACTION AND SPECTRUM OF ACTIVITY

The mechanism of action and spectrum of activity is same as that of colistin.

PHARMACOKINETICS (FIG. 1)

It is here that there are significant differences between colistin and polymyxin B. Polymyxin B is an active drug in itself unlike colistin, which is available as a prodrug. There is no renal excretion (first pass effect in the kidney) of the drug unlike colistin. Hence, the lag time between administration of polymyxin B and achievement of steady state levels and hence onset of antibacterial effect is shorter as compared to colistin. This may be of advantage in patients with septic shock where quick onset of action is desirable.

The distribution of the drug is similar to colistin with the exception of renal handling mechanisms. The drug is filtered by the glomeruli and extensively absorbed in the tubular epithelial cells. Very little drug is excreted in the urine. Hence, it is not useful for treatment of UTIs. The excretion of the drug is by undefined nonrenal mechanism. Hence, the drug does not need dose modification in patients with renal failure or on renal replacement therapy including continuous renal replacement therapy (CRRT).

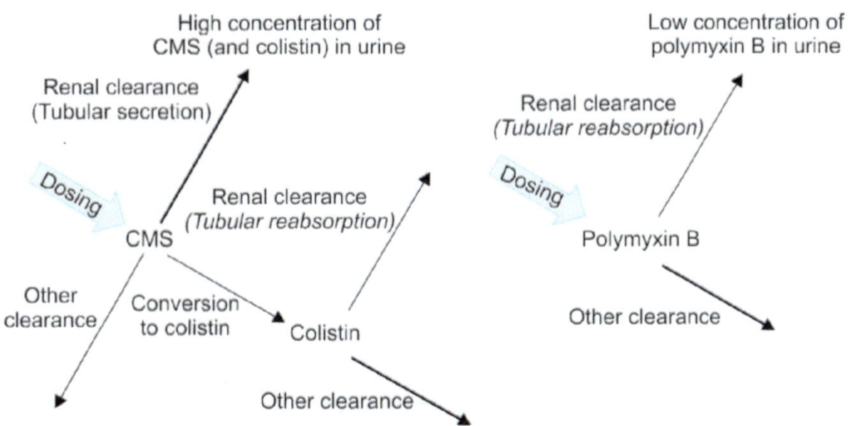

Fig. 1: Pharmacokinetics of colistin versus polymyxin B. (CMS: colistimethate)

CLINICAL USES

The clinical use of polymyxin B is same as that of colistin. However, experience is less than colistin. Since, it does not achieve good levels in the kidney and urine, it cannot be used for managing UTIs. However, it may be a superior drug in cases of septic shock since the pharmacokinetics is more predictable and time to achieve steady state level is less.

Unlike colistin, polymyxin B has found a unique use in direct neutralization of circulating endotoxins in patients with endotoxemia and septic shock. It is available as a plastic column containing polymyxin B-immobilized fiber fabric for adsorption and neutralization of endotoxins. First used in Japan, it is now available for use in 12 countries. Preliminary RCTs showed improved cardiac, renal, and mortality outcomes with use of this technology. However, the recently published randomized controlled blinded EUPHRATES (Evaluating the Use of Polymyxin B Hemoperfusion in a Randomized controlled trial of Adults Treated for Endotoxemia and Septic shock) trial conducted in the USA in 450 adults with septic shock and high circulating endotoxin activity, polymyxin B hemoperfusion compared with sham hemoperfusion did not significantly decrease 28-day mortality, 37.7% versus 34.5%, respectively.

DOSING AND ADMINISTRATION

Polymyxin B can be used intravenously, intramuscularly, intrathecally, and topically as polymyxin B sulfate. Each mg of polymyxin B base is equivalent to 10,000 IU of polymyxin B. According to the current recommended dosage, intravenous polymyxin B is to be used as a loading dose of 15,000–25,000 units per kg followed 12 h later by the same maintenance dose given 8–12 hourly. The intrathecal or intraventricular dose is 50,000 units. The drug has also been used via the inhalational route in dosage of 500,000 IU twice a day along with intravenous polymyxin B.

ADVERSE EFFECTS

Nephrotoxicity

There is considerable evidence to suggest that nephrotoxicity of polymyxin B is lower than that of colistin. Zavascki et al. summarized the overall incidence of AKI in patients treated with colistimethate (CMS) or polymyxin B. The incidences of AKI in CMS- and polymyxin B-treated patients, respectively, were 26.0% (10 of 39 patients) and 27.0% (8 of 30) in the study of Oliveira et al. 60.4% (64 of 106) and 41.8% (28 of 67) in the study of Akajagbor et al. 48.2% (40 of 83) and 23.1% (24 of 104) in the cohort without CF patients in the study of Phe et al. 38.9% (14 of 36) and 20.8% (20 of 96) in the study of Tuon et al. and 74.1% (60 of 81) and 46.1% (189 of 410) in the study of Rigatto et al. The exact reason for reduced nephrotoxicity is uncertain since the drug is extensively filtered and reabsorbed in the kidneys. It is believed that the handling of CMS by the kidneys and its conversion to colistin is the reason for increased nephrotoxicity of CMS.

Neurotoxicity

The incidence of neurotoxicity is higher with polymyxin B with chief side effects being weakness, paresthesia, ophthalmoplegia, dysphagia, and ataxia. There is also the risk of respiratory failure, if the drug is injected rapidly.

Other Adverse Effects

Other adverse effects include a small risk of congenital anomalies, pain upon intramuscular injection, hypersensitivity reactions, and bronchospasm with aerosolized administration.

TIGECYCLINE

INTRODUCTION

The main approach for developing new antibiotics in the past has been to modify existing drug classes to restore activity against bacteria that have become resistant to the previous generation of drugs. Tigecycline is the first in a new generation of tetracyclines, known as glycylcyclines, which have been developed to overcome the problems of resistance to earlier tetracyclines. It was approved by the US FDA for the treatment of a range of bacterial infections in June 2005. Although not yet approved for patients less than 18 years of age, its excellent safety and tolerability profile in adults suggest that it may be an important antimicrobial agent for children especially when therapeutic options are limited.

CHEMISTRY

The tetracycline nucleus consists of four linear fused tetracyclic rings, with a variety of functional groups attached at different positions. The glycylcyclines are obtained by adding N,N-dimethylglycylamido (DMG) substituent at the 9 position of minocycline and 6-demethyl-6-deoxytetracycline. Further modification of this structure led to the discovery of tigecycline (GAR-936), which is the 9-tert-butyl-glycylamido derivative of minocycline. Tigecycline is the only member of the glycylcyclines group of antibiotics, which has been approved for clinical use.

MECHANISM OF ACTION

Tigecycline, like the tetracyclines, acts by inhibiting bacterial protein synthesis. It binds to the A-site on 30S subunit of ribosome and blocks the entry of aminoacyl-transfer ribonucleic acid (tRNA) into the respective ribosomal binding sites. This prevents the incorporation of amino-acid residues into the elongating peptide chain. Although the mechanism of action of tigecycline is same as other tetracyclines, it has distinct advantages over the other members of the group. This is because tigecycline appears to assume a different steric conformation, owing to the large substituent at position 9. This results into high affinity of binding of tigecycline to the ribosome, and thus into evasion of the common ribosomal protection mechanisms that are associated with resistance to tetracyclines. Additionally, tigecycline has the property to evade common tetracycline efflux mechanisms.

SPECTRUM OF ACTIVITY

Tigecycline has a broad spectrum of antimicrobial activity, which includes aerobic and anaerobic gram-positive and gram-negative bacteria, as well as atypical pathogens. Specifically, tigecycline has been shown to possess excellent antimicrobial activity against methicillin-resistant *Staphylococcus aureus* (MRSA), Vancomycin-resistant Enterococci (VRE), and penicillin nonsusceptible *Streptococcus pneumoniae*. It has also demonstrated potent antimicrobial activity against extended-spectrum beta-lactamase (ESBL)-producing *Escherichia coli* and *K. pneumoniae*. Additionally, it constitutes one of the few potentially active agents against carbapenem-resistant *A. baumannii*, which typically exhibits resistance to all beta-lactam agents.

Though tigecycline has a wide spectrum of activity, it shows low activity against *Proteus* and is not active against *Providencia* species and *Pseudomonas aeruginosa*, due to the production in these organisms of chromosomally encoded resistance nodulation division (RND) type efflux pumps that recognize tigecycline as a substrate. Furthermore, the activity of this agent is not optimal against *B. cepacia*, *Stenotrophomonas maltophilia*, *Legionella pneumophila*, and certain members of the *Bacteroides fragilis* group.

DRUG RESISTANCE

Tigecycline is inherently not active against *Pseudomonas* species, *Proteus* species., *Providencia* species, and *Morganella morganii* due to the production in these organisms of chromosomally encoded RND type efflux pumps that recognize tigecycline as a substrate.

There have been recent reports of emerging tigecycline resistance among *Acinetobacter* species. In a prospective study conducted at PGI Chandigarh, which included isolates from urine of patients with complicated UTI, it was found that 14.2% isolates of *Acinetobacter calcoaceticus—A. baumannii* complex were resistant to tigecycline. Astonishingly, a study from Israel found 66% MDR *A. baumannii* had resistance to tigecycline. The mechanisms of resistance to tigecycline in *A. baumannii* should be elucidated; there may be a possible role of an efflux pump mechanism.

The increasing resistance to tigecycline is of great concern. Microbiological documentation prior to treatment with exact determination of tigecycline MIC is very important; some organisms with borderline susceptibility are difficult to eradicate and are prone to development of resistance on treatment.

PHARMACOKINETICS

A single intravenous tigecycline dose of 100 mg results in a C_{max} (peak serum concentration) of 0.85 to 1 mg/L, and an extended half-life of 27 h. In vitro plasma protein binding ranges from 71% to 89% at concentrations observed in clinical studies. The steady-state volume of distribution averages 7–9 L/kg. The large volume of distribution of tigecycline reflects the high penetration of this drug into tissues and low levels in the serum. In a study evaluating, the degree of tissue penetration of tigecycline in 104 patients undergoing various types of scheduled surgical interventions or lumbar puncture, it was found that the penetration of the drug was highest in bile, followed by gallbladder, colon, and lung tissue, whereas tigecycline exposure in bone, and synovial or cerebrospinal fluid was lower compared to serum.

Tigecycline is partially metabolized in the liver and the major elimination of unchanged drug and its metabolites is through biliary excretion into the gastrointestinal tract. The two major pathways of tigecycline metabolism in the liver consist of glucuronidation, and amide hydrolysis to *t*-butylaminoacetic acid and 9-amino-minocycline. None of the above products of tigecycline metabolism and degradation is considered to have significant pharmacological activity. In patients with severe hepatic impairment (Child-Pugh class C), the systemic clearance of tigecycline is decreased by approximately 55%, and the elimination half-life (is prolonged by approximately 43% compared to healthy subjects. So, in this group of patients (Child-Pugh class C), the maintenance doses of tigecycline should be reduced by 50%. Less than 15% of tigecycline is excreted unchanged in urine and renal clearance accounts for less than 20% of total clearance. Tigecycline kinetics in subjects with severe renal failure as well as in those with end-stage renal impairment treated by hemodialysis indicates that no dosage adjustment is required. It has also been shown that the amount of tigecycline removed by hemodialysis is minimal and the timing of administration of tigecycline with regard to the hemodialysis procedure does not appear to influence the tigecycline pharmacokinetics considerably.

PHARMACODYNAMICS

Regarding tigecycline, due to prolonged PAE against most pathogens, along with extensive volume of distribution, and prolonged elimination half-life in humans, the AUC/MIC ratio has been proposed as the most important predictor of clinical and microbiological efficacy.

Tigecycline, similarly to tetracyclines, exhibits in general a bacteriostatic pattern of antibacterial activity. However, this depends on the pathogen and strain examined, for example—tigecycline has demonstrated bactericidal activity against *S. pneumoniae* in several relevant studies.

CLINICAL APPLICATIONS OF TIGECYCLINE

Tigecycline was approved in 2005 by the US FDA and in 2006 by the European Medicines Agency (EMEA) for the treatment of complicated skin and skin structure infections (cSSSIs) and complicated intra-abdominal infections (cIAIs) in adults. In March 2009, the FDA approved tigecycline for the treatment of community-acquired pneumonia (CAP) caused by *S. pneumoniae* (penicillin-susceptible isolates), *H. influenzae* (beta-lactamase negative isolates) and *L. pneumophila*. Tigecycline is not currently approved for infections caused by MDR or XDR organisms; despite that, off-label use is increasing globally for indications such as nosocomial sepsis or septic shock, bacteremia and VAP in the critically-ill ICU patients. This is because of the appealing in vitro spectrum of tigecycline and the lack of other active antimicrobial agents against the XDR pathogens except for colistin.

Complicated Skin or Skin Structure Infections and Intra-abdominal Infections

Two phase-3, randomized, and double-blind studies evaluating the efficacy of tigecycline, compared with vancomycin plus aztreonam, were conducted in hospitalized patients with complicated skin or skin-structure infections. On analyzing the results, the overall clinical cure rates were similar (86.5% for tigecycline and 88.6% for vancomycin-aztreonam) in the two groups. Microbiological success rates were also comparable in the two treatment groups (86% vs 88%). Of note, tigecycline was as effective as vancomycin-aztreonam (78% vs 76%) in eradicating strains of MRSA. Moreover, all eight strains of *B. fragilis* isolated in the tigecycline treatment group were eradicated. In another open label randomized study, tigecycline was noninferior to therapy with aminopenicillin plus beta-lactamase inhibitor ± vancomycin for treatment of complicated skin or skin structure infections.

A pooled analysis of two phase-3, double-blind, randomized studies comparing tigecycline with imipenem-cilastatin in patients with cIAIs showed that overall, clinical cure rates were similar (86%) in the two treatment groups. Bacterial eradication rates were also similar between groups. In another randomized controlled trial, tigecycline was found to be noninferior to a combination of ceftriaxone and metronidazole for the same indication.

In summary, tigecycline has exhibited noninferiority to other standard treatments for cSSSIs and cIAIs. Although there are several antibiotic combinations that can be used to treat these infections, tigecycline is unique for its ability to be used as monotherapy for empirical coverage of various drug-resistant pathogens. But again, using this drug when other agents are available should preferably be avoided to preserve the shelf life of this drug for resistant strains, which are only susceptible to the polymyxins.

Pneumonia

Tigecycline has been compared with levofloxacin for the treatment of patients hospitalized for CAP, requiring intravenous antibiotics, in two multicenter, randomized, and double-blind clinical trials. At the test-of-cure evaluation (within 7–23 days after the completion of therapy), cure rates in the tigecycline treatment arms were not inferior compared to the levofloxacin treatment arms. In view of these positive results, tigecycline was approved for the treatment of CAP by FDA in 2009.

Apart from CAP, many cases of patients with nosocomial pneumonia treated with tigecycline have been reported in the biomedical literature, including cases caused by organisms like MDR *A. baumannii*, carbapenem-resistant *K. pneumoniae*, and MRSA. In a multicenter, randomized, double-blind study comparing tigecycline regimen (tigecycline ± ceftazidime ± aminoglycoside) with imipenem regimen (imipenem/cilastatin ± vancomycin ± aminoglycoside) in patients with nosocomial pneumonia, Freire et al. found significantly lower cure rates with tigecycline in VAP patients, and also more deaths occurred in VAP patients treated with tigecycline than imipenem. In non-VAP patients, tigecycline was noninferior to imipenem. In view of these discrepancies, the role of tigecycline in treatment of nosocomial pneumonia remains uncertain and it is currently not approved by FDA for this indication. However, in the real world setting, it may be used in combination with polymyxin for carbapenem resistant gram-negative pneumonia when no other susceptible drugs are available.

Other Indications

In the current era of MDR organisms, tigecycline is being increasingly prescribed for off-label indications like, nosocomial sepsis, septic shock, and bacteremia. However, this is of great concern because tigecycline is primarily a bacteriostatic agent with a very large volume of distribution. The steady-state serum concentrations achieved after a standard dosing with tigecycline are quite low relative to commonly used sensitivity breakpoints. So, in severe infections with high bacteremia risk, low serum levels combined with bacteriostatic rather than bactericidal activity may lead to an unfavorable microbiological response (higher noncure rates and delayed clearance of bacteremia).

Another problem with use of tigecycline for MDR infections is superinfection with organisms inherently resistant to tigecycline (i.e. *Proteus* species, *Providencia* species, *P. aeruginosa*). So, use of this drug as monotherapy should be restricted to patients with documented nonpseudomonal infections and an antipseudomonal agent should be added to empirical regimens in patients with risk factors for pseudomonal infections.

There are few reports of use of tigecycline for treatment of UTIs, however, there are concerns regarding its effectiveness because only 10–15% of an administered dose of the drug is excreted unchanged in the urine. The combination of tigecycline with piperacillin or tazobactam was found to be superior to the latter alone in a group of adult patients with hematologic malignancies and febrile neutropenia. In a small group of patients, it was found effective for the treatment of pyogenic vertebral osteomyelitis; however, when compared to ertapenem ± vancomycin for diabetic foot infections with and without osteomyelitis, it failed to meet the criteria for noninferiority. Also, data collected from three separate groups of patients treated for *Mycobacterium abscessus* and *M. chelonae* infections suggests that tigecycline could prove useful as an add on therapy for these difficult to treat patients.

Use in children

Tigecycline is not expected to be used in children less than 8 years of age because of possible bone and tooth discoloration, and therefore has not been tested in patients this young. Although the safety and effectiveness of tigecycline in pediatric patients below the age of 18 years have not been established and it is not approved by FDA for use in this age group, but, because of its excellent safety and tolerability profile in adults, tigecycline may be an important antimicrobial agent for children in selected cases.

A recent phase II, multicenter, open-label clinical trial was done in children aged 8–11 years with cSSSI, cIAI, and CAP to assess the pharmacokinetic properties, safety profile, and descriptive efficacy of tigecycline. The results of this trial showed that tigecycline was well tolerated in children and the clinical cure rates were acceptable. Nausea was the most frequent adverse event. This trial also suggested that tigecycline dose of ~1.2 mg/kg q 12 h be superior to the 1 mg/kg dose. However, further phase III trials are needed before the use of tigecycline can be established in children.

ADMINISTRATION AND DOSAGE

In view of a limited oral bioavailability, tigecycline is currently available as an intravenous formulation. The recommended regimen for adults is an initial loading dose of 100 mg followed by 50 mg every 12 h. Using a loading dose followed by multiple maintenance doses, the steady state of tigecycline is reached within 3 days. Recently, higher doses of tigecycline have been proposed to achieve better serum and tissue levels; 200 mg loading in adults with 100 mg 12 hourly as maintenance dose.

Though the safety and efficacy of tigecycline have not been established in children less than 18 years age, but it may be used with extreme caution in highly selective cases. The dosing recommended for children is—a loading dose of 1.5 mg/kg followed by 1 mg/kg (not to exceed 50 mg) every 12 h.

Tigecycline is available as a lyophilized powder in 50 mg vial strength (stored at 2–8°C). It is reconstituted with normal saline or 5% dextrose and given as an infusion in normal saline or ringer lactate (maximum concentration 1 mg/mL) over 30–60 min. Reconstituted solution may be stored at room temperature for up to 24 h and at 2–8°C for up to 48 h.

SAFETY PROFILE

All-cause Mortality

A meta-analysis of 13 RCTs comparing tigecycline with other active comparators demonstrated a significant increase in mortality and noncure rates with tigecycline. Overall, tigecycline was associated with a 0.7% absolute or 30% relative increase in mortality. The increased unfavorable outcomes with tigecycline therapy occurred for both FDA-approved as well as nonapproved indications. However, the greatest increase in risk of death with tigecycline was seen in patients with VAP, with baseline bacteremia. Based on these results, FDA has updated the Warnings and Precautions and Adverse Reactions sections of the tigecycline drug label to include information regarding increased mortality risk of this drug. The cause of excess death in these trials is often uncertain, but it is likely that most deaths are probably related to the severe infection for which tigecycline was used as a treatment.

Adverse Reactions

Tigecycline appears to have low potentials for organ toxicity. Nausea and vomiting are the most commonly encountered adverse effects associated with this drug, and they generally occur during the first 1–2 days of therapy. The majority of cases of nausea and vomiting associated with tigecycline are either mild or moderate in severity. Food may improve the tolerability of tigecycline, but decreasing the infusion rate of the drug has not been shown to be beneficial. Antiemetics have not been shown to be beneficial in decreasing the incidence of nausea and vomiting.

The frequent laboratory abnormalities observed in patients receiving tigecycline include thrombocytopenia, hyperbilirubinemia, elevated serum glutamate-oxaloacetate transaminase or serum glutamate-pyruvate transaminase (SGOT or SGPT), hypoproteinemia, anemia, prolongation of prothrombin time (PT), and activated partial thromboplastin time (aPTT). Isolated cases of significant hepatic dysfunction and hepatic failure have been reported in patients being treated with tigecycline.

Tigecycline is structurally similar to tetracycline-class antibiotics and may have similar adverse effects. Such effects may include permanent discoloration of the teeth in children less than 8 years of age, photosensitivity, pseudotumor cerebri, and antianabolic action (which can lead to increased blood urea nitrogen, azotemia, acidosis, and hyperphosphatemia). As with tetracyclines, pancreatitis has been reported with the use of tigecycline.

DRUG INTERACTIONS

Tigecycline is not a substrate, inhibitor, or inducer of common cytochrome P450 enzymes and is not highly protein bound. As a result of these properties, pharmacokinetic drug interactions are uncommon with tigecycline.

Concomitant administration of tigecycline and warfarin results in a decrease in clearance and an increase in C_{max} of warfarin. Though tigecycline does not significantly alter the effects of warfarin on international normalized ratio (INR) but, PT or other suitable anticoagulation test should be monitored if tigecycline is coadministered with warfarin.

MINOCYCLINE

INTRODUCTION

Minocycline belongs to the class of second-generation tetracyclines, originally introduced to combat infections resistant to older tetracyclines like those caused by *Staphylococcus* and gram-negative species. In view of decreasing use, its intravenous preparation was taken off the market in the US in 2005, but has been reintroduced in 2009. It is currently being explored for use against MDR or XDR organism especially *A. baumannii.*

CHEMISTRY

Minocycline is a semisynthetic derivative of tetracycline, first described in 1960. It has an additional diethylamino group at C-7 and no substituent at C-6. As a result of these chemical alterations, it enjoys better oral availability, a longer half-life and higher tissue penetration. At the same time, it may be shielded against some of the resistance mechanisms active against other tetracyclines.

The drug is available for both oral use as a tablet and intravenous use as a desiccated powder. The powder can be diluted with isotonic saline or dextrose solutions after reconstitution. Rapid infusion has to be avoided. An extended release oral preparation has also come into use recently.

MECHANISM OF ACTION

Like other tetracyclines, minocycline inhibits bacterial protein synthesis. It binds reversibly to the 30S subunit of the bacterial ribosome, thereby inducing a conformational change in the 16S ribosomal RNA that prevents the binding of the aminoacyl transfer RNA at the acceptor site and prevents elongation of the peptide chain. However, the binding being reversible, the action of the antibacterial is bacteriostatic.

SPECTRUM OF ACTIVITY

Among gram-positive organisms, minocycline is active against many strains of methicillin sensitive and resistant *S. aureus*, vancomycin intermediate and resistant *S. aureus* and coagulase negative staphylococci. It does not have consistent activity against enterococci. Gram-negative pathogens, which are susceptible, include *E. coli, Acinetobacter, Citrobacter, Enterobacter, K. pneumoniae, Serratia marcescens, and S. maltophilia*. It does not have activity against *P. aeruginosa.*

DRUG RESISTANCE

An important mechanism of resistance against tetracyclines in gram-negative organisms is the presence of efflux pumps, the most common of which is that encoded by *TetA* gene. Most of these efflux pumps are not active against minocycline with the exception of *TetB* gene. So much so that the absence of the gene has been shown to carry a high negative predictive value for minocycline resistance in *A. baumannii.*

On the other hand, the activity of tigecycline is affected by neither *TetA* or *TetB*. However, it does seem to be affected by resistance-nodulation-division-type efflux pumps. Importantly, these RND pumps do not affect susceptibility to minocycline.

PHARMACOKINETICS

Minocycline has good oral bioavailability, providing some leeway to interchange between intravenous and oral use. The plasma protein binding is around 76% with an elimination half-life of around 15–23 h. It has a greater tissue penetration than other tetracyclines owing to higher lipophilicity and achieves good levels in tissues including lung, liver, gallbladder, bile, prostate, and genitourinary organs. Cerebrospinal fluid levels have been found to be less than that in serum. The intravascular, lung, and CNS levels are superior to tigecycline.

The major route of elimination appears to be nonrenal with only 5–12% of the drug being recovered in the urine. The rest undergoes hepatic metabolism and eliminated by hepatobiliary circulation. Although, minocycline does not seem to get accumulated in renal failure, doses more than 200 mg daily may be associated with higher urea production in patients with CrCl less than 80 mL/min.

PHARMACODYNAMICS

Although available data seems to warrant more pharmacodynamics studies, analysis of in vitro modes seems to suggest that the ratio of the AUC of the free drug over the MIC is associated with an antibacterial effect.

CLINICAL USES

Data about clinical use of minocycline are predominantly derived from reports of small groups of patients and currently, randomized trials for the same are not available. However, whatever information is available, does place minocycline as an exciting option for treatment of both gram-positive and gram-negative infections while providing direction for further research.

Gram-positive Infections

Though minocycline has been found to be active against both methicillin sensitive and resistant *S. aureus,* its main role is in the treatment of MRSA infections of bone and joint as switchover therapy.

Gram-negative Infections

Minocycline is considered to be the second most active agent against *A. baumannii* in vitro. It has been used to treat respiratory infections, bloodstream, bone, and mixed infections. An analysis of seven retrospective studies including 126 adult patients with MDR *A. baumannii* infections, treated with oral or intravenous minocycline alone or in combination with other agents showed a clinical success rate of 78.2% with microbiological cure ranging between 50% to 89%. It can also be used for treatment of CRE infections in combination with polymyxins is susceptibility is demonstrated. The drug is also useful for treatment of melioidosis and infections with nonfermenters such as *Stenotrophomonas maltophilia* and *Elizabethkingia meningoseptica.*

DOSING AND ADMINISTRATION

The recommended initial dose of intravenous minocycline is 200 mg followed by 100 mg every 12 h. In pediatric patients with age more than 8 years of age, the dose is 4 mg/kg followed by 2 mg/kg every 12 h. The total dose should not exceed 400 mg in 24 h. The infusion should be given slowly, over 60 min after dilution. The recommended oral dose is same as the intravenous dose.

ADVERSE REACTIONS

Minocycline use may cause adverse effects common to tetracyclines, which include gastrointestinal upset, candidiasis, skin pigment changes, photosensitivity, CNS events, injection-site reactions, hepatotoxicity, and nephrotoxicity. Although it is not certain, if dosage adjustment is required, use in patients with significant renal impairment requires monitoring of blood urea and creatinine levels.

Minocycline should not be used in pregnant women because of evidence of teratogenicity and in children till 8 years of age because of risk of permanent tooth discoloration and impairment of bone growth. It may also cause dizziness, light-headedness, tinnitus, and decreased hearing. Other serious adverse effects include drug rash with eosinophilia and systemic symptoms and pseudotumor cerebri, especially if the patient complains of new onset headache or blurred vision.

DRUG INTERACTIONS

As tetracyclines decrease the plasma prothrombin activity, dose of anticoagulants may need to be reduced during concomitant use. Effectiveness of oral contraceptive drugs may also be decreased. As both isotretinoin and minocycline are associated with intracranial hypertension, their use together should be avoided. As the current formulation of intravenous minocycline contains magnesium sulfate, there is a risk of interaction with CNS depressants, cardiac glycosides, and neuromuscular blocking agents.

FOSFOMYCIN

INTRODUCTION

A search for alternative treatment strategies in view of the growing resistance among both gram-positive and gram-negative bacteria has resulted in a revival of interest in fosfomycin. Originally called phosphonomycin, it is an old antibiotic agent, discovered in Spain in 1969. It was reported to be produced by multiple *Streptomyces* species. While initially used orally for uncomplicated cystitis, it is now being looked upon as an effective bactericidal agent against many MDR and even XDR organisms. In 2011, it has been recommended as a first-line agent for acute uncomplicated UTI by the Infectious Diseases Society of America (IDSA) and the European Society for Clinical Microbiology and Infectious Diseases (ESCMID).

CHEMISTRY

Fosfomycin is not structurally related to any of the other known antibacterial groups in use. It is an analog of phosphoenolpyruvate (PEP) produced by *Streptomyces fradiae*, *S. viridochromogenes*, and *S. wedmorensis*. It may also be produced synthetically.

It is available as two oral formulations, namely fosfomycin tromethamine or trometamol and fosfomycin calcium as well as an intravenous preparation, fosfomycin disodium. Fosfomycin tromethamine tends to score over the calcium salt in terms of oral bioavailability. Commercially, fosfomycin tromethamine is available as a sachet with white granules while fosfomycin calcium comes as a tablet. The intravenous formulation comes as a powder, which can be dissolved in normal saline as well as dextrose.

MECHANISM OF ACTION

Fosfomycin is a bactericidal agent. It interferes with peptidoglycan chain synthesis during the formation of bacterial cell wall. It binds to the active site of the enzyme MurA and inhibits the formation of UDP N-acetylmuramic acid. The influx of the drug in the bacterial cell is regulated by two different pathways—(1) the constitutively expressed L-alpha-glycerophosphate system and (2) the hexose-6-phosphate transporter system, which is induced by glucose-6-phosphate. At the same time, fosfomycin may reduce the adherence of bacteria to both urinary and respiratory epithelial cells, as in the case of *S. pneumoniae* and *Haemophilus influenzae*.

Fosfomycin is also said to have immunomodulatory properties as it has been shown to affect the function of lymphocytes, neutrophils, and monocytes. Fosfomycin may also have antibacterial activity against biofilms especially in combination with fluoroquinolones and aminoglycosides. It may penetrate the biofilms better and at the same time, modify their structure, hereby facilitating the action of other agents.

SPECTRUM OF ACTIVITY

Fosfomycin is a broad spectrum antibiotic. Among gram-positive organisms, it is active against *Enterococcus faecalis* but not *E. faecium* including VRE, *S. aureus*, including MRSA, penicillin and cephalosporin resistant *S. pneumoniae* and *S. epidermidis*. Among gram-negative pathogens, *Salmonella* species, *Shigella* species, *E. coli*, *Klebsiella* and *Enterobacter* species, *Serratia* species, *Citrobacter* species, and *Proteus mirabilis* are susceptible. It has also been found to be active against *Neisseria gonorrhoeae*, *Listeria monocytogenes*, and *Helicobacter pylori*. Among anaerobes, it is active against *Peptococcus* species and *Peptostreptococcus* species but not against *Bacteroides* species. Notably, *Pseudomonas* species, *Acinetobacter* species, *B. cepacia*, *S. maltophilia*, *Mycobacterium tuberculosis* and *M. morganii* are intrinsically resistant to fosfomycin.

Susceptibility testing can be done by disk diffusion (using special media with glucose-6-phosphate), E test or automated methods. Here also there is discordance between the Clinical Laboratory Standards Institute (CLSI) and the European Committee on Antimicrobial Susceptibility Testing (EUCAST) breakpoints; the former denotes less than or equal to 64 as the susceptibility breakpoint and more than or equal to 256 as resistant; the latter denotes less than or equal to 32 and more than or equal to 64 as the corresponding breakpoints.

DRUG RESISTANCE

Resistance to fosfomycin can be both intrinsic and acquired. Following are the major mechanisms, which confer resistance both in vivo and in vitro:

- Reduced permeability to the drug
- Modification of the antibiotic target
- Antibiotic modification.

Reduction in the permeability of the cell is the main mechanism seen in clinical isolates. It is seen in *E. coli,* and is acquired via mutations in one of the two genes encoding the major transport systems utilized by fosfomycin—the glycerophosphate and the hexose-6-phosphate systems. However, strains with these mutations may have the disadvantage of not being able to use these carbohydrates for growth. Modification of the enzyme MurA, which is the target enzyme for fosfomycin, is a common mechanism for acquired resistance to the drug. Such acquisition of resistance is seen in *E. coli,* whereas *M. tuberculosis, Borrelia burgdorferi,* and *Chlamydia trachomatis* have naturally resistant enzymes. Increased synthesis of MurA may be another mechanism of antibiotic resistance. Microbes may produce enzymes that inactivate fosfomycin. Multiple such enzymes have been described till date and have been named as FosA, FosB, and so on.

PHARMACOKINETICS

Oral fosfomycin is rapidly absorbed. The bioavailability is around 40% for fosfomycin tromethamine versus 12% for the calcium salt, the latter getting inactivated by gastric acid. Metoclopramide, by enhancing gastric motility and coadministration with food may reduce serum levels.

Fosfomycin owing to its small size has been found to achieve clinically relevant levels in serum, kidneys, bladder wall, prostate, lungs, inflamed tissues, bone, cerebrospinal fluid, and heart valves. However, there is considerable interindividual variation in penetration into abscesses. Renal elimination of the drug accounts for about 95%, all via glomerular filtration and no tubular secretion. The half-life is between 4 h to 8 h, which may be increased in older patients and chronic kidney disease. The drug should be administered after each hemodialysis session. In patients on CRRT, the drug levels are similar to those in critically ill patients not on CRRT or even healthy individuals.

PHARMACODYNAMICS

Whether fosfomycin demonstrates, time or concentration-dependent killing may vary with the organism. In case of *S. aureus,* both mechanisms may be active, against *P. aeruginosa,* the drug may demonstrate time-dependent killing whereas against *E. faecium, E. coli, and P. mirabilis,* it may show concentration-dependent killing.

CLINICAL USES

Urinary Tract Infections

In European countries, oral fosfomycin has been in use for the treatment of both complicated and uncomplicated UTIs, whereas in the USA, it is FDA approved only for uncomplicated cystitis. The major advantages of oral fosfomycin include single dose usage that can achieve effective urinary concentrations that rapidly kill bacteria and reduce the chances of mutant selection. In a RCT involving 317 nonpregnant women with recurrent lower UTIs, it was found that the number of infections per patient per year and the time to first recurrence after 6 months of treatment was significantly lower in the fosfomycin group compared to the placebo group. According to a meta-analysis, the use of fosfomycin for treatment of cystitis in pregnant women was comparable in efficacy and associated with fewer adverse events to comparator antibiotics including quinolones, β-lactams, aminoglycosides, nitrofurantoin, and sulfonamides. Single dose treatment has also been found effective for prostatitis. However, this is not the place for fosfomycin therapy in the current era of MDR or XDR pathogens. It should be kept reserve for treatment of highly drug-resistant infections.

Other Infections

Intravenous fosfomycin, primarily in combination with other agents has been used in a multitude of infections including respiratory infections, septic arthritis, osteomyelitis, ear, nose and throat infections, meningitis or encephalitis, peritonitis, endocarditis, sepsis, eye infections, diabetic foot infections, and typhoid fever. It was often used after other antibiotics failed. The cure rate achieved was 81.1%. Recently, excitement with the drug has also been generated after it has been found to be effective in sepsis and nosocomial infections due to MRSA, carbapenem resistant *K. pneumoniae,* and other members of Enterobacteriaceae.

The current role of fosfomycin is in treatment of culture proven carbapenem-resistant fosfomycin sensitive infections as a companion drug to colistin or polymyxin B or drugs. Since resistance develops quickly, monotherapy should be avoided as far as possible. The drug should not be used as empiric therapy since it is not active against *Acinetobacter*, *Pseudomonas*, and many strains of *K. pneumoniae*. The drug can also be used as salvage therapy for serious MSSA or MRSA infections when alternative therapy has failed or is not tolerated.

Surgical Prophylaxis

Fosfomycin has been found to be an effective agent for preventing both gram-positive and gram-negative infections in the postoperative period after both urological and gastrointestinal procedures. While in the former, it has been compared with quinolones, a combination with metronidazole has been compared with similar combinations of doxycycline, ampicillin, and cephalothin in the latter. But here again, the use of fosfomycin for surgical prophylaxis should be avoided, if other drugs are active.

Inhaled Preparations

Fosfomycin delivered via the inhaled route has also attracted attention. In a double-blind, randomized, placebo-controlled trial with patients of CF and chronic *P. aeruginosa* infection, patients receiving a combination of inhaled fosfomycin or tobramycin showed less decline in their lung functions.

DOSING AND ADMINISTRATION

For uncomplicated cystitis in adults, a single oral dose of 3 g is considered adequate. For complicated UTI, a total of three doses given every 2–3 days are recommended. For oral administration, no dose modification is required in the elderly, pregnant or in case of hepatic or renal failure.

Parenteral fosfomycin can be given intravenously or sometimes, intramuscularly. The daily dose range in adults is 12–16 g, up to a maximum of 24 g, used in severe infections, given as 2–4 divided doses. It is to be administered as a slow infusion after dilution in 100 mL of normal saline. For estimated CrCls of 40, 30, 20, and 10 mL/min, a reduction to 70%, 60%, 40%, and 20% of the daily dose is recommended. There is no data regarding dose adjustment in the elderly and in hepatic impairment. A 2 g dose after each session should be administered in patients undergoing hemodialysis. In critically patients, it may be better to give more frequent, higher doses over the initial 24–48 h, followed by frequent, lower doses, guided by CrCl.

For pediatric patients, the dosing should be based on age and body weight. The recommended doses are—100 mg/kg in two divided doses for premature babies, 200 mg/kg in three divided doses in neonates, 200–300 mg/kg in three divided doses for infants up to 1 year (and up to 10 kg), and 200–400 mg/kg in three to four divided doses for children 1–12 years. Except in preterm neonates, a dosing interval of 6–8 h should be preferred over 12 h.

ADVERSE REACTIONS

Oral fosfomycin is usually well tolerated. Common adverse effects, which are generally not severe relate mainly to the gastrointestinal system. Headache, dizziness, weakness, back pain, upper respiratory tract symptoms, and vaginitis have also been reported. It can cause elevation of liver enzymes and alteration of almost all blood cell lines. Again, these are not a cause of concern usually. Opportunistic bacterial and fungal infections are associated with prolonged use.

Important adverse effects associated with intravenous administration include hypokalemia, hypernatremia, heart failure, hypertension, and injection site reactions. Hypersensitivity is a contraindication to administration of fosfomycin.

DRUG INTERACTIONS

Metoclopramide given concomitantly with fosfomycin may decrease its absorption and decrease serum levels by increasing gastrointestinal motility. Cholera vaccination should be avoided till about 14 days after completing a course of fosfomycin.

CONCLUSION

The drugs discussed in this chapter are our last line of defense against carbapenem resistant gram negative pathogens. Hence they should be used judiciously to prolong their shelf life especially when there are no effective options in the near future.

RECOMMENDED READING

1. Agwuh KN, MacGowan A. Pharmacokinetics and pharmacodynamics of the tetracyclines including glycylcyclines. J Antimicrob Chemother. 2006;58:256-65.
2. Alothman GA, Ho B, Alsaadi MM, et al. Bronchial constriction and inhaled colistin in cystic fibrosis. Chest. 2005;127:522-9.
3. Antibiotic treatment for cystic fibrosis. Consensus document. Report of the UK Cystic Fibrosis Trust Antibiotic Working Group, 2009. [online] Available from: http://www.cftrust.org.uk/aboutcf/publications/consensusdoc/ [Accessed, 2018].
4. Babinchak T, Ellis-Grosse E, Dartois N, et al The efficacy and safety of tigecycline for the treatment of complicated intra-abdominal infections: analysis of pooled clinical trial data. Clin Infect Dis. 2005;41:S354-66.
5. Bishburg E, Bishburg K. Minocycline—an old drug for a new century: emphasis on methicillin-resistant *Staphylococcus aureus* (MRSA) and *Acinetobacter baumannii.* Int J Antimicrob Agents. 2009;34:395-401.
6. Bishburg E, Shah M, Chan T. Use of intravenous minocycline for the treatment of methicillin-resistant Staphylococcus aureus (MRSA) and resistant gram-negative organisms: experience in a tertiary care hospital. Infect Dis Clin Pract. 2014;22:26-31.

7. Bogdanovich T, Adams-Haduch JM, Tian G, et al. Colistin-Resistant, *Klebsiella pneumoniae* Carbapenemase (KPC)-producing *Klebsiella pneumoniae* belonging to the international epidemic clone ST258. Clin Infect Dis. 2011;53(4):373-6.
8. Bucaneve G, Micozzi A, Picardi M, et al. Results of a multicenter, controlled, randomized clinical trial evaluating the combination of piperacillin/tazobactam and tigecycline in high-risk hematologic patients with cancer with febrile neutropenia. J Clin Oncol. 2014;32(14):1463-71.
9. Cai Y, Lee W, Kwa AL. Polymyxin B versus colistin: an update. Expert Rev Anti Infect Ther. 2015;13(12):1481-97.
10. Castanheira M, Mendes RE, Jones RN. Update on *Acinetobacter* species: mechanisms of antimicrobial resistance and contemporary in vitro activity of minocycline and other treatment options. Clin Infect Dis. 2014;59(suppl 6):S367-73.
11. Castañeda-García A, Blázquez J, Rodríguez-Rojas A. Molecular Mechanisms and Clinical Impact of Acquired and Intrinsic Fosfomycin Resistance. Antibiotics (Basel). 2013;2(2):217-36.
12. Chopra, I. Glycylcyclines: third-generation tetracycline antibiotics. Curr Opin Pharmacol. 2001;1:464-9.
13. Chopra I, Roberts M. Tetracycline antibiotics: mode of action, applications, molecular biology, and epidemiology of bacterial resistance. Microbiol Mol Biol Rev. 2001;65(2):232-60.
14. CLSI. 2015. Performance standards for antimicrobial susceptibility testing. Document M100-S25; twenty-fifth informational supplement. Clinical and Laboratory Standards Institute, Wayne, PA.
15. Colton B, McConeghy KW, Schreckenberger PC, et al. IV minocycline revisited for infections caused by multidrug-resistant organisms. Am J Health Syst Pharm. 2016;73(5):279-85.
16. Dalfino L, Puntillo F, Mosca A, et al. High dose, extended-interval colistin administration in critically ill patients: Is this the right dosing strategy? A preliminary study. Clin Infect Dis. 2012;54(12):1720-6.
17. Dellinger RP, Bagshaw SM, Antonelli M, et al. Effect of Targeted Polymyxin B Hemoperfusion on 28-Day Mortality in Patients With Septic Shock and Elevated Endotoxin Level: The EUPHRATES Randomized Clinical Trial. JAMA. 2018;320(14):1455-63.
18. Department of Health & Human Services. Letter to Wyeth Pharmaceuticals, Inc. Department of Health & Human Services. [online] Available from: http://www.accessdata.fda.gov/drugsatfda_docs/applett er/2009/021821s013,021821s017,021821s018ltr.pdf [Accessed December, 2018].
19. De Smet KA, Kempsell KE, Gallagher A, et al. Alteration of a single amino acid residue reverses fosfomycin resistance of recombinant MurA from *Mycobacterium tuberculosis*. Microbiology. 1999;145:3177-84.
20. Doan TL, Fung HB, Mehta D, et al. Tigecycline: a glycylcycline antimicrobial agent. Clin Ther. 2006;28(8):1079-106.
21. Dudhani RV, Turnidge JD, Coulthard K, et al. Elucidation of the pharmacokinetic/pharmacodynamic determinant of colistin activity against *Pseudomonas aeruginosa* in murine thigh and lung infection models. Antimicrob Agents Chemother. 2010;54:1117-24.
22. Durante-Mangoni E, Andini R, Signoriello S, et al. Acute kidney injury during colistin therapy: a prospective study in patients with extensively-drug resistant Acinetobacter baumannii infections. Clin Microbiol Infect. 2016;22(12):984-9.
23. Durante-Mangoni E, Signoriello G, Andini R, et al. Colistin and rifampicin compared with colistin alone for the treatment of serious infections due to extensively drug-resistant *Acinetobacter baumannii*: a multicenter, randomized clinical trial. Clin Infect Dis. 2013;57(3):349-58.
24. Ellis-Grosse EJ, Babinchak T, Dartois N, et al. The efficacy and safety of tigecycline in the treatment of skin and skin-structure infections: results of 2 double-blind phase 3 comparison studies with vancomycin-aztreonam. Clin Infect Dis. 2005;41:S341-53.
25. Falagas ME, Bliziotis IA, Tam VH. Intraventricular or intrathecal use of polymyxins in patients with Gram-negative meningitis: a systematic review of the available evidence. Int J Antimicrob Agents. 2007;29:9-25.
26. Falagas ME, Giannopoulou KP, Kokolakis GN, et al. Fosfomycin: use beyond urinary tract and gastrointestinal infections. Clin Infect Dis. 2008;46:1069-77.
27. Falagas ME, Karageorgopoulos DE, Dimopoulos G. Clinical significance of the pharmacokinetic and pharmacodynamic characteristics of tigecycline. Curr Drug Metab. 2009;10:13-21.

28. Falagas ME, Kasiakou SK. Colistin: the revival of polymyxins for the management of multidrug-resistant gram-negative bacterial infections. Clin Infect Dis. 2005;40:1333-41.
29. Falagas ME, Vouloumanou EK, Rafailidis PI. Systemic colistin use in children without cystic fibrosis: a systematic review of the literature. Int J Antimicrob Agents. 2009;33(6):503.e1-503.e13
30. Falagas ME, Vouloumanou EK, Samonis G, et al. Fosfomycin. Clin Microbiol Rev. 2016;29:321-47.
31. Freire AT, Melnykb V, Kimc MJ, et al. Comparison of tigecycline with imipenem/cilastatin for the treatment of hospital-acquired pneumonia. Diagn Microbiol Infect Dis. 2010;68:140-51.
32. Furtado GH, d'Azevedo PA, Santos AF, et al. Intravenous polymyxin B for the treatment of nosocomial pneumonia caused by multidrug-resistant Pseudomonas aeruginosa. Int J Antimicrob Agents. 2007;30(4):315-9.
33. Gales AC, Reis AO, Jones RN. Contemporary assessment of antimicrobial susceptibility testing methods for polymyxin B and colistin: review of available interpretative criteria and quality control guidelines. J Clin Microbiol. 2001;39:183-90.
34. Garg SK, Singh O, Juneja D, et al. Resurgence of Polymyxin B for MDR/XDR Gram-Negative Infections: An Overview of Current Evidence. Crit Care Res Pract. 2017;2017:3635609.
35. Garonzik SM, Li J, Thamlikitkul V, et al. Population pharmacokinetics of colistin methanesulfonate and formed colistin in critically ill patients from a multicenter study provide dosing suggestions for various categories of patients. Antimicrob Agents Chemother. 2011;55(7):3284-94.
36. Giamarellou H, Poulakou G. Pharmacokinetic and pharmacodynamic evaluation of tigecycline. Expert Opin Drug Metab Toxicol. 2011;7(11):1459-70.
37. Greig SL, Scott LJ. Intravenous Minocycline: A review in *Acinetobacter* infections. Drugs. 2016;76:1467-76.
38. Grégoire N, Aranzana-Climent V, Magréault S, et al. Clinical pharmacokinetics and pharmacodynamics of colistin. Clin Pharmacokinet. 2017;56(12):1441-60.
39. Gupta K, Hooton TM, Naber KG, et al. International clinical practice guidelines for the treatment of acute uncomplicated cystitis and pyelonephritis in women: A 2010 update by the Infectious Diseases Society of America and the European Society for Microbiology and Infectious Diseases. Clin Infect Dis. 2011;52:e103-20.
40. Gupta S, Govil D, Kakar PN, et al. Colistin and polymyxin B: a re-emergence. Indian J Crit Care Med. 2009;13(2):49-53.
41. Hendlin D, Stapley EO, Jackson M, et al. Phosphonomycin, a new antibiotic produced by strains of *Streptomyces*. Science. 1969;166(3901):122-3.
42. Iosifidis E, Antachopoulos C, Ioannidou M, et al. Colistin administration to pediatric and neonatal patients. Eur J Pediatr. 2010;169:867-74.
43. Jajoo M, Kumar V, Jain M, et al. Intravenous colistin administration in neonates. Pediatr Infect Dis J. 2011;30(3):218-21.
44. Joukhadar C, Klein N, Dittrich P, et al. Target site penetration of fosfomycin in critically ill patients. J Antimicrob Chemother. 2003;51:1247-52.
45. Karageorgopoulos DE, Kelesidis T, Kelesidis I, et al. Tigecycline for the treatment of multidrug-resistant (including carbapenem-resistant) Acinetobacter infections: a review of the scientific evidence. J Antimicrob Chemother. 2008;62(1):45-55.
46. Karbuz A, Özdemir H, Yaman A, et al. The use of colistin in critically ill children in a pediatric intensive care unit. Pediatr Infect Dis J. 2014;33(1):e19-24.
47. Karvouniaris M, Makris D, Zygoulis P, et al. Nebulised colistin for ventilator-associated pneumonia prevention. Eur Respir J. 2015;46(6):1732-9.
48. Kasbekar N. Tigecycline: A new glycylcycline antimicrobial agent. Am J Health Syst Pharm. 2006;63:1235-43.
49. Kaye KM, Kaye D. Polymyxins (polymyxin B and colistin). In: Mandell GL, Bennett JE, Dolin R (Eds). Mandell, Douglas, and Bennett's Principles and Practice of Infectious Diseases, 6th edition. Philadelphia: Churchill Livingstone; 2005. pp. 435-6.
50. Koch-Weser J, Sidel VW, Federman EB, et al. Adverse effects of sodium colistimethate. Manifestations and specific reaction rates during 317 courses of therapy. Ann Intern Med. 1970;72:857-68.

51. Koch-Weser J, Sidel VW, Federman EB, et al. Adverse effects of sodium colistimethate: manifestations and specific reaction rates during 317 courses of therapy. Ann Intern Med. 1970;72:857-68.
52. Kofteridis DP, Alexopoulou C, Valachis A, et al. Aerosolized plus intravenous colistin versus intravenous colistin alone for the treatment of ventilator-associated pneumonia: a matched case-control study. Clin Infect Dis. 2010;51:1238-44.
53. Kwa A, Kasiakou SK, Tam VH, et al. Polymyxin B: similarities to and differences from colistin (polymyxin E). Expert Rev Anti Infect Ther. 2007;5:811-21.
54. Kwa AL, Lim TP, Low JG, et al. Pharmacokinetics of polymyxin B1 in patients with multidrug-resistant Gram-negative bacterial infections. Diagn Microbiol Infect Dis. 2008;60(2):163-7.
55. Kwa AL, Tam VH, Falagas ME. Polymyxins: a review of the current status including recent developments. Ann Acad Med Singapore. 2008;37(10):870-83.
56. Landman D, Georgescu C, Martin DA, et al. Polymyxins revisited. Clin Microbiol Rev. 2008;21(3):449-65.
57. Lashinsky JN, Henig O, Pogue JM, et al. Minocycline for the Treatment of Multidrug and Extensively Drug-Resistant *A. baumannii*: A Review. Infect Dis Ther. 2017;6(2):199-211.
58. Lauf L, Ozsvár Z, Mitha I, et al. Phase 3 study comparing tigecycline and ertapenem in patients with diabetic foot infections with and without osteomyelitis. Diagn Microbiol Infect Dis. 2014;78(4):469-80.
59. Li J, Nation RL, Turnidge JD, et al. Colistin: the re-emerging antibiotic for multidrug-resistant Gram-negative bacterial infections. Lancet Infect Dis. 2006;6:589-601.
60. Lim LM, Neang Ly, Anderson D, et al. Resurgence of colistin: A review of resistance, toxicity, pharmacodynamics, and dosing. Pharmacotherapy. 2010;30(12):1279-91.
61. Linden PK, Paterson DL. Parenteral and inhaled colistin for treatment of ventilator-associated pneumonia. Clin Infect Dis. 2006;43 (Suppl 2):S89-94.
62. Lista F, Redondo C, Meilan E, et al. Efficacy and safety of fosfomycin-trometamol in the prophylaxis for transrectal prostate biopsy. Prospective randomized comparison with ciprofloxacin. Actas Urol Esp. 2014;38:391-6.
63. Lomovskaya O SD, Rubio-Aparicio D, Nelson K, et al. TetB testing and its absence identifies minocycline (MINO) susceptible isolates of Acinetobacter baumannii (ACB). Open Forum Infectious Disease. 2016;3:2043.
64. Matsumoto T, Tateda K, Miyazaki S, et al. Fosfomycin alters lipopolysaccharide induced inflammatory cytokine production in mice. Antimicrob Agents Chemother. 1999;43:697-8.
65. Matthews P, Alpert M, Rahav G, et al. Tigecycline 900 cSSSI Study Group. A randomized trial of tigecycline versus ampicillin-sulbactam or amoxicillin-clavulanate for the treatment of complicated skin and skin structure infections. BMC Infect Dis. 2012;12:297.
66. McGovern PC, Wible M, El-Tahtawy A, et al. All-cause mortality imbalance in the tigecycline phase 3 and 4 clinical trials. Int J Antimicrob Agents. 2013;41(5):463-7.
67. Michalopoulos A, Virtzili S, Rafailidis P, et al. Intravenous fosfomycin for the treatment of nosocomial infections due to carbapenem-resistant *Klebsiella pneumoniae* in critically ill patients: a prospective evaluation. Clin Microbiol Infect. 2010;16:184-6.
68. Michalopoulos AS, Livaditis IG, Gougoutas V. The revival of fosfomycin. Int J Infect Dis. 2011;15:e732-9.
69. Navon-Venezia S, Leavitt A, Carmeli Y. High tigecycline resistance in multidrug-resistant *Acinetobacter baumannii*. J Antimicrob Chemother. 2007;59:772-4.
70. Nguyen F, Starosta AL, Arenz S, et al. Tetracycline antibiotics and resistance mechanisms. Biol Chem. 2014;395(5):559-75.
71. Orwa JA, Govaerts C, Busson R, et al. Isolation and structural characterization of colistin components. J Antibiot. 2001;54:595-9.
72. Pankey GA, Steele RW. Tigecycline: A single antibiotic for polymicrobial infections. Pediatr Infect Dis J. 2007;26(1):77-8.
73. Pankey GA. Tigecycline. J Antimicrob Chemother. 2005;56:470-80.
74. Paul M, Daikos GL, Durante-Mangoni E, et al. Colistin alone versus colistin plus meropenem for treatment of severe infections caused by carbapenem-resistant Gram-negative ba*cteria: an open-label,* randomised controlled trial. Lancet Infect Dis. 2018;18(4):391-400.

75. Pereira GH, Muller PR, Levin AS. Salvage treatment of pneumonia and initial treatment of tracheobronchitis caused by multidrug-resistant Gram-negative bacilli with inhaled polymyxin B. Diagn Microbiol Infect Dis. 2007;58(2):235-40.
76. Polat M, Kara SS, Tapısız A, et al. Treatment of ventilator-associated pneumonia using intravenous colistin alone or in combination with inhaled colistin in critically ill children. Paediatr Drugs. 2015;17(4):323-30.
77. Prasad P, Sun J, Danner RL, et al. Excess deaths associated with tigecycline after approval based on noninferiority trials. Clin Infect Dis. 2012;54(12):1699-709.
78. Purdy J, Jouve S, Yan JL, et al. Pharmacokinetics and safety profile of tigecycline in children aged 8 to 11 years with selected serious infections: a multicenter, open-label, ascending-dose study. Clin Ther. 2012;34(2):496-507.
79. Qureshi ZA, Paterson DL, Potoski BA, et al. Treatment outcome of bacteremia due to KPC-producing *Klebsiella pneumoniae:* superiority of combination antimicrobial regimens. Antimicrob Agents Chemother. 2012;56:2108-13.
80. Qvist N, Warren B, Leister-Tebbe H, et al. Efficacy of tigecycline versus ceftriaxone plus metronidazole for the treatment of complicated intra-abdominal infections: results from a randomized, controlled trial. Surg Infect (Larchmt). 2012;13(2):102-9.
81. Rodrı´guez-Martı´*nez JM, Ballesta S,* Pascual A. Activity and penetration of fosfomycin, ciprofloxacin, amoxicillin/clavulanic acid and co-trimoxazole in *Escherichia coli* and *Pseudomonas aeruginosa* biofilms. Int J Antimicrob Agents. 2007;30:366-8.
82. Rodvold KA, Gotfried MH, Cwik M, et al. Serum, tissue and body fluid concentrations of tigecycline after a single 100 mg dose. J Antimicrob Chemother. 2006;58(6):1221-9.
83. Samonis G, Maraki S, Rafailidis PI, et al. Antimicrobial susceptibility of Gram-negative nonurinary bacteria to fosfomycin and other antimicrobials. Future Microbiol. 2010;5:961-70.
84. Sandri AM, Landersdorfer CB, Jacob J, et al. Population pharmacokinetics of intravenous polymyxin B in critically ill patients: implications for selection of dosage regimens. Clin Infect Dis. 2013;57(4):524-31.
85. Schafer JJ, Goff DA, Stevenson KB, et al. Early experience with tigecycline for ventilator-associated pneumonia and bacteremia caused by multidrug-resistant *Acinetobacter baumannii.* Pharmacotherapy. 2007;27(7):980-7.
86. Smith K, Leyden JJ. Safety of doxycycline and minocycline: a systematic review. Clin Ther. 2005;27(9):1329-42.
87. Stein GE, Craig WA. Tigecycline: A critical analysis. Clin Infect Dis. 2006;43:518-24.
88. Tamma PD, Lee CK. Use of Colistin in Children. Pediatr Infect Dis J. 2009;28(6):534-5.
89. Tanaseanu C, Bergallo C, Teglia O, et al. Integrated results of 2 phase 3 studies comparing tigecycline and levofloxacin in community-acquired pneumonia. Diagn Microbiol Infect Dis. 2008;61(3):329-38.
90. Taneja N, Singh G, Singh M, et al. Emergence of Tigecycline & Colistin resistant Acinetobacter baumanii in patients with complicated urinary tract infections in north India. Indian J Med Res. 2011;133:681-4.
91. Thamlikitkul V, Dubrovskaya Y, Manchandani P, et al. Dosing and Pharmacokinetics of Polymyxin B in Patients with Renal Insufficiency. Antimicrob Agents Chemother. 2016;61(1).
92. Townsend ML, Pound MW, Drew RH. Tigecycline: a new glycylcycline antimicrobial. Int J Clin Pract. 2006;60:1662-72.
93. Trapnell BC, McColley SA, Kissner DG, et al. Fosfomycin/tobramycin for inhalation in patients with cystic fibrosis with *Pseudomonas* airway infection. Am J Respir Crit Care Med. 2012;185:171-8.
94. Traunmüller F, Popovic M, Konz KH, et al. A reappraisal of current dosing strategies for intravenous fosfomycin in children and neonates. Clin Pharmacokinet. 2011;50(8):493-503.
95. US FDA. FDA Drug Safety Communication: Increased risk of death with Tygacil (tigecycline) compared to other antibiotics used to treat similar infections. [online] Available from: http://www.fda.gov/Drugs/DrugSafety/ucm224370.htm#.UH8JRVgnWAE.email [Accessed December, 2012].
96. Vardakas KZ, Rellos K, Triarides NA, et al. Colistin loading dose: evaluation of the published pharmacokinetic and clinical data. Int J Antimicrob Agents. 2016;48(5):475-84.

97. Vincent JL, Laterre PF, Cohen J, et al. A pilot-controlled study of a polymyxin b-immobilized hemoperfusion cartridge in patients with severe sepsis secondary to intra-abdominal infection. Shock. 2005;23:400-5.
98. Wallace RJ Jr, Dukart G, Brown-Elliott BA, et al. Clinical experience in 52 patients with tigecycline-containing regimens for salvage treatment of *Mycobacterium abscessus* and *Mycobacterium chelonae* infections. J Antimicrob Chemother. 2014;69(7):1945-53.
99. Zavascki AP, Nation RL. Nephrotoxicity of Polymyxins: Is There Any Difference between Colistimethate and Polymyxin B? Antimicrob Agents Chemother. 2017;61(3);e02319-16.
100. Zhanel GG, Homenuik K, Nichol K, et al. The glycylcyclines: a comparative review with the tetracyclines. Drugs. 2004;64:63-88.

Miscellaneous Antibacterial Drugs

14
Chapter

Baldev S Prajapati, Rajal B Prajapati

SULFONAMIDES

Introduction

The sulfonamide drugs were the first effective chemotherapeutic agents to be employed systematically for the prevention and cure of bacterial infections in human beings. Domagk and his colleagues (1938) while working on azo dyes demonstrated the efficacy of "Prontosil", a dye with a sulfonamide side chain in inhibiting the growth of streptococci both in vitro and in vivo. Domagk subsequently used prontosil in his daughter having streptococcal septicemia, which was fatal during those days. It was found that prontosil was broken down in the body to release sulfanilamide, which was the active antibacterial agent. Later on, several sulfonamides were produced and used extensively. However, because of rapid emergence of bacterial resistance and the availability of many effective and safer antibiotics, their use was declined. However, in the mid-1970s, the combination of trimethoprim (TMP) and sulfamethoxazole (SMX) became available, which resulted in increased use of sulfonamides for the treatment of specific microbial infections.

The antimicrobial agents containing a sulfonamide group are called sulfonamides. The sulfonamide group is also present in other nonantibacterial compounds like antidiabetic agent tolbutamide, diuretics like chlorothiazide, furosemide, and acetazolamide.

Classification

Sulfonamides employed for the treatment of systemic infections are subdivided depending upon their duration of action.

- Short-acting sulfonamides (4–8 hours) include sulfadiazine, sulfadimidine, sulfafurazole, and sulfisomidine.
- Intermediate-acting sulfonamides (8–12 hours) include SMX, sulfamoxole.
- Long-acting sulfonamides (approximately 7 days) include sulfadoxine, sulfamethopyrazine.
- Special purpose sulfonamides include sulfacetamide (ocular use), sulfasalazine (ulcerative colitis), mafenide, and silver sulfadiazine (burn dressing).
- Nonabsorbable sulfonamides such as phthalylsulfathiazole, succinylsulfathiazole, and sulfaguanidine have been banned in India.

Mechanism of Action

The compound sulfanilamide exhibits structural similarity to para-aminobenzoic acid (PABA) and hence competes with and probably substitutes for PABA in the bacterial mechanism. Folic acid derived from PABA is important in bacterial metabolism. Sulfonamides also inhibit the enzyme folic acid synthetase, which is involved in the conversion of PABA to folic acid. This causes folic acid deficiency resulting in injury to the bacterial cell. Such an injured or disrupted bacterial cell can be easily phagocytosed. Sulfonamides are ineffective in the presence of pus and tissue breakdown products that contain large amount of PABA. PABA can counter the bacteriostatic action of sulfonamides. It is also observed that sulfonamide-resistant microorganisms often show enhanced PABA synthesis.

Spectrum of Activity

Sulfonamides are primarily bacteriostatic against many gram-positive and gram-negative bacteria. However, bactericidal concentrations may be attained in urine. Sensitivity pattern among microorganisms have changed from time to time and place to place. In combination with other drugs that inhibit folic acid synthesis, sulfonamides are effective in malaria, toxoplasmosis, and pneumocystosis.

Therapeutic Uses

Systemic use of sulfonamides alone (without combination with TMP or pyrimethamine) is rare now.

Sulfadiazine has good penetration in brain and cerebrospinal fluid (CSF). It was the preferred compound for meningitis before availability of the modern and better antimicrobial agents.

- *Sulfadiazine*: For toxoplasmosis in combination with pyrimethamine (1 mg/kg/day) and folinic acid. Dosage of sulfadiazine is 100 mg/kg/day in two divided doses
- *Sulfamethoxazole*: Used in combination with TMP (see later)
- *Sulfisoxazole*: Ophthalmic solution, ointment
- *Sulfadoxine*: Along with pyrimethamine used for malaria
- *Sulfasalazine*: For ulcerative colitis and juvenile rheumatoid arthritis
- *Sulfacetamide*: 10%, 20%, and 30% eye drops, 6% eye ointment. For topical use in ocular infections due to susceptible bacteria and chlamydia including ophthalmic neonatorum
- *Silver sulfadiazine*: 1% cream. One of the most effective agents for prevention of infection of burn areas and chronic ulcers.

Adverse Effects

Common adverse effects due to sulfonamides are:

- Nausea, vomiting, and epigastric pain
- *Crystalluria*—Dose related
- Hematuria and anuria may develop
- *Hypersensitivity reactions*: Skin rashes, urticaria, and drug fever are common. Arthritis, serum sickness, and polyarteritis nodosa are infrequent. Photosensitization is known.

Stevens-Johnson syndrome and toxic epidermal necrolysis are common with long-acting agents. These are the most severe hypersensitivity reactions associated with sulfonamides, leading to death in some exposures
- Hepatitis
- Hemolysis in glucose-6-phosphate dehydrogenase (G6PD) deficiency individuals
- Neutropenia and other blood dyscrasias
- Kernicterus may be precipitated in newborns especially in premature babies.

Drug Interactions

Sulfonamides inhibit the metabolism of phenytoin, tolbutamide, and warfarin, thereby enhancing their actions. They displace methotrexate from binding sites and decrease its renal excretion, thus possibly increasing toxicity. Fixed dose combinations of sulfonamides and penicillin may cause serious hypersensitivity and are banned in India.

Contraindications

Sulfonamides are contraindicated in G6PD deficiency.

TRIMETHOPRIM–SULFAMETHOXAZOLE

The fixed dose combination of TMP and SMX is called co-trimoxazole. It contains a 5:1 ratio of SMX to TMP. The potency of this combination is expressed in terms of the TMP content. It was introduced in 1969.

Mechanism of Action and Relevant Pharmacology

It causes sequential block of folate metabolism. TMP is 50,000 times more active against bacterial dihydrofolate reductase than against the mammalian enzyme. Thus, human folate metabolism is not interfered at antibacterial concentrations of TMP. Individually both sulfonamide and TMP are bacteriostatic, but the combination becomes cidal against many organisms. Maximum synergism is seen when the organism is sensitive to both the components, but even when it is moderately resistant to one component, the action of the other may be enhanced. SMX was selected for combining with TMP because both have nearly the same plasma half-life. TMP adequately crosses blood–brain barrier and placenta, while SMX has a poor entry. Moreover, TMP is more rapidly absorbed than SMX. TMP is partly metabolized in liver and excreted in urine.

Spectrum of Activity

Many isolates of *Staphylococcus aureus* [both methicillin-susceptible *Staphylococcus aureus* (MSSA) and methicillin-resistant *Staphylococcus aureus* (MRSA)], and *Nocardia* are susceptible to co-trimoxazole. Certain strains of pneumococci group A streptococci, *Haemophilus*, *Enterobacter*, *Escherichia coli*, *Klebsiella*, *Salmonella*, and *Shigella* are also susceptible. It has no activity against *Pseudomonas aeruginosa*. It is active against *Toxoplasma gondii*, *Pneumocystis jiroveci*, and *Isospora*. It has no activity against strict anaerobes.

Resistance

Bacteria are capable of acquiring resistance to TMP mostly through mutational or plasmid-mediated acquisition of a dihydrofolate reductase having lower affinity for the inhibitor. However, resistance to the combination has been slow to develop compared to either drug alone. Widespread use of the combination has resulted in resistance in over 40% of pneumococci, *Haemophilus*, and group A streptococci. Resistance in *Shigella* is also considerable. Conversely, there is return of susceptibility in many strains of *Salmonella*. A fair number of extended-spectrum β-lactamase (ESBL) producing *Escherichia coli* isolates may also be susceptible to TMP-SMX.

Therapeutic Uses

- *Urinary tract infections (UTIs)*: Co-trimoxazole is useful for treatment of community-acquired acute or recurrent UTIs. It is recommended as prophylaxis for recurrent UTI. The TMP component is better suited as a prophylactic agent as compared to TMP-SMX, but is not available in India.
- *Infections in the immunocompromised*: Co-trimoxazole is the drug of choice for treatment of *Pneumocystis jiroveci* pneumonia and *Isospora* diarrhea in immunocompromised patients especially human immunodeficiency virus (HIV). It is also a second-line drug for toxoplasmosis. It is also effective as prophylaxis against *Pneumocystis jiroveci*, toxoplasmosis, recurrent bacterial infections, and nontyphoidal *Salmonella* infections in the immunocompromised particularly HIV.
- *Enteric fever*: Co-trimoxazole was widely used in therapy of enteric fever in the past. The emergence of multidrug-resistant enteric fever in the 1990s resulted in loss of its utility. However, recently there has been a reemergence of co-trimoxazole sensitivity and this drug may be a therapeutic option for outpatient therapy. A 12-week course eradicates carrier state of sensitive strains provided gallbladder is not involved.
- *Staphylococcal infections*: Owing to its activity against both MSSA and MRSA strains, it can be used as empiric therapy when susceptibility results are awaited. It can also be used to treat MRSA skin, soft tissue, bone, and joint infections. In certain circumstances, it may be used as IV preparation to treat MRSA bacteremia and meningitis.
- *Other conditions*: Co-trimoxazole is useful in therapy of brucellosis in children when doxycycline cannot be used. It is the drug of choice in treatment of nocardiosis. It is also the drug of choice for chronic therapy of melioidosis.
- *Nosocomial infections*: With increasing antimicrobial resistance in nosocomial infections, co-trimoxazole is being used to treat nosocomial infections due to extensively drug-resistant organisms including organisms like *Stenotrophomonas maltophilia*, *Chryseobacterium indologenes*, and other nonfermenters. It can be combined with colistin to treat carbapenem-resistant organisms that are susceptible to co-trimoxazole.
- The role of co-trimoxazole in treatment of respiratory tract infections both of the upper and lower respiratory tract as well as shigellosis and traveler's diarrhea is diminishing due to increasing resistance.

Preparations and Dosage

The drug is available as syrup with 40 mg of TMP/5 mL, single strength tablet with 80 mg of TMP and 400 mg of SMX, double strength tablet with 160 mg of TMP and 800 mg of SMX, and intravenous (IV) preparation as 16 mg of TMP/mL.

- 5–8 mg/kg of TMP or 25–50 mg/kg of SMX/day in two divided doses oral or IV
- 10 mg/kg/day in two divided doses of TMP for enteric fever
- 15–20 mg/kg/day in three to four divided doses of TMP for treatment of *Pneumocystis jiroveci* infection
- 5 mg/kg/day of TMP either single dose or in two divided doses daily, for three consecutive days in a week or every alternate day for prophylaxis against *Pneumocystis jiroveci* and *Toxoplasma gondii*
- 1–3 mg/kg/day of TMP in single dose for UTI prophylaxis.

Adverse Effects and Contraindications

See the section on sulfonamides.

CHLORAMPHENICOL

Chloramphenicol was discovered in 1948 from *Streptomyces venezuelae*. It was synthetically produced and marketed in 1949. The potential for aplastic anemia has resulted in marked decline of its use in current day practice.

Mechanism of Action

Chloramphenicol acts by interfering with synthesis of bacterial proteins. It inhibits protein synthesis by binding to 50S subunit of 70S ribosomes to prevent attachment of AA + RNA or to inhibit peptidyl transferase, required for formation of the peptide bond. At high doses, it can inhibit mammalian mitochondrial protein synthesis as well. Bone marrow cells are especially susceptible.

Spectrum of Activity

Chloramphenicol has a wide spectrum of antimicrobial activity. It has excellent activity against group A and B streptococci, *Haemophilus influenzae, Neisseria meningitidis, Bordetella pertussis, Shigella,* salmonellae, *Rickettsia,* chlamydia, mycoplasma, etc. It is inactive against mycobacteria, *Pseudomonas, Proteus,* and fungi.

Resistance

Intrinsic and acquired resistance occurs. Plasmid-mediated resistance is important, since cross-resistance to several antimicrobial agents like aminoglycosides, sulfonamides, and tetracycline is frequent. Resistance is due to hydrolyzing enzymes or target modification.

Clinical Pharmacokinetics

Pharmacokinetics of chloramphenicol has been characterized in neonates, infants, and children. Oral bioavailability is good, almost 80–90%. The drug is available as a lipid-soluble base or water-soluble ester of succinate (IV use) or palmitate (oral use). Both esters require to be hydrolyzed in the body to release the active form. The palmitate form probably gets hydrolyzed in the proximal part of small intestine and free base is rapidly absorbed. In the neonate, hydrolysis is less due to limited gastrointestinal (GI) lipase activity. The succinate form is probably hydrolyzed in the liver. In the newborns, the succinate ester hydrolysis is slower than in older infants and children and 36% gets excreted in the urine unchanged. When there is liver and renal dysfunction, the serum chloramphenicol levels show wide variations. This has been observed especially in sick neonates. The bioavailability of orally administered chloramphenicol palmitate is superior to that of succinate given intravenously. It seems that significant therapeutic advantage is observed when chloramphenicol palmitate is orally administered in children who can tolerate the drug by mouth.

The lipid solubility of chloramphenicol makes the drug diffuse widely in tissues and body fluids. CSF levels of the drug are nearly 50% of the serum concentration irrespective of the presence or absence of meningitis. In neonates and small infants when chloramphenicol is administered for meningitis, monitoring the drug levels is essential. The importance of monitoring increases when phenobarbitone or phenytoin or both are co-administered.

Therapeutic Uses

Therapy with chloramphenicol must be limited to infections for which the benefits of the drug outweigh the risks of the potential toxicities. When other antimicrobial drugs are available that are equally effective but potentially less toxic than chloramphenicol, they should be used.

Typhoid Fever

Chloramphenicol was widely used in therapy of enteric fever. By 1970s, resistance emerged which was plasmid-mediated and associated with resistance to other drugs like co-trimoxazole and ampicillin. Moreover with chances of developing blood dyscrasia and availability of modern, better, and safe antimicrobials specifically and third-generation cephalosporins, chloramphenicol lost its importance in therapy of enteric fever. But recently with re-emergence of chloramphenicol sensitivity, the scope for its use in enteric fever has emerged.

Bacterial Meningitis

Treatment with chloramphenicol produces excellent results in *Haemophilus influenzae* meningitis that are better than those achieved with ampicillin and equal to the third-generation cephalosporins. However, with the availability of third-generation cephalosporins, chloramphenicol has lost its top position in management of bacterial meningitis in young children. As it is very cheap, it can be used in nonaffording patients. Intramuscular preparations of chloramphenicol have been used to control the meningococcal epidemics in sub-Saharan Africa. In partially treated or chronic bacterial meningitis when the modern cephalosporins including ceftriaxone and other antibiotics have failed, chloramphenicol has been found effective. In this situation, it can be used with consent of parents.

Anaerobic Infections

Wound infections, pelvic, and brain abscesses caused by *Bacteroides fragilis* and other respond well to chloramphenicol. Excellent diffusibility of chloramphenicol is a management asset. Other therapeutic alternatives are metronidazole and clindamycin.

Rickettsial Diseases

The tetracyclines are usually the preferred agents for the treatment of rickettsial diseases. However, in children, patients with hypersensitivity to tetracyclines, in pregnant women, and in those with reduced renal functions, chloramphenicol is a suitable alternative.

Miscellaneous Uses

Nosocomial pathogens such as multidrug-resistant *Klebsiella pneumoniae and Escherichia coli* can often be treated successfully with chloramphenicol. Brucellosis, whooping cough, and *Mycoplasma pneumoniae* are other conditions in which chloramphenicol may be used as an alternative to other drugs.

Dosage

- 50–75 mg/kg/day in three divided doses orally
- 100 mg/kg/day in four divided doses IV.

Adverse Reactions

Bone Marrow Depression

Two forms of bone marrow involvement in chloramphenicol toxicity are known. One form is dose-related, reversible, and occurs usually during the course of treatment. The pathogenesis is assumed to be due to its ability to inhibit mammalian ribosomal protein synthesis. There is anemia, leukopenia, thrombocytopenia and increased serum iron, and free erythrocyte protoporphyrin. Keeping the serum level of chloramphenicol below 25 μg/mL will reduce the incidence of this toxic effect. The second type of bone marrow suppression is an idiosyncratic reaction and not dose-related. It is serious and irreversible. It may even appear sometime after discontinuation of the drug and may be fatal. Fortunately, the incidence of aplastic anemia is very uncommon with an incidence of 1 in 58,000 to 1 in 75,000.

To prevent deadly complications due to chloramphenicol, indiscriminate, prolonged use of the drug should be avoided. Peripheral smear should be examined at least twice a week during therapy. The treatment should be stopped if the leukocyte count drops below 4,000 cells/mm^3 or when the proportion of granulocytes is reduced below 40%. Discontinuation of chloramphenicol after the development of aplastic anemia does not prevent the relentless progress of the disorder.

Gray Baby Syndrome

This is another dangerous complication of chloramphenicol therapy with a high mortality rate, observed in neonates, especially in preterm babies, receiving large doses of the drug (100–200 mg/kg/day) and blood levels are more than 25 mg/L. The mechanism of high-level chloramphenicol toxicity is believed to be related to a disturbance of mitochondrial electron transport. Symptoms are pallid cyanosis, abdominal distension, hypothermia, and circulatory failure. The factors incriminated are: (1) the deficient conjugation of chloramphenicol in the liver. A low level of hepatic glucuronyl transferase enzyme activity in the first 2–3 weeks has been demonstrated and (2) immaturity of the renal tubules in the newborns leading to impairment of excretion of the free form of antibiotic. To avoid this complication, chloramphenicol should not be used in newborns, unless it is a must and level should not exceed 25 mg/L. The babies should be watched for early signs of toxicity.

Intolerance

This is relatively uncommon. However, skin rashes, drug fever, angioneurotic edema, exfoliative dermatitis, atrophic glossitis, and hemorrhages involving the skin, GI tract, and the bladder have been reported. Peripheral neuritis, headache, mental confusion, optic neuritis, internal ophthalmoplegia, and Herxheimer reaction are other rare adverse effects of chloramphenicol.

Interactions

Chloramphenicol inhibits phenytoin, tolbutamide, chlorpropamide, and warfarin metabolism. Phenobarbitone, phenytoin, and rifampicin enhance chloramphenicol metabolism and thereby reduces its concentration and failure of therapy may occur. Co-administration of chloramphenicol with cimetidine has been reported to increase potential for aplastic anemia.

TETRACYCLINES

The development of tetracycline antibiotics was the result of systematic screening of soil specimens collected from many parts of the world for antibiotic producing microorganisms. The first of these compounds, chlortetracycline, was introduced in 1948. All tetracyclines contain the four cyclic rings; the substitution of various groups at the R5, R6, or R7 positions of the nucleus varies antibacterial activity, absorption, and protein binding. For discussion on tigecycline and IV minocycline, see Chapter 13.

Classification

On the basis of chronology of development as well as for convenience of description, they may be divided into three groups.

Group I	*Group II*	*Group III*
• Tetracycline • Chlortetracycline • Oxytetracycline	• Demeclocycline • Methacycline • Lymecycline	• Doxycycline • Minocycline

Mechanism of Action

The tetracyclines are primarily bacteriostatic. They inhibit protein synthesis by binding to 30S ribosomes in susceptible organisms. Subsequent to such binding, attachment of aminoacyl-tRNA to the mRNA ribosomes complex is interfered with. As a result, peptide chain fails to grow. The sensitive organisms have an energy-dependent active transport process which concentrates tetracycline intracellularly. In gram-negative bacteria, tetracyclines diffuse through porin channels as well. The more lipid-soluble members such as doxycycline and minocycline enter by passive diffusion also. This may be the reason for their higher potency. The carrier involved in active transport of tetracyclines is absent in the host cells. Moreover, protein-synthesizing apparatus of host cells is less sensitive to tetracyclines. These two factors are responsible for the selective effect of tetracyclines on microbes. However, at very high concentrations, tetracyclines inhibit mammalian protein synthesis. The mechanism by which tetracyclines reduce lesions of acne vulgaris is not well-understood, but it appears to be the result of antimicrobial activity.

Spectrum of Activity

Tetracyclines have a broad spectrum of activity that includes most *Rickettsia*, chlamydia, *Mycoplasma* species, Spirochetes, and some gram-negative and gram-positive bacteria. All gram-positive and gram-negative cocci were originally sensitive, but now many *Streptococcus pyogenes*, *Staphylococcus aureus*, and enterococci have become resistant. Minocycline is still active against most *Neisseria gonorrhoeae* and *Neisseria meningitidis*. *Clostridia*, *Listeria*, *Leptospira*, corynebacteria, and *Bacillus anthracis* are inhibited by tetracyclines. *Vibrio cholerae*, *Yersinia pestis*, *Campylobacter*, *Helicobacter pylori*, *Brucella*, and many anaerobes are sensitive to tetracyclines.

Resistance

Intrinsic or acquired resistance to tetracyclines is due to decreased permeability as a result of mutation or presence of inducible plasmid-mediated resistance factors. Nearly complete cross-resistance is seen among different members of the tetracycline group. Partial cross-resistance between tetracyclines and chloramphenicol has been noted.

Clinical Pharmacokinetics

Few data are available in children. The older tetracyclines are incompletely absorbed from GI tract. They are better absorbed if taken empty stomach. Doxycycline and minocycline are completely absorbed irrespective of food. The predominant routes of excretion are renal and biliary. Therefore, any condition impairing renal or biliary functions would be expected to prolong the clearance of tetracyclines. Only doxycycline attains appreciable CSF concentrations. They are secreted in breast milk in amount sufficient to affect the suckling infant.

Therapeutic Uses

Although nearly all publications cite restriction of use in children younger than 9 years of age, most experts would prescribe a short course of 7–10 days duration of tetracycline in young children for serious or life-threatening infections in which tetracycline is a drug of choice, e.g. scrub typhus and spotted fever. A recent retrospective study concluded that doxycycline is safe in children of all ages as its affinity for teeth and bone is lower than other tetracyclines. Major indications for the tetracyclines are as mentioned in Table 1.

Dosage

- *Tetracycline hydrochloride*: 25–50 mg/kg/day orally 6 hourly
- *Oxytetracycline*: 7–10 mg/kg/day 6–12 hourly

TABLE 1: Major indications for tetracyclines.

Therapy of choice	*Effective therapy*
• Rickettsial infections • Brucellosis (with streptomycin, rifampicin) • Cholera • Acute epididymitis [sexually transmitted disease (STD)] • Granuloma inguinale • Leptospirosis • Pelvic inflammatory diseases • Relapsing fever	• Lyme disease • Acne • Anthrax • *Bordetella pertussis* • Chlamydia/*Mycoplasma*/*Legionella* infections • Rat bite fever • Tularemia • Companion drug with artemisinin/quinine for *falciparum* malaria.

- *Doxycycline*: 3–4 mg/kg/day (maximum 200 mg daily) 12 hourly; 6 mg/kg single dose up to maximum of 300 mg in children more than 8 years.

Adverse Reactions

Irritative Effects

Tetracyclines especially doxycycline can cause epigastric pain, nausea, vomiting, diarrhea, and esophageal ulcerations. Intramuscular injections of tetracyclines are very painful. Thrombophlebitis on IV route is known to occur.

Hepatic Toxicity

Fatty infiltration of liver and jaundice occur occasionally. Oxytetracycline and tetracycline are safer in this regard. Tetracyclines can precipitate acute hepatic necrosis in pregnant women.

Nephrotoxicity

This is mainly in the presence of existing kidney disease. Exposure to acidic pH, moisture, and heat favors degradation of tetracyclines. Such degraded products and outdated tetracyclines can cause proximal tubular damage and reversible Fanconi syndrome-like condition.

Photosensitivity

Sunburn like and other skin reactions on exposed parts are seen in some individuals. Distortion of nails occurs occasionally.

Teeth and Bones

Tetracyclines have chelating property. Calcium-tetracycline chelate gets deposited in developing teeth and bones. Brown discoloration, malformation, and susceptibility to caries are known problems with teeth. Given from mid-pregnancy to 5 months extrauterine life, the deciduous teeth are affected. Tetracyclines given between 3 months and 6 years of age affect permanent anterior dentition. Repeated courses are more damaging. Given during the late pregnancy or childhood tetracyclines can cause temporary suppression of bone growth. Doxycycline does not have these effects.

Miscellaneous

Antianabolic effect, increased intracranial pressure, vestibular toxicity, etc. are other known adverse effects of tetracyclines.

Drug Interactions

Aluminum, calcium, magnesium, and iron containing products or food can impair the absorption of tetracyclines. Interactions of tetracyclines are known with oral contraceptive pills, digoxin, rifampin, and loop diuretics. Anticoagulant effect of warfarin is enhanced while therapeutic action of penicillins is reduced.

METRONIDAZOLE

Metronidazole is the prototype of nitroimidazole introduced in 1959 for trichomoniasis and later found to be highly active against several protozoa and many anaerobic bacteria.

Mechanism of Action

Metronidazole is bactericidal, amebicidal, and trichomonacidal in action. After entering the cell by diffusion, its nitro group is reduced by certain redox proteins operative only in anaerobic microbes to highly reactive nitro radical, which exerts cytotoxicity by damaging DNA and other critical biomolecules. DNA helix destabilization and strand breakage have been observed in susceptible organisms. Aerobic environment attenuates cytotoxicity of metronidazole by inhibiting its reductive activation.

It has been found to inhibit cell-mediated immunity, to induce mutagenesis, and to cause radiosensitization.

Spectrum of Activity

Metronidazole is active against most obligatory anaerobic bacteria and many protozoa. Susceptible anaerobic bacteria include *Bacteroides fragilis, Clostridium, Peptococcus*, etc. *Gardnerella vaginalis* is also susceptible. *Actinomyces* are resistant. Facultative gram-negative bacilli, *Staphylococcus* and *Streptococcus* are resistant. Protozoa such as *Entamoeba histolytica, Trichomonas vaginalis*, and *Giardia lamblia* are inhibited by metronidazole.

Clinical Pharmacokinetics

Metronidazole is almost completely absorbed from the small intestine. It is widely distributed in the body, attaining therapeutic concentration in vaginal secretions, semen, saliva, and CSF. It is metabolized primarily in liver by oxidation and glucuronide conjugation. It is excreted in the urine. Its clearance is reduced markedly in neonates and infants in first 2–3 months of life.

Therapeutic Uses

Metronidazole has potent bactericidal activity against anaerobic bacteria and excellent tissue penetration, making it a mainstay of therapy for brain abscess, intra-abdominal infections, and other anaerobic closed space infections. Metronidazole is not used as monotherapy for any bacterial infection since infection involving anaerobic bacteria is typically polymicrobial. Metronidazole alone or in combination with other agents has been used successfully for prophylaxis in GI surgery, gynecologic surgery, or emergency appendicectomy. It was initially considered as the drug of choice for mild *Clostridium difficile* infection but the new guidelines recommend oral vancomycin as drug of choice for mild and severe *Clostridium difficile* infections. IV metronidazole is indicated in management of complicated *Clostridium difficile* infections along with oral vancomycin. It is also used in the management of necrotizing enterocolitis in preterm babies in dose of 15 mg/kg IV loading dose followed by 7.5 mg/kg per dose every 12 hours. Metronidazole has excellent CSF penetration and bactericidal activity. It is found effective in the treatment of anaerobic organisms causing meningitis or ventriculitis (traumatic, postsurgical, or nosocomial) and treatment of anaerobic brain abscess. Metronidazole in combination with other antibiotics and proton pump inhibitors has been used in treatment of *Helicobacter pylori*. It has been also found effective in treatment of parapharyngeal abscess, Ludwig angina, necrotizing fasciitis, and cellulitis.

It is effective therapy for bacterial vaginosis, trichomoniasis, intestinal amebiasis, and anaerobic and amebic liver abscess. Metronidazole is also effective against *Giardia lamblia* and *Balantidium coli*.

Dosage

- 15–20 mg/kg/day in three divided doses orally for 5 days for giardiasis
- 35–50 mg/kg/day in three divided doses orally for 10 days for amebiasis
- 20–30 mg/kg/day in four divided doses orally or IV for anaerobic infections.

Adverse Reactions

Side effects to metronidazole are relatively frequent but mostly nonserious.

- Anorexia, nausea, metallic taste (by both oral and parenteral administration), and abdominal cramps are the most common.
- Less frequent side effects are headache, glossitis, dryness of mouth, dizziness, rashes, and transient neutropenia.
- Prolonged administration may cause peripheral neuropathy, vertigo, ataxia, seizures, and other central nervous system (CNS) adverse effects.
- Thrombophlebitis if the solution is not well-diluted on IV therapy.
- Rare adverse effects include maculopapular skin rash, chest pain and palpitation, discoloration of urine, gynecomastia, and acute pancreatitis. Metronidazole has been shown to be mutagenic in vitro and carcinogenic in laboratory animals.

Contraindications

The drug is contraindicated in active neurological disease, blood dyscrasias, 1st trimester of pregnancy, and chronic alcoholism.

Drug Interactions

- A disulfiram-like intolerance to alcohol occurs among some patients taking metronidazole along with alcohol.

- Enzyme inducers like phenobarbitone and rifampicin may reduce its therapeutic effect.
- Cimetidine can reduce metronidazole metabolism, requiring reduction in its dosage.

LINCOSAMIDES

Although not related structurally to erythromycin or other macrolide compounds, the lincosamides (lincomycin and clindamycin) have similar mechanism of action and antimicrobial activity as macrolides.

Mechanism of Action

Lincomycin and clindamycin appear to inhibit RNA-dependent protein synthesis by binding to 50S ribosomal subunits, inhibiting peptide bond formation of susceptible organisms.

Spectrum of Activity

Clindamycin has the same spectrum of activity as lincomycin but is relatively more potent. Clindamycin is active against most gram-positive aerobic cocci including staphylococci (both MSSA and MRSA), *Streptococcus pneumoniae*, and other streptococci, even those resistant to penicillin. It is also active against many anaerobic organisms. Bacteroides fragilis may be resistant to clindamycin. Clindamycin also has activity against *Plasmodium*, *Pneumocystis*, and *Toxoplasma* species.

Resistance

Staphylococcal resistance to clindamycin can be induced in a stepwise manner in vitro. Clindamycin resistance confers complete cross-resistance with lincomycin and partial resistance with erythromycin.

Therapeutic Uses

Lincomycin should never be used because of adverse reactions and available alternatives. Clindamycin is effective therapy for moderate to severe infections due to aerobic gram-positive cocci and anaerobic bacteria. There is significant experience from infancy through adolescence for treatment of intra-abdominal, gynecologic, pelvic, and bone and joint infections. It is a superior agent in animal models of osteomyelitis, probably related to high concentration in bone, neutrophils, and macrophages. Clindamycin offers no advantage over penicillin G for treatment of uncomplicated, acute anaerobic upper and lower respiratory tract infection, but is superior to penicillin for treatment of chronic sinusitis, lung abscess, odontogenic, and parapharyngeal abscess. It is used as adjunctive therapy for necrotizing fasciitis due to its effect on reducing bacterial toxin production. For infections in a patient with hypersensitive to penicillin, clindamycin is an acceptable alternative drug for moderate to severe infections.

The ability of clindamycin to target ribosomal protein production has led its use in treatment of toxin-mediated infections caused by *Staphylococcus aureus* [toxic shock syndrome (TSS)] and *Streptococcus pyogenes* (toxic shock-like illness), either alone or in combination with cell wall active antibiotic agents.

Other uses of clindamycin include:
- Treatment of acne vulgaris
- Cerebral and ocular toxoplasmosis
- Adjunctive therapy for *falciparum* malaria
- Treatment of community-acquired MRSA infections of skin, soft tissue, bone, joint, and lung
- Therapy for *Pneumocystis jiroveci* resistant or intolerant to co-trimoxazole.

Dosage

- 20–30 mg/kg/day in four divided doses PO
- 20–40 mg/kg/day in three divided doses IV dilute for slow infusion over 30 minutes.

Adverse Reactions

Pseudomembranous colitis, initially reported to occur in upto 10% of adults with clindamycin, is much less common in children. Rapid infusion of undiluted lincosamides has led to cardiac arrest, presumably from a mechanism similar to quinidine. Other adverse effects of these compounds include increased serum hepatic enzymes, Stevens-Johnson syndrome, skin rashes, and eosinophilia.

Drug Interactions

Co-administration of clindamycin with gentamicin may increase nephrotoxicity. Clindamycin and lincomycin infusions potentiate effects of nondepolarizing neuromuscular blocking agents.

NITROFURANTOIN

Nitrofurantoin is one of the many synthetic *S. nitrofurans* derivatives, derived from pentosans obtained from corncobs, oat husks, and bran. Nitrofurantoin is more soluble in urine as compared to water due to presence of urea and creatinine in urine, resulting in high urinary drug levels.

Mechanism of Action

Nitrofurantoin is bacteriostatic, but may be bactericidal in high concentration in urine, following therapeutic doses. It appears that nitrofurantoin is reduced into active intermediates by bacterial enzymes, resulting in inactivation or alteration of ribosomal molecules and leading to inhibition of protein, DNA, RNA, and cell wall synthesis.

Spectrum of Activity and Resistance

Nitrofurantoin is active against several gram-positive and gram-negative organisms including *Staphylococcus aureus*, Group D *Streptococcus*, *Escherichia coli*, *Salmonella*, and *Shigella*. It is inactive against most isolates of *Pseudomonas aeruginosa*. Development of resistance has been reported rarely following prolonged therapy, cross-resistance with other agents has not been observed.

Clinical Pharmacokinetics

It is well-absorbed orally, rapidly metabolized in the liver and other tissues. Renal excretion accounts for 30–40% of elimination.

Therapeutic Uses

Its use is primarily as a urinary antiseptic agent and for prevention of recurrent UTIs. It may be used for treatment of cystitis where the microorganisms are resistant to other orally available agents but should not be used for treatment of tissue infection such as pyelonephritis. The drug is assuming greater importance in today's day and age with rising incidence of ESBL production in community-acquired UTIs.

Dosage

- 5–7 mg/kg/day in three to four divided doses
- 1–2 mg/kg/day in single bedtime dose as prophylaxis for UTI.

Adverse Reactions

Nausea, epigastric pain, and diarrhea are common GI adverse effects. Acute reaction with chills, fever, leukopenia, and hepatitis may occur occasionally. Pulmonary reactions in form of acute pneumonitis syndrome, subacute pulmonary syndrome with cough, dyspnea, pulmonary infiltrates, and pulmonary effusions as well as chronic pulmonary fibrosis are known following prolonged use of nitrofurantoin.

Drug Interactions

Nitrofurantoin antagonizes the antimicrobial effect of quinolones. Co-administration of nitrofurantoin with antacids may decrease bioavailability.

Contraindications

Individuals with impaired renal functions (since the drug will not be adequately concentrated in the urine) and children less than 3 months of age should not receive nitrofurantoin. It is contraindicated in G6PD deficiency.

RECOMMENDED READING

1. Abramson JS, Givner LB. Should tetracycline be contraindicated for therapy of presumed Rocky Mountain spotted fever in children less than 9 years of age? Pediatrics. 1990;86;123-4.
2. Hardman JG, Limbird LE, Gilman AG. Goodman and Gilman's The Pharmacological Basis of Therapeutics, 10th edition. New York: McGraw Hill; 2001.
3. Jacobs RF, Schutz GE, Young RA, et al. Antimicrobial agents. In: Long SS, Pickering LK, Prober CG (Eds). Principle and Practice of Pediatric Infectious Diseases. New York: Churchill Livingstone; 1997. pp. 1604-43.
4. Merchant SM, Vithlani NP. Current antibiotic usage, I: Penicillins, cephalosporins and chloramphenicol. Indian J Pediatr. 1986;53:25-36.

5. Merchant SM, Vithlani NP. Current antibiotic usage, II: Aminoglycosides, tetracyclines, erythromycin, vancomycin and sulfonamides. Indian J Pediatr. 1986;53:199-213.
6. Powell DA, Nahata MC. Chloramphenicol: new perspectives on an old drug. Drug Intell Clin Pharm. 1982;16:295-300.
7. Sack CM, Koup JR, Smith AL. Chloramphenicol pharmacokinetics in infants and young children. Pediatrics. 1980;66:579-84.
8. Saivin S, Houin G. Clinical pharmacokinetics of doxycycline and minocycline. Clin Pharmacokinet. 1988;15:355-66.
9. Salter AJ. Trimethoprim-sulfamethoxazole: an assessment of more than 12 years of use. Rev Infect Dis. 1982;4:196-236.
10. Tripathi KD. Sulfonamides, co-trimoxazole, and quinolones. In: Tripathi KD (Ed). Essentials of Medical Pharmacology, 5th edition. New Delhi: Jaypee Brothers Medical Publishers (P) Ltd; 2003. pp. 641-52.
11. Tripathi KD. Tetracyclines and chloramphenicol (broad-spectrum antibiotics). In: Tripathi KD (Ed). Essentials of Medical Pharmacology, 5th edition. New Delhi: Jaypee Brothers Medical Publishers (P) Ltd; 2003. pp. 668-77.

General Principles of Antimicrobial Therapy

15
Chapter

YK Amdekar

INTRODUCTION

Antibiotics are ideally prescribed for *treating bacterial infections*. In practice, it amounts to diagnosing bacterial infection reasonably correctly to ensure rational use of antibiotics. Antibiotics are also used for *prophylaxis of bacterial infections* in selective situations. It is important to strictly follow the standard protocols for prophylaxis. However, in clinical practice, antibiotics are most commonly used empirically. *Empirical use* is based on personal observation and practical experience. Empirical use of antibiotics may be scientifically acceptable if few prerequisites are judiciously met with. Therefore, it should be an endeavor of every physician to justify antibiotic prescription in general and specially in case of empirical use. It is ideal to document reasons for antibiotic prescription that would ensure rational practice.

DIAGNOSING ACUTE BACTERIAL INFECTION

Acute onset of fever is the hallmark of acute infection of varied etiology and hence *antibiotic therapy is generally not justified in any acute symptom that is not accompanied with fever*. Neonate and shock state may be an exception to this rule. However, the converse is not true in that *fever may not represent every time an acute bacterial infection*; it may be due to viral or parasitic infection, or it may result from a noninfective condition such as malignancy or systemic inflammatory disease. Central fever, heat fever, or drug fever may be other conditions leading to acute onset fever. Hence, it is important to differentiate acute bacterial infection from other causes of acute onset fever.

It is rational to consider that acute onset fever is commonly due to acute infection. It is also true that cause of infection is not generally evident within the first 2–3 days of fever. In such a situation, it is important to rule out seriousness or "emergency" whatever the cause may be. Change in behavior, reduced urine output, hemorrhagic or bullous skin rash, respiratory distress, and disproportionate tachycardia and tachypnea may pinpoint probable "emergency". It would need appropriate action and not just an antibiotic. Once "emergency" is ruled out at the onset of fever, it would be safe to observe further development without investigation or antibiotic. At this stage, parents must be counseled about observing for "red flag" symptoms (as mentioned earlier) indicating probable "emergency" and need for urgent medical attention. Close observation by parents and daily review by pediatrician over next 2–3 days would be the rational way forward at this juncture.

It is not easy to be sure about presence or absence of acute bacterial infection during initial days of presentation. However, if few principles are strictly followed, antibiotic misuse can be minimized to a great extent, if not totally avoided. Most of the time, clinical presentation can differentiate between acute bacterial and viral infections. Acute viral infection is disseminated throughout the system [upper respiratory tract infection (URTI) and lower respiratory tract infection (LRTI)], may affect multiple systems (respiratory and gastrointestinal), and spreads from and to other family members. Fever is usually high at onset, rhythmic every 4-6 hours in response to paracetamol, child is comfortable, and not sick during interfebrile state and fever usually settles by D3-4. In general, viral infections are self-limiting and do not need any specific antiviral antibiotic therapy. Oseltamivir should be reserved for suspected complicated or serious influenza viral infection. Acyclovir is used specifically in community herpes viral infections such as herpetic gingivostomatitis and varicella zoster. As against acute viral infection, acute bacterial infection is localized to one part of the system (acute tonsillitis does not present with running nose or chest signs and signs of pneumonia are mostly localized to one lobe of lung). Fever is generally moderate at the onset and peaks by D3-4 and child often continues to be sick even during interfebrile state. At this point, physical examination would mostly reveal localization as in case of pneumonia or meningitis. However, if suspected bacterial infection has no localizing symptoms or physical signs, typhoid is a possibility and blood culture should be ordered prior to starting appropriate antibiotic. Urinary tract infection (UTI) often present without localization but just with high fever in a sick child. Ideally, this should be suspected in sick-looking infant or toddler early in the course of fever. In malaria, fever is often erratic and child looks normal during interfebrile period. Classical rigors are often absent. Paucity of other symptoms and physical signs is common though splenomegaly and pallor, if present, is a strong clinical marker. It is important to confirm diagnosis of malaria to ensure rational therapy.

It is, thus, evident that diagnosis of acute bacterial infection is generally not possible for the first 2-3 days with the exception of *tonsillitis, otitis media, acute lymphadenitis, and bacillary dysentery*. Hence, antibiotic prescription for fever of acute onset is not justified on the first couple of days unless one of the abovementioned conditions are evident on physical examination. In the absence of definitive diagnosis during first 2-3 days of fever, *serious bacterial infections must be ruled out*, which is possible on careful physical examination. Serious bacterial infections where delay in instituting antibiotics would result in poor outcome include *meningitis, pneumonia, sepsis, UTI, and diphtheria*. In case of suspicion of any of these serious bacterial infections, suitable action is necessary in the form of appropriate tests and/or hospitalization *prior to antibiotic therapy*.

DIAGNOSING CHRONIC BACTERIAL INFECTION

Chronic bacterial infection such as tuberculosis (TB), chronic UTI, or chronic sinusitis can be suspected clinically and demands relevant investigations. Such chronic infection is not likely to worsen over next few days and there is always enough time on hand to confirm the diagnosis before starting antibiotic therapy. Antibiotic trial is not rational in these cases, as therapy may have to be continued for longer period even if patient becomes asymptomatic within few days. Ideally, bacteriological diagnosis must be attempted in chronic infection. Every pediatrician should attempt to confirm TB even in young children as gastric aspirate can be collected as outpatient procedure and sample subjected to GeneXpert MTB/RIF or TB culture. Chronic or recurrent UTI must be treated with antibiotics selected on the basis of urine culture sensitivity results. Chronic sinusitis is a difficult diagnosis to make and treatment is often controversial. Protracted bacterial bronchitis is another chronic bacterial infection that mimics asthma and diagnosis is confirmed ideally by bronchoalveolar lavage and treated with amoxicillin for 2–3 weeks.

PROPHYLACTIC ANTIBIOTIC THERAPY

Prerequisites for prophylactic antibiotic therapy include two key factors—(1) knowledge of specific infection against which prophylaxis is planned and (2) increased susceptibility of the host against that particular infection. Penicillin prophylaxis for rheumatic fever is a classical example of rational prophylactic therapy and so also is a neonate exposed to open TB in the mother. A person in immediate contact with meningococcal disease is another example of ideal prophylaxis. In all these conditions, prophylaxis is planned against specific infecting agent and hence choice and duration of prophylactic antibiotic therapy is clear. Perioperative administration of a narrow-spectrum antibiotic to prevent surgical site infections is another example of ideal prophylaxis. Routine prophylaxis using broad-spectrum antibiotics is irrational as it may lead to development of drug-resistant organisms.

EMPIRICAL ANTIBIOTIC THERAPY

There is a place for empirical antibiotic therapy in clinical practice. However, one must ensure that such therapy does not harm the patient by delaying correct diagnosis. Stringent prerequisites must be followed before considering empirical antibiotic therapy.

Young infants less than 3 months of age with high fever, undiagnosed fever in an immunocompromised patient, fever in a patient in the intensive care unit, and unaccounted fever in a child with heart defect (probability of subacute bacterial endocarditis) are high-risk situations for bacterial infection and should be treated with antibiotics but only after relevant investigations including bacteriological tests are sent to the laboratory. Minimum investigations include complete blood count (CBC), urinalysis, blood culture, and chest X-ray. Other tests may be considered in relevance to the probability of clinical diagnosis and include cerebrospinal fluid (CSF) examination. Viral infection with atypical progress such as persistent fever well beyond the appearance of skin rash in a child with measles may suggest secondary bacterial infection and necessitate an antibiotic. However, common viral infections rarely complicate with secondary bacterial infection.

CHOICE OF ANTIBIOTIC

It is based on probability of gram-positive or gram-negative bacterial infection as suggested by the age of the patient and site of infection. Drug resistance may not be the initial consideration in the treatment of community-acquired infections unless local epidemiology demands such a consideration. Multidrug-resistant typhoid fever or shigellosis is likely in the current scenario and an appropriate antibiotic may be chosen on the basis of antibiotic sensitivity pattern noted in the community. Multidrug-resistant tuberculosis (MDR-TB) is a serious problem and it is not rare to find response to first-line drugs during initial few weeks only to face worsening in patient's condition in spite of compliant therapy. Hence, choice of therapy should be ideally based on drug sensitivity tests. Most of the other community-acquired infections would respond to almost any antibiotic, though, with misuse of antibiotics, every infection has a chance to be resistant. It is important to choose an antibiotic, which has low potential to develop resistance such as amoxicillin for oral use or cefotaxime/ceftriaxone for parenteral use. Oral drug is always preferred unless patient's condition demands use of parenteral drug. In such a case, antibiotic available with both formulations may be the best choice so that one could shift to oral therapy with the same drug, once patient's condition stabilizes. Change from one parenteral drug to an oral drug of another class is not ideal.

Drug resistance plays heavily in the minds of the physicians; however, it should not be a serious contender in routine community-acquired infections. In stable conditions, there would always be time available to monitor response to an antibiotic, and hence choice of antibiotic should be restricted to first line of drugs. Addition of enzyme inhibitor to an antibiotic is an example of this (e.g. using amoxicillin-clavulanic acid instead of amoxicillin) for treatment of bacterial sinusitis and otitis media to cover for beta-lactamase producing *Haemophilus influenzae* or *Moraxella*. The combination may not be always needed. Besides, the cost of therapy increases considerably by addition of enzyme inhibitor.

Empiric therapy with high end broad-spectrum antibiotics is usually indicated for very serious infections where there may be no time to upgrade or for nosocomial infections or infections in immunocompromised individuals.

CHANGE OF ANTIBIOTIC

In case of failure of anticipated response, change of antibiotic may be considered after adequate trial for 3–4 days. Second antibiotic must be rationally chosen, as it should widen the bacterial cover beyond that offered by the first antibiotic. For example, if amoxicillin is used as a first antibiotic for community-acquired lower respiratory infection and has failed, second choice should essentially cover atypical organisms such as *Mycoplasma*/chlamydia that are not covered by amoxicillin. Macrolide would be the antibiotic of choice in such a case. Thus, higher generation or newer antibiotic is not necessarily the choice for a change. If second antibiotic fails, it is best to review the diagnosis. Invariably, wrong diagnosis is the cause of antibiotic failure and not the drug itself. Addition of another antibiotic, when first one fails, is not rational in acute bacterial infection. If first one has failed, it should be replaced.

COMBINATION ANTIBIOTIC THERAPY

It is irrational to use two antibiotics for a single infection in office practice. It may be necessary only in selective situations wherein unstable condition of the patient demands quick control and there is no clue to bacteriological diagnosis as happens in neonatal sepsis or suspected infection in immunocompromised patient. In such cases, time is the crucial factor to save life and it would be irrational not to use two antibiotics to widen the bacterial cover. TB must be treated with four drugs to take care of possible drug resistance to one or two first-line drugs.

Use of fixed drug combinations such as an antibiotic with antiparasitic drug is irrational. In children, acute dysentery is caused by bacterial infection and there is generally no co-infection with amebiasis. Similarly, antibiotic combined with lactobacillus or co-prescription with vitamin B complex is an exaggerated claim by pharmaceutical companies.

DURATION OF ANTIBIOTIC THERAPY

Duration of therapy depends upon the age, type of organism, and site of infection. Younger the age, more serious or disseminated the disease is, and is often caused by gram-negative organisms. Such a disease would require treatment for 2–3 weeks while therapy for a week may suffice for community-acquired infection in an older child. Deep-seated infection such as bone or joint infection may justify longer therapy.

IRRATIONAL ANTIMICROBIAL THERAPY AND ANTIBIOTIC RESISTANCE

Multiple factors are responsible for irrational therapy and increasing drug resistance. Poor patient compliance, aggressive marketing practices of pharmaceutical industry, self-medication, easy availability of antibiotics across the counter, substitution by chemists, substandard quality of drugs, and nonexistent control of drug regulation authorities are all responsible for increasing drug resistance. Use of antibiotics in agriculture and poultry are additional factors responsible for antibiotic resistance. However, irrational use by medical professionals is probably the main contributing factor for the current scenario. Most of the antibiotic misuse by medical professionals comes from diffidence and fear of missing serious bacterial infection and its direct consequences. Every practitioner is concerned with his or her individual patient and considers it safe to use antibiotic in almost every case. Fear of legal action makes many physicians prefer an error of commission to error of omission and hence, an antibiotic prescription gives them false sense of security. It is important to realize that such narrow vision in favor of an individual patient leads to spread of drug-resistant infections in the community, of which every individual patient is also a part.

It is not wrong clinical judgment as much as it is the negligence that is punished in the court of law. Poor communication with the patient and relatives and poor documentation of clinical opinion are the main reasons for legal problems. It is of utmost necessity that every physician documents his probable diagnosis and the basis for such a diagnosis before writing a prescription. If this is meticulously followed, irrational use of antibiotics would be minimal. In the court of law, such documentation would help in favor of the physician even in case of complications or poor outcome. Hence, legality should not be an excuse for irrational antibiotic use and "defensive" practice is not warranted. If physicians do not follow such an ideal practice, the time is not far when no antibiotic would work and community will be in danger of life even with so-called "benign" common infections.

CONCLUSION

In conclusion, if general principles of antimicrobial therapy were strictly followed, it would do immense good to the community. Problem of drug resistance is a result of our own wrongdoing and before the situation gets out of control, we need to act seriously. We all owe it to the community. Protocols and guidelines formulated by an official scientific organization would go a long way to give an impetus to rational use of antibiotics, as it would serve the community the best and also protect physicians from legal hassles.

RECOMMENDED READING

1. Bender MT, Niederman MS. Principles of antibiotic management of community-acquired pneumonia. Semin Respir Crit Care Med. 2016;37:905-12.
2. Dancer SJ. How antibiotics can make us sick: less obvious side effects of antimicrobial therapy. Lancet Infect Dis. 2004;4:611-9.
3. Doenberg SB, Chambers HF. Antimicrobial stewardship approaches in the intensive care unit. Infect Dis Clin North Am. 2017;31:513-24.
4. Douglas JE, Bennett GL. Principles and Practices of Infectious Diseases, 5th edition. New York: Churchill Livingstone; 2000.
5. Leone M, Bourgoin A, Cambon S, et al. Empirical antimicrobial therapy of septic shock patients: adequacy and impact on the outcome. Crit Care Med. 2003;31:462-7.
6. Long SS, Pickering LK, Prober CG. Principles and Practice of Pediatric Infectious Diseases, 2nd edition. New York: Elsevier; 2003.
7. Niederman MS. Appropriate use of antimicrobial agents—challenges and strategies for improvement. Crit Care Med. 2003;31:608-16.
8. Onufrak NJ, Forrest A, Gonzalez D. Pharmacokinetic and pharmacodynamic principles of anti-infective dosing. Clin Ther. 2016;38:1930-47.
9. Safdar N, Handelsman J, Maki DG. Does combination antibiotic therapy reduce mortality in gram negative bacteremia? A meta-analysis. Lancet Infect Dis. 2004;4:519-27.
10. Vora A, Krishnaprasad K. Guiding principles for the use of fluroquinolones in out-patient community setting of India: Panel consensus. J Assoc Physicians India. 2017;65:51-2.
11. Warren DK, Hill HA, Merz LR, et al. Cycling empirical antimicrobial therapy to prevent emergence of drug resistance. Crit Care Med. 2004;32:2450-6.
12. Weinstein L. Common sense (clinical judgment) in the diagnosis and antibiotic therapy of etiologically undefined infections. Pediatr Clin North Am. 1968;15:141-56.

Practicing Rational Antimicrobial Therapy

16

Chapter

Suhas Prabhu

INTRODUCTION

This chapter discusses the concepts introduced in the previous chapter in greater detail. The purpose is to reemphasize the same concepts and drive home the mechanism of rational antimicrobial practice.

Antibiotics are prescribed to treat bacterial infections. This is referred to as therapeutic use of antibiotics. But they must be used judiciously after a rigorous scientific approach, i.e. rationally (antibiotics are also used prophylactically for preventing infections in very selective situations, which are discussed in Chapter 32). Rational use of antibiotics means using a reasoned thought process firstly in deciding whether to use an antibiotic or not and secondly in choosing the most suitable antibiotic. Rational thought is also required before changing to a higher antibiotic (escalation) due to perceived nonresponse to the earlier one. A continued reappraisal of the route and duration of the therapy in a patient who is apparently responding to the antibiotic is also in order. Also when antibiotics have been started empirically, once a definitive diagnosis is made, therapy should be optimized by stepping down to the narrower spectrum antibiotic tailored to the identified pathogen (de-escalation).

Rational antimicrobial therapy requires answers to these questions:

- Is an antibiotic required at all?
- If so, which is the appropriate antibiotic of choice?
- Is the patient responding to the antibiotic chosen? If not, when to escalate and how?
- If the patient is responding well can we de-escalate to a different antibiotic?
- If a parenteral antibiotic is on, when should we switch to an oral antibiotic and to which one?
- How long to treat?

IS AN ANTIBIOTIC REQUIRED AT ALL?

Fever is probably the most common complaint for which a child is brought to a doctor and infection is no doubt the most common cause of fever. This has led to a reflex writing of an antibiotic prescription for every child who comes with fever. This is not rational. There is a four step process that one must follow before writing the antibiotic prescription for a patient with fever, by answering these four questions:

1. Is there definitely a fever?
2. Is the fever due to an infection?

3. Is the infection bacterial (not viral)?
4. Yes, the infection is bacterial, but does it need an antibiotic?

Only if the answer to all these questions is a "yes" then only one should prescribe an antibiotic.

Is there Definitely a Fever?

Fever is often reported by parents or caregivers on a subjective basis, by simply looking at the child's appearance or touching the forehead. This may be erroneous. While it is not prudent to summarily dismiss a parent's perception of fever, one should document the fever objectively by measuring it with a thermometer before labeling the child as being truly febrile.

Is the Fever due to an Infection? Fever ≠ Infection

All fevers are not due to infection. Fever may be due to environmental causes like overclothing of a young infant in the summer, severe exercise, dehydration in a neonate, and so on. Obviously, these conditions do not call for an antibiotic prescription. Fever may also be due to noninfectious condition like systemic lupus erythematosus (SLE) and other collagen vascular diseases, autoimmune hemolysis, hemophagocytic lymphohistiocytosis, Kawasaki's disease, and malignancies like leukemia just to name a few. These will not respond to antibiotics. So one must try and ensure that these nonmedical causes are not the cause of fever before prescribing an antibiotic. While some of them can only be diagnosed after tests, we should withhold antibiotics in nonserious patients where such conditions are suspected till the situation is clear.

Is the Infection Bacterial (Not Viral)?

The most common presentation of infection in children is fevers associated with a sore throat, nasal discharge and cough, or one associated with loose motions and abdominal pain. But one should remember that many (if not the majority) of these infections are viral and will therefore not require an antibiotic (there are only a few "antiviral" antimicrobials that are indicated like oseltamivir in influenza or acyclovir is herpes simplex encephalitis). The majority of nonspecific viral fevers [including most upper respiratory tract infections (URTIs), gastroenteritis cases, and the exanthematous fevers of childhood] do not require any antiviral drugs and definitely will not benefit from the administration of antibiotics. Antibiotics do not prevent bacterial superinfections in viral infections. Clinical clues that can help one to distinguish viral from bacterial infections and certain "spot diagnoses" of bacterial infections have been described in the previous chapter.

Yes, the Infection is Bacterial, But does it Need an Antibiotic?

All bacterial infections do not need an antibiotic for a cure. Some are self-limiting and antibiotics do not improve either the rate or chances of recovery. In toxigenic bacterial diarrheas, like that due to enterotoxigenic *Escherichia coli* (ETEC) or *Staphylococcus*, antibiotics are not indicated. Similarly, acute otitis media in an immunocompetent child over 2 years of age does not mandate an antibiotic at least for the first 48 hours. Many of them will respond to other measures alone like nasal drops, decongestants, analgesics, etc. Paronychia responds to simple removal of the nail and superficial pyodermas or infected abrasions in nonsick children require only a local antiseptic.

WHICH ANTIBIOTIC SHOULD BE USED?

Therapeutic use of antibiotics is done under two circumstances:

1. *Empirical therapy:* This is resorted to when it is reasonably certain that there is a bacterial infection requiring an antibiotic but it has not been detected or isolated yet. Antibiotic treatment may be started empirically based on reasonable possibilities for the organism and its possible sensitivity.
2. *Definitive therapy:* The organism is clearly identified and its sensitivity is known (by culture or molecular methods).

Empirical Therapy

Empirical therapy is guesswork; but it has to be reasoned guess.

A reasoned and educated guess is required to answer this question. The choice of empiric therapy depends on the likely pathogens or likely susceptibility, prior antibiotic therapy, severity of infection, site of infection, and host comorbidities. While it is always good to do this exercise, when choosing an empiric antibiotic; adherence to country specific guidelines also serves the purpose. It is because these guidelines are formulated based on local data about etiology and susceptibility.

What are the likely Organisms in the Patient under Consideration?

The answer to this question requires knowledge of the relative distribution of causative organisms in a particular clinical situation. For example, we should know that the organisms causing pneumonia in preschool age group are viruses, *Streptococcus pneumoniae, Haemophilus influenzae,* and *Moraxella catarrhalis.* These account for about 80% of all such cases. So we can safely choose an antibiotic like amoxicillin that will cover these organisms to treat a 3-year-old nonserious child with pneumonia. The possible pathogens may be different in special clinical situations and that needs to be considered while making empirical choices. For example, in a human immunodeficiency virus (HIV)-infected child with severe immunosuppression and not on cotrimoxazole prophylaxis, *Pneumocystis* becomes an important likely cause of pneumonia, in a child with cystic fibrosis, it may be *Pseudomonas* and in an infant with severe acute malnutrition or pyoderma, one must remember that it may be *Staphylococcus aureus.* So the empiric choice will be different in each of these cases to cover the respective organisms.

What is the likely Antibiotic Sensitivity of those Organisms?

The second factor that needs to be considered is the drug sensitivity of the likely organisms under consideration. In the example given above, if a large percentage of *H. influenzae* and *M. catarrhalis* are likely to be β-lactamase (BL) producers then the correct empiric choice of antibiotic will be not amoxicillin, but amoxiclav.

Now, it is important to remember that antibiotic resistance patterns vary temporally and also from area to area. For example, fluoroquinolones were very effective for salmonella in the 1990's but are ineffective today. So while ciprofloxacin was life-saving in a case of typhoid fever then, it will fail miserably today. Similarly, the geographical needs to be taken into account. A significant percentage of nosocomial gram-negative infections in India are extended-spectrum BL (ESBL) producing necessitating the use of BL-beta-lactamase inhibitor (BLI) combinations and carbapenems for empiric therapy of healthcare-associated infections. Conversely, ESBL rates are very low in Scandinavian countries where cephalosporins do the job very well.

It is therefore incumbent on us to have this knowledge of the possible pathogens in a clinical given situation and the current pattern of drug resistance in our geographical area to make the correct empiric choice of antibiotic.

What is the Severity of Infection?

A very important consideration in empiric antibiotic therapy is the severity of the infection and the general condition of the patient. If the infection is very severe and consequently the child is very sick (or also if the child is immunocompromised) the antibiotic(s) chosen must cover almost all the possible organisms taking into account their possible drug susceptibilities. This is because, one may not have a second chance to change or escalate the antibiotic before the child succumbs to the infection. This may mean that the initial empiric choice of antibiotic is very broad spectrum or even a combination of two such antibiotics.

However, in majority of cases and especially in the outpatient clinic, one has the luxury of having an opportunity to correct the error of choosing a wrong antibiotic that does not cover the organism in question, by change or escalation after a couple of days. This is quite safe as the child is unlikely to become seriously ill before that time, even if the antibiotic chosen is not effective. This approach allows us to start an empiric antibiotic that has narrower coverage than in the previous case of the critically ill patient. For example, in a patient with otitis media or sinusitis who is not sick and toxic, one can start with amoxicillin and escalate to amoxiclav only if there is no improvement.

It has two advantages:
1. It allows us to keep the more potent antibiotics in reserve for possible escalation in the few who do not respond to the first choice.
2. It is beneficial for antimicrobial stewardship as stronger antibiotics are used less often and are therefore less likely to induce bacterial resistance to them. This then helps to preserve their potency for deserved use in the severely ill truly drug resistant cases.

Other Factors

These include prior antibiotic therapy. If a patient has received some antibiotics and has not responded empiric therapy should consist of those agents, which will cover what the earlier did not. Of course one must rule out other causes of nonresponse—alternative diagnosis or collection of pus that needs drainage, etc. Attention to the site of infection is important and one should choose antibiotics that penetrate the affected site, e.g. the central nervous system (CNS), urine, and biliary tract. Attention to host comorbidities is important. For example, in a patient with renal dysfunction one must avoid nephrotoxic antibiotics as far as possible. Some antibiotics are contraindicated in neonates or young infants. However, one must remember that when pushed to the wall, treatment of infection takes precedence over host comorbidities. In immunocompromised hosts more aggressive therapy is needed since the host defense mechanisms are not operating and antibiotics have to do the entire job.

Dose and Route of Antibiotics

Adequate attention should be paid to the dosing. Dose should be calculated per kg body weight and should not exceed the ceiling dose. Higher doses may be needed for serious infections (meropenem is dosed as 40 mg/kg for serious infections versus 20 mg/kg/dose for less serious infections). Some antimicrobials may need a loading dose, e.g. colistin, polymyxin B, vancomycin, tigecycline, fluconazole, etc. Dose modification should be done if indicated for renal impairment, but the first dose is always the full dose. Pharmacodynamic properties of antibiotics have to be taken into account, e.g. once daily dosing for aminoglycosides, frequent dosing, and continuous infusion for BL. The route chosen depends on severity of infection, parenteral route (intravenous) is the choice for serious infections.

Definitive Therapy

Definitive therapy seems straightforward as we have an organism isolated and its drug sensitivity available (by culture or other methods). But it is not that simple. An organism grown on culture is to be considered as the true pathogen only after we have excluded the three Cs—(1) contaminant, (2) commensal, and (3) colonizer.

Positive Culture ≠ Definite Infection

1. *Contaminant* is an organism that (as the name suggests) has contaminated the culture. It may be from the patient's (or healthcare provider's) skin, use of unsterile equipment, or sometimes by careless handling of the culture material during transport or in the laboratory. Naturally, as this was not in the patient's body in the first place treating this would be irrational.
2. *Commensal* is an organism that normally resides in certain sites in the patient's body and is not the pathogen, i.e. not the cause of the infection. Some examples of nonsterile sites in the patient body from which commensals can be grown in the laboratory are the throat or the urine.
3. *Colonizer* is an organism that is present on an artificial structure in the patient's body like an endotracheal tube, a urinary catheter, or an indwelling line. These organisms that are present and therefore grown may simply be harmlessly growing there and not necessarily causing disease. It is a challenge sometimes to distinguish them from true pathogens.

It is only after these three imposters of a true pathogen are excluded that a decision is made to treat the organism that has been isolated or identified with an appropriate antibiotic. The choice of the agent has to be thoughtfully decided instead of just picking up any one labeled as "sensitive" on the laboratory report. It should preferably be of the narrowest spectrum to reduce collateral damage (e.g. for methicillin sensitive *S. aureus,* cloxacillin or cefazolin is preferred to coamoxiclav). If minimum inhibitory concentration (MIC) values are available, they should also be taken into account while choosing the antibiotic (the antibiotic with the lowest MIC—breakpoint ratio should be chosen). The antibiotic chosen should reach the site of the infection in adequate amounts to cure the infection in the dosage employed (e.g. BL-BLI combinations cannot be used for treating CNS infections since the BLI does not cross the blood brain barrier). The host's comorbidities like hepatic and renal dysfunction or circulatory status are additional factors that can affect the choice of the drug to be used or its dosage or route. If the child is on multiple other drugs, drug interactions also need to be taken into account before making a final decision.

The dose and route have to be taken note of as discussed earlier.

ESCALATION OF ANTIBIOTICS

What is Escalation?

Escalation is changing over from the current antibiotic(s) to another one (or more) antibiotic which is/are more potent, i.e. has/have a broader spectrum. The decision to escalate should to be based on clinical as well as laboratory criteria. But if the patient is not doing well when the antibiotic choice has been definitive (i.e. based on a culture sensitivity report), one should look for the possibility of a complication or additional diagnosis instead of blindly escalating the antibiotic. The question of escalation is more frequent and the choice more difficult when the earlier choice of antibiotic has been empirical. In such cases, if prior cultures have been sent, escalation may be required once the organism is identified by culture or molecular methods and found to be resistant to the antibiotic chosen empirically.

Escalation is not possible beyond a certain limit. If the patient is already receiving one or more very broad-spectrum antibiotic(s), (e.g. meropenem and vancomycin with colistin), the question of escalation does not arise. Therefore, starting very broad-spectrum antibiotics empirically for every patient is counterproductive as it leaves no room for escalation, if the patient does not respond to them.

When to Escalate?

Quite obviously, it should be done when the patient has not responded. Objective proof of nonresponse is by positive culture showing an organism demonstrating resistance to the antimicrobial in use. If one has such a report in hand, escalation is justified.

However, such a situation is rare. More often, the nonresponse has to be judged on clinical grounds. In that case, it is important to decide the parameters for judging clinical nonresponse. This can be done rationally only with a thorough knowledge of the clinical course expected even when the patient is on the correct antibiotic treatment. For example, in a case of enteric fever, one should be aware that defervescence may take up to 1 week and not escalate the antibiotic just because the patient is febrile 4 or 5 days after administration of a correctly chosen drug. Similarly, nonresolution of a pulmonary consolidation on X-ray in a patient who is otherwise clinically better, is not a good reason for escalation as we know that X-ray shadows after an acute pneumonia may take weeks to resolve. Another example is a case of pulmonary tuberculosis (TB) which would be labeled as resistant only if the sputum (or gastric aspirate) remains positive after 8 weeks of therapy.

On the other hand, a child with acute otitis media who is still febrile and in pain on 3rd day of an empirically chosen antibiotic calls for escalation. Similarly, a child with bacillary dysentery, who is still febrile and/or has visible blood in the stool after 2 days of antibiotic therapy, requires a change in his treatment. So also a neonate with bacterial sepsis whose clinical parameters or acute phase reactants have shown no improvement after 48 hours of a chosen course of antibiotics requires escalation. But it is important to allow sufficient time for the antibiotics chosen to act, (generally at least 48 hours) before giving up and deciding to change them.

When not to Escalate?

Escalation is generally not justified before 48 hours of the current antibiotic regimen is over, if the choice of empiric therapy was rational and well thought out. The exception is of course, if the patient becomes seriously ill, e.g. he or she develops septic shock. Changing antibiotics very frequently, like on a daily basis, without any objective data of resistance is irrational and must be deplored.

Escalation is also not justified, if the repeat culture shows the same organism with the same sensitivity. In these cases, escalation of the antibiotic may not be the answer. The nonresponse may be due to pharmacological reasons like nonadherence, inadequate dosage, or drug-drug interaction (like giving an oral fluoroquinolone with an antacid that hinders its absorption form the gut). Or there may be some other reason for failure—e.g. collection of pus (abscess or empyema), presence of dead tissue (like a sequestrum), or a foreign body like an indwelling catheter. Attention to these problems and continuation of the same antibiotic in the correct dose will suffice to effect a cure.

Escalation may also not be required, if the patient improves with empiric therapy and the cultures yield a resistant organism. For example, a child with urinary tract infection may have responded to third generation cephalosporins, while the urine culture grows ESBL producing organism. Here the *in vivo* response has happened because of concentration of the drug in the urine, which is higher than the MIC. Such patients should, however, be followed up carefully for relapse or late failures. One must also remember the 60/90 rule of antibiotic susceptibility testing. An organism designated as resistant to a particular antibiotic responds 60% of the times compared to 90% of the times with a sensitive antibiotic. This is because the breakpoints for defining resistance are very conservative and overestimate resistance. There may, however, be an exception to this rule. For example newborns or immunocompromised patients may need escalation of antibiotics based on the culture report even if they may have shown some clinical response.

How is Escalation Done?

It can be done in a variety of ways:

- Changing to a more potent molecule, e.g. from third generation cephalosporins or BL-BLI combination to carbapenems. While changing antibiotics to a more potent one, it is still important to make a rational choice rather than just starting any very broad-spectrum drug. This requires one to think of the possible organisms causing the infection in that particular case and which of these would have failed to respond to the antibiotic used. For example, if a child with acute otitis media has not responded to amoxicillin, one should think that there is possibly infection with a BL producing organism like *H. influenzae* and step up to a drug (like coamoxiclav) that will specifically cover such organisms and not just any broad spectrum antibiotic such as linezolid or ciprofloxacin.
- Adding another antibiotic of a different class, e.g. adding clarithromycin to amoxicillin in a school age child with pneumonia. In this last example, escalation is achieved by adding a new antibiotic while continuing the old one. This is because the macrolide added is required to cover atypical organisms like mycoplasma which are not attacked by the BL antibiotic amoxicillin. This is justified in community acquired pneumonia as the causative organism is hardly ever identified by culture or other means, i.e. the treatment is empirical. But generally speaking, especially when backed by a positive culture, escalation calls for replacement of the old drug with the new one.

DE-ESCALATION OF ANTIBIOTICS

What is De-escalation?

De-escalation is a method of narrowing empiric therapy. This has to be based on both culture reports and clinical improvement. The decisive factor for confidence in the success of de-escalation is a positive identification of the causative organism and its sensitivity pattern. Only then is it safe to de-escalate without jeopardizing the patient's safety and risking a relapse of the infection.

Why De-escalate?

It is human tendency to not "rock the boat". The usual refrain is "my patient is doing so well on the current combination of broad-spectrum antibiotics. Why take a chance and try to reduce or change the antibiotics being given?" But while it is tempting to continue and complete a course of antibiotics on which the patient has shown good improvement, it is noteworthy to remember that de-escalation of antibiotic therapy has multiple benefits. And de-escalation, properly done results in treatment outcomes that are noninferior to continuing on the previous therapy.
Some of the benefits of de-escalation are:

- Decrease in antibiotic related adverse events and super infection. By stepping down to a narrower spectrum antibiotic, you can prevent secondary infection with a "super-bug" that would be resistant to the broad-spectrum drug that the patient would be on.
- Cost savings! The narrower spectrum, more specific antibiotic is likely to be cheaper than the broad-spectrum combinations.
- Multidrug resistant (MDR) bugs in the hospital environment are reduced. This occurs by reduction of environmental exposure to broad-spectrum antibiotics. We need to remember that whenever an antibiotic is administered to even one patient, because of spillage at the time of preparation or administration and release into the environment via excreta of the patient, the hospital flora gets repeatedly exposed to these powerful antibiotics and they become resistant to them over a period of time. Also of course, the patient's normal gut organisms also get exposed to these antibiotics and can become resistant. When these environmental or gut organisms cause a nosocomial infection in the patient (or in the next patient), treatment becomes difficult as these will be resistant to the broad-spectrum antibiotics.

When to De-escalate?

While de-escalation is desirable, it has to be timed correctly. If done too early, the patient's infection may worsen and if done too late, the benefit will only be marginal. The timing of de-escalation has to be based both on clinical as well as some laboratory criteria. One point at which this can be easily done is when the result of the culture arrives. Take the example of a young infant admitted with septic shock and started (correctly so) on broad-spectrum combination of meropenem and amikacin. If after 2 days of this therapy, his blood culture report shows *S. pneumoniae* sensitive to all BL antibiotics, it is easy to confidently de-escalate to ampicillin or ceftriaxone. All of us are also familiar with the "de-escalation" of antitubercular therapy from four drugs to three after 2 months of therapy are over. Of course, this should be done only if the patient is clinically better and repeat sputum for acid-fast bacilli (AFB) is negative.

How to De-escalate?

De-escalation can be done in a variety of ways. One simple example is by dropping one of two (or more) antibiotics started. If one has started ceftriaxone and amikacin in a 7-week-old child with pyogenic meningitis and the culture report shows *S. pneumoniae*, the amikacin can be safely omitted. Or take the example of a school age group child with a severe community-acquired pneumonia started on ceftriaxone and a macrolide. If evidence for *Mycoplasma* is obtained [such as immunoglobulin M (IgM), enzyme-linked immunosorbent assay (ELISA) or cold agglutinins positive] the ceftriaxone can and should be omitted. One example of this is stepping down from a combination of cloxacillin and vancomycin to cloxacillin if the culture throws up methicillin sensitive *S. aureus* (MSSA). At other times, de-escalation is done by shifting to another antibiotic of narrower spectrum of the same or other class. For example, a patient started on meropenem for a suspected resistant gram-negative infection is switched to ceftriaxone, if the report shows susceptibility.

SWITCHING FROM PARENTERAL TO ORAL ANTIBIOTICS

Why Switch?

The switch from parenteral to oral therapy has to be timed correctly and the right choice of oral antibiotic has to be made. Some infections such as those of bone and joints and deep tissue abscesses require prolonged antibiotic therapy for several weeks. The financial costs, social problems, and medical risks of prolonged hospitalization are well known. Persisting with intravenous administration of antibiotics necessitates prolongation of the hospital stay with all these associated problems and risks (the exception of course is outpatient parenteral therapy, but this is practically possible only, if the antibiotic can be given in once a day dose). Hence, the treating clinician must consider discharging the child on oral medication as soon as it is safely possible.

When to Switch?

For common infections like enteric fever, an oral switch (and discharge) can be done as soon as the patient is afebrile. For other infections like osteomyelitis, specific guidelines exist to decide the timing of the switchover, which can be as early as 4–7 days in milder cases. This would include absence of fever, normal C-reactive protein (CRP), near normal counts, and a declining erythrocyte sedimentation rate (ESR). In the presence of retained sequestrum, an abscess or a foreign body, oral switch will have to delay till resolution of these issues. Caution also needs to be exercised, if the patient is immunocompromised in any way.

One important fact to remember is that an antibiotic given parenterally achieves a much higher concentration in the plasma (and by consequence, at the site of the infection) than the same one given orally. This is particularly so for the BL group of antibiotics where oral dosing results is plasma levels only around 10% of those achievable by intravenous route with standard dosing. So certain clinical situations where high tissue levels of antibiotic are required for complete clinical cure, switching to oral route might result in clinical failure, and must be avoided. Examples of these are pyogenic meningitis, neonatal sepsis, febrile neutropenic children, and bacterial endocarditis. In such cases, it is mandatory to complete the antibiotic course by parenteral route.

Types of Parenteral to Oral Switch

The change can happen in three different ways.

1. *Sequential:* In this, the injectable antibiotic is replaced with the same molecule in oral formulation, e.g. amoxicillin, ciprofloxacin, linezolid and metronidazole.
2. *Switch:* Changing from an intravenous preparation to an oral compound from the same class with (almost) the same spectrum. For example, ceftriaxone to oral cefixime for enteric fever.
3. *Step-down:* Here we change from an injectable antibiotic to an oral agent in another class or to a different medication where the spectrum of activity may not be exactly the same. Usually, the oral antibiotic used to replace the injectable one is of a narrower spectrum

than the injectable one. So this is actually an example of parenteral to oral switch with simultaneous de-escalation. Some examples of this type of step-down are discharging a child with community-acquired pneumonia treated with ceftriaxone on oral amoxicillin or a child with community-associated (CA)-MRSA cellulitis who responded to injectable vancomycin is sent home on oral cotrimoxazole.

Prerequisites for Switch

There are certain prerequisites for a successful parenteral to oral switch. First of all, the patient should have an intact and functioning gastrointestinal tract. Children with protracted vomiting, paralytic ileus, or malabsorption are obviously not suitable candidates for oral antibiotic therapy. As most of these patients had some serious illness to start with, proper completion of the antibiotic course is essential to prevent a relapse or other complications. So, one needs to ensure that the parent or care-taker is completely familiar with the oral medication, its dose and method of administration and he or she can be depended on to adhere to the therapy. It is always prudent to give the first few doses of the oral drug under supervision in the hospital before discharge so that this competence is demonstrated and any doubts addressed before transferring the onus of continued therapy to the parent. It is also wise to call the patient for frequent follow-ups, not just to monitor the progress of the recovery, but also to check on whether the doses are being correctly given at home. In critical cases, the outpatient oral therapy should be done under direct supervision as is done in directly observed treatment short course (DOTS) for TB. In critical cases, therapeutic drug monitoring should be done (if available) to ensure adequate serum levels of the antibiotic at prescribed oral dosages.

HOW LONG TO TREAT?

This obviously depends on the type of infection. For some infections such as cystitis even 3 days therapy may be needed while others like endocarditis may need therapy for 6 weeks. It is important to adhere to standard guidelines while making this decision of duration of therapy. However, the general trend in today's era is to shorten therapy for infections. This is in the interest of antimicrobial stewardship. For example, studies have shown that treatment of intra-abdominal infections with good source control for 4–7 days, ventilator-associated pneumonia for 8 days, gram-negative blood stream infections for 7 days, and pyelonephritis in adults for 7 days is as good as longer regimens. Conversely, new data recommends treatment of bacterial sinusitis for 10–14 days against shorter therapy to prevent relapses. New data also recommends use of procalcitonin normalization or reduction as criteria to stop therapy. This is especially important in today's era of MDR or extensively drug-resistant (XDR) pathogens, which are treated with toxic antibiotics where even a couple of day's reduction of therapy can pay huge dividends in terms of cost and adverse effects.

CONCLUSION

In conclusion, antibiotic therapy is a complex process and should not be embarked upon carelessly. The goal of achieving optimum therapy with assured clinical cure for the patient along with the least cost and side-effects calls for a fair amount of rational thought. The thought process has to start even before the first antibiotic is written, to decide whether it is needed or not in the first place. The choice of agent to be used, whether definitive or empirical, should not be haphazard but chosen after a logical thought process outlined above. It does not end with making the first empirical or definitive choice correctly. One needs to repeatedly cross check the appropriateness of the choice with the results of investigations and the patient's clinical condition on a continuous basis. The initial choice of antibiotic may need to be changed (escalated or de-escalated) for optimizing therapy. A switch to outpatient oral therapy with the appropriate antibiotic is also required and has to be timed right.

Rational antibiotic therapy is the mainstay of antibiotic stewardship. It will help to ensure that the current set of available antibiotics continue to remain potent and serve us well in fighting infections for many more years to come.

RECOMMENDED READING

1. Bradley JS, Nelson JD. Nelson's Pediatric Antimicrobial Therapy, 19th Edition. United State: American Academy of Pediatrics; 2013.
2. Camargo FA. The de-escalation concept and antibiotic de-escalation: a missed opportunity? Shock. 2013;39:29-31.
3. Deresinski S. Principles of antibiotic therapy in severe infections: optimizing the therapeutic approach by use of laboratory and clinical data. Clin Inf Dis. 2007;45(suppl 3):5177-83.
4. Krogstad P. Osteomyelitis. In: Feigin RD, Cherry JD, Demmler-Harrison GD, Kaplan SL (Ed). Textbook of Pediatric Infectious Diseases, 6th Edition. PA, USA: Saunders Elsevier; 2009. pp. 725-42.
5. Le Saux N, Howard A, Barrowman NJ, et al. Shorter courses of parenteral antibiotic therapy do not appear to influence response rates for children with acute hematogenous osteomyelitis: a systematic review. BMC Infect Dis. 2002;2:16-25.
6. Leung AKC, Wong AHC. Acute Otitis Media in Children. Recent Pat Inflamm Allergy Drug Discov. 2017;11:32-40.
7. Masterton RG. Antibiotic de-escalation. Crit Care Clin. 2011;27(1):149-62.
8. Menezes GA, Harish BN, Khan MA, et al. Antimicrobial resistance trends in blood culture positive *Salmonella* Paratyphi A isolates from Pondicherry, India. Indian J Med Microbiol. 2016;34(2):222-7.
9. Sharma S. Tuberculosis. In: Parthasarathy A (Ed). Textbook of Pediatric Infectious Diseases. Delhi: Jaypee Brothers Medical Publishers; 2013. pp. 246-56.
10. Sierra A, Lopez P, Zapata MA, et al. Non-typeable *Haemophilus influenzae* and *Streptococcus pneumoniae* as primary causes of acute otitis media in Colombian children: a prospective study. BMC Infect Dis. 2011;11:4.
11. Traa BS, Walker CLF, Munos M, et.al. Antibiotics for the treatment of dysentery in children. Int J Epidemiol. 2010;39(suppl 1):i70-4.
12. Van de Beek D, Cabellos C, Dzupova O, et al. ESCMID guideline: Diagnosis and treatment of acute bacterial meningitis. Clin Microb Inf. 201;22(Suppl 3):S37-62.
13. Yewale V. Management of typhoid fever including MDRTF. In: Ganguly N, Kundu R, Ghosh TK (Eds). Multi-drug resistant pediatric infections. Delhi: CBS Publishers and Distributors; 2009. pp. 22-8.

Antimicrobial Therapy in Acute Gastroenteritis

17
Chapter

Shinjini Bhatnagar, Tanu Singhal

INTRODUCTION

Antimicrobial therapy is required in only a small percentage of children with acute gastroenteritis since most infections especially in children below 5 years are viral (Table 1). However, as maintenance of hydration and correction of dehydration take precedence over all other modes of therapy in the management of childhood diarrhea, it is also discussed.

REVISED RECOMMENDATIONS FOR TREATMENT OF ACUTE DIARRHEA

The revised World Health Organization (WHO) and Indian Academy of Pediatrics (IAP) recommendations for treatment of acute diarrhea are use of reduced osmolarity oral rehydration salt (ORS) for treating dehydration and maintaining hydration, and twice required daily allowance (RDA) of elemental zinc for at least 14 days.

Reduced Osmolarity Oral Rehydration Salt

The new improved reduced osmolarity ORS recommended for all ages and all types of diarrhea by the WHO, Government of India, and the IAP contains 75 mmol/L of sodium and 75 mmol/L of glucose with an osmolarity of 245 mOsm/L. These recommendations are based on a recent meta-analysis, which included 12 large randomized controlled trials. Use of reduced osmolarity ORS was associated with a significant 39% reduction in need for intravenous (IV) fluids, 19% reduction in stool output and 29% lower incidence of vomiting as compared with the standard

TABLE 1: Etiology of acute diarrhea.

Pathogen	*Incidence*
Rotavirus	25–30%
Enterotoxigenic *E. coli* (ETEC)	20%
Shigella	5–10%
Enteropathogenic *E. coli* (EPEC), Locally adherent *E. coli*, *Campylobacter*, *Salmonella*	5–7%
Giardia lamblia, *Entamoeba histolytica*	<2%
Vibrio cholerae	5–10%

WHO ORS (sodium 90 mEq/L glucose 110 mmol/L, osmolarity 311 mOsm/L). The need for IV fluids is considered an important outcome measure as in many peripheral health facilities, where IV therapy may not be available; reducing the need for unscheduled IV therapy would reduce the risk of death from dehydration. It was also found to be as effective in adults and children with cholera. The safety data in patients with cholera, while limited, is reassuring.

Zinc in the Treatment of Diarrhea

Based on studies in India and other developing countries there is sufficient evidence to recommend zinc in the treatment of acute diarrhea as adjunct to oral rehydration. Studies have shown that zinc supplemented children had 16% [95% confidence interval (CI) 11-22%] faster recovery from diarrhea with a 34% (95% CI 17–48%) reduction in the odds of acute episodes lasting more than 7 days and the total stool output was reduced by 24% (95% CI 2–41%) as compared to the placebo group. Importantly, zinc supplementation has shown to reduce the incidence and severity of diarrhea in the subsequent 2–3 months after supplementation has been stopped. All studies showed that the effect of zinc did not vary significantly with age, nutritional status assessed by anthropometry or the type of zinc salt used—zinc sulfate, zinc acetate, or zinc gluconate. The results of the most recent meta-analyses are consistent with the previous data.

Therapeutic benefits of zinc administration during diarrhea are biologically plausible because of its effects on various components of the immune system and its direct gastrointestinal (GI) effects. Zinc is said to improve absorption of water and electrolytes by helping in early regeneration of intestinal mucosa, restoration of enteric enzymes, and enhancing humoral and cellular immunity. Zinc has been also shown to have antisecretory properties in malnourished guinea pigs.

The WHO recommends that 20 mg per day of zinc supplementation should be given once or twice daily for 10–14 days starting as early as possible after onset of diarrhea in children older than 6 months. Although more evidence is required, it is recommended that infants less than 6 months should be given 10 mg per day. These recommendations have been endorsed by the IAP and the pharmaceutical industry has responded positively by marketing formulations that contain only zinc. Iron containing formulations should not be used with zinc as it may interfere with zinc absorption.

ANTIMICROBIAL DRUGS

Antimicrobial drugs are not required for routine treatment of acute diarrhea because most episodes are caused by pathogens for which antimicrobial drugs are not effective (Table 1). Rotavirus is responsible for 20–25% of diarrhea episodes in children aged 6–24 months visiting treatment facilities and for 15% of cases in the same age group in the community. It causes patchy blunting of intestinal villi with some reduction of mucosal disaccharidases, which return to normal within 2–3 weeks. The diarrhea is watery, and is usually associated with vomiting and low-grade fever. Antimicrobials are not recommended as the diarrhea is self-limiting with the median duration being about 8 days and can be effectively treated with oral rehydration fluids and continued feeding. Enterotoxigenic *E. coli* (ETEC) is another major cause of diarrhea and is responsible for up to 25% of all diarrheas in children from developing countries. ETEC does not invade the mucosa or damage the brush border but manifests with watery diarrhea by producing heat labile (LT) and/or heat stable (ST) enterotoxins that induce secretion of fluids and electrolytes. Antibiotic therapy does not offer any significant clinical benefit, as the diarrhea is self-limiting. The mainstay of treatment is oral rehydration fluids and continued feeding.

When should antimicrobials be given for treatment of acute diarrhea?

The only specific clinical indications for use of antimicrobial agents where they have been found to be useful include:

- Suspected cholera with severe dehydration
- Bloody diarrhea (probably shigellosis)
- Serious associated non-GI infections, e.g. pneumonia, septicemia, meningitis, urinary tract infection, etc.

CHOLERA

The mainstay of therapy for cholera is rehydration with oral rehydration solution (for some dehydration) or IV Ringer's lactate (for severe dehydration). In a recent Cochrane review evaluating 39 trials with 4,623 participants, antimicrobials used as an adjunct to oral or IV rehydration therapy have shown reduction in the duration of diarrhea by 1.5 days, stool output by 50%, requirement of IV fluids by 40%, and time of excretion of *Vibrio cholerae* by 3 days. Antibiotics like tetracycline (12.5 mg/kg four times a day for a period of 3 days), erythromycin (12.5 mg/kg given four times a day for 3 days), cotrimoxazole [trimethoprim (TMP) 5 mg/kg or sulfamethoxazole (SMX)25 mg/kg twice a day for 3 days], and furazolidone (1.25mg/kg four times a day for 3 days) have been used effectively in the past. TMP SMX and furazolidone are no longer recommended due to resistance. Four times dosing of tetracycline and erythromycin for 3 days is cumbersome and associated with GI side effects. The relatively newer options include single dose doxycycline or ciprofloxacin, and azithromycin 20 mg/ kg single dose. There is rising incidence of resistance to quinolones in South Asia. Studies on doxycycline show that it has less affinity for calcium as compared to tetracyclines and is safe for infants, children, and pregnant women. Rates of resistance to azithromycin are the lowest at present. The Global Task Force on cholera control in its publication in May, 2018 has recommended antimicrobial therapy with doxycycline as the first choice (300 mg single dose in adults including pregnant women and 2–4 mg/kg single dose in children) for cholera with severe dehydration or in immunocompromised patients or those where the purge rate is not reducing in the initial few hours, if the local strain is susceptible. Alternative options include ciprofloxacin or azithromycin (20 mg/kg single dose or 1 g). The dose of ciprofloxacin in South Asia has been recommended to be increased to 15 mg/kg twice daily for 3 days to counter the increasing minimal inhibitory concentrations (MICs). The use of antimicrobials for prophylaxis of cholera in contacts or during outbreaks is not recommended.

BLOODY DIARRHEA

Definition

The episode is termed bloody diarrhea or dysentery when visible blood is present in the stool. Terms like bloody diarrhea, dysentery, bacillary dysentery, and invasive diarrhea are often used interchangeably. Bloody diarrhea refers to any episode of diarrhea with visible red blood and does not include melena or episodes, where blood streaks are present on the surface of formed stool. Episodes where blood is identified by microscopic examination or biochemical tests are not defined as bloody diarrhea. Classical textbook definition of dysentery means bloody diarrhea accompanied with fever, abdominal cramps, tenesmus, and mucoid stools. However, in clinical practice all these accompanying features may not always be present. Bacillary dysentery is used for dysentery caused by Shigella and distinguishes shigellosis from amoebic dysentery (not a common cause of dysentery in children). The term bacillary dysentery is usually used synonymously with infection due to Shigella; though other bacteria can also cause dysentery and not all Shigella infections are associated with visible blood and mucous in stool. Dysentery or bloody diarrhea can also be seen with other bacterial pathogens including nontyphoidal salmonella, Enteroinvasive *E. coli*, Enterohemorrhagic *E. coli*, *Campylobacter*, and *Yersinia*. It is estimated that Shigella causes 5–10% of all childhood diarrhea and 30–50% of all cases of dysentery.

Antimicrobial Therapy in Bloody Diarrhea

Rationale for Antimicrobial Therapy

Antimicrobial therapy is the mainstay of treatment in bloody diarrhea and is targeted toward Shigella as it is the most common cause of bloody diarrhea. Prompt antimicrobial therapy decreases associated mortality, reduces the duration of anorexia and malabsorption, and hastens elimination of Shigella from the stool. It is recommended that absorbable, systemically effective antimicrobials agents should be used as Shigella invades the intestinal mucosa and multiplies within the submucosa.

Choice of Antimicrobials

The choice of antimicrobial as advised by the WHO depends on the local resistance patterns and is crucial since evidence suggests that use of an ineffective drug may actually exacerbate the disease by destroying the normal intestinal flora that compete with *Shigella* for nutrition.

Antimicrobial resistance is a serious problem with *Shigella* all over the world and especially in India. The period between 1940 and 1980 saw stepwise evolution of resistance to sulfonamides, cotrimoxazole, tetracyclines, ampicillin, and finally nalidixic acid. In the late 1980's, quinolones emerged as the preferred drug for managing shigellosis; excellent results were seen with even single doses and even in multidrug-resistant (MDR) *S. dysenteriae* type 1. However, indiscriminate use and over the counter availability led to rapid development of resistance to quinolones. Scores of studies from various parts of India have reported quinolone resistance rates ranging from 50% to 90%. Resistance to third generation cephalosporins in *Shigella* mediated by production of extended spectrum beta-lactamase enzymes is on the rise as well. Sporadic cases of azithromycin resistance have been reported from Bangladesh.

Choices for antimicrobial therapy in India include quinolones, cefixime, azithromycin, and ceftriaxone and are compared in Table 2. Pivmecillinam is also effective but not available in India. Ampicillin, cotrimoxazole, and nalidixic acid are not recommended owing to high resistance rates; amoxicillin, first and second generation cephalosporins, and aminoglycosides are not recommended despite in vitro susceptibility.

The patient should be called back after 2 days for evaluation. The signs of improvement include disappearance of fever, less blood in stool, passage of fewer stools, improved appetite, decreased abdominal pain, and return to normal activity. If signs of improvement are present then the same antimicrobial should be given for 5 days. If there is no improvement in 2 days the antimicrobial therapy should be changed to an alternative effective antimicrobial. If there is no

TABLE 2: Antimicrobial therapy for bloody diarrhea.

Drug	*Adults*	*Children*	*Comments*
Ciprofloxacin	500 mg twice daily	• 15 mg/kg twice daily • Not approved by DCGI for <18 years	Drug of choice worldwide but not in India due to rising resistance rates
Azithromycin	500 mg day 1 and then 250 mg	12 mg/kg day 1 and then 6 mg/kg	• Prolong QT interval • Limited trial data • Lack of breakpoints • Rapid development of resistance
Cefixime	200 mg twice daily	10 mg/kg/day	• Inadequate trial data but performs well in clinical practice • Resistance emerging
Ceftriaxone	2–4 g daily	50–100 mg/kg/day	Preferred drug for inpatient treatment

(DCGI: Drug Controller General of India)

improvement with the second antimicrobial, the diagnosis should be reviewed, stool sent for culture and susceptibility testing and antiamoebic therapy with metronidazole may be tried.

Other Causes of Bloody Diarrhea

Other uncommon causes of bloody diarrhea are *Campylobacter jejuni*, *Schistosoma*, Salmonella, enteroinvasive and enterohemorrhagic *E. coli*. All these pathogens require special laboratory procedures for isolation. New multiplex polymerase chain reaction (PCR) tests (Biofire film array GI panel that tests for 20 odd GI pathogens including viruses, bacteria, and protozoa) are now available that can help diagnose these infections. However, the panel is very expensive and therapeutic implications of diagnosis are limited. This panel may be useful in the immunocompromised patients. Infection with *C. jejuni* responds to early treatment with an effective antimicrobial, e.g. erythromycin, but most episodes recover by the time the laboratory diagnosis is made. Antimicrobial therapy in Salmonella infection may prolong the carriage of the pathogen.

High Risk Cases of Dysentery

Risk factors for death are greatest among infants, nonbreastfed, dehydrated, or malnourished children. History of convulsions or measles and presence of unconsciousness, hypo-, or hyperthermia at first contact are indicators of severe illness and these children are at greater risk of dying. Such children should be referred to the hospital for treatment. Those with severe malnutrition should be additionally screened and treated for associated sepsis.

When to Consider Amoebic Dysentery?

Young children should not be routinely treated for amoebiasis, as it is an infrequent cause of bloody diarrhea in children. The incidence of disease with *Entamoeba histolytica* increases with age and most episodes are in adults. Amoebiasis should be considered only if two different antibiotics usually effective for *Shigella* in the area have been given sequentially without showing signs of clinical improvement, or if a microscopic examination of fresh stool done in a reliable laboratory shows trophozoites of *E. histolytica* containing red blood cell (RBC). Amoebic dysentery should be treated with metronidazole given at 10 mg/kg/dose three times a day for 5–10 days. This should be followed by diloxanide furoate for eradication of the cysts for a period of 10 days (Dose in children more than 12 years, adolescents and adults is 500 mg thrice daily for 10 days, for children below 12 years 20 mg/kg/day in three divided doses). Presence of cysts of *Entamoeba histolytica* is not an indication for treatment as usually these are nonpathogenic *E. dispar* cysts.

Supportive Care

Supportive care is very essential while treating dysentery. This includes treating dehydration, associated fever, other systemic infections (such as pneumonia or urinary tract infection), convulsions, metabolic complications, and rectal prolapse. Adequate calorie dense feeding should be continued. WHO and IAP recommend daily dose of 20 mg of elemental zinc (as zinc sulfate, or zinc acetate or zinc gluconate) once daily for 10–14 days (10 mg per day for infants below 6 months) in children up to 5 years of age. Drugs for symptomatic relief, abdominal and rectal pain should preferably be avoided, as they can increase severity of illness.

GIARDIASIS

Treatment for *Giardia* is definitely indicated if *Giardia* cysts *or* trophozoites are identified in stool or duodenal fluid. Giardiasis is treated with 5 mg/kg/dose of metronidazole given three times a day for 5 days. Tinidazole can also be given as a single dose (50 mg/kg orally; up to a maximum of two doses). The adverse effects and treatment failures to these drugs have given rise to the need for alternative antigiardial agents. There is some evidence to suggest that albendazole and mebendazole are equally effective and better tolerated than metronidazole. There is recent preliminary evidence from a randomized controlled trial in Egypt that nitazoxanide (nitrothiazolyl-salicylamide derivative, dose 12–47 months 100 mg 12 hourly × 3 days; 4–11 years 200 mg 12 hourly × 3 days) was significantly better in achieving earlier recovery from diarrhea as compared to a placebo. However, there was no clinical difference when 110 children were randomly treated with nitazoxanide or metronidazole. There is presently limited evidence from randomized controlled trials to recommend routine treatment with nitazoxanide for giardiasis. Additionally, the cost of treatment with nitazoxanide is almost seven times higher than that with metronidazole.

INFECTION WITH UNUSUAL PATHOGENS

Cryptosporidium parvum is an intracellular protozoa causing watery, nonbloody diarrhea often accompanied with fever, vomiting, and anorexia. It is an important cause of community acquired and persistent diarrhea in children with normal immune function where the disease is self-limiting with a mean duration of diarrhea of 10 days. Chronic high volume diarrhea leading to malnutrition, extraintestinal manifestations, and sometimes death are features of immunocompromised children [chiefly human immunodeficiency virus (HIV)-infected children] with cryptosporidiosis. Diagnosis is established by performing a modified acid-fast bacilli (AFB) stain on the stool sample. Supportive therapy is the mainstay of treatment of cryptosporidium infection in immunocompetent children. Nitazoxanide is presently the only Food and Drug Administration (FDA) approved treatment available for children 1–11 years of age with normal immune function. The optimum therapy for cryptosporidiosis in HIV-infected children is prompt initiation of combination antiretroviral therapy with fluid, electrolyte, and nutrition support. The role of nitazoxanide in treating cryptosporidiosis in immunocompromised children is not clear but 2 weeks of therapy is recommended. Paromomycin a nonabsorbable aminoglycoside is another are other drug that has shown to have potential benefits in HIV-infected individuals with cryptosporidiosis but is not available in India.

Other protozoan parasites including *Isospora belli* and Microsporidia may cause severe diarrhea in immunocompromised patients and can be diagnosed by AFB staining of stool specimens. *I. belli* responds well to treatment with cotrimoxazole.

CLOSTRIDIUM DIFFICILE COLITIS

Clostridium difficile is an anaerobic spore bearing gram positive bacillus that colonizes the gut of around 2% of healthy individuals. This colonization rate increases with hospitalization due to acquisition from the hands of healthcare workers and the environment. In the presence of risk factors such as antimicrobial therapy, infection with *C. difficile* can occur. While use of nearly any antibiotic may result in *C. difficile* toxin production, β-lactam antibiotics (e.g. cephalosporins and penicillins), and clindamycin are most commonly implicated. Pathogenesis is through production of toxin A and B. Clinical symptoms range from mild to severe consisting of mild self-limiting diarrhea to a toxic megacolon. Bloody diarrhea is unusual in *C. difficile.*

Clostridium difficile infection (CDI) is significantly more common in adults than in children. In fact asymptomatic carriage of toxigenic *C. difficile* is very common in neonates, infants, and toddlers younger than 2 years and hence current guidelines from the Infectious Disease Society of America (IDSA) recommend not testing for *C. difficle* unless all other infectious and noninfectious causes are excluded. Diagnosis should be considered in children older than 2 years with diarrhea and risk factors such as prolonged hospitalization, antimicrobial therapy, immunosuppression, inflammatory bowel disease, and presence of gastrostomy or jejunostomy tube. The diagnostic tests currently recommended are an assay for glutamate dehydrogenase (GDH) as a screening test and then a toxin assay as a confirmatory test for patients who are GDH positive. The sensitivity of the toxin assay is around 70–80%. Alternatively, a *C. difficile* PCR, which is now available on the Xpert platform with a turnaround time of 2 hours can also be used.

Discontinuing antibiotics, if possible is the most important component of therapy. Probiotics provide no benefit in treatment of established *C. difficile* disease. As per current guidelines, children with an initial nonsevere CDI episode can be treated with either oral vancomycin 10 mg/kg/dose 6 hourly (maximum 125 mg 6 hourly) or oral metronidazole 7.5 mg/kg/ dose 8 hourly for 10 days. Vancomycin is preferred for patients with severe CDI. In complicated CDI (with shock and megacolon) a combination of oral vancomycin with IV metronidazole may have to be used. Relapses of infection should be treated with vancomycin for 10–14 days, and second recurrence may need prolonged tapering course of vancomycin for up to 4–6 weeks and even fecal microbiota transplantation.

Strict contact isolation of affected patient, use of gloves and antimicrobial soap for hand hygiene (*C. difficile* spores are resistant to alcoholic hand rub) and cleaning the environment with sodium hypochlorite are crucial to prevent nosocomial transmission. Primary prevention of *C. difficile* entails antibiotic stewardship, proper hand hygiene, good environmental disinfection protocols, and use of dedicated patient care equipment. A recent meta-analysis showed that probiotics (*Lactobacillus acidophilus* or *Saccharomyces boulardii*) reduced the incidence of *C. difficile* by 60% in adults and children particularly those at high risk for CDI.

ASSOCIATED NONGASTROINTESTINAL INFECTION

All children, particularly infants less than 3 months of age or those severely malnourished, should be carefully screened for non-GI infection, e.g. pneumonia, septicemia, meningitis, and urinary tract infection. Early detection and appropriate treatment of associated systemic infection in malnourished children can reduce the mortality significantly.

OTHER DRUGS THAT ARE INEFFECTIVE IN DIARRHEA AND CAN ALSO CAUSE SIDE EFFECTS

Antidiarrheal Agents

Agents like adsorbents (kaolin, pectin, activated charcoal, and bismuth subcarbonate), motility suppressants (opiates, opiate-like compound tincture of opium, camphorated tincture of opium or paregoric, codeine, diphenoxylate with atropine, and loperamide hydrochloride) are not indicated in the routine treatment of acute diarrhea. Motility suppressants decrease intestinal peristalsis and delay the elimination of the causative organisms. Their use in infants can be particularly dangerous causing paralytic ileus, respiratory depression, abdominal distension, bacterial overgrowth, and sepsis.

The antisecretory properties of the new synthetic enkephalinase inhibitor, racecadotril, are attributed to inactivation of endogenous enkephalins and secreted by myenteric and submucous plexus in the digestive tract. This compound differs from μ-opiate receptor agonists like loperamide and diphenoxylate because its antisecretory mechanisms are independent of effects on intestinal motility. This drug has been evaluated in a small number of children and adults with diarrhea in randomized controlled trials with varying results. The benefit of this drug for treatment of acute diarrhea has not been documented to an extent and in a manner that is required to recommend its use. We need more evidence of its efficacy and safety from well-designed randomized controlled studies done in our settings.

Combination Therapy

Several combinations of antibacterial agents and of antibacterials with antidiarrheals are available. They offer no extra clinical benefit as compared to a properly selected single antibacterial agent for the small proportion of diarrheal illness where indication for their use exists. Combination therapy can promote overgrowth of harmful resistant bacteria and the antimotility agents that are often a part of these combinations may delay excretion of invasive pathogens. Some drug combinations containing metronidazole group of drugs can induce further vomiting.

PROBIOTICS

The role of probiotics in treatment of acute diarrhea in children is controversial. Several recent randomized controlled trials conducted in developed or developing countries have not shown any benefit of probiotics including *Lactobacillus* or *Saccharomyces* in reducing the severity of acute gastroenteritis. However, certain meta-analysis has demonstrated such benefits. Therefore, the jury is still out as far as probiotics and acute gastroenteritis is awaited. There is more robust data demonstrating the efficacy of probiotics in preventing and treating antibiotic associated diarrhea.

CONCLUSION

Oral rehydration salt remains the mainstay of therapy during acute diarrhea and zinc as an adjunct as an additional modest benefit in the reducing the stool volume and duration of diarrhea. Antimicrobials should be restricted to children with bloody diarrhea, cholera with severe dehydration, for associated non-GI infections especially malnourished children or infants less than 3 months and for definitely proven amoebiasis and giardiasis.

RECOMMENDED READING

1. Amadi B, Mwiya M, Musuku J, et al. Effect of nitazoxanide on morbidity and mortality in Zambian children with cryptosporidiosis: a randomised controlled trial. Lancet. 2002;360:1375-80.
2. Basualdo W, Arbo A. Randomized comparison of azithromycin versus cefixime for treatment of shigellosis in children. Pediatr infect Dis J. 2003;22:374-7.
3. Bhatnagar S, Bhandari N, Mouli UC, et al. Consensus statement of IAP National Task Force: status report on management of acute diarrhea. Indian Pediatr. 2004;41:335-48.
4. Bhattacharya SK, Sur D. An evaluation of current shigellosis treatment. Expert Opin Pharmacother. 2003;4:1315-20.
5. Bhutta ZA, Bird SM, Black RE, etc. Therapeutic effects of oral zinc in acute and persistent diarrhea in children in developing countries; pooled analysis of randomized controlled trials. Am J Clin Nutr. 2000;72:1516-22.
6. Cezard JP, Duhamel JF, Meyer M, et al. Efficacy and tolerability of racecadotril in acute diarrhea in children. Gastroenterology. 2001;120:799-805.
7. Florez ID, Veroniki AA, Al Khalifah R, et al. Comparative effectiveness and safety of interventions for acute diarrhea and gastroenteritis in children: A systematic review and network meta-analysis. PLoS One. 2018;13(12):e0207701.
8. Freedman SB, Williamson-Urquhart S, Farion KJ, et al. PERC PROGUT Trial Group. Multicenter trial of a combination probiotic for children with gastroenteritis. N Engl J Med. 2018;379(21):2015-26.
9. Global Task Force on Cholera Control. Technical note. Use of antibiotics in treatment and control of cholera. [online] Available from: https://www.who.int/cholera/task_force/use-of-antibiotics-for-the-treatment-of-cholera.pdf [Accessed December, 2018].
10. Goldenberg JZ, Lytvyn L, Steurich J, et al. Probiotics for the prevention of pediatric antibiotic-associated diarrhea. Cochrane Database Syst Rev. 2015;(12):CD004827.
11. Goldenberg JZ, Yap C, Lytvyn L, et al. Probiotics for the prevention of *Clostridium difficile*-associated diarrhea in adults and children. Cochrane Database Syst Rev. 2017;12:CD006095.
12. Ianiro G, Rizzatti G, Plomer M, et al. Bacillus clausii for the treatment of acute diarrhea in children: a systematic review and meta-analysis of randomized controlled trials. Nutrients. 2018;10(8). pii:E1074.
13. Khan WA, Seas C, Dhar U, et al. Treatment of shigellosis: V. Comparison of azithromycin and ciprofloxacin. A double blind, randomized, controlled trial. Ann Intern Med. 1997;126:697-703.
14. Kosek M, Alcantara C, Lima AA, et al. Cryptosporidiosis: an update. Lancet Infect Dis. 2001;1:262-9.
15. Leibovici-Weissman Y, Neuberger A, Bitterman R, et al. Antimicrobial drugs for treating cholera. Cochrane Database Syst Rev. 2014;(6):CD008625.
16. Lukacik M, Thomas RL, Aranda JV. A meta-analysis of the effects of oral zinc in the treatment of acute and persistent diarrhea. Pediatrics. 2008;121:326-36.
17. Martin JM, Pitetti R, Maffei F, et al. Treatment of shigellosis with cefixime: two days vs. five days. Pediatr Infect Dis J. 2000;19:522-6.
18. McDonald LC, Gerding DN, Johnson S, et al. Clinical Practice Guidelines for *Clostridium difficile* Infection in Adults and Children: 2017 Update by the Infectious Diseases Society of America (IDSA) and Society for Healthcare Epidemiology of America (SHEA). Clin Infect Dis. 2018;66:987-94.

19. Ortiz JJ, Ayoub A, Gargala G, et al. Randomized clinical study of nitazoxanide compared to metronidazole in the treatment of symptomatic giardiasis in children from Northern Peru. Aliment Pharmacol Ther. 2001;15:1409-15.
20. Pengsaa K, Sirivichayakul C, Pojjaroen-anant C, et al. Albendazole treatment for Giardia intestinalis infections in school children. Southeast Asian J Trop Med Public Health. 1999;30:78-83.
21. Schnadower D, Tarr PI, Casper TC, et al. Lactobacillus rhamnosus GG versus placebo for acute gastroenteritis in children. N Engl J Med. 2018;379:2002-14.
22. Taneja N, Mewara A. Shigellosis. Epidemiology in India. Indian J Med Res. 2016;143:565-576
23. White AC Jr, Chappell CL, Hayat CS, et al. Paromomycin for cryptosporidiosis in AIDS: a prospective, double blind trial. J Infect Dis. 1994;170:419-24.
24. WHO. (2005). The treatment of diarrhea. A manual for physicians and other senior health workers. 2005 WHO/CDD/SER/80.2. [online] Available from: http://apps.who.int/iris/handle/10665/43209 [Accessed December, 2018].
25. WHO. Guidelines for the control of shigellosis, including epidemics due to *Shigella dysenteriae* type 1 2005. [online] Available from: URL: http://apps.who.int/iris/bitstream/10665/43252/1/924159330X.pdf?ua=1&ua=1 [Accessed December, 2018].
26. WHO. Reduced osmolarity oral rehydration salts (ORS) formulation. A report from a meeting of experts jointly organized by UNICEF and WHO. New York, USA; UNICEF House; 2001.
27. Yereli K, Balcioglu IC, Ertan P, et al. Albendazole as an alternative therapeutic agent for childhood giardiasis in Turkey. Clin Microbiol Infect. 2004;10:527-9.

Antimicrobial Therapy in Intra-abdominal Infections

18

Chapter

Suhas Prabhu

INTRODUCTION

The term intra-abdominal infection generally refers to infections of the several solid organs and the peritoneal cavity. When the infection is located within the peritoneal space, it is called peritonitis, a fairly common and dangerous entity in children. Another important infection is liver abscess, which may be bacterial or amoebic. A third condition that will be covered here is infections of the biliary tract. Infections within the bowel (gastroenteritis) are covered in Chapter 17. Infections of the retroperitoneal space such as psoas abscess or pyelonephritis are, strictly speaking, outside the abdomen, and are not covered here.

ACUTE APPENDICITIS

This is the most common intra-abdominal infection faced in clinical practice. The usual causative organisms are gram negative (*E. coli* and *Klebsiella*), anaerobes, and enterococci. Therapy includes source control with appendicectomy and antimicrobials.

Need for Appendicectomy

There have been several randomized controlled trials comparing appendicectomy with only antibiotic therapy in acute uncomplicated (nonperforated) appendicitis in children and adults.

A recently conducted meta-analysis included five studies, 404 patients with uncomplicated appendicitis (aged 5–15 years). Nonoperative treatment was successful in 152 of 168 patients (90.5%), which was noninferior to the group treated with surgery. Subgroup analysis showed that the risk for treatment failure in patients with appendicolith increased. Another meta-analysis included 147 children (nonoperative treatment) and 173 children (appendectomy) with 1 year follow-up. Percentage of children experiencing complications ranged from 0% to 13% versus 0–17% for nonoperative and appendectomy, respectively. Nonoperative treatment avoided an appendectomy in 62–81% of the children after 1 year follow-up. A large randomized controlled trial for acute uncomplicated appendicitis in children is in the offing. But meanwhile one can consider conservative management in children older than 5 years with acute uncomplicated or nonperforated appendicitis without an appendicolith.

Antibiotic Therapy

Acute Appendicitis with Surgery

In acute uncomplicated appendicitis, where surgery is planned, ceftriaxone and metronidazole are administered as surgical prophylaxis. If the appendix is not perforated, then 24 hours of therapy is sufficient. If the appendix has perforated then antibiotics need to be continued till normalization of fever, white blood cell (WBC) count, and gastrointestinal (GI) functioning (4–5 days).

Acute Uncomplicated Appendicitis without Surgery

Here therapy with ceftriaxone or cefotaxime with metronidazole for a period of 4–5 days till normalization of clinical and inflammatory parameters is indicated.

Acute Complicated Appendicitis with Perforation, Peritonitis, or Septic Shock

Here treatment may include beta-lactam-beta-lactamase inhibitor (BL-BLI) combinations or carbapenems in sick patients and is discussed in the section on secondary peritonitis.

PERITONITIS

The peritoneal space extends from the floor of the pelvis to the under surface of the diaphragm and is divided by the mesentery into two major compartments. In addition, it extends into several recesses like the lesser sac, the subphrenic space, the left and the right paracolic gutters, and the pouch of Douglas (in females). In each of these sites, the infection may be segregated to form localized intraperitoneal abscesses, but the antibiotic choices for these cases remain the same as for generalized peritonitis. Chronic low-grade peritoneal infections such as tuberculous peritonitis also occur but those are not addressed here and treatment options discussed here refer only to the acute infections.

Acute peritonitis can be caused by a variety of organisms. They may reach there via the bloodstream (or rarely by transmural bacterial translocation from the intestine) or via direct penetration into the peritoneal cavity. The former is called primary peritonitis and the latter is referred to as secondary peritonitis. All peritonitis cases require inpatient treatment and intravenous antibiotics. Supportive care includes maintenance of homeostasis with attention to dehydration, acidosis, electrolyte imbalance, hypotension, and hypoxia.

Primary Peritonitis

Primary peritonitis (or spontaneous bacterial peritonitis) is seen most commonly in patients with chronic ascites as can happen in nephrotic syndrome or portal hypertension due to cirrhosis of liver or extrahepatic portal hypertension including Budd–Chiari syndrome. Presentation is usually fever, abdominal pain, abdominal distension, and diarrhea. Diagnosis is established by ascitic tap. At least 20 mL of the ascitic fluid should be inoculated in aerobic and anaerobic culture bottles for better isolation. The most common pathogen in primary peritonitis in the past used to be *Streptococcus pneumoniae,* but its incidence is declining (at least in the West) possibly due to increasing use of antibiotics and pneumococcal vaccination. Other causative gram-positive organisms are group A streptococci, enterococci (<5% of cases), and staphylococci. Gram-negative organisms, such as *Escherichia coli, Enterobacter, Klebsiella,* or *Acinetobacter* account for about half the cases especially in patients with liver disease. Anaerobic infections are not common as the oxygen content of ascitic fluid is quite high.

In the setting of nephrotic syndrome associated primary peritonitis, where *Pneumococcus* is the likely offender ceftriaxone is the drug of choice. Since the incidence of drug resistance in *Pneumococcus* in nonmeningeal infections in India is infrequent routine addition of vancomycin is not recommended. In the setting of chronic liver disease associated primary peritonitis where gram-negative pathogens predominate, choices for empiric therapy include ceftriaxone or cefotaxime, BL-BLI combinations such as piperacillin tazobactam or cefoperazone sulbactam or even carbapenems. The choice depends on the severity of illness and risk factors for infection with drug resistant bacteria including prior antibiotic therapy or hospitalization, etc. The high prevalence of resistance to quinolones in India precludes their use. Aminoglycosides should be avoided, if possible due to risk of precipitating hepatorenal syndrome. Antibiotic therapy for 5 days is sufficient in patients with quick response and uncomplicated course. It may be longer in those with bacteremia, delayed response. Procalcitonin may be used to guide the duration of antibiotic therapy.

Secondary Peritonitis

Secondary peritonitis is more common and the usual route of entry of the pathogens is from a ruptured hollow viscus, usually the bowel. By far the most common condition is a ruptured appendix. Other causes are gangrene and perforation of the bowel following intussusception, volvulus, etc. necrotizing enterocolitis, and failure of surgical intestinal anastomosis. It is then obvious that the infecting pathogens are the bowel flora. These pathogens are mainly gram-negative organisms mostly *E. coli, Klebsiella,* anaerobes (*Bacteroides* species), and less commonly enterococci. Peritonitis due to penetrating abdominal injury is due to organisms from the environment or the patient's skin (like *Staphylococcus aureus*). In either case, one should remember that secondary peritonitis is likely to be polymicrobial and this calls for antibiotics with a broader spectrum of coverage and might even require a combination of antibiotics. Adequate surgical management including repair of ruptured bowel and drainage of pus is the cornerstone for management. If the patient is too sick for surgical intervention, ultrasonography or computed tomography (USG or CT)-guided drains can be inserted to drain the pus.

Rational choices include a combination of a third generation cephalosporin such as ceftriaxone or cefotaxime with metronidazole. Alternatively one can use monotherapy with a BL-BLI combination such as cefoperazone-sulbactam or piperacillin-tazobactam. The advantages of these drugs include coverage of extended-spectrum beta-lactamase (ESBL) producing organisms, which are now increasingly being recognized as cause of intra-abdominal infections even in patients from the community. Since anaerobic cover is good, metronidazole is not required. In patients with severe intra-abdominal infections with septic shock, where adequate source control may not be immediately possible empiric therapy with carbapenems (meropenem or imipenem or ertapenem) may have to be initiated with an option to de-escalate later when susceptibility results are available. Polymyxins or tigecycline should be used only for patients with demonstrated carbapenem resistant organisms or highly antibiotic experienced patients with history of prolonged hospitalization. Routine empiric coverage for *Enterococcus* and *Candida* is not required. Isolation of Candida along with other organisms from pus cultures after a ruptured viscus does not merit antifungal therapy. Antifungals are indicated, if there is pure culture of candida or in the presence of acute necrotizing pancreatitis or in patients with a positive biomarker (beta-D-glucan) and not responding to antibacterial therapy. Isolation of candida, and other multidrug resistant pathogens from indwelling drains usually indicate colonization or contamination and does not generally merit change of therapy.

Recent trials have demonstrated that patients with mild or moderate peritonitis who have undergone adequate source control treated for 4 days had comparable outcomes to those who were treated till vital signs and GI continuity had returned (mean of 8 days). Patients with severe peritonitis need to be treated till there is resolution of fever, leukocytosis, and ileus or till procalcitonin concentrations have normalized.

HEPATIC OR LIVER ABSCESS

Hepatic abscesses may be due to bacterial pathogens [pyogenic liver abscess (PLA)] or *E. histolytica* [amoebic liver abscess (ALA)]. ALA is not a true abscess because it consists of necrotic tissue and blood with necrotic wall. If this gets infected by another organism then it becomes a true abscess. Most of the liver abscesses in children are pyogenic (70–80%). PLA can result from hematogenous spread through the hepatic artery, ascending infection from the biliary tract or from the intestine through the portal circulation and sometimes by direct penetration. Occurrence of PLA must arouse suspicion of an immunocompromised state like chronic granulomatous disease (CGD) or other primary immunodeficiencies.

In PLA in children, the most common organism is *S. aureus,* but other aerobic and anaerobic organisms can also cause PLA. They include *Peptostreptococcus, Bacteroides fragilis,* and other *Bacteroides* species, microaerophilic streptococci, *E. Coli,* Klebsiella of the highly mucoid phenotype, *Salmonella, Brucella,* and even *M. tuberculosis.* In immunocompromised patients, fungi including candida should also be considered.

Whenever possible a diagnostic aspiration of the abscess should be considered and specimens sent for aerobic and anaerobic culture along with smear examination for trophozoites. Serology for *Entamoeba histolytica* [enzyme-linked immunosorbent assay (ELISA) or hemagglutinin inhibition test] has good negative predictive value for ALA. Blood cultures should also be sent. Surgical drainage by insertion of a pigtail catheter should be considered for large abscesses (> 6 cm in diameter or those in the left lobe of the liver or where there is the likelihood of impending rupture due to thin rim between the abscess and surface of the liver parenchyma). Surgical drainage is more crucial for pyogenic as compared to amoebic abscess.

Antimicrobial Therapy

It is sometimes not possible to differentiate between amoebic and PLA at onset of illness in spite of the theoretical differences in clinical presentation, serology, and USG. Hence, combined treatment is started and continued till differentiation is made (if at all). To cover aerobic and anaerobic organisms, a combination of third generation cephalosporin (ceftriaxone or cefotaxime), and metronidazole may be considered for initial management. This regime provides cover for *S. aureus*, aerobic gram-negative pathogens, anaerobes, and amoebiasis. In case of failure of this first-line combination or in very sick patients or when there is greater possibility of gram-negative pathogens (such as patients with cholangitis) a suitable second-line of therapy is with piperacillin tazobactam or carbapenems with metronidazole (to cover for *E. histolytica*).

Antibiotic therapy for PLA depends on whether drainage has been achieved. Duration of therapy is guided by normalization of clinical and inflammatory parameters and stabilization of abscess size on USG and can vary from 2–4 weeks. It must be noted that the abscess may persist for months on radiology and does not merit continuation of antibiotics.

About 10 days of metronidazole is recommended for ALA followed by an oral course of a cysticidal agent like diloxanide furoate to prevent relapses (*see* chapter 17). The dose of metronidazole for ALA is 10–15 mg/kg 8 hourly.

BILIARY TRACT INFECTIONS

Infection of the biliary tract is referred to as cholangitis and may be associated with significant morbidity and mortality. In adults cholelithiasisis is the most common cause of cholangitis but this is rare in children. Common causes in children are biliary atresia or choledochal cyst with subsequent bile stasis. Ascending infections from the gut can result following surgical interventions like instrumentation or Kasai's procedure for extrahepatic biliary atresia. Gram-negative gut flora lead the pack of pathogens with *E. coli* being the most common organism isolated. Enterococcus and anaerobes are also frequently seen. Anaerobes are particularly important when there is a biliary enteric anastomosis.

Blood and bile cultures should be sent, if possible.

Treatment

Appropriate broad-spectrum antibiotics and attention to fluid and electrolyte management and liver dysfunction are crucial in this condition. It is important to remember that chance of the infection being polymicrobial is doubled to 90% in patients following instrumentation or surgery. Patients in this group also have a higher likelihood of having a positive blood culture. Biliary drainage is essential, if there is obstruction to bile drainage. This can be achieved by open surgery, endoscopic, or transbiliary drainage.

The choice of empiric antimicrobial therapy is determined by the underlying cause for cholangitis, local susceptibility patterns, prior antibiotic therapy, degree of sickness, and also biliary penetration of antibiotics. Antibiotics with the best biliary penetration include piperacillin tazobactam, ciprofloxacin, tigecycline, ceftriaxone, coamoxiclav, metronidazole, and cefoperazone sulbactam. The carbapenems (meropenem or imipenem), aminoglycosides, and colistin have lower biliary penetration. There is increasing resistance to third generation cephalosporins and high resistance to ciprofloxacin in the Indian scenario.

Keeping these factors in mind ceftriaxone with or without metronidazole (if biliary enteric anastomosis is present) or monotherapy with piperacillin tazobactam is the choice for empiric therapy. Piperacillin tazobactam has excellent biliary penetration, covers ESBL and anaerobes as well as enterococcus to a certain extent. In patients with nosocomial infections, those with failure of previous therapy or those with drug resistant pathogens, higher antibiotics including carbapenems, linezolid (for resistant enterococcus), tigecycline, and polymyxins may be needed.

Antibiotic therapy for 4–7 days is sufficient, if adequate surgical drainage has been achieved but in patients where drainage is not possible 2 weeks may be required.

CONCLUSION

The usual causative agents of intra-abdominal infections are *E. coli* and anaerobes. Accordingly, first-line therapy is a third generation cephalosporin with metronidazole and second-line is BL-BLI combinations such as piperacillin tazobactam or cefoperazone sulbactam. Surgical drainage is of paramount importance. The duration of antibiotic therapy can be limited to as short as 5 days where adequate source control has been achieved.

RECOMMENDED READING

1. Dever JB, Sheikh MY. Review article: spontaneous bacterial peritonitis--bacteriology, diagnosis, treatment, risk factors and prevention. Aliment Pharmacol Ther. 2015;41:1116-31.
2. Ferreira MA, Pereira FE, Musso C, et. al. Pyogenic liver abscess in children: Some observation in Le Espirito Santo state. Brazil Arg Gasteroenterol. 1997:34:49-54.
3. Gorter RR, The SML, Gorter-Stam MAW, et al. Systematic review of nonoperative versus operative treatment of uncomplicated appendicitis. J Pediatr Surg. 2017;52:1219-27.
4. Guitter V, Menager C, Missotte I, et al. Hepatic liver abscess in childhood: retrospective study about 33 cases observed in New-Caledonia between 1985 and 2003. Arch Pediatr. 2004;11(9):1046-53.
5. Hendricks MK, Moore SW, Millan AS. Epidemiological agents of liver abscesses in children in Western Cape Province of South Africa. J Tropical Pediatr. 1997:43(2):103-5.
6. Huang L, Yin Y, Yang L, et al. Comparison of antibiotic therapy and appendectomy for acute uncomplicated appendicitis in children: a meta-analysis. JAMA Pediatr. 2017;171:426-34.
7. Khotaii G. Pyogenic liver abscess in children. A long time hospital experience. Aeta Medica Iranica. 2004;42:55-60.
8. Kioumis IP, Kuti JL, Nicolau DP. Intra-abdominal infections: considerations for the use of carbapenems. Expert Opin Pharmacother. 2007;8(2):167-82.
9. Kumar AS, Sharma AK. Pyogenic liver abscess in children - South Indian experience. J Ped. Surg. 1998:33(3):417-21.
10. Levison ME, Bush LM. Peritonitis and intraperitoneal abscesses. In: Mandell BL, Bennett JE, Dolin R Mandell (Eds). Douglas & Bennett's Principles and Practice of Infectious Diseases, 7th edition Churchill Livingstone: Elsevier; 2010. pp. 1011-32.
11. Patra K, Prabhu SV, Pai B, et al. Case Files of the Hinduja hospital: liver abscess. Pediatr Infect Dis. 2009;1:85-95.
12. Prabhu SV. Intra-abdominal infections. Chapter 3:10. In: Parthasarathy A (Ed). Textbook of Pediatric Infectious Diseases. New Delhi: Jaypee Brothers Medical Publishers; 2013. pp. 190-6.
13. Rerknimitr R, Fogel EL, Kalayci C, et al. Microbiology of bile in patients with cholangitis or cholestasis with and without plastic biliary endoprosthesis. Gastrointest Endosc. 2002;56:885-9.
14. Tain Yl, Lin G, Cher TW. Microbiological spectrum of septicemia and peritonitis in nephrotic children. Pediatr Nephrol. 1999;13:835-7.

Antimicrobial Therapy in Upper Respiratory Tract Infections

19
Chapter

Nupur Ganguly, Jaydeep Choudhury, Suchi Acharya

INTRODUCTION

Upper respiratory tract infections (URTIs) are the most common illnesses affecting children. URTIs can broadly be classified into:

- Rhinosinusitis
- Pharyngitis
- Otitis media
- Croup or epiglottitis.

They can be caused both by virus and bacteria, but majority are of viral etiology. Most common viral cause of URTI is rhinovirus, respiratory syncytial virus (RSV), parainfluenza and influenza virus, Human metapneumovirus, adenovirus, Coronavirus, Epstein–Barr virus, and herpes simplex virus. Viral URTI is self-limiting and antibiotics have no role in their management. However, due to difficulty in differentiating viral from bacterial etiology many a time empirical antibiotics are used or misused giving rise to antibiotic resistance. Decreasing antibiotic use is an important focus of antibiotic stewardship.

The main bacterial etiologic agents of URTIs in children are Group A beta hemolytic streptococci (GABHS), *Streptococcus pneumoniae, Haemophilus influenzae,* and *Moraxella catarrhalis.* Other pathogens causing URTI include mycoplasma, pertussis, and *Corynebacterium diphtheriae.*

ANTIMICROBIAL RESISTANCE IN BACTERIAL PATHOGENS CAUSING URTI

The GABHS is universally susceptible to penicillin.

Streptococcus pneumoniae develops resistance to aminopenicillin (e.g. amoxicillin) by altering the penicillin binding proteins (PBP) and not by production of beta-lactamase. Thus, use of higher doses of amoxicillin (80–90 mg/kg/day) helps in overcoming this resistance but not addition of clavulanic acid. Recent use of beta-lactam antibiotics (within 3 months), extremes of age (< 2 years and >65 years), and day-care center attendance are risk factors for drug resistant *S. pneumoniae* (DRSP). Though in the Western countries about 25–50% of *S. pneumoniae* are penicillin resistant, most Indian isolates are still sensitive to penicillin. Hence, standard doses of amoxicillin suffice in most cases. There is high prevalence of resistance in *S. pneumoniae* to macrolides (30–40%).

With *H. influenzae* and *N. catarrhalis,* there is alternate mechanism of resistance to aminopenicillin. They produce β-lactamase, which directly degrades the β-lactam ring of aminopenicillin. Here increasing the dose will be of no help but adding β-lactamase inhibitor like clavulanate can overcome the resistance. Alternatively using a β-lactamase stable antibiotic like cefuroxime or cefpodoxime will be able to kill these organisms. A significant proportion of *H. influenzae* (25–30%) and most *Moraxella* isolates (95%) are beta-lactamase producing and resistant to amoxicillin. The prevalence of macrolide resistance in these pathogens also approaches 30–40%.

ACUTE RHINOSINUSITIS (COMMON COLD)

Rhinosinusitis is one of the most common conditions treated by primary care providers. Like other upper respiratory infections (URI), rhinosinusitis is usually a viral infection. It predominantly affects the nasal part of the respiratory mucosa. Most children below 5 have 3–8 colds per year.

The usual presenting features of common cold include sore throat, runny or blocked nose, and cough with or without systemic symptoms including fever and malaise. The term influenza like illness is used when there are systemic signs such as fever and malaise along with the upper respiratory symptoms.

Antimicrobial therapy is not indicated for viral URTI. These illnesses are best treated with symptomatic therapy including paracetamol, nasal saline drops, rest, oral fluids, humidification, and certain home remedies such as honey, ginger, etc. In selected cases, oral and nasal decongestants and antitussives such as dextromethorphan or codeine may be used. The patients should be warned about symptoms, which herald complications including breathing difficulty, persistent fever beyond 4–5 days, or ear pain.

The use of oseltamivir in patients with influenza when started within 48 h of onset reduces duration of symptoms by 1 day, viral shedding or infectiousness and may reduce the risk development of complications. Empiric therapy with oseltamivir may be considered in patients with influenza like illness during an ongoing outbreak, if they are at high risk of complications such as pregnant women, those with comorbidities and the immunocompromised.

ACUTE BACTERIAL SINUSITIS

Acute sinusitis is defined pathologically by transient inflammation of the mucosal lining of the paranasal sinuses lasting less than 30 days. It can be both viral and bacterial in origin. The viral infections are self-limiting. Common cold is the trigger for acute sinusitis; 0.5–5% of common colds are complicated by development of acute bacterial sinusitis.

The diagnosis of bacterial sinusitis is made on clinical criteria—(1) persistence and nonimprovement of symptoms and signs of acute rhinosinusitis beyond 10 days, (2) worsening of symptoms or signs including new onset fever, headache, or increase in nasal discharge following a typical viral URI that lasted 5–6 days and was initially improving (double sickening), or (3) acute onset of high fever with facial pain or purulent nasal discharge for at least 3–4 days. Mere presence of purulent nasal discharge in the first few days of an URTI can occur with viral etiology and does not merit antibiotics.

The principal bacterial pathogens implicated in bacterial sinusitis include *S. pneumoniae, H. influenzae,* and *M. catarrhalis. Staphylococcus aureus* is an uncommon pathogen but its increasing prevalence is a real cause of concern. Early identification of bacterial sinusitis is beneficial to prevent the rare but life-threatening complications such as meningitis, cavernous sinus thrombosis, and orbital cellulitis.

Choice of Antibiotic

In Disease of Mild-to-moderate Severity

Approximately 80% of children with acute bacterial sinusitis will respond to treatment with amoxicillin. Use of amoxicillin as first-line therapy in suspected cases of acute bacterial sinusitis is desirable because of its general effectiveness, safety, tolerability, low cost, and narrow spectrum. The usual dosage in children mild-to-moderate uncomplicated acute bacterial sinusitis is 30–40 mg per kg per day in two or three divided doses. It must be mentioned here that DRSP in nonmeningeal isolates is uncommon in India. Hence, routine use of high dose amoxicillin is not indicated. Most patients will respond within 48–72 hours. If the patient does not improve, the antimicrobial is ineffective or the diagnosis of sinusitis is incorrect.

In Case of Severe Disease or Patients Who do not Respond to Initial Therapy with Amoxicillin

In this setting, we need to cover for beta-lactamase producing *H. influenzae* and *Moraxella*. The drug of choice is coamoxiclav dosed as 30–40 mg/kg of the amoxicillin component per day in two to three divided doses. Other oral options include cefuroxime, cefpodoxime, or cefdinir. In patients who are acutely ill with vomiting or poor oral intake, ceftriaxone may be given @ 75 mg/kg/day.

For Patients, Who are Allergic to Amoxicillin

For nontype I hypersensitivity options include cefdinir (14 mg/kg per day in one or two doses) or cefuroxime (30 mg/kg per day in two divided doses) or cefpodoxime (10 mg/kg once daily) or a combination of cefixime (10 mg/kg/day in two doses) with clindamycin (20–30 mg/kg/day in two doses).

For type 1 hypersensitivity the recommended option is respiratory fluoroquinolone (levofloxacin 10 mg/kg or moxifloxacin 10 mg/kg once daily).

Duration of Therapy

The recent guidelines from the American Academy of Pediatrics (APP) recommend therapy for 10–14 days in children as shorter therapies have been associated with increased risk of relapse.

Adjuvant Therapy

Adjuvant therapies such as saline nasal irrigation, antihistamines, and decongestants to supplement antimicrobial therapy have not been thoroughly investigated, and the AAP makes no recommendations for their use. Likewise, the use of antibiotic prophylaxis to prevent recurrent episodes of acute bacterial sinusitis has not been evaluated and no recommendations are made for its use. Risk factors for sinusitis should be looked for; a common risk factor in today's era is allergic rhinitis or adenoid hypertrophy. Appropriate management for the same should be instituted including use of intranasal steroids.

PHARYNGITIS

It affects the mucosa of the throat resulting in a predominant symptom of pain that may be associated with headache, fever, and general malaise and can be of viral or bacterial etiology. Among bacterial etiologies, GABHS is the most important and needs antibiotic treatment to prevent the nonsuppurative (rheumatic fever, which has become less common) and suppurative (especially peritonsillar abscess) complications, decrease person-to-person spread, and to shorten symptom duration. Other rare bacterial pathogens causing pharyngitis are *Corynebacterium diphtheriae* and *Neisseria gonorrhoeae*, where antibacterial therapy is indicated. Viruses causing pharyngitis are influenza, parainfluenza, corona, adeno, rhino, EBV, herpes simplex, etc. Except mononucleosis, viral pharyngitis is generally mild.

Group A beta hemolytic streptococcal pharyngitis usually affects children between 5 and 15 years of age and is characterized by sudden onset of fever, sore throat with pain during swallowing. Examination findings include tonsillopharyngeal erythema and exudates, palatal petechiae, tender anterior cervical adenopathy, and sometimes scarlatiniform rash. The positive predictive value of these signs for streptococcal sore throat is around 60%. Other causes of exudative pharyngitis include EBV, adenovirus, and *C. diphtheriae*. Hence confirmation of diagnosis by rapid antigen test or throat swab culture is desirable but not always possible. Repeat clinical evaluation sometimes helps in diagnosis. One can also use clinical scoring systems such as modified McIssac criteria. Presence of features indicative of viral etiology including coryza, conjunctivitis, cough, hoarseness, diarrhea, ulcerations, and viral exanthema have good negative predictive value for GABHS pharyngitis and here diagnostic testing and antimicrobial therapy are not indicated.

Drug of Choice

Penicillin is the drug of choice for GABHS with its narrow spectrum and few adverse effects. Although penicillin V is the drug of choice, it is not readily available. Ampicillin or amoxicillin is equally effective and is a suitable option in children. Prompt administration of penicillin therapy shortens the clinical course, decreases the incidence of suppurative sequelae, the risk of transmission, and prevents acute rheumatic fever even when given within 9 days after onset of illness.

Recommendations for antimicrobial therapy for Group A streptococcal pharyngitis are shown in Table 1.

Recurrent Pharyngitis

A repeat episode of pharyngitis following an episode of GABHS can be due to three possibilities—(1) inadequate therapy, (2) acquisition of new infection from contact or community, and (3) intercurrent viral pharyngitis. Mere isolation of GABHS from the throat swab does not indicate bacterial etiology as this may represent viral pharyngitis in a person who is a chronic carrier. Here attempt to differentiate viral from bacterial etiology should be made on clinical features as discussed earlier. If antibiotics are indicated then antibiotics which have better eradication rates should be chosen as discussed in Table 2. Current guidelines do not recommend tonsillectomy for repeated episodes of GABHS pharyngitis.

TABLE 1: Therapeutic options for GABHS pharyngitis recommended by American Heart Association and American Academy of Pediatrics.

Drug	*Dose*	*Duration*
Penicillins		
Penicillin V (oral)	Children <27 kg: 250 mg two to three times daily; Children >27 kg, adolescents, and adults: 500 mg twice daily	10 days
Amoxicillin (oral)	50 mg/kg once daily/ 25 mg/kg twice daily (maximum 1g once/ 500 mg twice daily)	10 days
Benzathine penicillin (intramuscular)	Children <27 kg: 600, 000 U; Children >27 kg, adolescents, and adults: 1, 200, 000 U	Once
For individuals allergic to penicillin		
Non type 1 hypersensitivity		
Cephalexin	20 mg/kg twice daily (max 500 mg twice daily)	10 days
Cefadroxil	30 mg/kg once daily (max 1 g once daily)	
Type 1 hypersensitivity		10 days
Clindamycin (oral)	20 mg/kg per day divided in three doses (maximum 300 mg/dose or 900 mg per day)	
Azithromycin (oral)	12 mg/kg once daily (maximum 500 mg)	5 days
Clarithromycin (oral)	15 mg/kg per day twice daily (maximum 250 mg twice daily)	10 days

TABLE 2: Treatment regimens for recurrent pharyngitis or chronic carriers.

Drug	*Dose*	*Duration*
Coamoxiclav	40 mg/kg/day of amoxicillin in two doses (maximum 2 g/ day)	10 days
Clindamycin	20 mg/kg/day in three divided doses (maximum 300 mg/dose)	10 days
Oral Penicillin V	50 mg/kg/day in four doses (max 2 g/day in four doses)	10 days
OR		
Benzathine penicillin	600,000 units (<27 kg)/ 1,200,000 units (>27 kg)	Single dose
AND		
Rifampicin	20 mg/kg/day (max 600 mg) single dose	Last 4 days of therapy

ACUTE OTITIS MEDIA

Otitis media is an acute URTI that affects the respiratory mucosa of the middle ear cleft. In developed countries otitis media is the most common indication for antibiotic prescribing and surgery in young children. Otitis media is best regarded as a spectrum of disease. The most important conditions are:

- *Otitis media with effusion (OME):* OME is a condition with presence of fluid in the middle ear for at least 8 weeks in the absence of signs and symptoms of acute infection. OME is the most common form of otitis media. It can occur spontaneously as a component of rhinosinusitis or following an episode of acute otitis media (AOM).

- As per updated guidelines from the AAP, AOM is defined as either (1) moderate or severe bulging of the tympanic membrane or (2) new onset otorrhea not due to otitis externa or (3) mild bulging of the tympanic membrane and recent onset of ear pain or erythema of the tympanic membrane.
- Chronic suppurative otitis media (CSOM) is defined as discharge through a perforated tympanic membrane for longer than 2–6 weeks.

Most children experience at least one episode of AOM peaking between 6 and 12 months of age. Pathogenesis in OME and AOM is multifactorial, both bacterial and viral. Bacterial infections with common respiratory pathogens (*S. pneumoniae, H. Influenzae,* and *M. catarrhalis*) often follow a viral illness. Viral etiology includes RSV and influenza virus. Mycoplasma is also an etiology in bullous myringitis. The pain associated with AOM resolves within 24 hours in 60% cases and within 3 days in 80%. But AOM is less likely to resolve spontaneously in children younger than 2 years. Complications include CSOM, mastoiditis, labyrinthitis, facial palsy, meningitis, intracranial abscess, and lateral sinus thrombosis. These complications have reduced with the use of antibiotics. Complications are uncommon with OME.

A major challenge is to distinguish between AOM and *OME as antimicrobial treatment for OME is usually not indicated.* Purulent ear discharge of recent origin is most likely to be AOM, but the difficulty arises in AOM without perforation. To support the diagnosis of AOM in a child with middle ear effusion, it should be accompanied by ear pain, fever, hearing loss, and discharge.

Indications for Antibiotics

Factors that determine need for antimicrobial therapy include:

- The age of the child
- Whether the disease is unilateral or bilateral
- Whether disease is severe (temperature 39° C or higher OR severe otalgia OR otalgia persisting for more than 48 hours).

Antibiotic therapy is definitely indicated in:

- Any child with otorrhea or
- Severe disease
- Bilateral AOM in children below the age of 24 months
- Acute otitis media in children below 6 months.

All other situations (children older than 24 months with nonsevere AOM whether unilateral or bilateral) or children between 6 months and 24 months with nonsevere unilateral AOM can be managed with watchful waiting for 48–72 hours with use of anti-inflammatory drugs including paracetamol or ibuprofen and use antibiotics, if there is failure to improve with conservative management. The new guidelines from AAP are less conservative and allow for antibiotic administration upfront in these groups of patients as well on physician discretion.

Drugs of Choice (Table 3)

Principles of therapy are same as for acute bacterial sinusitis with amoxicillin at 30–40 mg/kg/day being the preferred drug for nonsevere disease and coamoxiclav being the drug of choice for severe disease. Single dose ceftriaxone @ 50 mg/kg may be used in children who are vomiting or where compliance is an issue.

TABLE 3: Antibiotics used in acute otitis media and their doses.

Drugs	*Dosage*	*Comments*
Amoxicillin	40–50 mg/kg/day, given orally in two divided doses	First-line drug. Safe, effective, and inexpensive
Amoxicillin/clavulanate	40 mg of amoxicillin per kg per day; 6.4 mg of clavulanate per kg per day, given orally in two divided doses	Second-line drug. For patients with recurrent or persistent acute otitis media, those taking prophylactic amoxicillin, those who have used antibiotics within the previous month, and those with concurrent purulent conjunctivitis
Azithromycin (one dose)	30 mg per kg, given orally	For patients with penicillin allergy. One dose is as effective as longer courses
Azithromycin (3-day course)	20 mg per kg once daily, given orally	For patients with recurrent acute otitis media
Azithromycin (5-day course)	5–10 mg per kg once daily, given orally	For patients with penicillin allergy (type 1 hypersensitivity)
Cefdinir	14 mg per kg per day, given orally in one or two doses	For patients with penicillin allergy, excluding those with urticaria or anaphylaxis to penicillin (i.e. type 1 hypersensitivity)
Cefpodoxime	30 mg per kg once daily, given orally	For patients with penicillin allergy, excluding those with urticaria or anaphylaxis to penicillin (i.e. type 1 hypersensitivity)
Ceftriaxone	50 mg per kg once daily, given intramuscularly or intravenously. One dose for initial episode of otitis media, three doses for recurrent infections	For patients with penicillin allergy, persistent or recurrent acute otitis media, or vomiting
Cefuroxime	30 mg per kg per day, given orally in two divided doses	For patients with penicillin allergy, excluding those with urticaria or anaphylaxis to penicillin (i.e. type 1 hypersensitivity)
Clarithromycin	15 mg per kg per day, given orally in three divided doses	For patients with penicillin allergy (type 1 hypersensitivity). May cause gastrointestinal irritation
Clindamycin	20–30 mg per kg per day, given orally in three divided doses	For patients with penicillin allergy (type 1 hypersensitivity)

Duration of Treatment

The optimal duration of treatment of AOM is uncertain. There are two schools of thought. One advocates treatment for 10 days and the other for 1–7 days. Studies comparing these two durations of treatment are inconclusive. For children below 2 years and for children with severe disease treatment for 10 days is recommended. For mild-to-moderate disease in children aged 2–5 years, duration recommended is 7 days and for those 6 years or older 5 day course is appropriate.

Persistent Acute Otitis Media

If there is no clinical improvement within 48–72 hours, the patient must be reassessed to confirm the diagnosis, exclude other causes of illness, and initiate antibiotic therapy in those on symptomatic treatment alone. Patients who are already taking antibiotics should be changed to second-line therapy. Options include high-dose amoxicillin or clavulanate and cephalosporins (cefuroxime and cefpodoxime). Parenteral ceftriaxone administered daily over 3 days is useful in children with emesis. For children who do not respond to second-line antibiotics, clindamycin and tympanocentesis are appropriate options. Although it is not approved for use in children, levofloxacin is effective in children who have persistent or recurrent AOM.

Recurrent Acute Otitis Media

It is defined as having at least three episodes of AOM in a period of 6 months, or four or more episodes in 12 months. The microbiology is often more complex than in occasional episodes of AOM, but the most common bacteria are nevertheless *S. pneumoniae, H. influenzae,* and *M. catarrhalis*. Most children with recurrent AOM improve with watchful waiting and overgrow this as they grow old. Although antibiotics like penicillin and amoxicillin (with or without clavulanic acid) prophylaxis may reduce recurrence, there are no widely accepted recommendations for antibiotic choice or duration of treatment. Other preventive measures include pneumococcal vaccination, adenoidectomy, avoiding cigarette smoke exposure, and breastfeeding.

CROUP OR EPIGLOTTITIS

Croup is a common clinical illness in preschool children. The incidence peaks in the second year of life. Viral agents are the principal factors responsible for laryngotracheobronchitis. Of these parainfluenza viruses head the list, followed by influenza A and B, RSV, adenovirus, and measles. Croup can be due to involvement of the structures surrounding the vocal cord. When it involves structures above the cord, i.e. epiglottis then the condition is known as acute epiglottitis. Involvement of the vocal cord and structures below it is termed laryngitis, laryngotracheitis or laryngotracheobronchitis depending upon the extent of inflammation.

Presentations include a barking cough and inspiratory stridor. The diagnosis is based on clinical assessment. Traditionally, the most important differential diagnosis has been acute epiglottitis though incidence of this condition has fallen dramatically with the widespread use of vaccination against type b *H. influenzae* in western countries. It is still important to consider the possibility because of vaccine failure and poor vaccine coverage in developing countries. In epiglottitis, lateral neck radiograph shows enlarged epiglottitis (thumb sign), ballooning of the hypopharynx, and normal subglottic structures. X-ray has moderate sensitivity and specificity. The best method of diagnosis is to visualize the epiglottis after intubation. Intubation may precipitate laryngeal spasm and hence laryngoscopy should be performed in suspected cases only when facilities for intensive care are available.

As laryngotracheobronchitis is primarily viral in origin, antibiotics have no role; main stay of therapy includes airway management, nebulized epinephrine, and corticosteroids. In case of airway obstruction, stabilization of airway is critical.

Role of Antibiotics

In epiglottitis, ceftriaxone in a dose of 80–100 mg/kg/day in two divided doses or cefotaxime 50–180 mg/kg/day in four divided doses is given parenterally till culture reports are available. Other option is amoxicillin clavulanate. Combined ampicillin and sulbactam or clavulanic acid may be used as another alternative. The patient should improve immediately following intubation with disappearance of respiratory distress and cyanosis.

Duration of Therapy

Antibiotics should be continued for 7–10 days.

ROLE OF POLYMERASE CHAIN REACTION IN DIAGNOSIS OF UPPER RESPIRATORY TRACT INFECTION

Multiplex polymerase chain reaction (PCR) is an emerging technology for detection of respiratory bacterial and viral pathogen in a single test. Commercial tests such as the FilmArray respiratory panel from Biofire is available that detects multiple pathogens including influenza, parainfluenza, RSV, adenovirus, rhinovirus, Enterovirus, H. metapneumovirus, Coronavirus, pertussis, mycoplasma, and chlamydia. These tests are often used in the resource-replete setting for distinguishing bacterial from viral infections and thus practice antimicrobial stewardship. Detection of influenza helps in making the decision to treat with oseltamivir.

However, the use of these tests routinely in healthy children is controversial. The cost is a major issue and so is the inability to distinguish colonization from true infection. Hence in our setting, the use of these tests should be limited to severely immunocompromised patients such as those who are on intense cancer chemotherapy for leukemia or those who are undergoing hematopoietic stem cell transplant where detection of RSV, parainfluenza, adenovirus, influenza can help in instituting appropriate antivirals (ribavirin for RSV and parainfluenza, cidofovir for adenovirus, and oseltamivir for influenza), isolation, administration of intravenous immunoglobulin (IVIG) and also decisions about delay in conditioning or chemotherapy.

CONCLUSION

Interventions to control URTI in children can be divided into four basic categories—(1) immunization against specific pathogens, (2) early diagnosis and treatment, (3) nutrition, and (4) hygiene. Most URTIs are viral and do not merit antibiotics. Antibiotics do not prevent bacterial superinfection. Antibiotics are indicated for acute bacterial sinusitis, acute suppurative otitis media (ASOM), and streptococcal sore throat. Amoxicillin is the drug of choice for all; in severe or nonresponsive sinusitis and otitis media coamoxiclav may be used. Third-generation cephalosporins should be used sparingly. Macrolides are usually ineffective due to high prevalence of resistance in the causative pathogens but are still widely abused. Widespread use of vaccines against measles, diphtheria, pertussis, *Haemophilus influenza* type b (Hib), pneumococcus, and influenza has substantially reduced the incidence of URTIs in children in developed countries.

RECOMMENDED READING

1. American Academy of Pediatrics, Committee on Infectious Diseases. Red Book: Report of the Committee on Infectious Diseases, 27th edition. Elk. Grove Village: American Academy of Pediatrics. 2006.
2. Arguedas A, Dagan R, Pichichero M, et al. An open-label, double tympanocentesis study of levofloxacin therapy in children with, or at high risk for, recurrent or persistent acute otitis media. Pediatr Infect Dis J. 2006;25:1102-9.
3. Behrman RE. Textbook of pediatrics, 19th edition. Philadelphia: WB Saunders Company; 2011.
4. Casey JR, Pichichero ME. Symptomatic relapse of group A beta-hemolytic streptococcal tonsillopharyngitis in children. Clin Pediatr (Phila). 2007;46(4):307-10.
5. Chow AW, Benninger MS, Brook I, et al. Infectious Diseases Society of America. IDSA clinical practice guideline for acute bacterial rhinosinusitis in children and adults. Clin Infect Dis. 2012;54(8):e72-112.
6. Gerber MA, Baltimore RS, Eaton CB, et al. Prevention of rheumatic fever and diagnosis and treatment of acute Streptococcal pharyngitis: a scientific statement from the American Heart Association endorsed by the American Academy of Pediatrics. Circulation. 2009;119:1541-51.
7. Gerber MA. Group A *Streptococcus.* In: Kliegman M (Ed). Nelson Textbook of pediatrics, International editions 18, Vol. 182. India: Elsevier; 2007. pp. 1135-9.
8. Lieber JJ, Epiglottitis. Ferri's Clinical Advisor: Instant Diagnosis and Treatment. London: Mosby; 2005. pp. 295-3.
9. Lieberthal AS, Carroll AE, Chonmaitree T, et al. The diagnosis and management of acute otitis media. Pediatrics. 2013;131:e964-99.
10. Morris PS, Upper respiratory tract infections (including otitis media). Pediatr Clin N Am. 2009;56: 101-17.
11. Shenoy PA, Chawla K, Vishwanath S, et al. Microbiological characterization of *Haemophilus influenzae* isolated from patients with lower respiratory tract infections in a tertiary care hospital, South India. J Clin Diagn Res. 2016;10(5):DC31-4.
12. Shulman ST, Bisno AL, Clegg HW, et al. Clinical practice guideline for the diagnosis and management of group A streptococcal pharyngitis: 2012 Update by the Infectious Diseases Society of America. Clin Infect Dis. 2012;55(10):e89.
13. Singh J, Sundaresan S, Manoharan A, et al. Serotype distribution and antimicrobial susceptibility pattern in children ≤5 years with invasive pneumococcal disease in India - A systematic review. Vaccine. 2017;35:4501-9.
14. Steinhoff MC. Invasive *Haemophilus influenzae* disease in India: a preliminary report of prospective multihospital surveillance. IBIS (Invasive Bacterial Infections Surveillance) Group. Pediatr Infect Dis J. 1998; 17(9Suppl):S172-5.
15. Verghese VP, Veeraraghavan B, Jayaraman R, et al. Increasing incidence of penicillin- and cefotaxime-resistant *Streptococcus pneumoniae* causing meningitis in India: Time for revision of treatment guidelines? Indian J Med Microbiol. 2017;35(2):228-36.
16. Weber SM, Grundfast KM. Modern management of acute otitis media. Pediatr Clin North Am. 2003;50:399-411.
17. Zoorob R, Sidani MA, Fremont RD, et al. Antibiotic use in acute upper respiratory tract infections. Am Fam Physician. 2012;86:817-22.

Antimicrobial Therapy in Lower Respiratory Tract Infections

20
Chapter

Prawin Kumar, Sushil Kabra

INTRODUCTION

Pneumonia is the leading cause of mortality among infectious diseases and a common cause of morbidity in children under 5 years of age. The epidemiology of community-acquired pneumonia (CAP) varies widely between different regions and countries. The estimated incidence of pneumonia is 0.22 and 0.015 episodes per child-year in low- and middle-income and high-income countries, respectively. There were 108 million new episodes in the year 2015 and most of these occurred in sub-Saharan Africa and South East Asia regions. Despite global decrease in under 5-year mortality in last 3 decades, pneumonia accounts for 1 million deaths in children in 2015, which is about 16% of total deaths in this age group. In India, the burden of CAP in children under 5 years of age is estimated to be 3.6–4.0 million episodes in the year 2010 and of these 30.7–32.0 episodes per 1,000 child year were recognized as severe pneumonia. Overall, the largest number of children death due to pneumonia occurred in India where annually 0.35–0.37 million children die from CAP under 5-years of age (13–16% of under 5 mortality in India, 30% of global deaths due to pneumonia).

ANTIMICROBIAL THERAPY FOR COMMUNITY-ACQUIRED PNEUMONIA

Introduction

Administration of appropriate antibiotics in the early course of pneumonia alters the outcome of illness particularly when the causative agent of pneumonia is a bacterium. Antibiotics may not have any role in pneumonia caused by viruses except for influenza. Unnecessary antibiotics administration in children apart from increased risk of adverse effects may lead to selection of resistant organisms and thus may promote serious illness in the future. However, in view of the public health implications of better outcome of pneumonia by early administration of antibiotics and inability to conclusively clinically differentiate between bacterial and viral pneumonia, antibiotics are administered to all children with pneumonia. Differentiation between viral and bacterial pneumonia is also not possible by complete blood counts, acute phase reactants like C-reactive protein (CRP), and chest X-ray (CXR). Procalcitonin level appears to be a more effective biomarker, but is limited by the lack of precise cut off level, which can differentiate bacterial from viral infection. In view of the difficulty and cost associated with identification of etiological agents, the choice of antibiotic in most cases of CAP is empiric. In children with severe disease requiring hospitalization, in those with poor response, underlying disease, and immunocompromised status, an attempt should be made to identify the etiological agent.

Blood cultures should be sent in all hospitalized children with CAP (positivity rates are 10–15%). CXR should be done for all inpatients but not recommended for outpatients. Other tests such as mycoplasma serology and multiplex polymerase chain reaction (PCR) in nasopharyngeal swab for viruses are expensive and not routinely indicated. During influenza outbreaks, throat swab or nasopharyngeal swab for flu PCR can be sent in hospitalized patients.

Since, antimicrobial therapy in CAP is mostly empirical, the factors that may help in selection of appropriate empirical antibiotics include knowledge of etiological agents, sensitivity of pathogens to antibiotics, severity of the disease, immune status, nutritional status, previous antimicrobial usage, history of previous hospitalization, duration of illness, associated complications, and cost and safety of antibiotics.

Etiological Agents

The etiology of CAP varies for different age groups. In neonates, etiologic agents include gram-negative enteric bacteria, *Streptococcus pneumoniae* and *Chlamydia trachomatis*. A recent community-based study from South Asia, detected respiratory syncytial virus (RSV) (6.5%) and ureaplasma (2.8%) as the most common pathogens causing sepsis in babies below age 60 days. In children between the ages 2 months and 5 years, viruses predominate; in developing countries, bacterial infections are probably commoner than viral. Viruses have been isolated in nasopharyngeal aspirates of children below five years of age with pneumonia in 44–49% cases. The most common viral pathogen is RSV; others are influenza, parainfluenza, Human metapneumovirus, Coronavirus, adenovirus, and rhinovirus. Currently, the most common bacterial pathogen isolated in under 5 children with pneumonia are *S. pneumoniae* (30–50%) followed by *Haemophilus influenzae* (10–30%), *S. aureus*, and *Klebsiella pneumoniae*. Atypical organisms like *Mycoplasma pneumoniae* and *Chlamydia pneumoniae* are emerging pathogens for CAP in preschool-aged children. The main pathogens of CAP in older children and adolescents are *S. pneumoniae* followed by mycoplasma.

Coinfection with two or more microbial agents is 10–40% in hospitalized patients, which is more common than previously thought. Pertussis should be considered in all children with CAP, especially if immunizations are not complete. *Mycobacterium tuberculosis* may also cause CAP in children.

Sensitivity of Pathogen

Antibiotic resistance in pneumococci is an emerging problem all over the world. The mechanism of drug resistance is by changing the cell wall protein, which is the binding site for beta-lactam antibiotics. Higher doses of beta-lactams can overcome this type of resistance. Addition of beta-lactamase antagonist (like clavulanic acid) has no effect as production of beta-lactamase is not the basis for resistance. Review of recent studies addressing the problem of pneumococcal resistance reveals the very low prevalence of resistance to penicillin in nonmeningeal isolates [<1%, with revised Clinical Laboratory Standard Institute (CLSI) breakpoints], but high level of resistance to macrolides (25–30%) and cotrimoxazole (> 90%). Since penicillin resistance is very low, standard doses of amoxicillin (30–40 mg/ kg/day) suffice. Resistance in *H. influenzae* type b (Hib) to ampicillin in a recent study evaluating lower respiratory tract isolates was 10%. Resistance in invasive Hib isolates to ampicillin, macrolides, and cotrimoxazole in the IBIS (invasive bacterial surveillance) study conducted two decades ago was around 40%. Macrolide resistance in atypical organisms such as chlamydia, mycoplasma, and legionella is not reported in India. Thus, macrolides are the drug of choice for pneumonia due to atypical organisms. Newer quinolones such as levofloxacin have an advantage of good coverage for *S. pneumoniae, H. influenzae,* and atypical organisms. However, levofloxacin is also one of the important components in the treatment of multidrug-resistant tuberculosis. Therefore, it should be avoided in CAP in children when other effective antimicrobial agents are available.

Severity of Illness

In most circumstances, microbial etiology of pneumonia remains similar despite varying degree of severity of illness. However, it is logical to select the most appropriate antibiotics that have lesser chance of failure in more severe disease (Table 1 and Box 1 for categorization of severity of illness).

Underlying Disease

Identification or knowledge of underlying disease is also important for selection of antibiotics. Some underlying diseases predispose a patient to pneumonia due to specific organisms. Children with hemoglobinopathies or nephrotic syndrome are more susceptible to pneumococcal infections. A child with cystic fibrosis is likely to have infections due to *Staphylococcus, H. influenzae,* or *Pseudomonas* species. Immune deficiency whether primary or secondary predisposes a child to infections due to unusual opportunistic organisms. Pneumonia in human

TABLE 1: Diagnosis and assessment of severity of pneumonia in children aged 2 months–5 years with cough or difficult breathing.

Clinical category	*Essential features*
No pneumonia: Cough and cold	No fast breathing and no indicators of severe pneumonia
Pneumonia	Fast breathing for age with or without chest indrawing with oxygen saturation >92%
Severe pneumonia	Pneumonia with presence of any of the general danger sign (not able to breastfeed or drink, persistent vomiting, convulsions, or central cyanosis or lethargic or unconscious, stridor in a calm child or severe malnutrition, or severe respiratory distress, e.g. head nodding)

BOX 1: Criteria for respiratory distress in children with pneumonia.

Signs of respiratory distress:

- Tachypnea, respiratory rate, breaths/min
  - Age 0–2 months ≥60
  - Age 2–12 months ≥50
  - Age 1–5 years ≥40
  - Age >5 years ≥20
- Dyspnea
- Retraction (suprasternal, intercostal, or subcostal)
- Grunting
- Nasal flaring
- Apnea
- Altered mental status
- Pulse oximetry measurement <90% room air

immunodeficiency virus (HIV) infection may be due to gram-negative bacilli, *Pneumocystis jirovecii* (PCP) and fungi in addition to usual pathogens. The progression of disease is rapid in immunodeficient patients hence most efficient antibiotics combinations are used as first-line treatment in immunocompromised host.

In a neutropenic child with pneumonia, causative organisms include gram-negative bacilli (especially *Pseudomonas*), *Staphylococcus*, *Aspergillus* in addition to common pathogens such as *S. pneumoniae* and *H. influenzae*.

Nutritional Status

The etiology of pneumonia in malnourished children is generally similar to that in well-nourished children, with an added predisposition for gram-negative organisms and *Staphylococcus aureus*. Pneumonia in malnourished children may progress to severe disease rapidly. The symptoms of pneumonia may be masked in severely malnourished children possibly due to a blunted inflammatory response. In a study on malnourished children with pneumonia, fast breathing had a sensitivity of 61% and specificity of 79% compared to sensitivity of 79% and specificity of and 65% in well-nourished children. The required respiratory rate (RR) for malnourished children stood about 5 breaths/min less than that for well-nourished children. Since they are a high-risk group, malnourished children with severe malnutrition with nonsevere pneumonia by definition should be treated as severe pneumonia or should have RR cut off of 5 breaths/min less than that is defined for pneumonia in children less than 5 years by World Health Organization (WHO).

Previous Antibiotics

History of antibiotics in the current episode or in the recent past (previous 2–4 weeks) may give an idea about possible resistant organisms. If a patient had received repeated courses of antibiotics; patient's microbial flora may be resistant to those antibiotics and a different set of antibiotics should be chosen.

History of Hospitalization

The microbial flora of a patient usually changes to gram-negative bacilli after hospitalization hence it should be considered as the etiology of pneumonia with history of hospitalization. If it is a *Staphylococcal pneumonia*, it may be due to a resistant strain [healthcare-acquired methicillin-resistant *Staphylococcus aureus* (HA-MRSA)].

Duration of Illness

A short duration of the illness suggests a possible bacterial or viral etiology. A longer duration of the illness (>2 weeks) suggests a possibility of infection due to *M. tuberculosis* or atypical organisms or certain viral infections like adenovirus, etc.

TREATMENT OF PNEUMONIA

For treatment purposes, pneumonia may be classified as (1) community-acquired, without risk factors, and (2) pneumonia with risk factors. Both these can be further classified as nonsevere and severe illness. The common risk factors associated with adverse outcome in pneumonia include young age, severe malnutrition, underlying illness (congenital heart disease, immunodeficiency, patient on cancer chemotherapy, organ dysfunction, and bronchiectasis), recent hospitalization, and received a course of antibiotic in past 2–4 weeks.

Indications for Hospitalization

Children with danger signs should be hospitalized. Indication for hospitalization in children is summarized in Box 2.

Indication for Intensive Care Unit Admission

Some of the children with CAP may need pediatric intensive care unit (ICU) care, the indication for shifting the child with CAP in ICU is summarized in Box 3.

Choice of Antimicrobials for CAP (Table 2)

Antibiotics for CAP without Risk Factors in Children 2 Months–5 Years of Age

Nonsevere pneumonia can be managed on ambulatory basis. The drug of choice is amoxicillin. Though other agents including coamoxiclav, or second (cefuroxime) or third-generation cephalosporins (cefpodoxime or cefprozil or cefdinir) are also effective, they are more expensive and not more efficacious. Therefore, amoxicillin is the drug of choice for nonsevere CAP. Due to high prevalence of resistance in *S. pneumoniae* and *H. influenzae* and rarity of atypical organisms in this age group macrolides are not recommended as first-line therapy.

BOX 2: Factors determining the need for hospital admission.

- Age younger than 2 months
- Toxic appearance
- Hypoxemia
- Oxygen saturation less than 92%
- Cyanosis
- Respiratory difficulty
- Apnea
- Grunting
- Flaring of the nostrils
- Dehydration, vomiting, or poor feeding
- Immunocompromised status
- Failure to respond to oral antibiotics
- Inadequate observation or supervision by family

BOX 3: Indications for intensive care unit admission.

- Partial pressure of oxygen (PaO_2) or fraction of inspired oxygen (FiO_2) <250
- Need for mechanical ventilation
- Chest X-ray showing bilateral, multilobar pneumonia with increase in the size of the opacity >50% in the 48 hours prior to admission
- Hypotension
- Vasopressor requirement
- Acute renal failure

TABLE 2: Therapy for pneumonia.

	Outpatient	*Inpatient*
Neonates	Cefotaxime or ampicillin and gentamicin or amikacin Macrolide if chlamydia or pertussis	
<5 years (*Pneumococcus, H. influenzae* type B, and viruses)	Amoxicillin	• Coamoxiclav • Cefuroxime • Ceftriaxone
>5 years (pneumonia and mycoplasma)	Amoxicillin or macrolide	• Ampicillin or coamoxiclav • Ceftriaxone • With or without macrolide
Suspected methicillin-resistant *Staphylococcus aureus*	Add vancomycin or linezolid or teicoplanin	
Suspected gram-negative pathogens	Ceftazidime or piperacillin tazobactam or ciprofloxacin with or without aminoglycoside	
Suspected influenza	Add oseltamivir	

Children with *severe pneumonia* need hospitalization. The first-line antibiotic in children with severe pneumonia who need hospitalization is amoxiclav or a third or second-generation cephalosporin like ceftriaxone or cefuroxime. If methicillin-resistant *Staphylococcus* is suspected then vancomycin or teicoplanin should be added.

Antibiotics for CAP with Presence of Risk Factors in Children 2 Months–5 Years of Age

The antibiotics are decided on basis of individual patient's characteristics, risk factors, and severity of pneumonia. Broadly speaking a child with *nonsevere pneumonia* may be treated with oral cefuroxime or coamoxyclav. In case of deterioration or failure of therapy or *severe disease,* the second-line antibiotic for these patients may be intravenous third-generation cephalosporins (antipseudomonal agent if *Pseudomonas* is suspected) with or without an aminoglycoside with or without anti-MRSA drug like vancomycin or teicoplanin or linezolid.

CAP in Infants Less than 2 Months of Age

They should be hospitalized and treated with a combination of intravenous third-generation cephalosporin like cefotaxime and gentamicin as it will cover both gram-negative and gram-positive bacteria. Ampicillin can replace the cephalosporin, if group B streptococci are suspected. If meningitis is also suspected, third-generation cephalosporin should be used. If chlamydia is suspected than macrolides are recommended.

CAP in Children above 5 Years of Age

The etiology of pneumonia above 5 years of age is similar to that of adults including *M. pneumoniae, C. pneumoniae,* and *S. pneumoniae.* A recent retrospective cohort study compared beta-lactam monotherapy with combination of beta-lactam and macrolide antibiotics. Results suggest that children receiving combination (Beta-lactam and macrolide antibiotics) had lesser duration of hospital stay but no difference in relapse rates in children above 5 years of age. There are no large studies documenting etiology of pneumonia in children above 5 years of age from

India. Till we have more studies that document burden of pneumonia due to *Mycoplasma,* treatment of *nonsevere pneumonia* for this age group may be similar to that of children below 5 years of age. Therefore, amoxicillin is the drug of choice. If a patient does not improve with antibiotics or there are clinical features pointing toward infections due to atypical organism (protracted course, extra respiratory manifestations such as rash and dropping hemoglobin) macrolide therapy can be initiated. For *severe pneumonia* that needs hospitalization intravenous penicillin or ampicillin or ceftriaxone is the drug of choice. One may consider adding macrolide therapy empirically to this set of patients at the outset (especially if the patient is hypoxic) or if there is no response to initial antibiotics or investigations are suggestive of an atypical organism.

Doses of Amoxicillin in CAP

If we go through different international guidelines, the daily dose of amoxicillin in CAP varies from 40–50 mg/kg to 90–100 mg/kg with higher dosage recommended in areas with higher risk for penicillin-resistant pneumococcus. The breakpoints for defining penicillin resistance in pneumococcus have been revised; for nonmeningeal isolates the susceptibility breakpoint is 2 and the resistance breakpoint is 8. With these breakpoints, the prevalence of resistance in nonmeningeal isolates is around 1%. Therefore, it is advisable to continue using 40–50 mg/kg/day of oral amoxicillin in India at present. However, physician or pediatrician treating children with CAP should be aware about a possibility of penicillin-resistant pneumococcal disease, and if suspected, should increase doses of amoxicillin to 80–90 mg/kg/day. When these agents are used intravenously, the recommended dose is 80–100 mg/kg/day which automatically takes care of penicillin resistance.

Oral versus Intravenous Initial Antibiotic Therapy for CAP

It is rational to use oral antibiotic in the treatment of nonsevere CAP in children 2–59 months of age, who are able to tolerate orally and do not have any general danger signs. There are increasing evidences for use of oral antibiotics in severe pneumonia also in some children with specific characteristics. Systematic reviews of studies that used oral amoxicillin in children with severe pneumonia without hypoxia suggests that such patients can be managed on ambulatory basis with oral antibiotics. Two cluster randomized controlled trials (RCTs) also suggest that oral amoxicillin may be equal or superior to standard treatment (referral and injectable antibiotics in hospital) for children with severe pneumonia without hypoxia. Therefore, children with pneumonia with chest indrawing without hypoxia can be managed with oral antibiotics on ambulatory patients provided that parents are willing to bring the child to healthcare facility on deterioration in clinical condition. Intravenous antibiotic therapy is warranted, if the child has disturbed consciousness, improper swallowing, frequent vomiting, suspected drug malabsorption, and in newborn.

Need for Empirical Antiviral drug Oseltamivir

Influenza contributes toward 5–10% of all acute respiratory infections. While there is controversy about the efficacy of oseltamivir in influenza without lower respiratory tract involvement or without risk factors in reducing hospitalization or deaths the situation is different when a child has lower respiratory tract involvement due to suspected influenza. Hence in children with CAP during an ongoing influenza outbreak or when clinical features suggest influenza; early use of oseltamivir along with antibacterials is recommended. If available, the throat swab can be sent for PCR testing but oseltamivir should be started without waiting for the results and continued even if the swab is negative (since the test has a sensitivity of only 70%).

Response to Antimicrobial Therapy and Monitoring

Clinical improvement may take up to 48–96 hours; fever can last 2–4 days, leukocytosis usually resolves by day 4, abnormal physical findings may persist more than 7 days. Most nonsevere CAP shows clinical resolution of symptoms in 2–3 days. Radiographs may worsen even though clinical picture is improving and CXR usually returns to normal (occasionally leaving some haziness) within 6 weeks in patients and hence follow-up X-ray is not recommended to look for recovery. Therefore, careful monitoring of children with CAP is important to assess failure or response to treatment.

The monitoring strategy of child with CAP will depend upon whether the child is being treated on ambulatory basis or hospitalized (Flowcharts 1 and 2).

Switching from Parenteral to Oral Antibiotics

Child can be shifted oral antibiotics when the child has improved as indicated by general well-being, absence of chest indrawing, no requirement of supplementation of oxygen, and accepting orally. Most children with severe CAP may be ready to switch to oral antibiotics by 2–4 days.

The choice of oral antibiotics will depend on the parenteral antibiotics, which the child is receiving. If child is on intravenous penicillin, the child should be shifted on oral amoxicillin,

Flowchart 1: Monitoring of child with community-acquired pneumonia (CAP) treated on ambulatory basis.

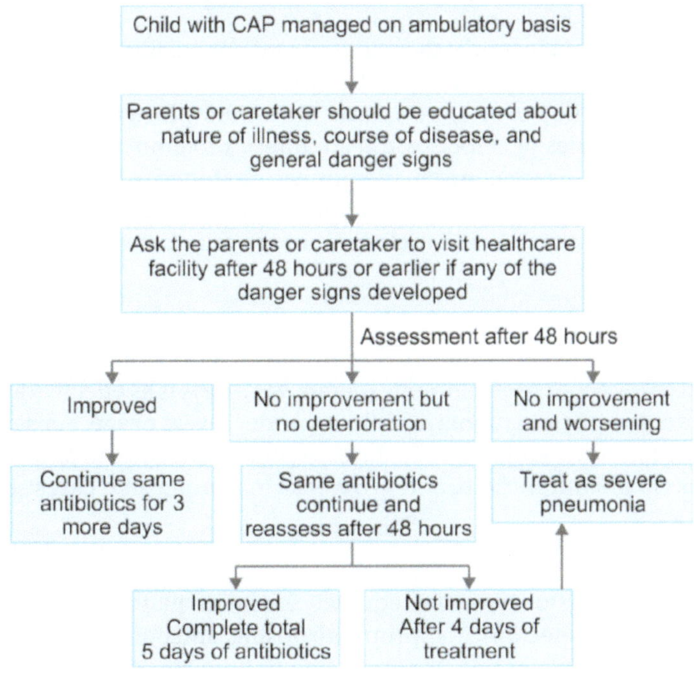

Flowchart 2: Monitoring of hospitalized child with CAP.

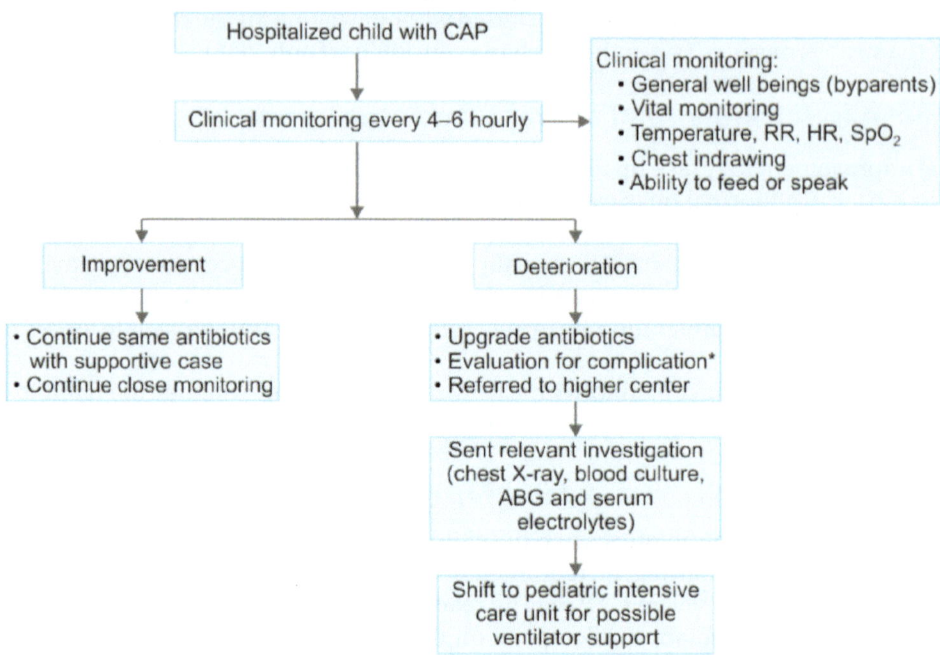

*Empyema thoracis, pneumothorax, infection in other part of body or acute respiratory distress syndrome (ARDS)

(CAP: community-acquired pneumonia; HR: heart rate; RR: respiratory rate; SpO_2: peripheral oxygen saturation; ABG: arterial blood gas)

if receiving intravenous cephalosporin then shift to oral amoxicillin (in a child above 5 years), coamoxyclav (in a child below 5 years since *H. influenzae* is a possibility), second-generation cephalosporin (cefuroxime) or cefpodoxime. One must, however, remember that the pharmacodynamic properties of cefpodoxime are inferior to amoxicillin and ceftriaxone and failures can occur. Intravenous vancomycin therapy can be shifted to oral linezolid. It is desirable to observe the child for next 24 hours after switching over to oral antibiotics. The total duration of antibiotics remains same and should include duration of intravenous antibiotics also.

Duration of Therapy

The usual duration of therapy is 5 days. Two multicenter RCTs from India and Pakistan have demonstrated that a short course of antibiotic therapy for 3 days is as effective as a 5 days therapy for WHO defined nonsevere pneumonia in children under 5-year of age. For severe pneumonia, total duration of antibiotics should be 7–10 days. In pneumonia due to *Staphylococcus,* a total duration of 2 weeks in uncomplicated, and 4–6 weeks in complicated cases should be given.

Causes of Failure to Improve

The possible causes of failure to respond adequately are inadequate therapy, which may be due to inappropriate antibiotic selection, inappropriate dosing, and poor compliance. It can also be due to development of complications like empyema or lung abscess. If there is impaired host defense mechanism, or there is development of drug resistance in the community there may be delayed response or poor response. Nonbacterial CAP has longer course than expected. Pre-existing disease like cystic fibrosis, primary ciliary dyskinesia, or bronchiectasis may take longer duration than usual course to improve.

EMPYEMA THORACIS

The most common cause of pediatric empyema is *S. pneumoniae* followed by *S. aureus*. The development of empyema should be suspected in children with pneumonia who complain of chest pain or who fail to improve after 48–72 hours for treatment or deteriorate after initial improvement. The diagnosis of a pleural collection can be confirmed by a CXR or an ultrasonography (USG) of the chest. Patients with a collection that occupies more than half of the hemithorax and who continue to have fever should have a pleural tap performed. Pleural fluid analysis that suggests empyema includes turbid fluid or pus, organisms on Gram stain, pH less than 7.0, sugar less than 40 mg/dL, LDH more than 1,000 IU/L, or lactate more than 45 mg/dL. It should be sent for culture in both aerobic and anaerobic blood culture bottles.

Antimicrobial therapy should be continued. The most crucial aspect of empyema is establishing drainage. A chest tube should be inserted. Some patients fail to improve despite insertion of a chest tube; this is generally due to loculations or very thick fluid. These patients may need additional interventions such as instillation of intrapleural fibrinolytics or video-assisted thoracoscopic surgery (VATS). If the locules are thin, intrapleural urokinase in a dose of 3,000 units/kg/ day in 1–2 divided doses (maximum dose of 100,000 units and concentration of 1,000 units/mL) can be used. If the fluid is thick, then VATS may be needed. A recent RCT showed equal efficacy of intrapleural urokinase and VATS in management of pediatric empyema. Approach to empyema is depicted in Flowchart 3.

Flowchart 3: Approach to empyema.

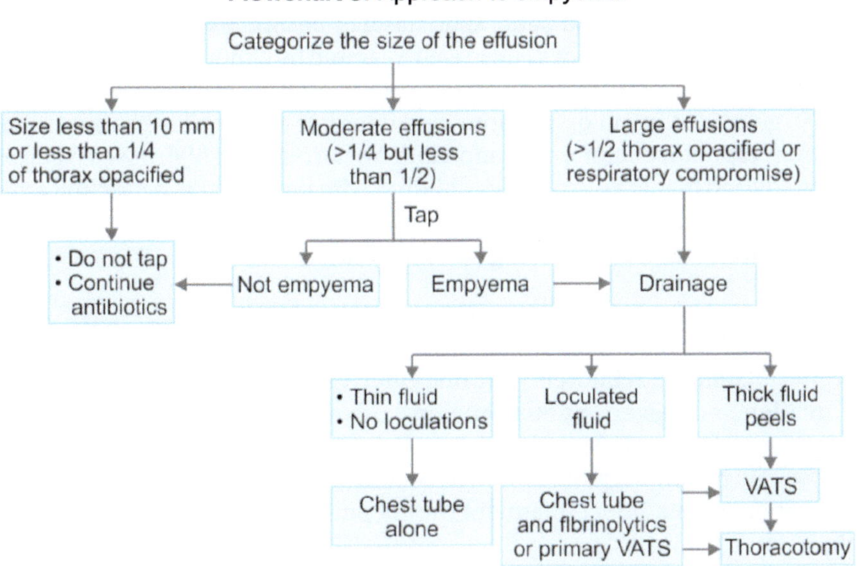

(VATS: video-assisted thoracoscopic surgery)

SUPPORTIVE THERAPY

Children should be given supportive therapy for the associated problems. Children with pneumonia may have fever, poor intake, vomiting, electrolyte abnormalities, hypoxia, and respiratory failure. The antibiotics require some time to produce a response. Fever should be treated with paracetamol in doses of 10–15 mg/kg/ dose. It can be repeated every 4-6 hourly. Cough is common symptom associated with pneumonia. Cough suppressants should be avoided. Common household remedies like *tulsi,* ginger, and honey may be given to the child. If there is bronchospasm, inhaled bronchodilators can be prescribed. Most of the vomiting may be associated with cough and does not require specific treatment. Persistent vomiting may be managed with antiemetics. However, before starting antiemetics, it is advisable to rule out other causes of vomiting including central nervous system (CNS) infection, acidosis, or intestinal problems.

Associated comorbid conditions like diarrhea, congenital heart diseases, and immunodeficiency are associated with high case fatality. Children with congenital heart diseases require careful monitoring for fluid and electrolyte balance as these patients may develop congestive heart failure. Children with diarrhea may need more fluids for correction of dehydration and ongoing losses. In malaria, endemic area, a possibility of malarial infection presenting as pneumonia or malaria as comorbid condition should be kept in mind. There may be hyponatremia due to syndrome of inappropriate antidiuretic hormone secretion (SIADH). A careful monitoring and restriction of fluid is the intervention required in most cases.

Hypoxia may be present in children with severe pneumonia. Hypoxia if untreated may be associated with increased case fatality rates. It is difficult to identify hypoxia by clinical features alone and pulse oximetry must be resorted to. Oxygen should be administered to children with tachypnea (RR >70/min), chest indrawing, poor feeding, cyanosis, or oxygen saturation ($SaO_{2)}$ readings below 90-92%. Oxygen may be administered by nasal prongs, nasopharyngeal tubes (low flow, i.e. 1–2 L/min); or oxygen hood or facemask (both high flow 4–8 L/min). Small children tolerate oxygen with hood better than nasal or nasopharyngeal cannula or facemask. Nasal cannula after cutting the prongs is also well tolerated by children. Noninvasive monitoring of hypoxia by saturation monitoring is well-accepted method. However, it should be kept in mind that SaO_2 gives idea about oxygenation and does not give any idea about carbon dioxide (CO_2). Even with respiratory failure, saturation may be normal with high flow oxygen inhalation. Therefore, it is advised that in critically sick children with pneumonia, a baseline arterial blood gas (ABG) should be done and subsequently monitored with SaO_2. With clinical deterioration, a repeat ABG for documentation of rising CO_2 is desirable.

ROLE OF MICRONUTRIENTS IN THE TREATMENT OF CAP

It has been postulated that children with micronutrient deficiency may be associated with increased incidence of severe pneumonia and adverse outcome. Initial reports suggest improved outcome of pneumonia when zinc was used as adjunct treatment. However, a large RCT and a systemic review suggest no beneficial role of zinc in pneumonia. Similarly, vitamin A supplementation as an adjunct treatment during pneumonia has not improved outcome of pneumonia.

ROLE OF STEROIDS IN THE TREATMENT OF PNEUMONIA

The role of systemic corticosteroids in pediatric CAP has been evaluated in past. Two retrospective studies demonstrate that there was greater odd for rehospitalization in children with CAP who received steroid as an adjunct therapy. However, there is evidence in favor of systemic steroid when used along with antibiotics in *Pneumocystis carinii* pneumonia (PCP) with hypoxia or occasionally in severe *Mycoplasma pneumonia*. Till date, systemic steroid is not recommended as standard of care for children with CAP.

PROGNOSIS OF COMMUNITY-ACQUIRED PNEUMONIA

Most children with CAP recover with recommended treatment. About 10% of children with pneumonia may have severe disease requiring hospitalization. In a prospective study factors associated with failure of first-line antibiotics and prolonged hospital stay included lack of breastfeeding, overcrowding at home, and abnormal chest X-ray. Children presenting with cyanosis are at increased risk of requiring ventilator support. Children at risk of death had head nodding at presentation, altered sensorium, abnormal leukocyte counts, and pallor.

CONCLUSION

Pneumonia is the leading cause of mortality and common cause of morbidity in children below 5 years of age. In developing countries, bacterial infections are the most common cause of pneumonia, *S. pneumoniae* is the most common bacterial pathogen identified. Administration of appropriate antibiotics in the early course of pneumonia alters the outcome of illness. Oral amoxicillin is the drug of choice in nonsevere pneumonia and pneumonia with chest indrawing without hypoxia. All children with severe pneumonia with hypoxia and very severe pneumonia need to be hospitalized and treated with parenteral antibiotics.

RECOMMENDED READING

1. Adegbola RA. The etiology of pneumonia in malnourished and well-nourished Gambian children. Pediatr Infect Dis J. 1994;13:975-82.
2. Awasthi S, Agarwal G, Singh JV, et al. Effectiveness of 3-day amoxicillin vs. 5-day co-trimoxazole in the treatment of non-severe pneumonia in children aged 2–59 months of age: a multi-centric open labeled trial. J Trop Pediatr. 2008;54:382-9.
3. Donà D, Luise D, Da Dalt L, et al. Treatment of community-acquired pneumonia: are all countries treating children in the same way? A Literature Review. Int J Pediatr. 2017;2017:4239268.
4. Farooqui H, Jit M, Heymann DL, et al. Burden of Severe Pneumonia, Pneumococcal Pneumonia and Pneumonia Deaths in Indian States: Modelling Based Estimates. PLoS One. 2015;10:e0129191.
5. GBD 2015 LRI Collaborators. Estimates of the global, regional, and national morbidity, mortality, and etiologies of lower respiratory tract infections in 195 countries: a systematic analysis for the Global Burden of Disease Study 2015. Lancet Infect Dis. 2017;17:1133-61.
6. Haider BA, Lassi ZS, Ahmed A, et al. Zinc supplementation as an adjunct to antibiotics in the treatment of pneumonia in children 2 to 59 months of age. Cochrane Database Syst Rev. 2011;(10):CD007368.
7. Haider BA, Saeed MA, Bhutta ZA. Short-course versus long-course antibiotic therapy for non-severe community-acquired pneumonia in children aged 2 months to 59 months. Cochrane Database Syst Rev. 2008;(2):CD005976.

8. Invasive Bacterial infection Surveillance (IBIS) Group, INCLEN. Prospective multicentre hospital surveillance of *Streptococcus pneumoniae* disease in India. Lancet. 1999;353:1216-21.
9. Jefferson T, Jones M, Doshi P, et al. Oseltamivir for influenza in adults and children: systematic review of clinical study reports and summary of regulatory comments. BMJ. 2014;348:g2545.
10. Kabra *SK, Lodha R, Baroor S*, et al. Etiology of acute lower respiratory tract infection. Indian J Pediatr. 2003;70:33-6.
11. Kabra SK, Singhal T, Verma IC. Rational use of antibiotics. Indian J Pediatr. 2001;68 (Suppl3):S5-7.
12. Kumar KJ, Ashok Chowdary KV, Usha HC, et al. Etiology of community acquired pneumonia among children in India with special reference to atypical pathogens. Lung India. 2018;35:116-20.
13. Kumar P, Medigeshi GR, Mishra VS, et al. Etiology of acute respiratory infections in infants: a prospective birth cohort study. Pediatr Infect Dis J. 2017;36:25-30.
14. Kumar RM, Kabra SK, Singh M. Efficacy and acceptability of different modes of oxygen administration in children: implications for a community hospital. J Trop Pediatr. 1997;43:47-9.
15. Lodha R, Kabra SK, Pandey RM. Antibiotics for community- acquired pneumonia in children. Cochrane Database Syst Rev. 2013;6:CD004874.
16. Lodha R, Randev S, Kabra SK. Oral Antibiotics for community-acquired pneumonia with chest indrawingin children aged below five years: a systematic review. Indian Pediatr. 2016;53:489-95.
17. Maitreyi RS, Broor S, Kabra SK, et al. Rapid detection of respiratory viruses by centrifugation enhanced cultures from children with acute lower respiratory tract infections. J Clin Virol. 2000;16:41-7.
18. Marhuenda C, Barceló C, Fuentes I, et al. Urokinase versus VATS for treatment of empyema: a randomized multicenter clinical trial. Pediatrics. 2014;134;e1301-7.
19. Mathew JL. Vitamin A supplementation for prophylaxis or therapy in childhood pneumonia: a systematic review of randomized controlled trials. Indian Pediatr. 2010;47:255-61.
20. Pandey A, Choudhary R, Nisar N, et al. Acute respiratory tract infections in Indian children with special reference to Mycoplasma pneumoniae. J Trop Pediatrics. 2000;46:371-4.
21. Patel AB, Bang A, Singh M, et al. A randomized controlled trial of hospital versus home based therapy with oral amoxicillin for severe pneumonia in children aged 3–59 months: The India CLEN Severe Pneumonia Oral Therapy (ISPOT) Study. BMC Pediatrics. 2015;15:186.
22. Principi N, Esposito S. Biomarkers in pediatric community-acquired pneumonia. Int J Mol Sci. 2017;18. pii: 447
23. Shenoy PA, Chawla K, Vishwanath S, et al. Microbiological Characterization of *Haemophilus influenzae* isolated from patients with lower respiratory tract infections in a tertiary care hospital, South India. J Clin Diagn Res. 2016;10:DC31-4.
24. Singh J, Sundaresan S, Manoharan A, et al. Serotype distribution and antimicrobial susceptibility pattern in children ≤5 years with invasive pneumococcal disease in India - A systematic review. Vaccine. 2017;35(35 Pt B):4501-9.
25. The WHO Young Infant Study Group. Bacterial etiology of serious infections in young infants in developing countries: results of multicenter study. Pediatr Infect Dis J. 1999;18 (suppl):S17-22.
26. Tramper-Stranders GA. Childhood community-acquired pneumonia: a review of etiology- and antimicrobial treatment studies. Paediatr Respir Rev. 2018;26:41-8.
27. Verghese VP, Veeraraghavan B, Jayaraman R, et al. Increasing incidence of penicillin- and cefotaxime-resistant *Streptococcus pneumoniae* causing meningitis in India: Time for revision of treatment guidelines? Indian J Med Microbiol. 2017;35:228-36.
28. Weiss A, Hall M, Lee G, et al. Adjunct corticosteroids in children hospitalized with community-acquired pneumonia. Pediatrics. 2011;127:e255-63.

Antitubercular Therapy

21
Chapter

Varinder Singh, Tanu Singhal

INTRODUCTION

Tuberculosis (TB) is still the most frequent infectious cause of death in the world even though 130 years have elapsed since the pathogen was identified and six decades since antituberculosis drugs were discovered. India accounts for more than 25% of incident cases of TB in the world. About 40% of the Indian population is infected with TB bacillus; every year 1.8 million Indians develop TB, of which 0.8 million are infectious. The death rate for all forms of TB in India (excluding HIV) in the year 2010 was 26 (confidence interval, 17–39) per 100,000 population. Almost 3.4 million Indian children have TB disease of which 40% contract disease by the age of 6 and 80% by the age of 16 years. It has been assumed that 10% of the actual total TB caseload in India is amongst children. Childhood TB is an indicator of recent transmission and thus serves as a sentinel event. Reliable and adequate data on the burden of all forms of TB, amongst children in India, is not available.

Children are not only at higher risk of developing the disease but also are more likely to develop the severe form of the disease. Proper identification and treatment of infectious cases in a community will reduce burden of childhood TB. Till such time, the profession shall need to focus on proper management of pediatric cases to prevent morbidity and handicap due to the disease.

HISTORICAL BACKGROUND

Since Ehrlich's original concept of chemotherapy based on selective staining by dyes, attempts had been made to find chemotherapeutic agents for TB. Sanocrysin—a gold salt, sulphones, vitamin D, and nicotinamide [from which several current antituberculosis drugs, including isoniazid (INH) and ethionamide were subsequently developed as analogs] were used. During this phase, treatment approaches included rest for the patient in sanatorium and rest for the affected portion of the lung by collapse therapy through operative procedures on the chest wall (thoracoplasty) and the injection of air into the pleural cavity (artificial pneumothorax).

This was followed by the advent of INH, streptomycin, and other drugs in the 40s and later. A combination of these drugs for as long as 18 months was used till as recently as the early 1980s. Although these regimens were effective if properly used, the actual failure rates were quite high because of poor compliance among patients.

The availability of rifampin in the 1970s and the reutilization of pyrazinamide ushered in the era of "Short Course" chemotherapy enabling TB to be cured in 6-month time. Rifampin, in combination with INH and streptomycin for 9 months, led to cure rates of almost 100% with relapse rates of less than 5% in patients with pulmonary TB. However, the impact of this new approach was not merely the shortening of duration alone but also the capability of the intensive initial multidrug therapy to effectively manage existing resistance to INH and many other nonrifampin drugs.

However, this initial advantage has been lost to an extent due to usage of unregulated and poor TB regimens with these potent drugs. Both, the medical profession as well as mankind has not learnt from past mistakes and the nonchalant use of the short course drug therapy has led to complex problems and issues surrounding the treatment of TB infection and disease. The threat of increasing INH and polydrug resistance has necessitated a 4-drug regimen using rifampin (R), INH (H), pyrazinamide (Z), and ethambutol (E) as the front-line therapy. Treatment of TB in the setting of multidrug resistance (INH and rifampin), coinfection with HIV/transplantation can be challenging. This chapter shall focus on the basic principles and current regimens for treating children using short course chemotherapy (SCC).

PRINCIPLES OF CHEMOTHERAPY FOR TUBERCULOSIS

Aims of Chemotherapy

- To cure patients of TB by the shortest duration of drug administration
- To prevent death from TB or late effects of disease
- To prevent relapse of disease
- To prevent emergence of drug resistance
- To reduce transmission of disease

Several biologic characteristics of *M. tuberculosis* have led to a hypothesis concerning the action of various drugs and drug combinations. *M. tuberculosis*, the causative organism of TB, is a slow growing bacterium with doubling time of about 20 hours, and it can also enter a phase of dormancy, which is drug refractory. The tubercle bacilli can be killed only in the replication phase when they are metabolically active. Mitchison described four subpopulations of bacilli in a host, depending upon their metabolic activity.

Bacilli Subpopulation (Mitchison Hypothesis)

The postulated differences in the metabolism of these bacilli present in different lesions make them variably susceptible to the various front-line drugs despite having no true resistance. The proportion of these subpopulations of bacilli differs with the type of lesion and there, probably, is a constant shift between these subpopulations.

These subpopulations include:

- *Rapidly growing/multiplying bacilli*: Because *M. tuberculosis* is an obligate aerobe, activity rates vary with oxygen supply. Bacilli are active and replicate freely where oxygen tension is high. A neutral or alkaline pH also promotes metabolic activity and growth. Environmental conditions for growth are optimal in cavities, leading to a very large bacterial population.
- *Slow growing (intracellular)*: This represents the bacilli present within the macrophages at inflamed sites where pH is low.
- *Spurters*: These represent the group of bacilli in the caseous material, which are slowly dividing due to low oxygen concentration and neutral pH.

- *Dormant*: This represents the bacilli, which are dormant due to adverse environment. This period of dormancy can be very prolonged. As drugs largely do not act upon these types of bacteria, they are the usual cause of subsequent relapse.

Children with primary pulmonary TB and patients with only extrapulmonary TB are infected with a much smaller numbers of tubercle bacilli, because the cavitary population is not present.

Another important bacteriologic consideration for the treatment of TB is the presence of naturally occurring drug-resistant mutants (primary resistance) in bacillary populations, even before chemotherapy is started. Although the population of bacilli as a whole may be considered "drug susceptible," a subpopulation of drug-resistant mutants occurs at a fairly predictable mean frequency of about 10^{-6} bacterial replications, but varies among drugs:

- Streptomycin: 10^{-5}
- Isoniazid: 10^{-8} to 10^{-9}
- Ethambutol: 10^{-6}
- Rifampin: 10^{-8}

A cavity containing 10^9 tubercle bacilli has thousands of drug-resistant organisms; a closed caseous lesion with 10^6 bacilli has few or none. Cross-resistance does not occur naturally. Fortunately, the chance occurrence of resistance to one drug is unrelated to that for any other drug. Thus, when three to four effective drugs are used in combination for treatment of TB, there are negligible chances of emergence drug resistance. For an organism to be "naturally" resistant to two drugs (primary multidrug resistance) the population size would have to be 10^{11} to 10^{16}, which is rare in clinical practice. Most clinical cases of multidrug resistance are due to sequential selection of resistant organisms on sequential poor therapy or else due to transmission of multidrug resistant (MDR) infection from an infectious case, as is more common in children.

The combination of bacterial population size and drug-resistant mutations explains why a single antitubercular drug cannot cure multibacillary disease like cavitary TB. The major biologic determinant of antitubercular therapy is the size of the bacillary population. In adults with pulmonary cavities and children with extensive pulmonary infiltrates there are many bacilli that are resistant to at least one of the first-lines drugs mandating the use of more than two antituberculosis drugs. A single effective drug would select for emergence of a dominantly resistant population. Children with limited primary pulmonary TB and patients with extrapulmonary TB have lower bacterial load where the presence of significant numbers of drug-resistant mutants shall be more reflective of the prevalence of resistance in the infectious pool rather than the occurrence of natural mutants. In case, the prevalence of resistance in the community is low then therapy with two bactericidal drugs may suffice while in the presence of high-drug resistance one may need to use more numbers of bactericidal drugs. This is an important issue in order to prevent amplification of drug resistance.

Types of Antitubercular Drugs

Antitubercular drugs may have several different activities as some drugs are bactericidal while others are bacteriostatic. Their action on various subpopulations of bacilli also differs thus accounting for differences in their sterilizing activity, bactericidal activity, and prevention of emergence of resistance (Fig. 1). On the basis of animal experiments and clinical trials, Mitchison classified and graded antitubercular drugs into three categories.

1. *Drugs with sterilizing activity:* The sterilizing activity is the ability to kill all the bacilli in tubercular lesions as rapidly as possible. Because the speed of killing becomes progressively

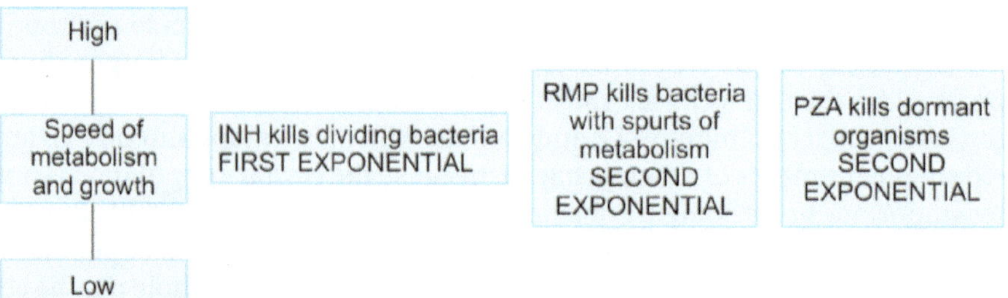

Fig. 1: The hypothesis on the action of drugs according to their speed of growth at the start of treatment. INH kills multiplying bacilli. Rifampin (RMP) kills bacilli when there are spurts of metabolism. PZA is the only drug, which kills dormant bacilli.
(INH: isoniazid; PZA: pyrazinamide)

slow during chemotherapy, sterilizing activity really measures the speed with which the last few viable bacilli are killed. In general, sterilizing activity indicates the suitability of an agent for use in intensive therapy of short-course regimens. Rifampin and pyrazinamide have the greatest sterilizing activity.

2. *Drugs with early bactericidal activity:* The bactericidal action refers to the ability of the drug to kill dividing *M. tuberculosis*. These drugs induce a rapid decrease in the number of living bacilli in the sputum at the beginning of treatment, rapidly reduce the bacillary load and quickly convert the sputum cultures to negative, thus reducing the infectivity of the patient. INH is the most effective drug in this category as it kills 90% of the bacilli in the first few days of treatment. Rifampin has also good early bactericidal activity.
3. *Drugs with resistance prevention activity*: These agents when combined with others can prevent the emergence of resistant mutants to the companion drug. This is dependent on the ability of the agent to inhibit growth, analogous to bacteriostatic activity. INH and rifampin are the most effective in this category. Ethambutol has been shown to potentiate this action of other drugs like INH.

Short-course Chemotherapy

The short-course regimens usually consist of two phases: An initial intensive phase of 2 months using three or more drugs, followed by a continuation phase of two drugs given for several months. The intensive initial phase is designated to eliminate quickly many logs of tubercle bacilli in all three populations, whereas the continuation phase slowly eliminates the several logs that remain. Rifampin and pyrazinamide form the backbone of modern chemotherapy. Rifampin is particularly effective against mycobacteria in closed caseous lesions, which are active in intermittent short spurts of only a few hours. Pyrazinamide was discovered to have very potent activity against organisms coated in an acid environment, especially those inside macrophages. Clinical studies indicate that it contributes to early sterilization and extends its maximum effect during the initial phase of therapy rather than throughout the full course of treatment. INH and rifampin are most commonly used in the continuation phase because they kill bacilli in all three populations.

All regimens shorter than 12 months are called as short-course and always have rifampin and INH as their basic components; and to bring down this treatment period to less than 9 months. Pyrazinamide needs to be added in the initial period called intensive phase. Shorter duration of antituberculosis chemotherapy is desirable as it improves adherence, decreases period of exposure to potentially toxic drugs and being potent it increases the likelihood of early bacteriologic killing thus decreasing period of infectiousness on therapy.

Regimens using INH, rifampin, pyrazinamide, and streptomycin during the initial (2 months), followed by INH and rifampin in the continuation phase (4 months), (2SHRZ/4HR) routinely yielded cure rates of greater than 98% and relapse rates less than 3%. This regimen was pioneered in the late 1980s for adults with TB in Singapore and its efficacy and low toxicity confirmed by later studies in other countries. SCC has also been shown in clinical trials to be effective in treating extrapulmonary TB in adults.

There have been recent efforts to shorten further the duration of treatment of drug-sensitive pulmonary TB in adults. Randomized controlled trials where moxifloxacin/gatifloxacin/ofloxacin were substituted for ethambutol/INH to see if treatment could be shortened further to 4 months were however not successful.

Intermittent Regimens for Tuberculosis

Few key events in the early 90s resulted in global awakening to resurgence of TB and prompted intensifications of global efforts for control and management of TB with the impetus coming largely from the observation of epidemiological anomalies in the USA, where there were increasing notification rates and reports of serious outbreaks of MDR-TB from hospitals in New York City and Miami.

This acted as a strong stimulus to World Health Organization (WHO) and other international agencies to focus attention on the global TB problem. Also, problems with adherence to chemotherapy regimens and drug-resistance prompted the need for simple, shorter, more effective and compliant regimens and thus, began rediscovery of short-course intermittent regimens that could be given under observation.

The scientific basis of intermittent chemotherapy is the long generation time (18–21 hours) of the tubercle bacilli and lag period after chemotherapy when a culture of *M. tuberculosis* was exposed to an antitubercular drug. When the drug was washed out after 24 hours, the organisms did not begin multiplying immediately. Their numbers continued to fall for some time before re-multiplication began. This period when the drug was not available and before organisms begin multiplying is called "lag phase." It is variable with the type of drug and the length of exposure to drug. It is possible to prevent further growth of bacilli if the next dose is given before the end of the lag period and this is the basis of intermittent therapy. Most of the antituberculosis drugs except thiacetazone, have a lag phase and can be given intermittently. Intermittent therapy should always be given under supervision and not as self-administration, simply because there is no scope for any further decrease in the doses received by the patient.

Directly observed therapy (DOT) under which the patient actually consumes the drug in front of treatment supervisor, was being followed under Revised National Tuberculosis Program. WHO and the Government of India recommended thrice weekly DOT regimens under Revised National Tuberculosis Program for the country.

However, rising incidence of drug resistance, relapses and failures with intermittent therapy has caused a rethink in this policy. Another reason for doing away with intermittent regimen was the unwanted severe consequence of missing even a few doses a month in the intermittent regimen. The patient used to receive 13 doses a month (on thrice weekly basis). A drop of even three doses a month meant a reduction of 23% in total drug intake which was definitely not desirable as it would promote drug resistance.

Chemotherapy of Childhood Tuberculosis

Childhood TB differs from adult TB in several ways that have treatment implications, *viz.*

- Lack of cavitary lesions in primary disease.
- Smaller bacterial population, hence less chances of secondary resistance while receiving therapy, even if compliance is poor.
- Propensity for extrapulmonary disease especially disseminated disease and meningitis.
- Higher dosage of medication tolerated.
- Low rates of adverse reactions to medications and therefore, fewer interruptions in therapy.
- Pediatric dosage forms not always available.
- Noncompliance rate as high as 50%.

Before 1980, guidelines for the treatment of TB in children were derived mainly from studies of adults with TB. Subsequently, various SCC trials for childhood TB were undertaken with different chemotherapy regimens. Most of the currently recommended regimens lay stress on SCC for children as well. This usually includes an intensive initial phase of 2 months with three or four drugs to be followed by a continuation phase containing two drugs. Rifampin, INH, and pyrazinamide form the backbone of initial regimens. The current consensus amongst experts is to use an additional fourth drug if the prevalence of initial INH resistance in a community is 5% or more. Ethambutol is usually recommended as the fourth drug though some still use streptomycin. With increasing experience in usage of ethambutol in pediatric cases, confidence has now been reposed in this drug as oral formulation makes it safer, easier, and cheaper than injectable streptomycin.

A systematic review on the impact of initial drug resistance on treatment outcome with standardized first-line treatment showed that the risk of failure as well as relapse was higher in the presence of initial resistance to INH. This came from pooled data of 33 trials involving more than 2,000 patients with INH monoresistance. The failure rates in patients with INH resistance were 9–45%. Lower failure rates in INH resistant cases were seen with daily therapy and more number of drugs in the regimen. Hence, three key changes emerged in the management of TB in India and countries with high prevalence of INH resistance:

- WHO therefore recommended against the omission of ethambutol in intensive phase for any new patient in countries where the elevated levels of primary INH resistance (>4%) have been reported and there is lack of routine testing for INH resistance. The Revised National TB Control Program (RNTCP) in India had, therefore in 2012, done away with the 3-drug regimen (category III). While in countries where the initial INH resistance in new cases is 4% or below, the paucibacillary cases like EP and smear negative pulmonary are still given 3-drug (RHZ) initial regimen. This has made the hitherto differentiation between smear negative and smear positive pulmonary cases (or an effort to differentiate paucibacillary cases from others) less relevant for treatment categorization.
- Till a few years ago, the continuation phase usually contained rifampin and INH for duration of 4 months except for patients with like meningeal, disseminated or bone TB where the recommendation was 7–10 months of continuation phase. However, the increasing incidence of INH monoresistance in India meant that those patients with such INH monoresistance would be receiving a single effective drug [Rifampicin (RMP)] in the continuation phase. Hence the current recommendation is to administer four drugs (as before) in the intensive phase but add the third drug, ethambutol, for the entire duration of the continuation phase.
- Starting December 2016, the RNTCP [with the approval of the Indian Academy of Pediatrics (IAP)] moved to daily therapy for childhood and adult TB to be introduced in a phased manner all over the country.

Hence, the current recommendation therefore is four drugs (HRZE) daily for 2 months in intensive phase and three drugs (HRE) daily for the treatment of all forms of drug-sensitive pediatric and adult TB.

Usually, all the antitubercular drugs are given orally as there are only limited choices for parenteral administration. Aminoglycosides and quinolones are the only drugs currently available for parenteral administration. However, all the oral forms of drugs can be given through nasogastric tubes. Suspension form of drugs can be made and are available for the ease of administration. The emergence of newer pharmacokinetic data has led to an upward revision of the drug dosages for childhood TB.

ESTABLISHING A MICROBIOLOGIC DIAGNOSIS OF TUBERCULOSIS

The revised guidelines stress the need to establish a microbiologic diagnosis of TB in all children. This is to ensure accurate diagnosis and also to enable susceptibility testing in case drug resistance is suspected. This can be done by sputum examination in older children, induced sputum following nebulization with hypertonic saline or bronchodilators or gastric aspirate. Bronchoalveolar lavage may be done if resources permit. Patients with extrapulmonary TB should undergo fluid examination and biopsies. The material obtained should be processed for Ziehl–Neelsen (ZN) stain and if resources permit for acid-fast bacilli (AFB) culture.

Polymerase chain reaction (PCR) had long held promise for rapid diagnosis of TB. But the initial assays were cumbersome, inaccurate and. Welcome developments were automated molecular methods including cartridge-based nucleic acid amplification testing (CBNAAT) and line probe assay that became available for rapid confirmation of *M. tuberculosis*. Additionally, they offered rapid detection of RMP and (in case of the line probe assay to other drugs) resistance. Earlier, these techniques were resorted to in children with suspected drug-resistant TB. But it was realized that the short turnaround time of the CBNAAT combined with sensitivity greater than that of Z-N staining and the "bonus" information of RMP resistance was of great advantage. The current recommendations therefore are to use CBNAAT whenever and wherever possible in every case where a sample is sent for Z-N smear and AFB culture.

RECOMMENDED REGIMENS

While several recommendations including consensus protocols have been made in the past, the latest recommendations now approved are discussed. Table 1 details the recommended regimens for management of various forms of childhood TB. A patient is considered as "new" case (having received treatment for less than 4 weeks) or a retreatment case (previously treated completely or, partially but for more than 4 weeks, in other words, relapse, failure, and defaulters). In fact, the regimen for the retreatment category is also under consideration and is at best a holding regimen. Efforts should be made to quickly subject these patients to drug susceptibility testing by molecular methods and transition them to treatment of drug-susceptible TB or drug-resistant TB as the case may be. It is equally important to decide the form of TB—pulmonary or extrapulmonary. Disease of organs where the penetration of drugs may not be so adequate like in bones or across meninges, require prolonged continuation phase. IAP and RNTCP do not advise use of streptomycin instead of ethambutol for new cases.

As discussed earlier, the new guidelines recommend daily therapy for all patients with TB. The doses of the antitubercular drugs in children are discussed in Table 2. Use of fixed drug combinations is recommended by the WHO and the RNTCP since they are easy to administer,

TABLE 1: Treatment categories and regimens for childhood tuberculosis.

Category of treatment	*Type of patients*	*TB treatment regimens*
New cases (previous category 1 and 3)	• New bacteriologically diagnosed TB • New clinically diagnosed TB • New extrapulmonary TB	2HRZE and 4HRE
Retreatment category (previous category 2)	• Microbiologically confirmed recurrent • Microbiologically positive failure • Microbiologically positive treatment after default • Others	2SHRZE + 1HRZE+ 5HRE

H = Isoniazid, R = Rifampicin, Z = Pyrazinamide, E = Ethambutol, S = Streptomycin

Intermittent therapy for childhood tuberculosis is being phased out by the RNTCP in favor of daily therapy.

Pulmonary TB refers to disease involving lung parenchyma. Extrapulmonary TB refers to disease involving sites other than lung parenchyma. If both pulmonary and extrapulmonary sites are affected, it will be considered as pulmonary for registration purposes. Extrapulmonary TB involving several sites should be defined by most severe site.

New Case: A patient who has had no previous antitubercular treatment (ATT) or for less than 4 weeks.

Recurrence: Patient declared cured/completed therapy in past and has evidence of recurrence.

Treatment after default: A patient who has taken treatment for at least 4 weeks and comes after interruption of treatment for 2 months and has active disease.

Failure to respond: A case of pediatric TB who fails to have bacteriological conversion to negative status or fails to respond clinically or deteriorates after 12 weeks of compliant intensive phase shall be deemed to have failed response, provided alternative diagnoses/ reasons for non-response have been ruled out.

Others: Cases who are smear negative or extrapulmonary but considered to have relapse, failure to respond or treatment after default or any other case which do not fit the above definitions.

TABLE 2: Currently recommended doses of antitubercular drugs.

	Rifampicin	*Isoniazid*	*Ethambutol*	*Pyrazinamide*	*Streptomycin*
Range daily dose in mg/kg/day (average)	10–20 (15)	7–15 (10)	15–25 (20)	30–40 (35)	15–20 (20)
Ceiling dose/day in mg	600	300	1,600	2,000	1,000

no scope for missing one or more of the combination drugs and reduced risk of emergence of resistance. However, FDC's with the right ratio of the drugs should be used.

ROLE OF CORTICOSTEROIDS AS ADJUNCTIVE THERAPY IN TUBERCULOSIS

In acute overwhelming TB there is significant host response associated with tissue inflammation and fibrous proliferation. The heightened host response can lead to a poor clinical outcome in cases with acute respiratory failure, acute respiratory distress syndrome, and involvement of extrapulmonary sites such as meninges, pericardium, adrenals, and peritoneum. Corticosteroid agents are beneficial in the management of TB in children when the host inflammatory response contributes significantly to tissue damage or impaired function.

The addition of systemic corticosteroid therapy to TB regimens has been found useful in some clinical settings. These include:

- *TB meningitis*: This is an absolute indication for prescription of steroids. Meta-analysis shows reduced mortality and neurodeficit with use of steroids. The dose is 2 mg/kg day of prednisone (0.4 mg/kg/day of dexamethasone) for 4 weeks followed by tapering over 4 weeks. In some patients with excessive inflammatory response, slower tapering over months may be needed.

- *Pericardial TB*: There is some data to suggest that use of steroids reduces the risk of pericardial constriction and reaccumulation of effusion.
- Miliary disease with alveolar-capillary block and hypoxemia.
- Tuberculomas with raised intracranial pressure.
- Endobronchial TB with localized emphysema or collapse-consolidation lesions.
- *Pleural effusion*: Not indicated unless massive and bilateral.
- *Peritoneal TB*: The role of steroids in reducing the risk of adhesive intestinal obstruction is uncertain.
- Potts spine with neurodeficit or severe pain.
- Adrenal insufficiency.
- Severe drug-related hypersensitivity reactions.
- Paradoxical reactions causing severe morbidity such as tuberculomas with perilesional edema, enlarging lymph nodes with compression of nearby structures, etc.

It may be useful to mention that although corticosteroid is helpful in certain patients, they should not be prescribed injudiciously due to its potential to cause dissemination of TB. For most situations, prednisolone 2 mg/kg/day for the initial 4 weeks and tapering doses for the next 2–4 weeks may be sufficient.

ROUTINE USE OF B6

The principal toxic effects of INH are peripheral neuritis and hepatitis. Peripheral neuritis resulting from competitive inhibition of pyridoxine utilization is a rare event in children on INH therapy. Therefore, the use of supplementary pyridoxine is not necessary routinely. However, special consideration should be given to those who have one or more of the following conditions: HIV coinfection, severely malnourished, chronic renal or liver disease, pregnancy, and pre-existing peripheral neuropathy. In such situations pyridoxine is used to prevent and treat central and peripheral nervous system side effects of INH in a dose of 25–50 mg/day.

ROLE OF SURGERY

Treatment of TB is mainly medical. Surgery may have an adjunctive role to play in certain cases and should be done after few weeks of adequate anti-TB therapy. Surgery is indicated in patients with Potts spine with neurodeficit, in hydrocephalus due to tuberculous meningitis (TBM) (to place VP shunt), pericardiectomy for constrictive pericarditis, lobar resection for sequelae such as bronchiectasis and finally in MDR/extensively drug resistant (XDR) TB for resection of diseased lobe.

MONITORING OF PATIENT ON TREATMENT

It is important to monitor the patient for:

- Response to treatment
- Treatment adherence
- Occurrence of side effects.

Monitoring for Response to Therapy

Clinical: The clinical improvement in a patient on antitubercular treatment (ATT) is the mainstay of assessing the response to therapy. Symptomatic improvement should be assessed on each clinic visit especially at the end of the initial phase and in subsequent follow-up, by judging the improvement of fever, decrease in cough, weight gain, improved appetite and subjective well-being, and decrease in lymph node size. Majority of the patients show clinical improvement in symptoms and signs within a few weeks' time usually by 2–4 weeks and definitely by 8 weeks. Worsening after 4 weeks of treatment or nonresolution of symptoms by 8 weeks is considered failure of therapy. Causes of nonresponse include nonadherence, improper doses, alternative diagnosis, comorbidities/coinfections/intercurrent infections, paradoxical reactions, and finally drug resistance. Follow-up visits need to be scheduled every 4 weeks for the duration of treatment and subsequently every 3–6 months for next 2 years particularly in children with serious disease such as congenital TB or meningitis, or those with extensive residual chest radiographic findings at the end of chemotherapy.

Radiological: The patients who are improving should be assessed for resolution of the radiological abnormalities at the end of therapy. Patients who do not show optimum improvement, radiographs should be repeated at end of intensive phase. In patients, who show increase or little change in radiological shadows coupled with inadequate clinical response, the intensive phase should be extended by 4 more weeks. All efforts need to be made to isolate and determine the drug sensitivity of the mycobacteria from the patient. The patients showing improvement after extended intensive therapy can be put on continuation phase or else the patient is investigated for treatment failure and drug-resistant TB. Normal chest radiograph appearance is not a necessary criterion for discontinuation of therapy in children treated for primary pulmonary disease. After completion of therapy, hilar adenopathy may be present for months to few years.

Microbiological: To monitor treatment outcome, it is recommended by RNTCP that all patients with pulmonary TB should have repeat sputum/gastric aspirate smears performed at the end of initial phase of treatment to detect conversion to negative status among those who were initially positive and to detect early failures in those who were AFB negative. To verify treatment success, additional sputum examinations are recommended at least once before stopping treatment. Sensitivity tests for all available drugs if possible need to be performed for any new patient whose sputum is still positive at the end of the intensive phase of treatment, and for any patient suspected to be at risk of being drug resistant, e.g. relapsed cases, defaulters.

Treatment Adherence

A simultaneous check on treatment adherence along with response to treatment is needed. It could be undertaken by asking the patient directly, by a pill count or prescription check and by asking for the color of the urine. Patients should be evaluated monthly and should be given only enough medicine for the interval between evaluations. As far as possible, all patients must be on Directly Observed Treatment, Short course (DOTS). The arrangements for observation of therapy must be arranged either at the nearby health facilities, family practitioner or by a responsible person/relative. The patients not on directly observed therapy should be followed up more regularly and must be made aware of his follow-up appointments to ensure compliance with treatment. To strengthen patient adherence, the patient and the caregiver should always be educated about the illness and treatment, and regularly motivated during the course of treatment. Efforts should be made for prompt defaulter tracing. Often the complete treatment of a patient may entail socioeconomic assistance and advice for the family.

It must be emphasized that routine hospitalization of TB patients is not required to ensure completion of treatment while those with serious sickness and complications may need to be admitted.

One of the reasons for poor adherence is drug stock outs or inability to buy drugs. RNTCP in India introduced the unique feature of the free patient-wise drug boxes (PWB) for all adult and pediatric cases registered with them. These "ready-to-use" PWBs containing a patient's complete course of standardized drug therapy are made available to every registered patient with TB with the patient's name on it. This improves patient care, adherence, and ensures complete treatment of every registered patient as the drug outages on treatment are obviated. The anti-TB drugs for pediatric patients are available in the form of two generic PWBs and the different weight bands are covered by mixing and matching these PWBs. The boxes contain strips of blister combi-packs with each combi-pack containing all the drugs to be consumed by the patient on a given visit. This mechanism of drug delivery ensures that the treatment of a registered case gets never interrupted due to drug outages and the risks for drug errors are few.

Drug Toxicity Monitoring and Management

Rates of adverse reactions to antituberculous drugs among children are low. The important side effects, which have clinical implications, include hepatotoxicity, ocular toxicity, and skin hypersensitivity reactions. All patients should be monitored clinically for adverse reactions during the period of chemotherapy. They should be informed about symptoms of common adverse reactions to the medications they are receiving. Children taking ethambutol require regular monitoring of visual acuity and color discrimination. Routine biochemical monitoring is usually not required.

Minor Side Effects

Minor side effects, such as gastrointestinal intolerance, mild skin rash, pruritus, or flushing, are best managed by reassurance and symptomatic treatment and the patient should be encouraged to continue antituberculosis treatment. Nonsteroidal anti-inflammatory drugs (NSAIDs) provide symptomatic relief for pyrazinamide-related arthralgia. Skin rashes can usually be managed by withholding the causative drug and if it is really necessary to reintroduce the drug, the patient should undergo desensitization.

Hepatitis

The factors that may decide hepatotoxicity include acetylator phenotype, doses and combination of antituberculosis drugs (ATDs), malnutrition, and severity of disease. Pyrazinamide is the most hepatotoxic followed by INH and then RMP.

As the anti-TB drugs are hepatic enzyme inducers, asymptomatic biochemical derangement is common and not considered as hepatitis unless the enzymes exceed 5 times the normal range. However, if patient develops jaundice/vomiting or other signs of liver dysfunction during therapy, it is considered hepatitis irrespective of enzyme levels. The patient should also be investigated for the possibility of intercurrent viral hepatitis.

The drugs are withheld till the serum bilirubin becomes normal and the enzymes also start touching the normal range. Rechallenge is best done in a place where liver function can be carefully monitored. The drugs should be reintroduced every 4–7 days in the order of RMP, followed by INH and then pyrazinamide. Pyrazinamide should not be reintroduced if the hepatitis was severe (enzymes more than 500). If the period without drugs is likely to be prolonged, and the patient is sick and requires treatment, at least two other drugs (e.g. streptomycin, ethambutol, and fluoroquinolones) should be given until it is determined whether the offending drug can be resumed. Drugs causing hepatitis on rechallenge should be stopped and substituted with other drugs. All patients who require alteration from the standard regimen should be referred to experienced physicians.

Other Side Effects

Clinical manifest neuritis in children on INH therapy due to pyridoxine deficiency is very rare. If at all it occurs, it manifests as pins and needle sensation in hands and feet. It is treated with pyridoxine 25–50 mg/day. Ocular toxicity due to ethambutol may occur in up to 5% of patients if doses are between 25 mg/kg/day and 50 mg/kg/day. However, it is rare in doses of 15–20 mg/kg/day. The toxicity results in reversible optic neuritis, blurred vision, and alteration in color vision. In young children if ethambutol toxicity is suspected they should be monitored by electroretinogram (ERG) in consultation with an eye specialist. However, in older patient regular monitoring of color vision is sufficient.

The development of the following conditions contraindicates further use of the offending drug:
- Thrombocytopenia, shock and/or renal failure due to RMP.
- Visual impairment due to ethambutol.
- Eighth nerve damage from streptomycin.
- Steven-Johnson syndrome.

Interruption of Treatment

Patient compliance is crucial factor in treatment failure and the development of acquired drug resistance. It is very important to realize that the emergence of multidrug-resistant tuberculosis (MDR-TB) is always a manmade problem and failure of the patient to complete the prescribed course completely and adequately is one of the reasons. In general, if it is certain that the patient was taking all medications correctly prior to interruption, then (s)he can be managed as per the guidelines for treatment after interruption shown in Table 3. Whenever treatment is interrupted for more than 2 weeks, the child should be reassessed clinically and radiologically, with

TABLE 3: Managing patients with interruptions in treatment.

Duration of therapy	*Duration of interruption*		*Decision*
Up to 4 weeks	*<2 weeks*		Resume original regimen
	>2 weeks		*Reassess and start treatment again*
4–8 weeks	*<2 weeks*		Resume original regimen
	2–8 weeks		Extend intensive phase by 1 month more
	>8 weeks		*Consider Category II if diagnosis is still Tuberculosis*
>8 weeks	*<2 weeks*		Resume original regimen
	>2 weeks	Review activity	• *No active disease*: Continue same treatment • *Active disease*: Category II therapy

bacteriological examination, wherever possible. In all such cases the resumption of treatment must be preceded by evaluation for activity and investigating the causes for nonadherence. The pediatrician should not merely restart the treatment but also enable the completion of treatment by addressing issues related to nonadherence in the first instance. Addressing issues like side effects of the therapy (real or perceived), cost involved as well as educating about the need for a complete treatment even after the symptoms abate may help adherence. Both the child as well as the caregivers must be involved in decision making for re-initiating treatment.

DRUG-RESISTANT TUBERCULOSIS

Introduction

Drug resistance in TB has become an important public health problem because of selection of strains resistant to potent drugs like rifampin and INH leading to failure of first-line drugs. It is primarily a microbiological diagnosis. Documentation of the level of drug resistance in the community is important in order to monitor the impact of RNTCP program over time and to ensure that the treatment regimens are appropriate. Various types of drug resistance are described below:

- *Monodrug resistance*: Resistance to any first-line anti-TB drug (HRZES)
- *MDR-TB:* It is caused by strains of *Mycobacterium tuberculosis* that are resistant to at least INH and RMP with or without resistance to other first-line drugs.
- *Polyresistance*: Strains of *Mycobacterium tuberculosis* that are resistant to combination of drugs other than both isoniazed and rifampicin are called polyresistant.
- *XDR-TB*: Infection by MDR strains of *Mycobacterium* with additional resistance to any newer fluoroquinolone and one of the three second line injectable drugs amikacin, kanamycin or capreomycin, is labelled as XDR-TB.
- *Pan-drug or totally drug-resistant tuberculosis* (*TDR-TB*) is caused by strains of *Mycobacteria* resistant to all known antitubercular drugs that can be tested in the laboratory.

The treatment of drug-resistant TB is challenging because of the complexity of the drug regimens, adverse drug reactions, secondary to second-line antitubercular drugs, and social and financial constrains to treatment. Most of the drug resistance in children is primary resistance, i.e. due to acquisition of a drug-resistant strain from an adult contact rather than secondary resistance (acquisition of resistance following inappropriate or incomplete treatment). Thus drug-resistant TB in children is usually a sentinel event. It reflects on poor management of the infectious pool, usually the adult patients. In general, the pattern of drug resistance in children tends to mirror that found in the adult patients in the same population.

When to Suspect Drug Resistance?

The following situations mandate evaluation for drug resistance:

- Failure to respond 4–8 weeks after initiation of appropriate anti-TB therapy
- Contacts of adults with drug-resistant TB
- Previous history of treatment for TB either complete/incomplete
- Children with HIV.

All patients with suspected drug-resistant TB should undergo extensive microbiologic tests including CBNAAT, line probe assays, and AFB culture even if it is by invasive methods.

Treatment of INH Monoresistance

The current recommendations for treatment of INH monoresistance is with three drugs RZE for 6–9 months. Fluoroquinolones (levofloxacin and moxifloxacin) may be added for extensive disease.

Treatment of Multidrug-resistant TB/Rifampicin Monoresistance/ Extremely Drug-resistant TB

This is complex situation. Second-line drugs are very expensive and the response to treatment is much poorer among those who are susceptible to first-line drugs. Even though the children tolerate the second-line drugs better than the adults, yet the adverse effects with these are much higher than with the first-line drugs. The average cost of treatment in children would approximate to more than 60 times the cost of treatment with the first-line drugs, and this is one of the biggest hurdles in treatment of drug-resistant cases. Therefore treatment of drug-resistant TB should always be in consultation with an expert. The basic principles in treatment of MDR-TB include:

- Sending molecular tests and AFB culture and phenotypic susceptibility tests to all first- and second-line drugs before starting therapy.
- Use of empiric regimen based on local susceptibility patterns in that area/susceptibility of the contact/previous drug regimen. At least 4–5 new drugs to which the isolate is likely to be susceptible should be used till susceptibility reports are available.
- One or two drugs should never be added to a failing regimen.
- The correct doses should be used and need for compliance stressed.
- The therapy should be modified based on susceptibility. If any first-line drugs are susceptible they should be added but not counted.
- Patient should be monitored closely for adherence, treatment response, and drug side effects.
- Treatment should be continued for the optimum duration.

Changes in Treatment Approaches for MDR-TB over Time

Conventional: The conventional classification of drugs for treatment of MDR-TB is represented in Table 4. The principles were to use five effective drugs, one from group A, one from group B, 2–3 from group C, and drugs from group D only if group A, B and C did not add up to five drugs. Injectables were an integral part of the regimen. The total duration of recommended therapy was 18–24 months after culture conversion and injectables 5 times per week for 6–8 months. Based on these principles the empiric regimen for MDR-TB in India was consisting of ethionamide, cycloserine, levofloxacin, pyrazinamide, ethambutol, and kanamycin. The WHO later in its recommendations in 2016 recommended that in children with mild disease the injectables could be avoided.

The problems with this regimen was the prolonged duration and toxicity associated with the injectables. Also in hotspots of MDR-TB in India like Mumbai where resistance to pyrazinamide, ethambutol, ethionamide, and quinolones was significant, the regimen is likely to be poorly efficacious and at risk of converting MDR to XDR-TB. Hence a one size fits all approach cannot work for MDR-TB and attention to an individual's own drug susceptibility is extremely important. Soman and Singhal et al. demonstrated very good outcomes with individualized susceptibility based therapy.

TABLE 4: Classification of drugs used for MDR/XDR-TB.

Group	*Conventional grouping*	*New grouping*
Group A	• Moxifloxacin • Levofloxacin • Gatifloxacin	• Moxifloxacin • Levofloxacin • Bedaquiline • Linezolid
Group B	• Amikacin • Capreomycin • Kanamycin	• Clofazimine • Cycloserine/Terizidone
Group C Other core second-line agents	• Ethionamide/ Prothionamide • Cycloserine/Terizidone • Clofazimine • Linezolid	• Ethambutol • Delamanid • Pyrazinamide • Meropenem/Imipenem with clavulanate • Amikacin/Streptomycin • Ethionamide/Prothionamide • PAS
Group D agents	• D1 • Pyrazinamide • Ethambutol • High dose isoniazid • D2 • Delamanid • Bedaquiline • D3 • PAS • Imipenem/Meropenem with amoxicillin clavulanate • Thioacetazone	

(MDR; multidrug resistant; PAS: para-aminosalicylic acid; XDR-TB: extensively resistant tuberculosis)

Shorter regimens for MDR-TB: Randomized trials from Bangladesh and Africa with shorter regimens of 9–12 months compared to conventional regimens showed equivalent efficacy at lower cost and lower toxicity. A prototype regimen consisted of prothionamide, high-dose INH, moxifloxacin, clofazimine, amikacin, pyrazinamide and ethambutol for 4–6 months followed by moxifloxacin, PZA, E, and clofazimine for 3–4 months. Hence, the WHO in its guidelines recommended that these regimens can be used in the treatment of MDR-TB including children with the following exceptions:

- Those with history of previous treatment with second-line drugs
- Those with resistance to any drugs in the regimen with the exception of INH
- Those with disseminated/meningeal disease or those with HIV and extrapulmonary TB.

The applicability of these regimens to the Indian setting is debatable owing to high prevalence of resistance to the component drugs.

New all oral regimens for treatment of MDR-TB: Globally, including in the WHO there has been a movement for a paradigm shift in the treatment of TB. This has resulted from the following events:

- An individual patient data meta-analysis has been recently published in the Lancet. This involved 50 datasets from 25 countries, with 12,030 patients treated for pulmonary MDR-TB. Of the drugs analyzed, levofloxacin, moxifloxacin, linezolid, and bedaquiline were associated with greater treatment success and reduced death. Clofazimine and the carbapenems were associated with significantly improved treatment success but not reduced death. Pyrazinamide, streptomycin, amikacin, cycloserine, and terizidone were associated with modest benefits, but only in patients with susceptible isolates, whereas the use of kanamycin, capreomycin, ethionamide, prothionamide, para-aminosalicylic acid, macrolides and amoxicillin-clavulanic acid (when used without carbapenems) were associated with no significant benefit or significantly worse outcomes.

- The efficacy of shorter regimens in treatment of TB.
- The efficacy of new drugs bedaquiline and delamanid in treatment of MDR and even XDR-TB.
- The ototoxicity seen in 25% of patients treated with the aminoglycosides.

Based on this the WHO published a rapid advice statement suggesting a paradigm shift in the treatment of drug-resistant TB. The key features of this statement include a regrouping of medicines into three categories with levofloxacin/moxifloxacin/bedaquiline and linezolid in Group A, cycloserine/terizidone/clofazimine in Group B and the rest of the other drugs used for MDR-TB including delaminid in Group C (Table 4). The principles of constructing a new longer MDR regimen involve choosing all available drugs from Group A and B if susceptible and add other drugs from Group C only if Group A and B drugs cannot be used. Also, the statement advises against use of drugs like pyrazinamide/ethambutol unless susceptibility is documented. If injectables are recommended then amikacin/streptomycin is preferred to kanamycin/capreomycin. Other factors governing choices include preference of oral over injectable agents; the results of drug-susceptibility testing (DST); the reliability of existing DST methods; population drug resistance levels; history of previous use of the medicine in a patient; drug tolerability; and potential drug-drug interactions. Finer details of these regimens are yet awaited.

There are several concerns with extrapolating these recommendations to the Indian setting; representation of Indian data in this meta-analysis, the good outcomes noted with the erstwhile Group C drugs in current regimens, the side effects associated with prolonged linezolid therapy, the poor CNS penetration of bedaquiline, applicability to extrapulmonary and meningeal TB being some of them. The applicability of these regimens to young children is also contentious. Bedaquiline is currently approved above the age of 18 (may be used in children weighing above 12 years and above weight 33 kg), while delamanid is approved in children 6 years and above. Trials with these drugs in younger children are underway. This leaves children below age 3–5 where older long MDR-TB regimens based on susceptibility data of the index case or the contact may have to be used. Paradoxically, this is the group where it is most difficult to detect drug side effects including injectable associated ototoxicity or linezolid induced neuropathy/optic neuritis.

Hence till there is more data about the efficacy of new therapy and recommendations from the RNTCP, practitioners should continue to use the pre-existing conventional regimens for treatment of MDR/XDR-TB. At the same time consideration should be given to more liberal use of linezolid/clofazimine and restriction of use of aminoglycosides in mild disease. Efforts should also be made to procure new drugs like bedaquiline or delamanid for patients with XDR-TB. The doses and side effects of commonly used drugs in MDR-TB are detailed in Table 5.

EXTRAPULMONARY TUBERCULOSIS

Controlled trials of various forms of extrapulmonary TB are virtually nonexistent. In most reports extrapulmonary forms have been combined with pulmonary cases and are often not analyzed separately. Extrapulmonary TB is associated with lower bacillary burden than pulmonary disease, therefore, extrapulmonary disease generally can be treated with standard short-course regimens that are effective for pulmonary disease. Owing to the serious implication of relapsed

TABLE 5: Drugs used for MDR-TB.

Drug	*Daily dose and route*	*Maximum dose*	*CSF penetration*	*Adverse effects/comments*
Ethionamide	10–20 mg/kg/d, Oral, qod/bd	750 mg	Good	Gastric intolerance, hepatitis, hypothyroidism
Prothionamide	10–20 mg/kg/d, oral, qod	750 mg	Good	Gastric intolerance, hepatitis
Kanamycin	15–20 mg/kg/d, IM Inj, qod	1,000 mg	Poor	Auditory and vestibulo-toxicity
Amikacin	15–20 mg/kg/d, IM Inj, qod	1,000 mg	Poor	Auditory and vestibulo-toxicity, nephrotoxic
Capreomycin	15 mg/kg/d IM qod	1,000 mg	Poor	Audiotoxicity, nephrotoxicity
Cycloserine	15 mg/kg/d, Oral, qod	750 mg	Good	Psychosis, depression, seizures, pyridoxine deficiency
Levofloxacin	15–20 mg/kg/d qod	1000 mg	Good	Arthropathy Seizures
Moxifloxacin	10–15 mg/kg/day qod	400– 600 mg	Good	
Para amino–salicylic acid (PAS)	150–300 mg/kg/d, oral, qod/bd	12,000 mg	Inflamed meninges	Gastric intolerance, hepatitis, hypothyroidism
Clofazimine	2–5 mg/kg/day qod	100 mg	Poor	Hyperpigmentation
Linezolid	10 mg/kg/d qod	600 mg	Good	Peripheral neuropathy Thrombocytopenia
Bedaquiline (above 12 years/ more than 33 kg)	400 mg daily for 2 weeks and then 200 mg thrice weekly for 22 weeks	400 mg	Poor	Increased QT interval Liver impairment
Delamanid	7–23 kg: 25 mg bd 24–34: 50 mg bd 35 kg: 100 mg bd < 7 kg: 1.5–2 mg/kg bd	200 mg	Good	Increased QT interval

(CSF: cerebrospinal fluid; MDR-TB; multidrug-resistant tuberculosis)

disease at sites of potentially limited drug penetration, most clinicians treat miliary, meningeal, and skeletal TB for 9-12 months. Adjunctive therapy with steroids and surgery should be considered when indicated.

CONGENITAL TUBERCULOSIS

Congenital TB is defined as TB occurring in an infant as a result of infection with *M. tuberculosis* during intrauterine life. It can occur after maternal bacteremia at different stages in the course of tubercular disease. Postnatal TB, on the other hand, is usually acquired from a mother, other close family member, or caregiver with cavitary TB. In 1935, Beitzke suggested criteria for distinguishing congenital from postnatally acquired TB. Cantwell and coworkers revised these criteria making it more appropriate. According to them, the infant with congenital TB must have *proven tuberculous* lesions and *at least one* of the following:

- Lesions in the first week of life
- A primary hepatic complex or caseating hepatic granulomas
- Tuberculous infection of the placenta or the maternal genital tract
- Exclusion of the possibility of postnatal transmission by a thorough investigation of contacts, including the infant's hospital attendants.

Usually these infants should be treated as severely sick patients using 4-drug regimen discussed earlier. The response to treatment is slower as compared to older children. Although the optimal duration of therapy has not been established, many experts treat infants with congenital TB for about 9–12 months because of the decreased immunologic capability of the young infant. Current recommendations however suggest that 6 months maybe adequate. Clinical experience suggests that the drugs in usual doses are effective and safe in young infants.

TUBERCULOSIS AND HIV

Introduction

Impact of coinfection with HIV and TB is however more complex as it is bidirectional. HIV and TB intersect each other at various levels and fueling each other. As a consequence of coinfection, TB accelerates the natural history of HIV, leading to early death. This is supported by the evidence that HIV DNA levels are higher in the involved segments of lung and decline with treatment. Thus, patients not on antiretroviral therapy (ART) may be at disadvantage if TB treatment or diagnosis is delayed due to enhanced HIV replication. On the other hand, HIV infection greatly increases the risk of active TB in children coinfected with *M. tuberculosis* by 10 times as compared to those without coinfection (~10% per year). Chemoprophylaxis is thus an important strategy for prevention of disease in such individuals. Hence, WHO/NACO (National AIDS Control Organization) and RNTCP recommend screening all HIV infected patients for TB and all TB patients for HIV.

Clinical presentation of TB coinfection is similar to as in non-HIV infected children, though extrapulmonary involvement is more common. Severely immunocompromised children are more likely to have extensive/disseminated disease. The diagnosis is more difficult as the disease manifestations of TB mimic those of HIV and other infections, radiology is not specific, AFB negativity is common and tuberculin skin test positivity is very low.

Treatment

The basic principles of treatment of TB in HIV infected individuals are:

- Use of the standard regimen for 6 months followed by 6 months of INH preventive therapy.
- Initiation of antiretroviral therapy 2–8 weeks after starting anti-TB therapy. This should be 2 weeks if the CD4 count is very low. This delay in starting ART is to reduce pill burden, prevent adverse events due to combined anti-TB and anti HIV-drugs and finally to reduce the risk of development of immune reconstitution syndrome.
- Address the issues of drug interactions between rifampicin and anti-HIV drugs. The main interaction is the reduction of drug levels of protease inhibitors and nevirapine due to the enzyme inducing effect of rifampicin. There is now enough data to suggest that rifampicin should be a component of the anti-TB regimen since non-rifampicin-based regimens

are associated with poorer outcomes. Hence, the ART regimen should be modified. In children below 3 years the recommended ART regimen is two NRTI (zidovudine/abacavir with lamivudine) and super boosted lopinavir and ritonavir. In children older than 3 years efavirenz with two NRTI as mentioned earlier is recommended. Other alternative inferior options include a triple NRTI regimen (zidovudine, lamivudine, abacavir) or high-dose nevirapine with two NRTI.

- Monitor the patient for development of immune reconstitution syndrome (IRIS) due to restoration of immunologic activity. This syndrome manifests as clinical worsening with either apparent increase in disease at the initial site or development of new sites. The risk of IRIS is higher in patients with low baseline CD4 count, extensive TB disease and rapid immunologic/virologic response. IRIS is a diagnosis of exclusion and other reasons for worsening including new opportunistic infections or drug resistance should be excluded by appropriate tests. Mild IRIS can be treated with symptomatic therapy like paracetamol. Severe IRIS may necessitate the use of short-term steroids at 1–2 mg/kg/day. The anti-TB or anti-HIV medications should not be stopped.

CHEMOPROPHYLAXIS

Basics

Chemoprophylaxis of TB/treatment of latent infection involves usage of one or more anti-tubercular drugs in persons already infected or suspected of being infected with TB in order to prevent occurrence of active disease in future. Thus it prevents occurrence of disease in already infected individual and thereby decreasing the potential future source of infection.

Children and adults in close contact with an adult suspected of having infectious pulmonary TB are at risk for infection. The risk varies with various factors including type of disease in the host, whether the smear is positive, closeness of contact, cough hygiene, and administration of treatment. Though the risk is highest with smear positive contacts, even smear negative contacts can transmit disease. Studies have shown latent infection in 50% of contacts of an adult with pulmonary TB while clinical disease in around 4% of the contacts.

The average lifetime risk of developing disease in an individual with TB infection is 10%. The risk of disease is higher with young age (50% in infants and around 10–25% in children aged 2–5 years). The risk is 10 times more in HIV infected individuals. The risk of development of disease is highest just after the infection has occurred and gradually decreases with time. Recent converters are usually defined as individuals whose tuberculin test reaction increased by at least 6 mm, from less than 10 mm to more than 10 mm within past 2 years. Children, particularly those with a history of a recent contact with an infectious case or recent tuberculin convectors are at special risk of developing full-blown disease.

Indications for Chemoprophylaxis/Treatment of Latent Infection

The indications for chemoprophylaxis differ between countries depending on endemicity. In countries with low endemicity, treatment of all latently infected people is recommended since the chances of reinfection are low and the approach is cost effective. However in countries with high endemicity including India the priority is to administer chemoprophylaxis to those at highest risk of disease/severe disease. Therefore, children form a major group requiring preventive treatment. A pre-requisite for chemoprophylaxis is to rule out active disease by appropriate history, clinical examination and if indicated radiology. Current indications for chemoprophylaxis include:

- All children less than 6 years of age who are in contact of an infectious case irrespective of their nutrition or tuberculin skin tests (TST) status.
- All TST positive children who are receiving immunosuppressive therapy (e.g. children with nephrotic syndrome, acute leukemia, etc.).
- A child born to mother who was diagnosed to have TB in pregnancy/after delivery.
- All HIV-infected children (1) between the ages of 1–5 years irrespective of contact (2) history of contact with infectious TB or a positive TST of more than or equal to 5 mm irrespective of age.

Which Drug to Use?

Isoniazid has been the standard chemoprophylactic drug for decades since large randomized controlled trials have shown its efficacy in preventing disease. INH appears to be more effective for children than adults, with several large clinical trials demonstrating risk reduction by 70% to 90%. Also, the risk of INH-related hepatitis is minimal in infants, children and adolescent, who generally tolerate the drug better than adults. A 9-month regimen has superior efficacy than a 9 month regimen. The AAP currently recommends a 9-month course of INH with effectiveness of over 90%. However, among patients with average compliance, 6-month treatment appears to yield the best benefit risk ratio. Hence the WHO/RNTCP recommends a 6-month regimen. The dosage is 10 mg/kg body weight daily therapy.

Recently, many new regimens for preventive therapy have been advocated. These include combination of INH and rifampicin for 3–4 months, rifampicin alone for 3–4 months or combination of weekly rifapentine with daily INH for 3 month. The advantages of these regimens are better compliance due to shorter duration with similar efficacy. However, these have still not become standard of care in India and are awaiting approval from the RNTCP.

Chemoprophylaxis for Contact of MDR

This is a contentious issue. There are some trials from South Africa that have demonstrated efficacy of an alternative regimen but a recent meta-analysis found insufficient evidence to recommend the same. Hence, at present the consensus is to with hold any chemoprophylaxis and closely follow up these children for 2 years.

Management of a Neonate Born to a Mother Who had Tuberculosis in Pregnancy/Post-delivery

The current guidelines recommend prophylaxis of babies who are born to mothers who had TB in pregnancy (even if they have been successfully treated) or those who have been exposed soon after birth. The babies should be evaluated carefully for congenital TB. If negative, INH at the rate of 10 mg/kg/day should be started for next 6 months. Bacillus Calmette-Guérin (BCG) can be given along with INH. Separation of the mother and infant is no longer considered mandatory once therapy is started. Separation should occur only if the mother is ill enough to require hospitalization, if she has been or is expected to become nonadherent to her treatment, or if she is infected with a drug resistant strain of *M. tuberculosis*.

TREATMENT OF BCG-ASSOCIATED COMPLICATIONS

BCG-associated local complications are not uncommon and usually consist of local abscess formation or suppurative/nonsuppurative lymphadenitis. These usually happen if BCG is given subcutaneously or following vaccination at an older age. Most of these regress spontaneously over weeks or months. In some cases local aspiration may be needed. Rarely excision is required. There is no role of administering anti-TB therapy/erythromycin for local BCG-related complications.

Disseminated BCG infection (BCGiosis) occurs in babies with immunodeficiency disorders including HIV/severe combined immunodeficiency disorder (SCID) who have been administered BCG vaccine. The presentation is with fever, failure to thrive, disseminated lymphadenopathy, and hepatosplenomegaly. Diagnosis is by culture of affected tissue or blood. The Xpert does not differentiate between TB/BCG and neither do the usual tests such as MPT 64. Differentiation of *M. bovis* from *M. tuberculosis* needs specialized PCR-based tests. Treatment is with antitubercular drugs including INH, rifampicin, ethambutol, quinolones, and aminoglycosides for 12–18 months. *M. bovis* is inherently resistant to pyrazinamide.

CONCLUSION

- Try to establish bacteriologic diagnosis as far as possible.
- The aim of antituberculosis treatment is to: Cure the patient in as short a time as possible; prevent death or late effects from disease; prevent relapse; prevent emergence of drug resistance; and to protect community from infection.
- Intensive SCC is better than traditional two-drug regimens due to faster sterilization and bactericidal action, shorter duration over which patient noncompliance can occur, less expense on monitoring of treatment, lower failure and relapse rate, and broader coverage of possible drug-resistant *M. tuberculosis*.
- The current recommendation calls for a 6-month regimen for pulmonary TB in children with an intensive phase of 2-months of daily HRZE, followed by 4-months of HRE, given supervised daily.
- In general extrapulmonary TB in children should be treated in the same way as pulmonary TB, except bone and joint disease and meningitis for which there are inadequate data to support limiting the therapy to 6-months. Increase of the continuation phase to 7–10 months is prudent in these cases.
- Routine biochemical monitoring is not required, however, monthly physician-patient contact is required to ensure compliance and assess for toxicity and efficacy of therapy.
- Patient compliance is a crucial factor in treatment failure and the development of acquired drug resistance. Whenever possible, TB treatment should be administered as directly observed therapy.
- Both the physician and the patient share responsibility for successful treatment.
- Adjunctive use of steroids and surgery should be considered in special circumstances.
- Diagnosis and treatment of drug-resistant TB is highly specialized and should be in consultation with an expert.

RECOMMENDED READING

1. Ahmad N, Ahuja SD, Akkerman OW, et al. Treatment correlates of successful outcomes in pulmonary multidrug-resistant tuberculosis: an individual patient data meta-analysis. Lancet. 2018;392:821-34.
2. Baba H, Shinkai A, Izuchi R, et al. Controlled clinical trial of 4-6 months regimens of chemotherapy for pulmonary tuberculosis. Bull Int Union Tubercle. 1984;59:26-9.
3. Bloch AB, Snider DJ. How much tuberculosis in children must we accept? Am J Pub Health. 1986;76:14-5.
4. British Thoracic Research Committee. Short-course chemotherapy for tuberculosis of lymph nodes: a controlled trial. Br Med J. 1985;290:1106-8.
5. British Thoracic Society. A controlled trial of 6-month chemotherapy in pulmonary tuberculosis. Final Report: Results during the 36 months after the end of chemotherapy and beyond. Br J Dis Chest. 1984;78:330-6.
6. Cantwell MF, Shehab ZM, Costello AM, et al. Brief report: congenital tuberculosis. N Eng J Med. 1994;330:1051-4.
7. Centers for Disease Control and Prevention. Treatment of Tuberculosis. American Thoracic Society, CDC, and Infectious Diseases Society of America. MMWR. 2003;52:1-74.
8. Cotton MF, Schaff HS, Hesseling AC, et al. HIV and childhood tuberculosis: the way forward. Int J Tuberc Lung Dis. 2004;8:675-82.
9. Dingley HB. Short-term chemotherapy in tuberculosis in children. Ind J Tub. 1981;29:48.
10. Dutt AK, Moers D, Stead WW. Short-course chemotherapy for extrapulmonary tuberculosis: nine years experience. Ann Intern Med. 1986;104:7-12.
11. D'Esopo ND. Clinical trials in pulmonary tuberculosis. Am Rev Respir Dis. 1982;125(Suppl):85.
12. East and Central African/British Medical Council Fifth Collaborative Study. Controlled clinical trial of 4 short course regimens of chemotherapy (three 6 month and one 8 month) for pulmonary tuberculosis: Final report. Tubercle. 1986;67:5-15.
13. Getahun H, Matteelli A, Chaisson RE, et al. Latent *Mycobacterium tuberculosis* infection. N Engl J Med. 2015;372(22):2127-35.
14. Graham SM, Daley HM, Banerjee A, et al. Ethambutol in tuberculosis: time to reconsider. Arch Dis Child. 1998;79:274-8.
15. Grosset J. Bacteriologic basis of short course chemotherapy for tuberculosis. Clin Chest Med. 1980;1:231-41.
16. Grosset JH. Present status of chemotherapy for tuberculosis. Rev Infec Dis. 1989;11(suppl 2):342-47.
17. Iseman MD. Treatment of multidrug-resistant tuberculosis. New Engl J Med. 1993;329:784-91.
18. Lew W, Pai M, Oxlade O, et al. Initial drug resistance and tuberculosis treatment outcomes: systematic review and meta-analysis. Ann Intern Med. 2008;149(2):123-34.
19. Mitchison DA. The action of antituberculous-drugs in short course chemotherapy. Tubercle. 1985;66:219-25.
20. Mitchison DA. The diagnosis and therapy of tuberculosis during the past 100 years. Am J Respir Crit Care Med. 2005;171:699-706.
21. Moore DP, Schaaf HS, Nuttall J, et al. Childhood tuberculosis guidelines of the Southern African Society for Paediatric Infectious Diseases. South Afr J Epidemiol Infect. 2009;24(3):57-68.
22. Mukherjee JS, Rich ML, Socci AR, et al. Programmes and principles in treatment of multidrug resistant tuberculosis. Lancet. 2004;363:474-81.
23. O, brien RJ. Hepatotoxic reaction to antituberculous drugs: adjustments to therapeutic regimen. JAMA. 1991;265:3323.
24. RNTPC Status Report Central TB Division, Ministry of Health and Family Welfare, Delhi. (2012). TB India 2012. [online] Available from https://tbcindia.gov.in/showfile.php?lid=3141 [Accessed January 2019].
25. Singapore Tuberculosis Service/British Medical Research Council. Long-term follow up of a clinical trial of six month & four month regimens of chemotherapy in treatment of pulmonary tuberculosis. Am Rev Respir Dis. 1986;133:779-83.

26. Singhal T, Rodrigues C, Soman R, et al. Satisfactory outcomes in children with MDR tuberculosis in Mumbai with individualized susceptibility based treatment. Program and abstracts of the 51st Annual Meeting of the Infectious Diseases Society of America, San Francisco, California, USA, Oct 2-6; 2013 [Abstract # 1658].
27. Singh V. Tuberculosis in children: some issues. Health Millions. 1995;21:27-8.
28. Snider DE, Caras GJ, Koplan JP. Preventive therapy with isoniazid: Cost effectiveness of different duration of therapy. JAMA. 1986;25:1579-83.
29. Snider DE, Graczyk J, Bek E, et al. Supervised six-month treatment of newly diagnosed pulmonary tuberculosis using isomiazid, rifampin, and pyrazinamide with and without streptomycin. Am Rev Respir Dis. 1984;130:1091-6.
30. Soman R, Pillai P, Madan S, et al. Successful management of drug resistant tuberculosis using individualised DST. J Assoc Physic India. 2014;62:567-71.
31. Starke JR. Multidrug therapy for tuberculosis in children. Pediatr Infect Dis J. 1990;9:785-93.
32. Starke JR. Childhood tuberculosis: ending the neglect. Int J Tuberc Lung Dis. 2002;6:373-74.
33. Working Group on Tuberculosis, Indian Academy of Pediatrics (IAP). Consensus statement on childhood tuberculosis. Indian Pediatr. 2010;47(1):41-55.
34. World Health Organization. (2011). Global tuberculosis control: WHO Report 2011. [online] Available from http://www.who.int/iris/handle/10665/44728 [Accessed January 2019].
35. World Health Organization. (2018) Rapid Communication: Key changes to treatment of multidrug- and rifampicin-resistant tuberculosis (MDR/RR-TB). [online] Available from https://www.who.int/tb/publications/2018/rapid_communications_MDR/en/. [Accessed January 2019].
36. World Health Organization. Rapid Advice: *Treatment of tuberculosis 1 in* children. Geneva, Switzerland: WHO Press; 2010.

Antimicrobial Therapy in Enteric Fever

22
Chapter

Digant Shastri, Tanu Singhal

INTRODUCTION

Enteric fever is endemic in many developing countries due to poor sanitation and substandard water supply. *Salmonella typhi/paratyphi A/B/C* (now termed as *Salmonella enterica serotype typhi or Salmonella enterica serotype paratyphi)* is the infecting organism. Infections due to *Salmonella typhi* (typhoid fever) are the most common, but with increasing immunization coverage with the typhoid Vi vaccine, cases of paratyphoid fever (*Salmonella paratyphi A*) are on the rise. It is estimated that India has 2.1–3.4 million cases of typhoid and paratyphoid each year and typhoid contributed to 9.7% of all febrile inpatients. With increasing multidrug and quinolone resistance in *Salmonella typhi/paratyphi*, therapy of enteric fever is becoming more complicated and expensive.

Timely and appropriate management of typhoid fever can reduce both morbidity and mortality. The crux is choice of the appropriate antimicrobial therapy. Patients with persistent vomiting, inability to take oral feed, severe diarrhea, and abdominal distension usually require parenteral antibiotic therapy preferably in a hospital. Close medical follow-up is necessary to look for development of complications or treatment failure or relapse of disease.

ANTIMICROBIAL RESISTANCE IN *SALMONELLA TYPHI/PARATYPHI*

Lack of a reliable point-of-care test to diagnose typhoid fever results in presumptive antimicrobial therapy for typhoid in patients with undifferentiated febrile illness. This presumptive therapy based on the most appropriate antimicrobial for the circulating clade of *S. typhi* drives the resistance pattern. The antimicrobial susceptibility is a dynamic process. It changes with time and varies in different regions. The introduction of chloramphenicol in the 1940s was followed by development of resistance within the next 2 years. However, it was not until 1972 that chloramphenicol-resistant typhoid fever became a major problem. Chloramphenicol resistance was associated with high-molecular-weight, self-transferable, HI plasmids. These *S. typhi* strains were also resistant to sulfonamides, tetracycline, and streptomycin, but amoxicillin and trimethoprim–sulfamethoxazole remained effective alternative drugs. Toward the end of the 1980s and 1990s, *S. typhi* developed resistance simultaneously to all the drugs that were then used as first-line treatment (chloramphenicol, trimethoprim, sulfamethoxazole, and ampicillin). Outbreaks of infections with these strains occurred in India, Pakistan, Bangladesh, Vietnam, Middle East, and Africa. Fluoroquinolones were introduced in the late 1980s and early 1990s and produced very good results. However, the past two decades has seen a progressive increase in the minimal inhibitory concentrations (MICs) of ciprofloxacin in *S. typhi* and *paratyphi* and eventual development of quinolone resistance. Resistance rates to quinolones now approach 90% in many cities in India. With the emergence of quinolone resistance there has also been a return in sensitivity to first-line antibiotics, such as chloramphenicol, cotrimoxazole, and ampicillin. However, concerns of toxicity have precluded their widespread use and beta-lactams, such as ceftriaxone and cefixime are now used as first-line agents for therapy of enteric fever. Decrease susceptibility to azithromycin has been reported though no extensively drug-resistant (XDR) strain resistant to azithromycin has been reported.

Increase in MICs to ceftriaxone in *Salmonella* in India has been reported and so has been high-level resistance to ceftriaxone (MIC, 64 mg per liter). An outbreak of MDR *S. typhi* that was also resistant to ceftriaxone occurred in Sindh province of Pakistan in November 2016. More than 1,000 cases have been confirmed till date. The outbreak is caused by the H58 clade, a multidrug-resistant haplotype of *S. typhi* that is common in Asia and areas of Africa. The resistance seen in the Pakistan outbreak is mediated by genes on chromosome and plasmid that confer resistance to all the main antimicrobials that have been considered first-line drugs to treat typhoid fever during the past 70 years including chloramphenicol, ampicillin, cotrimoxazole, fluoroquinolones, and ceftriaxone. This outbreak was treated with combination therapy with meropenem and azithromycin.

Fortunately however as of now most *Salmonella enterica* isolates from India remain susceptible to the third-generation cephalosporins and azithromycin. However, the antimicrobial arsenal for typhoid is receding. *S typhi* can transform from multidrug-resistant (MDR) to XDR in a single step by acquisition of a plasmid. The XDR strain can spread globally. The growing antimicrobial resistance (AMR) may shift the treatment of suspected enteric fever from outpatient settings, where more than 90% of patients with typhoid are typically treated, to inpatient settings, thereby overwhelming hospitals in places where nosocomial infections with drug-resistant bacteria are common. The cost and effect on health systems in countries where typhoid is endemic could be devastating.

Another point worth mentioning is discordance between in vitro and in vivo susceptibility in *Salmonella enterica*. Though *Salmonella* shows in vitro susceptibility to aminoglycosides and second-generation cephalosporins, these agents are not associated with good in vivo responses and should not be used to treat enteric fever.

DRUGS IN ENTERIC FEVER

Cephalosporins

Ceftriaxone

Ceftriaxone is currently the preferred drug for inpatient therapy and severe enteric fever. The recommended dose is 75–100 mg/kg/day (maximum 4 g/day) as single or two doses. The average fever clearance time is around 1 week. Clinical failure defined as persistent symptoms or development of complications necessitating further antimicrobial treatment (in spite of the strain being susceptible) has been reported in 5–10%. The relapse rate is around 5–10% and depends on duration of therapy. A randomized controlled trial by Bhutta et al. demonstrated relapse rates of 15% with 7 days treatment versus 5% with 14 days therapy. Hence, 14 days therapy is recommended. However, the course of therapy may be completed with oral third-generation cephalosporins once complications have resolved, defervescence is achieved and oral intake is satisfactory. In some patients biliary sludging can occur during therapy and if symptomatic may warrant change in treatment. Cefotaxime in a dose of 150–200 mg/kg/day in three divided doses can be used instead of ceftriaxone.

Cefixime

This oral third-generation cephalosporin is used for outpatient therapy of enteric as well as a switch over drug from ceftriaxone. Trials have shown superior efficacy to quinolones and chloramphenicol in areas where there is high prevalence of resistance to these antibiotics and comparable efficacy to ceftriaxone. The dose of cefixime is not standardized and doses ranging from 10 to 20 mg/kg/day have been used in various trials. Since *Salmonella* is an intracellular pathogen and has high MICs to cefixime higher doses (20 mg/kg/day, max 1,200 mg/day) are preferred. The mean fever clearance time is around 1 week with rates of clinical failure and microbiologic failure ranging from 5 to 15 and 0.5 to 5%, respectively. Relapse rates range from 1 to 10% in various studies. At least 2 weeks of treatment should be given.

Cefpodoxime

This oral third-generation cephalosporin has similar gram-negative coverage as cefixime but superior gram-positive activity than cefixime; the dose is yet not standardized. Probably higher doses in the range of 10–20 mg/kg would be required. In the absence of good efficacy data, the use of this drug in management of enteric fever is not recommended.

Ampicillin/Cotrimoxazole and Chloramphenicol

These were the first-line antibiotics against enteric fever till widespread drug resistance made them redundant. However with the return of sensitivity to first-line drugs they are now potential therapeutic options.

Ampicillin/Amoxicillin

High doses (ampicillin 200 mg/kg/day and amoxicillin 100 mg/kg/day) in 3–4 divided doses have to be administered for a total of 14 days or at least 5–7 days after defervescence has occurred. Defervescence takes at least 1 week and failure rates (in spite of strain being susceptible) range from 5 to 12%. Relapse rates reported are 1–5%. Problems with ampicillin/amoxicillin include the high pill burden, poor oral tolerability, and high incidence of diarrhea.

Chloramphenicol

This was considered the gold standard for treatment of enteric fever in the past. In patients with susceptible strains, 50–75 mg/kg/day in four divided doses produces rapid defervescence (mean fever clearance time 5 days). Recommended duration of therapy is 14 days or at least 5–7 days after defervescence has occurred. Relapse and fecal carriage rates are higher with chloramphenicol as compared to other drugs and range from 4 to 8% in various studies. The main limitation with use of chloramphenicol is the chance of aplastic anemia. This nondose dependent, nonreversible, and idiosyncratic reaction occurs at an incidence rate of 1 in 20,000 to 1 in 40,000 treatment courses. This rare but often fatal adverse effect is responsible for reluctance to use this drug even though there is return of sensitivity to chloramphenicol when other effective/less toxic drugs are available.

Cotrimoxazole

The recommended dose and duration is 10 mg/kg/day of trimethoprim (TMP) for 14 days. The mean time to defervescence is 6 days and relapse rates are low (0.5–5%). However, clinical failure rates range from 5 to 15% despite susceptible strains. This is the cheapest drug for enteric; however, the concern is adverse skin reactions especially Steven Johnson's syndrome. This drug may have an important role to play in the current era of evolution of ceftriaxone resistance. This drug has been successfully used to treat ceftriaxone-resistant enteric fever in Mumbai where there was clinical failure with beta lactam/beta lactamase inhibitor (BL-BLI) combinations, carbapenems, and azithromycin (Singhal T, unpublished data).

Aztreonam

This monobactam with exclusive gram-negative activity has been reported to be effective in therapy of enteric in a dose of 50–100 mg/kg/day in three divided doses for 7–14 days. The average defervescence time is 6 days with very low relapse and fecal carriage rates. However, clinical failure rates can be as high as 5–15%. Trials have reported longer time to defervescence as compared to ceftriaxone and chloramphenicol. The main role of aztreonam is in management of severe/complicated enteric in patients with serious allergy to the cephalosporins.

Quinolones

In the era of quinolone susceptibility, quinolones produced the most dramatic responses in patients with enteric with average time to defervescence being 4 days and almost 0 relapse and fecal carriage rates. Ciprofloxacin and ofloxacin were used in doses of 10–20 mg/kg/day and 5–7 days therapy was sufficient. The usual MICs of *Salmonella* to ciprofloxacin in this era were 0.0004–0.004 mg/mL. However, with rising MICs (currently around 0.2–1 mg/mL) and increasing quinolone resistance, clinical failure with quinolones is common. Therefore, quinolones in standard doses most not be used as empirical therapy for enteric in these areas. There is insufficient data on the efficacy of newer quinolones (levofloxacin, gatifloxacin, moxifloxacin) against *S.typhi/paratyphi*. Conversely if the isolate is nalidixic acid sensitive, the quinolones are the most effective drugs and may be used as the drugs of first choice for both inpatient/outpatient therapy.

Azithromycin

This newer macrolide with very high intracellular penetration has been recommended in therapy of enteric fever. Randomized controlled trials have shown efficacy equal to intravenous ceftriaxone and superior to chloramphenicol and ofloxacin in patients with *Salmonella* resistant to these drugs. Average time to defervescence is reported as 4.4 days with very low fecal carriage and relapse rates (0–3%). All this makes azithromycin a promising drug for enteric fever.

Possible limitations of azithromycin include no information on efficacy in severe typhoid/inpatient therapy and marked variability in the doses used in various clinical trials. Another issue is duration of therapy. If defervescence occurs by day 6, can therapy be stopped by day 7? The proponents of azithromycin believe that because of high tissue penetration, stopping azithromycin will still ensure adequate intracellular levels for a long time; many clinicians would however be uncomfortable stopping the drug immediately after defervescence. The other issue with use of azithromycin is prolongation of the QT interval and cardiac arrhythmia.

Beta-lactam/Beta-lactamase Inhibitor Combinations and Carbapenems

Beta lactam/beta-lactamase inhibitor combinations including cefoperazone sulbactam/ piperacillin tazobactam are indicated for ceftriaxone-resistant enteric fever in sick patients. The maximum doses should be used initially and then therapy switched to oral options including azithromycin/cotrimoxazole. The role of indigenous combinations including ceftriaxone sulbactam/ceftriaxone tazobactam is uncertain in this setting due to absence of susceptibility breakpoints and efficacy data. In seriously sick patients with ceftriaxone-resistant enteric fever, carbapenems including meropenem/imipenem may be needed.

However, these drugs should be kept reserve for culture confirmed ceftriaxone-resistant cases. They should not be used routinely for escalation of therapy in case of nonresponse to ceftriaxone (discussed later).

CHOICE OF EMPIRICAL THERAPY (TABLE 1)

This is the situation where enteric is clinically suspected but where cultures have not been sent, or results are as yet not available or when cultures are negative. Choice of empirical therapy is guided by various factors including severity of the illness, inpatient/outpatient therapy, presence of complications, and local sensitivity patterns of *S.typhi/paratyphi*. At present oral cefixime is the preferred drug for empirical therapy in outpatients. The alternative option is azithromycin. Advantages of azithromycin include shorter therapy leading to better compliance and reduce relapses. However, it may be better to keep it as a reserve drug in case ceftriaxone resistance becomes widespread. For empirical therapy in severe illness/presence of complications/ inpatient treatment the drug of first choice is ceftriaxone. In patients with history of severe penicillin/cephalosporin allergy aztreonam may be used.

ROLE OF STEROIDS IN ENTERIC FEVER

Trials done around three decades ago advocated the use of high-dose dexamethasone in an initial dose of 3 mg/kg and then 1 mg/kg 6 hourly for 48 hours for patients with myocarditis, encephalopathy or shock. However, there is no recent data to support the use of such high-dose steroids in enteric fever. Use of steroids to hasten defervescence should also be avoided since it produces a false sense of security and can increase relapse rates.

TABLE 1: Treatment of enteric fever.

Type of treatments	*First line*	*Second line*
Outpatient treatment	Cefixime @ 20 mg/kg/day for 14 days (max 1200 mg)	Azithromycin 10–20 mg/kg/day for 7–10 days (max 1,000 mg) Cotrimoxazole 10 mg/kg/day of TMP for 14 days (max 640 mg of TMP)
Inpatient treatment	Ceftriaxone @ 100 mg/kg/day (max 4,000 mg)	Aztreonam 100 mg/kg/ day for 14 days (max 6 g) IV cotrimoxazole @ 10 mg/kg/day of TMP for 14 days (max 640 mg of TMP) IV azithromycin 10–20 mg/kg/day (max 1,000 mg) IV ampicillin 100 mg/kg/day (6,000 mg)

MODIFICATION OF THERAPY

If cultures are positive then therapy should be modified as per culture sensitivity if indicated. Parenteral treatment should be continued till defervescence has occurred, oral intake has improved and complications resolved. Thereafter therapy can be switched to oral to complete the requisite duration of therapy (14 days with beta-lactams/7–10 days with azithromycin).

NONRESPONSE TO THERAPY

The usual time to defervescence in enteric fever is around 5–7 days. Nonresponse in patients with suspected/confirmed enteric is a common clinical problem. Here assessment of response is extremely important. In patients, where the diagnosis of enteric fever is not culture confirmed a thorough search for an alternative diagnosis should be made. If the diagnosis is culture confirmed and the strain is susceptible to the antibiotic being administered causes of nonresponse include:

- *Delayed response*: Here the fever still continues though is less intense than before. Toxicity is less and oral intake has improved. These patients can be managed by continuing the same treatment.
- *Therapeutic failure*: Here there is failure despite in vitro susceptibility to the drug. Defined as persistent fever even 7 days after initiating therapy. Occurs in 5–10% of cases and can be due to poor intracellular penetration of the drug (*Salmonella* is an intracellular pathogen). This should be managed by switching to a drug from a different class, e.g. switching from ceftriaxone/cefixime to azithromycin/cotrimoxazole.
- *Development of complications*: This may include hepatic/splenic abscesses or osteomyelitis. Careful imaging is needed. These patients need prolonged therapy with antibiotics.
- *Drug fever*: Presents as recurrence of fever after an initial response. There may be eosinophilia. The patient is nontoxic. It is a diagnosis of exclusion.
- *Thrombophlebitis*: A common cause of persistent fever in hospitalized patients and those who are switched to outpatient parenteral therapy (OPAT).
- *Coinfections*: This is rare but possible.
- *Hemophagocytic syndrome*: This should be suspected if there is persistent fever with drop in hemoglobin (Hb)/white blood cell (WBC)/platelet count with hepatitis and splenomegaly. Confirmation is by estimation of serum ferritin, fasting triglycerides, and bone marrow examination. Many a time the hemophagocytic lymphohistiocytosis (HLH) resolves with antimicrobial therapy and may not need immunosuppression.

COMBINATION THERAPY

Increasing resistance and prolonged time to defervescence is prompting several clinicians to use combination therapy for enteric fever in hope of bringing about early defervescence and possibly preventing relapses. The most common combination used in clinical practice is cefixime/ceftriaxone with azithromycin. Cefixime and ofloxacin is also used but is actually not combination therapy since ofloxacin has no activity in the current era of quinolone resistance.

Some retrospective data showed no benefit of combination therapy over monotherapy. However, there is a recent trial conducted in adults in Nepal with culture confirmed typhoid fever who were randomized into four groups: Cefixime monotherapy (400 mg); ceftriaxone monotherapy (2,000 mg); cefixime and azithromycin (400 + 500 mg), and ceftriaxone and azithromycin (2 g + 500 mg) for 7 days. The logic of using this combination was using the beta-lactam for extracellular clearance and the macrolide for intracellular clearance. The results indicated shorter fever clearance time in the combination group (88 hours) as against 95 hours in the monotherapy group. The microbiologic clearance on day 3 of therapy was faster with the combination group (96%) as against 83% in the monotherapy group. However, whether using two drugs to reduce the duration of fever by 7 hours is justified remains to be seen. Azithromycin is an important drug if ceftriaxone resistance spreads and thus should not be used indiscriminately. Hence, more data is needed especially on impact of combination therapy on drug resistance and relapses before it can be routinely recommended.

THERAPY OF RELAPSES

The relapse rate varies with the type of drug and is most common with beta-lactams (ceftriaxone, cefixime) especially if shorter duration of therapy or inadequate doses are used. Relapses are however generally milder and respond well and quickly to the same drug as used for primary therapy. Hence, broadly speaking relapses may be satisfactorily treated with the same drug as used for primary therapy but in right doses and for the right duration. However, if the isolate is nalidixic acid sensitive and quinolones were not used for primary therapy, they should be used for treatment of the relapse. Azithromycin may also be a good therapeutic option for relapse treatment.

CONCLUSION

Enteric fever is a common clinical problem in India with evolving resistance. The emphasis should be on establishing a microbiologic diagnosis by sending blood cultures. The usual choice of drugs includes cefixime/ceftriaxone/azithromycin. Appropriate doses for the right duration should be used. Routine use of combination therapy should be avoided.

RECOMMENDED READING

1. Bhutta ZA, Khan IA, Molla AM. Therapy of multidrug-resistant typhoid fever with oral cefixime vs. intravenous ceftriaxone. Pediatr Infect Dis J. 1994;13:990-4.
2. Bhutta ZA, Khan IA, Shadmani M. Failure of short-course ceftriaxone chemotherapy for multidrug-resistant typhoid fever in children: a randomized controlled trial in Pakistan. Antimicrob Agents Chemother. 2000;44:450-2.
3. Chinh NT, Parry CM, Ly NT, et al. A randomized controlled comparison of azithromycin and ofloxacin for treatment of multidrug-resistant or nalidixic acid-resistant enteric fever. Antimicrob Agents Chemother. 2000;44:1855-9.
4. Frenck RW Jr, Mansour A, Nakhla I, et al. Short-course azithromycin for the treatment of uncomplicated typhoid fever in children and adolescents. Clin Infect Dis. 2004;38:951-7.
5. Frenck RW Jr, Nakhla I, Sultan Y, et al. Azithromycin versus ceftriaxone for the treatment of uncomplicated typhoid fever in children. Clin Infect Dis. 2000;31:1134-8.
6. Feder HM Jr, Osier C, Maderazo EG. Chloramphenicol: A review of its use in clinical practice. Rev Infect Dis. 1981;3:479-91.
7. Girgis NI, Sultan Y, Hammad O, et al. Comparison of the efficacy, safety and cost of cefixime, ceftriaxone and aztreonam in the treatment of multidrug-resistant Salmonella typhi septicemia in children. Pediatr Infect Dis J. 1995;14:603-5.

8. Hoffman SL, Punjabi NH, Kumala S, et al. Reduction of mortality in chloramphenicol-treated severe typhoid fever by high-dose dexamethasone. N Engl J Med. 1984;310(2):82-8.
9. Jog S, Soman R, Singhal T, et al. Enteric fever in Mumbai–clinical profile, sensitivity patterns and response to antimicrobials. J Assoc Physicians India. 2008;56:237-40.
10. John J, Van Aart CJ, Grassly NC. The burden of typhoid and paratyphoid in India: systematic review and meta-analysis. PLoS Negl Trop Dis. 2016;10:e0004616.
11. Klemm EZ, Shakoor S, Page AJ, et al. Emergence of extensively drug-resistant *Salmonella enteric* serovar typhi clone harboring a promiscuous plasmid encoding resistance fluroquinolones and third generation cephalosporins. MBio. 2018;9(1):1-10.
12. Kundu R, Ganguly N, Ghosh TK, et al. IAP Task Force Report: Management of enteric fever in children. Indian Pediatr. 2006;43:884-7.
13. Parry CM, Hien TT, Dougan G, et al. Typhoid fever. N Eng J Med. 2002;347:1770-82.
14. Parry CM. The treatment of multidrug-resistant and nalidixic acid-resistant typhoid fever in Viet Nam. Trans R Soc Trop Med Hyg. 2004;98:413-22.
15. Pokharel BM, Koirala J, Dahal RK, et al. Multidrug-resistant and extended-spectrum beta-lactamase (ESBL)–producing Salmonella enterica (serotypes typhi and paratyphi A) from blood isolates in Nepal: surveillance of resistance and a search for newer alternatives. Int J Infect Dis. 2006;10:434-8.
16. Rodrigues C, Shenai S, Mehta A. Enteric fever in Mumbai, India: The good news and the bad news. Clin Infect Dis. 2003;36:535.
17. Saha SK, Talukder SY, Islam M, et al. A highly ceftriaxone-resistant Salmonella typhi in Bangladesh. Pediatr Infect Dis J. 1999;18:387.
18. Sekar U, Srikanth P, Kindo AJ, et al. Increase in minimum inhibitory concentration to quinolones and ceftriaxone in salmonellae causing enteric fever. J Commun Dis. 2003;35:162-9.
19. Soe GB, Overturf GD. Treatment of typhoid fever and other systemic salmonelloses with cefotaxime, ceftriaxone, cefoperazone, and other newer cephalosporins. Rev Infect Dis. 1987;9:719-36.
20. Zmora N, Shrestha S, Neuberger A, et al. Open label comparative trial of mono versus dual antibiotic therapy for typhoid fever in adults. PLoS Negl Trop Dis. 2018;12(4):e0006380.

Antimicrobial Therapy in Urinary Tract Infections

23
Chapter

Pankaj Deshpande

INTRODUCTION

Urinary tract infections (UTIs) are one of the common infections seen in childhood. While various studies will show different numbers, the general figure of 6 to 8% of children having UTI in childhood is agreed upon. In a 2008 systematic review, approximately 7% of children 2–24 months of age presenting with fever without a source and 8% of children 2–19 years of age presenting with possible urinary symptoms were diagnosed with a UTI. Repeated episodes of pyelonephritis (upper UTI) are very likely to cause parenchymal damage to the renal tissue and hence cause long-term consequences such as renal dysfunction and hypertension.

Upper UTI indicates pyelonephritis (infection affecting the renal parenchyma) while lower UTI is the term for cystitis (infection limited to the bladder). While the symptoms may make it a bit easier to differentiate in older children and adolescents with high fever, vomiting and loin pain suggesting pyelonephritis, it is clinically virtually impossible to differentiate between upper and lower UTI in infants and younger children. Hence, it is prudent to consider most UTIs in infants and younger children as upper UTIs.

ETIOLOGY

Urinary tract infections in children are mostly ascending infections. Gram-negative organisms are the common causative organisms. Most UTIs are caused by *E. coli*, followed by *Proteus*, *Klebsiella*, and *Pseudomonas*. Gram-positive organisms isolated on culture, especially in boys should make one wonder about obstructive pathology in the urinary tract. *Staphylococcus* may be isolated. *Candida* may also be seen in immunocompromised hosts or babies who have been in hospital and on multiple antibiotics for a long time. Here it may be a colonizer and not a true pathogen. Viral infections of the urinary bladder (viral cystitis) can also occur and the most well-known one is viral hemorrhagic cystitis caused by enteroviruses or adenovirus.

With the rampant use of antibiotics, UTIs by resistant organisms are on the rise and extended beta lactamase producing (ESBL) bacterial infections are difficult to treat as there is a limited stock of oral antibiotics that can be used. A recent study from the Institute of Child Health, Chennai found 40% of organisms causing community-acquired UTI as being ESBL producers. Further, there were no identifiable risk factors that were significantly associated with ESBL production.

BASICS OF THERAPY

Once the diagnosis of UTI is suspected with suggestive symptoms and pyuria either on microscopy or dipstix, *urine culture sample should be given*. After the urine culture sample is given, an appropriate antibiotic can be started. There is no point in doing a urine culture after starting antibiotics. It is surprising to note positive growth in cultures after antibiotics are started making one wonder about contamination. Also, a negative culture on antibiotics will not allow one to make the diagnosis of UTI with certainty and definitely not rule it out. Sending urine cultures is particularly important in today's era of multidrug resistant infections.

ROUTE OF ADMINISTRATION

In most children, therapy can be started with an oral antibiotic. If the child looks sick or toxic, has persistent vomiting (unable to take medications), or is suspected to have a drug resistant UTI or if no response is seen after 48 to 72 hours of oral antibiotics, the child will require admission for intravenous antibiotics (IV antibiotics). In neonates and very young infants (less than 3 months age), IV antibiotics should be the preferred mode of administration as these babies can become septic fairly quickly.

EMPIRIC ANTIBIOTIC (TABLE 1)

The choice of antibiotic should be based on likely susceptibility and previous antibiotic use. The concentration of the antibiotic in the urine is also a very important factor influencing antibiotic use. Certain antibiotics including macrolides, tetracyclines, chloramphenicol, and polymyxin B do not attain any appreciable concentration in the urine.

Choice of Oral Antibiotic

The usual choices include co-amoxiclav, cephalexin, and cefixime. Quinolones are not the preferred antibiotic for empiric therapy in infants and young children due to high prevalence of resistance and also that, they are not legally approved by Drug Controller General of India (DCGI). Surprisingly susceptibility to co-trimoxazole in the current era of ESBL producers is even better than the beta lactams.

TABLE 1: Choice of empiric antibiotics for urinary tract infection.

Setting	*Choice*
Outpatient therapy	Co-amoxiclav, cephalexin, cefixime
For inpatient therapy, but low likelihood of drug resistant pathogens	Cefotaxime/Ceftriaxone/IV Co-amoxiclav
For inpatient therapy High-risk of resistant pathogens, very sick patient or nonresponse to first line	Beta-lactam beta-lactamase inhibitor combinations (cefoperazone sulbactam/ piperacillin tazobactam) *or* Carbapenems (ertapenem/imipenem/meropenem)

Choice of Intravenous Antibiotics

The first line here is third-generation cephalosporins including ceftriaxone/cefotaxime/co-amoxiclav. However in neonates/infants and children where there is history of previous antibiotic use or known infection/colonization with ESBL-producing Gram-negative bacteria or there is nonresponse to the first-line antibiotics, beta-lactam beta-lactamase inhibitor (BL-BLI) combinations including piperacillin tazobactam/cefoperazone sulbactam may be used. Rarely carbapenems may be indicated in septic shock. The use of aminoglycosides for empiric therapy should be generally avoided due to their nephrotoxicity.

MODIFICATION OF THERAPY

The child should be monitored for clinical response such as resolution of fever, toxicity, and dysuria. The urine culture and sensitivity report become available by 72 hours after giving the sample. If de-escalation can be practiced it should be done; e.g. changing from amoxiclav/cefixime to ampicillin if the report so indicates (remember *Klebsiella* is inherently resistant to ampicillin). If the child has shown a clinical response, then there is no need to escalate antibiotics even if there is *in vitro* resistance to the antibiotic being administered. This is because most antibiotics will achieve a very high concentration in the urine so that the organisms are killed despite *in vitro* resistance (see chapter 2). So, completing the course with the same antibiotic is logical. These patients should however be carefully monitored for a relapse or late treatment failure.

If there has been no clinical response by 72 hours, then the child should be reassessed to make sure that the diagnosis of UTI is right. One should also look for other causes preventing response. These include obstructive causes in the urinary tract, anomalies of the urinary tract, renal abscesses, etc. The urine culture report should also be carefully interpreted for resistance to the currently administered antibiotics. Such patients will need admission (if not already admitted) and change in antimicrobial therapy along with other adjunct measures.

Once the child is afebrile and tolerating oral food well, IV antibiotics can be changed to oral antibiotics to complete the course. This should be done on the basis of susceptibility. The problem is oral switchover for infections with ESBL pathogens which have been treated with BL-BLI combinations. If the isolate is susceptible to co-trimoxazole/quinolones, the same can be used. Nitrofurantoin cannot be used for switchover even if it is susceptible since it does not achieve adequate tissue levels. An option is to use once daily aminoglycosides for the required duration of antibiotics. However, these are associated with nephrotoxicity and ototoxicity and should be avoided in patients with pre-existent renal dysfunction. If used, the serum creatinine should be carefully monitored. If aminoglycosides cannot be used then the BL-BLI combinations (cefoperazone sulbactam) or ertapenem can be continued on an OPD basis.

DURATION OF THERAPY

The duration of therapy for upper UTI/pyelonephritis is 10–14 days. This includes IV and oral antibiotics. Patients with renal abscesses will need 3–4 weeks of treatment. In clear cases of cystitis in older children and adolescents even 3–5 days of therapy is adequate.

Once clinical response is seen there is no need to repeat the urine examination. If at all it is done, a microscopy will help to demonstrate reduction in the pyuria. There is no need to chase away every last pus cell!! Also, there is absolutely no need to repeat a urine culture at the end of therapy. There are so many patients who continue to receive multiple prolonged courses of antibiotics chasing the organisms in the repeat urine culture when the child is completely asymptomatic. These are contaminated samples and should never be treated. It is harmful in the long run as we are exposing these antibiotics to organisms for prolonged periods inviting resistance.

OTHER ASPECTS OF THERAPY

There are other important aspects to address regarding management of UTI apart from antimicrobial therapy. There are very good defense mechanisms that prevent us all getting urine infections. Unless there is a disturbance in these local factors, UTI is unlikely. These local factors are bowel bladder disturbances.

One of the common causes of UTIs is constipation. It has been shown that addressing this problem reduces the risk of UTIs. Temporary relief of constipation is pointless. It usually needs prolonged therapy to clear out the large intestine and rectum and establish a pattern for the child. This will include modification of the diet.

The bladder washes out all organisms that ascend the urethra. Urine staying in the bladder for more than 4 hours will allow the organisms to settle and multiply. The inner lining/mucosa of the bladder has protective properties and repeated voiding helps to prevent UTIs. Children should be encouraged to void at least 6 to 8 times a day. Constipation causes infrequent voiding thereby worsening the cycle.

Infrequent voiding is usually a consequence of poor fluid intake. This compounds the problem of constipation and bladder voiding. Thus, it is easy to see how simple factors like these will predispose to UTIs. One of the other important aspects to remember is that children are forever in a hurry as they do not want to miss out on things happening around them. Hence the tendency is to leave voiding till the last minute and then rush in and out of the toilet. If the post void residue of a child more than 3 years is greater than 20 mL, the risk of UTIs is higher. A child has to be encouraged to void appropriately and if greater than 6 years should be taught double voiding to empty the bladder. Attention to simple matters like this prevents most UTIs and recurrence of UTIs.

EVALUATION OF A CHILD WITH A UTI

Investigations recommended for a child with first UTI are shown in Table 2. Patients with recurrent UTI (more than 2 UTI in 6 months) will need all investigations including ultrasound (US) scan, dimercaptosuccinic acid (DMSA), and possibly a micturating cystourethrogram (MCUG) as well.

RECURRENT UTI

Recurrence of UTI is said to be present if UTI occurs after finishing therapy. A repeat UTI occurs in about one-third to half of the children who have suffered a UTI. Causes include structural

TABLE 2: Investigations recommended for a child with first urinary tract infection.

Age	*Investigations recommended*
Less than 1 year	US scan, DMSA and MCUG
1–6 years	US scan, DMSA
More than 6 years	US scan

(DMSA: dimercaptosuccinic acid; MCUG: micturating cystourethrogram; US: ultrasound)

abnormalities of the urinary tract/bladder bowel dysfunction, constipation, etc. Hence these children need evaluation as mentioned above and antibiotic prophylaxis if indicated. Attention to constipation and voiding issues is also important as discussed earlier. In boys, circumcision reduces the recurrence of UTIs remarkably. Circumcision reduced the risk of recurrence of UTIs by 90% or so. And the risk of developing the first UTI is also much lower in circumcised boys as compared to uncircumcised boys. Yet there are confounding factors and it is not recommended to subject every boy to a circumcision. After addressing the bowel bladder factors mentioned above, one can use a mild steroid cream for 2 weeks to help relieve physiologic phimosis, if present and be vigilant for recurrence of UTIs. If there are no further UTIs, no intervention is required. Despite these measures, if there are frequent UTIs (2 in 6 months) then circumcision would be helpful.

RESISTANT UTI

In recent times, it is often noted that UTIs occur with organisms that seem to be resistant to most antibiotics. This may create a dilemma in the clinics. One should first assess whether it is a UTI. Most contaminant organisms seem to show such pattern. If the child has responded clinically to the oral/IV antibiotic prescribed (in terms of absence of fever and urinary symptoms), there is no need to go hunting for the "best" antibiotic and the same antibiotic should be continued to *finish* the course. As explained earlier this may occur because the urinary concentration of the antibiotic is much higher.

If it is indeed a true resistant UTI with clinical nonresponse, high-end antibiotics including BL-BLI combinations and carbapenems may be needed. Nosocomial UTIs followed placement of indwelling catheter can be highly resistant including to carbapenems. These may need to be treated with reserve drugs such as colistin/fosfomycin. Catheter-associated UTI are discussed in greater detail in Chapter 30.

Resistance can be prevented by:

- Treating UTIs only when suspected and confirmed
- Completing the course of antibiotics
- Keeping prophylaxis duration short or not using it unless really indicated
- Not using prophylaxis for unindicated conditions like pelvi-ureteric junction obstruction.

PROPHYLAXIS

One of the ways of preventing UTIs relied mainly on using a small dose of an antibiotic to prevent growth of pathogenic organisms. However, recent literature has suggesting a large rethink in this field and there is good evidence to support change of practice.

The premise was that infants and children diagnosed with any grade of VUR (vesicoureteral reflux) were at increased risk for recurrent UTIs and therefore required antibiotic prophylaxis to prevent UTIs and long-term sequelae like hypertension and renal failure. There were very few studies to assess this and as the definitions of UTI were not stringent, the efficacy of prophylaxis was probably overestimated.

The American Academy of Pediatrics Subcommittee on Urinary Tract Infections had published guidelines in 2011. Their meta-analysis of six studies for children less than 24 months of age did not show a significant benefit of antibiotic prophylaxis, either in infants without VUR or in those with grades I-IV VUR. If one reviews the Cochrane meta-analysis of 12 studies or recent studies like the Randomised Intervention for Children with Vesicoureteral Reflux (RIVUR trial) along with older studies like Montini et al. or PRIVENT trial, it is generally noted that the results are varied as there was heterogeneity in the study design for all. There was a small benefit noted but it was noted that prophylactic antibiotics would have to be prescribed for long periods in many children (two years for nine children) to prevent recurrent UTIs in 1 child! More importantly, all trials found a similar low rate of worsening of renal scarring in both *cases and controls*. This would beg the question about how effective prophylaxis really is as there seems no evidence of it preventing renal scarring or long-term sequelae. So long-term prophylaxis given for years together in the past (up to 5 or 7 years) certainly is not advocated. Managing the simple factors like constipation seem far better in preventing UTIs. There are several other disadvantages of prophylactic antibiotics. Apart from the possibility of adverse effects, though the number is quite small, it increases the risks of allowing the bacteria to develop resistance to these antibiotics. Losing any further antibiotics because of resistance will be detrimental to treating UTIs when it actually matters. Also, the drudgery of taking antibiotics daily cannot be underestimated and even in the studies mentioned above, the non-compliance rate was more than 25%. Thus, outside of a study setting the compliance of taking daily prophylactic antibiotics can drop to as much as 64% as demonstrated so many years ago. So what good are these antibiotics if they are not taken anyway?

For our local Indian setting, prophylaxis can be offered to infants with VUR as the risk of UTIs is higher in that age group and investigations are not yet complete. However, beyond the first year, prophylaxis should not continue for more than 6 months after the last UTI. This includes children with high grade VUR. The idea is that local problems like bowel bladder dysfunction should be treated so that prophylaxis can be stopped in 6 months. Also, as the child gets older, diagnosing a UTI is that much easier and hence prophylaxis may not be needed (also see chapter 32).

An ideal agent for prophylaxis should have no adverse effects and not change the bowel and periurethral flora along with being cheap. The two agents widely recommended for prophylaxis include trimethoprim-sulfamethoxazole (Trimethoprim dose 2 mg/kg daily) or nitrofurantoin (1–2 mg/kg daily). They do not change the periurethral flora. However, the former carries the risk of severe adverse reaction like Steven–Johnson syndrome and the last is frankly unpalatable inducing vomiting in most children.

Cephalosporins (cephalexin) have also been used as a prophylactic agent (15 mg/kg daily) but these are broad-spectrum antibiotics and hence change the bowel and periurethral flora. Hence UTIs occurring on these agents tend to be with more pathogenic or resistant bacteria. However, they can be used in children where the other two agents cannot be used (e.g. in young infants).

Prophylactic agents are not required in children with pelvi-ureteric junction obstruction, posterior urethral valves patients a few months after surgery or neurogenic bladder patients on regular catheterization.

LONG-TERM OUTCOME

We started off by mentioning that treating UTIs are important because of long-term sequelae. However recent data suggests that recurrent UTIs occurring in children with normal kidneys do not seem to lead to long-term sequelae irrespective of whether they lead to minor scarring or not! Diverting our attention to only VUR and UTIs has allowed the real culprit to go undetected. Renal dysplasia, where the kidneys are not formed normally at birth is the condition that will lead to long-term grief for the kidneys. These children are not sick and are perfectly normal with a normal activity. Ultrasound of the kidneys may actually show normal kidneys with subtle changes like loss of corticomedullary differentiation. DMSA scan is more likely to show abnormalities with diffuse reduced uptake and unfortunately, they are likely to be reported as scarring in the kidneys. Irrespective of the presence of VUR or recurrent UTI, these children are more likely to drop their renal function as the body size grows and often around puberty, the phase of maximum growth, the kidney function will drop drastically. Chasing and fixing VUR will not change the outcome in these children. Simple tests will help evaluate whether the renal function is intact.

It is amazing to note that most children with UTIs have never had a serum creatinine checked though they may have had MCUG and other tests done. Regular monitoring of serum creatinine [and calculating estimated glomerular filtration rate (eGFR) for every child] to ensure normal renal function and looking for proteinuria by a urine protein creatinine ratio are simple measures to detect this condition. These tests have to be regularly done (once a year) along with the blood pressure. This will help to reduce the massive load of children who end up on dialysis as adults and not just using antibiotics and treating VUR. Let us all work toward this.

RECOMMENDED READING

1. Bader M, McCarthy L. What is the efficacy of circumcision in boys with complex urinary tract abnormalities? Pediatr Nephrol. 2013;28:2267-72.
2. Balasubramanian S, Kuppuswamy D, Padmanabhan S, et al. Extended-spectrum beta-lactamase-producing community-acquired urinary tract infections in children: Chart Review of Risk Factors. J Glob Infect Dis. 2018;10(4):222-5.
3. Craig JC, Williams GJ. Denominators do matter: It's a myth-urinary tract infection does not cause chronic kidney disease. Pediatrics. 2011;128(5):984-5.
4. Hari P, Bagga A. Antimicrobial prophylaxis for children with vesicoureteral reflux. N Engl J Med. 2014;371(11):1071-2.
5. Indian Society of Pediatric Nephrology. Revised Statement on Management of Urinary Tract Infections. Indian Pediatr. 2011;48:709-17.
6. Krzemien G, Szmigielska A, Artemuik I, et al. False positive urine cultures in children under two years of age-own research. Dev Period Med. 2014;18(2):203-8.
7. Paintsil E. Update on recent guidelines for the management of urinary tract infections in children: the shifting paradigm. Curr Opin Pediatr. 2013;25:88-94.
8. Robinson JL, Finlay JC, Lang ME, et al. Prophylactic antibiotics for children with recurrent urinary tract infections. Pediatr Child Health. 2015;20(1):45-7.
9. Shaikh N, Morone NE, Bost JE, et al. Prevalence of urinary tract infection in childhood: A meta-analysis. Pediatr Infect Dis J. 2008;27(4):302-8.
10. Silver SA, Baillie L, Simor AE. Positive urine cultures: A major cause of inappropriate antimicrobial use in hospitals? Can J Infect Dis Med Microbiol. 2009;20(4):107-11.
11. Smyth AR, Judd BA. Compliance with antibiotic prophylaxis in urinary tract infection. Arch Dis Child. 1993;68(2):235-6.
12. Subcommittee on Urinary Tract Infection, Steering Committee on Quality Improvement and Management, Roberts KB. Urinary tract infection: clinical practice guideline for diagnosis and management of the initial UTI in febrile infants and children 2 to 24 months. Pediatrics. 2011;128(3):595-610.
13. The Rivur Trial Investigators. Antimicrobial prophylaxis for children with vesicoureteral reflux. N Engl J Med. 2014;370(25):2367-76.

Antimicrobial Therapy in Skin and Soft Tissue Infections

24
Chapter

Dhanya Dharmapalan

INTRODUCTION

The skin forms a primary defensive barrier of the body that protects it from microbial invaders present in the environment. The skin has two primary layers--epidermis and dermis. The thin epidermis resists external chemical erosion and can regenerate easily while the thick dermis contains vascular structures, nerves, and adnexal structures like sweat glands, hair follicles, and sebaceous glands.

The entry of these microbes can occur in following ways:

- Through breaks in the skin as in wounds, intravenous sites, insect bites, and excoriated dermatitis.
- Through erosion of skin as in keratolytic actions of fungal dermatophytes or by production of exfoliative toxins by *Staphylococcus* from inside leading to localized bullous impetigo or widespread staphylococcal scalded syndrome in neonates.
- Through inability to defend locally as in those deficient in CD4 T-cell function, for example, opportunistic skin infections in acquired immunodeficiency syndrome patients.

BACTERIAL INFECTIONS

Epidermal Infections: Impetigo and Ecthyma

Impetigo is the most common bacterial infection and is caused by *Staphylococcus aureus* or *Streptococcus pyogenes*. Face and extremities are the commonly affected sites. The nonbullous impetigo/impetigo contagiosa lesions are initially maculopapular which rupture soon into erosions covered by the classical honey-colored crusts. Bullous impetigo is caused by exfoliative toxin of *Staphylococcus aureus* and is characterized by fragile bullae which rupture to ooze yellow fluid and form annular rims of scale with central erythema. It is mostly found on the trunk, axilla, and extremities, and in intertriginous areas. Both impetigo types heal within 2–3 weeks without scarring.

Ecthyma is an ulcerated form of bullous impetigo and is usually caused by *S. pyogenes*. It initially presents as a vesicle that develops into a shallow "punched out" ulcer with adherent brown-black crusts. The lower extremities are commonly affected. Unlike impetigo, it heals with scarring.

Management of Epidermal Infections

Topical antibiotics such as mupirocin/fusidic acid or retapamulin applied twice a day for 5 days are recommended for few lesions. Oral antibiotic therapy is recommended for multiple lesions, recurrent lesions, and for impetigo with large bullae. Options include cloxacillin or cephalexin or cefadroxil for duration of 7 days. Co-amoxiclav though effective is relatively broad-spectrum due to its effect on the gut Gram-negative and anaerobic flora and should be avoided. Clindamycin is a good choice for suspected community-associated methicillin-resistant *Staphylococcus aureus* (CA-MRSA) lesions. Cotrimoxazole may be used in suspected MRSA but is not useful for streptococcal infections.

Dermal Infections: Cellulitis and Necrotizing Fasciitis

Cellulitis presents as warm, red, and painful local part of skin due to inflammation of the connective tissue. It commonly occurs after a break in the skin and is predominantly caused by Gram-positive organisms like *Staphylococcus aureus* and *S. pyogenes*. It may be polymicrobial in immunosuppressed patients or in penetrating injuries. *H. influenzae* type B, *Pneumococcus*, and *Pseudomonas* are other causes in young children. Cellulitis frequently occurs on the head and neck in children, but is also found on the scalp, perianal areas, and sites of traumatic wounds, bruises, and bites. The condition may be associated with systemic signs like fever, regional lymphadenopathy, and lymphangitis. Management is discussed later.

Necrotizing fasciitis is classified into three types based on microbiological etiology:

Type 1 (polymicrobial) as seen in diabetic patients (Meleney's and Fournier's gangrene)

Type 2 monomicrobial mostly caused by *S. pyogenes, S. aureus, Clostridium perfringens,* Vibrio species and *Klebsiella*

Type 3 caused by fungal infections like zygomycetes in immunocompromised patients.

Children mostly have monomicrobial type of necrotizing fasciitis due to *S. pyogenes* following chicken pox.

The consistent early feature of necrotizing fascitis is pain disproportionate to the swelling or erythema. On palpation, the tenderness extends beyond the area of apparent involvement due to spread along the facial planes. Since the infection occurs in deep fascia, margins on involvement are not distinct. There may be associated hypotension, organ dysfunction, leukocytosis, hyponatremia, and hyperglycemia. Necrotizing fasciitis can be confused with cellulitis and certain scoring systems can be used for differentiation if in doubt. Necrotizing fasciitis unlike cellulitis is a surgical emergency and should be treated with urgent radical surgical debridement. Antibiotic management is discussed later.

Follicular Infections – Folliculitis, Furunculosis and Carbunculosis

Folliculitis is infection of hair follicle. Furuncles are deeper hair follicle associated infection extending into the subcutaneous tissue where a small abscess forms. *Carbuncles* involve several adjacent hair follicles, with extensive tissue inflammation and formation of a coalescent mass. The most common causative agent is *Staphylococcus aureus*. Multiple furuncules are often seen in immunocompromised children with functional neutrophil disorder such as hyperimmunoglobin E syndrome and Job syndrome. Carbuncles are common in obesity, diabetes mellitus, severe atopic dermatitis, impaired neutrophil function, and prolonged corticosteroid use.

Management of Dermal and Follicular Infections

The recent Infectious Diseases Society of America (IDSA) guidelines (2014) on skin and soft tissue infections classify treatment of purulent (carbuncle, folliculitis, and abscess) and nonpurulent infections (cellulitis, erysipelas, and necrotizing fasciitis) based on severity to guide clinical management. The likelihood of *S. aureus* and possibly CA-MRSA as a pathogen is higher in the purulent group while nonpurulent infections are primarily streptococcal. Mild infections are those without systemic signs, moderate those with systemic signs, and severe are those with failed incision and drainage plus oral antibiotics or those with severe systemic signs of infection such as temperature more than 38°C, tachycardia, tachypnea or abnormal white blood cell count (<12,000 or <400 cells/μL), or immunocompromised patients.

For purulent infections, culture sensitivity is strongly recommended for moderate and severe cases. Mild infections require incision and drainage alone, moderate require addition of an oral antibiotic cephalexin/cloxacillin. In case the prevalence of MRSA is high, an agent which covers CA-MRSA like doxycycline/clindamycin or cotrimoxazole is recommended instead of the beta lactams. However, in clinical practice/real world scenario where the exact burden/likelihood of CA-MRSA is often unknown, therapy with beta lactams can be started and changed depending on the response or results of culture sensitivity. In severe cases, parenteral therapy with cloxacillin/cefazolin is recommended. Addition of anti-MRSA drug such as vancomycin, teicoplanin, linezolid upfront should also be considered in toxic patients. Daptomycin which covers methicillin susceptible *Staphylococcus aureus* (MSSA) and MRSA equally well can be used for monotherapy. The other recommended drugs effective for monotherapy are ceftaroline/delafloxacin and telavancin which are presently not available in India. Therapy should be modified once culture results are available.

For nonpurulent infections (cellulitis and necrotizing fasciitis), blood cultures or cultures of aspirate/swab/biopsy of cellulitis should be sent in severe infections or underlying immunocompromised conditions. Oral antibiotics suggested for mild infections are cephalexin, cloxacillin, and clindamycin for a duration of at least 5 days. For moderate infections, intravenous ceftriaxone or clindamycin or cefazolin is recommended. For severe infections including necrotizing fasciitis, urgent surgical reference with surgical debridement and empirical treatment with a beta lactam [ceftriaxone, carbapenem, β-lactam-β-lactamase inhibitor (BL-BLI) combination depending on the setting) with clindamycin (for its toxin inhibition effect/anaerobic activity), and an anti-MRSA drug (vancomycin/teicoplanin) should be given for a broad coverage. One can also replace the clindamycin and vancomycin/teicoplanin combination with linezolid that has both anti-MRSA and antitoxin activity. Once the tissue cultures are available, therapy should be modified. Definitive treatment for *S. pyogenes* or *Clostridium* infections is combination of penicillin/ceftriaxone and clindamycin.

FUNGAL INFECTIONS

Tinea Infections

The disease resulting from dermatophytic infection is called tinea. Tinea infections are further classified based on the body part affected, for example: Tinea capitis is dermatophyte infection of the head, tinea pedis of the foot, tinea unguium of nails, tinea cruris of genitals, and tinea corporis of the trunk. Tinea capitis can manifest as scaly patches with alopecia with black dots at follicular orifices that represent hairs breaking at the scalp, an inflamed boggy mass called kerion and cup-shaped crusts (scutula) grouped together to appear like piece of honeycomb called favus. Oral antifungals are the mainstay for symptomatic tinea capitis. Tinea unguium due to *T. rubrum* causes nail bed infection leading to nail pitting and onycholysis. Tinea pedis manifests with cracking and fissuring in the webbing between the toes. Tinea corporis presents as pruritic annular red and scaly patches on the trunk.

Management of Tinea Infections

Due to excessive use of over the counter antifungal creams there are reports of increasing resistance in tinea from India, compromising treatment options.

Topical antifungals are indicated for treatment of limited disease of body and genital area. Topical antifungals commonly used are clotrimazole 1%, miconazole 1% (available as cream or lotion) twice daily application for 4–6 weeks, and terbinafine available as powder, cream twice daily for 2 weeks (4 weeks in tinea pedis). Newer antifungals are luliconazole, available as 1% cream formulation, approved for once daily application for 1–2 weeks for dermatophytic infections. It has a good safety profile and works for resistant tinea infections. Microemulsion preparations of amphotericin B, terbinafine, and griseofulvin have been reported to have excellent clinical results due to their better bioavailability. However, there are concerns if topical amphotericin can promote antibiotic resistance considering its crucial use in invasive fungal infections.

Systemic antifungals are indicated in case of extensive involvement and patients who fail topical therapy. Tinea capitis and tinea unguium are unlikely to resolve without oral antifungals.

Oral antifungals commonly used are terbinafine, griseofulvin and fluconazole, and itraconazole. Griseofulvin is absorbed better after a fatty meal and is given in the dose of 10–20 mg/kg (max. dose 500 mg per day). The dose of fluconazole is 6 mg/kg daily (max. 400 mg) or 8 mg/kg weekly (150–300 mg in adults). The dose of terbinafine is 62.5 mg daily for 10–20 kg, 125 mg daily for 20–40 kg, and 250 mg daily for those above 40 kg and in adults. Itraconazole is dosed at 2.5–5 mg/kg/day (200 mg once or twice daily). Studies show higher cure and lower relapse rates with terbinafine as compared to the azoles. In refractory cases combination therapy with terbinafine and itraconazole has also been used.

The dose and duration depend on the site of infection and the antifungal used. For tinea corporis, tinea pedis and tinea cruris treatment with terbinafine is indicated for 2 weeks, with weekly fluconazole for 4 weeks and daily griseofulvin for 4–8 weeks. For tinea capitis, treatment with terbinafine is for 2–4 weeks, itraconazole for 4 weeks, daily fluconazole for 3–6 weeks, weekly fluconazole for 8–12 weeks and daily griseofulvin for 6–8 weeks. For finger nail infection, duration is 6 weeks and for toe nails it is 12 weeks. If weekly fluconazole is used then treatment needs to be given for 3–6 months for finger nail infection and 6–12 months for toe nail infections with 50% cure rate.

It is also important to advise against sharing of towels and clothings, and in case of tinea capitis, avoid sharing of hair care tools.

Candida Dermatitis

It occurs mostly in moist and occluded sites such as axilla and groins. Diaper dermatitis is commonly caused by candida. It is characterized by confluent erythematous rash with satellite lesions.

Management of Candida Dermatitis

The most commonly used topical antifungal medications for candida dermatitis are nystatin, miconazole, clotrimazole, ketoconazole for at least 2 weeks. Low-potency topical corticosteroids may be used in conjunction to treat associated pruritus, pain, and burning. In severe cases with maceration oral antifungals like fluconazole 6 mg/kg once, then 3 mg/kg per day (max. 100 mg/day) can be used for 2–6 weeks or until signs and symptoms have resolved.

PARASITIC INFECTIONS

Scabies

Scabies is caused by the mite *Sarcoptes scabei*. The clinical manifestation of classical scabies is itching and erythematous papules occur due to hypersensitivity reaction to the mites and their products such as eggs, saliva, and feces. The itching tends to worsen at night. Burrows are usually located between the fingers, in the flexure of the wrist, elbows or armpits, or on the genitals. In infants burrow may be also found on head and neck. Nodular scabies is a less common manifestation characterized by erythematous, extremely pruritic, papules 5 or 6 mm in diameter. Crusted scabies or Norwegian scabies is a rare condition caused by the host response to control the mite, resulting in hyperinfestation with millions of mites, severe inflammation, and hyperkeratotic reaction. It is seen more in immunocompromised conditions.

Management of Scabies

Five percent topical permethrin is applied to the whole body including webs and fingers from neck to toes, usually for hours, often overnight and then washed off. For infants the lotion should be applied to the face as well. A repeat application is recommended after 1 week. It is better to avoid use of permethrin in less than 3 months of age.

Benzyl benzoate 10% may be applied once daily at night on 2 consecutive days, with a repeat treatment cycle after 7 days. Topical sulphur (6–33%) precipitated in petroleum jelly is recommended in neonates and young infants and is applied overnight for three consecutive days.

Ivermectin is useful in community outbreaks of scabies, crusted scabies and in recurrent infections. It is used in 200 µg/kg single dose followed by a repeat dose after 1–2 weeks. It should be avoided in children less than 15 kg. Crusted scabies should be treated with combination of oral ivermectin and topical permethrin.

Nodules can be treated with once- to twice-daily application of a potent topical steroid for 2–3 weeks or intralesional injection of a corticosteroid such as triamcinolone acetonide (5–10 mg/mL). Secondary bacterial infections need to be treated with topical or oral antibiotics, depending on severity. Itching may need antihistaminics.

Pediculosis Capitis

It is the most common ectoparasitic infection causing infestation of the hair and scalp by Pediculus humanus capitis (the head louse). It manifests as intense pruritus caused due to saliva injection by lice during feeding. Lice can be visualized by inspection of scalp or combing with fine-toothed comb.

Management of Pediculosis Capitis

Wet combing: Mechanical removal of lice by wet combing is an alternative treatment. This however requires multiple sessions of hair combing for several weeks.

Permethrin cream (1%) is applied to wet hair that is first shampooed with a nonconditioning shampoo and then towel dried. It is left on for 10 minutes and then rinsed off. Permethrin leaves a residue on the hair to kill nymphs emerging from 20% to 30% of the eggs not killed with the first application. A reapplication is suggested after 10 days.

Malathion lotion (0.5%) is applied to dry hair, left to air dry, then washed off after 8–12 hours, with instructions not to use any heat source for drying. It should be reapplied in 7–9 days if live lice are still seen. Safety is not established in young children less than 6 years and is contraindicated in less than 2 years.

There is increasing reports of drug resistance to both permethrin and malathion lotion. Lack of adherence or reinfestation should be considered before concluding on treatment failure. Alternative topical therapy or single dose ivermectin 200 μg/kg repeated in 2 weeks can be tried in treatment failures.

RECOMMENDED READING

1. Banerji A. Scabies. Paediatr Child Health. 2015;20(7):395-8.
2. Brodell LA, Rosenthal KS. Skin structure and function: The body's primary defense against infection. Infect Dis Clin Pract. 2008;16(2):113-7.
3. Gilbert DN. Sanford Guide for Antimicrobial Therapy 2018. Sperryville, VA: Antimicrobial Therapy, Inc.; 2018.
4. Pai V, Ganavalli A, Kikkeri NN. Antifungal resistance in dermatology. Indian J Dermatol. 2018;63(5): 361-8.
5. Sahoo AK, Mahajan R. Management of tinea corporis, tinea cruris, and tinea pedis: A comprehensive review. Indian Dermatol Online J. 2016;7(2):77-86.
6. Stevens DL, Bisno AL, Chambers HF, et al. Infectious Diseases Society of America: Practice guidelines for the diagnosis and management of skin and soft tissue infections: 2014 update by the Infectious Diseases Society of America. Clin Infect Dis. 2014;59(2):e10-52.
7. Verma P, Namdeo C. Treatment of pediculosis capitis. Indian J Dermatol. 2015;60(3):238-47.
8. White TC, Findley K, Dawson Jr TL, et al. Fungi on the skin: Dermatophytes and malassezia. Cold Spring Harb Perspect Med. 2014;4:a019802.
9. Zundel S, Lemaréchal A, Kaiser P, et al. Diagnosis and treatment of pediatric necrotizing fasciitis: A systematic review of the literature. Eur J Pediatr Surg. 2017;27(2):127-37.

Antimicrobial Therapy in Skeletal Infections

25
Chapter

Winsley Rose

INTRODUCTION

Bone and joint infections (osteomyelitis and septic arthritis) cause significant morbidity in infants and young children though there has been substantial reduction in mortality with advances in pharmacological therapy. Since the pathogenesis, microbiology, and treatment approaches are by and large similar for both osteomyelitis and septic arthritis; and concurrent osteomyelitis and septic arthritis are frequent in children, they are considered together in this chapter. Tuberculous osteomyelitis, an important cause of chronic osteomyelitis, is dealt with elsewhere in this book.

EPIDEMIOLOGY

Septic arthritis and osteomyelitis are more common in the younger age group especially in children less than 5 years of age. Boys are more likely to be affected than girls. Lower limb osteomyelitis involving the tibia or femur accounts for over 50% of osteomyelitis although any bone may be involved. Most children with acute bone and joint infections do not have underlying predisposing factors. However, some subgroups of children are at an increased risk: immunocompromised children (diabetes, malignancy, HIV, steroid use, malnourished), sickle cell disease, premature infants and those chronic illnesses requiring frequent venesection. Recent systemic infection (37%) and blunt trauma (29%) have been reported frequently in children with osteomyelitis.

MICROBIOLOGY

Staphylococcus aureus is the most common cause of osteomyelitis. Methicillin-resistant *S. aureus* (MRSA) including community-acquired MRSA is on the rise and is of considerable concern. Association of the Panton–Valentine leukocidin (PVL) gene with MRSA may explain the high virulence of MRSA.

However, in children less than 4 years of age, osteomyelitis is also caused by streptococci (*Streptococcus pneumoniae, Streptococcus pyogenes, Streptococcus agalactiae* (Group B *Streptococcus*) and Gram-negative organisms (*Kingella kingae, Haemophilus influenzae*). Implementation of the *Haemophilus influenzae* type b (Hib) vaccine in the national immunization programs has resulted in dramatic decline in infections due to this organism in young children. *Kingella kingae* is another important Gram-negative organism causing skeletal infections which is difficult to grow on culture. Molecular detection methods may have to be used in culture negative patients to make a microbiological diagnosis of *Kingella kingae*.

The etiology in neonates is even more diverse and reflects the organisms causing neonatal sepsis. Causes include group B *Streptococcus*, resistant Gram-negative bacteria, coagulase-negative staphylococci, *S. sureus* and *Candida*. *Salmonella* is an important cause of osteomyelitis in patients with sickle cell anemia. *Staphylococcus epidermidis* is often isolated in infections associated with implants. *Pseudomonas aeruginosa* causes osteomyelitis due to penetrating foot injury by direct inoculation and is almost never associated with hematogenous osteomyelitis. Brucella causes osteomyelitis, spondylitis, and arthritis in patients with exposure to animals/ animal products. *Gonococcus* is another cause in sexually active adolescents.

TREATMENT

Successful treatment of bone and joint infections in children depends upon the early initiation of appropriate antimicrobial therapy and surgical drainage wherever needed. If acute osteomyelitis has associated abscess (intraosseous, subperiosteal and/or soft tissue), it would require drainage and devitalized bone would require surgical removal. Joint aspiration or arthrotomy is important in the treatment of septic arthritis.

Choice of Empiric Antimicrobial Therapy

The choice of empiric therapy for both acute osteomyelitis and septic arthritis depends upon the age, immunization status, the underlying medical condition, and the clinical condition of the child; and the resistance patterns for the most common causative organisms in the community. Blood cultures (at least one set) should always be sent before initiating antibiotics. If imaging suggests, diagnostic aspiration of local collections should also be done before initiating antimicrobials. However, delay in performing a biopsy or aspiration for definitive diagnosis should not delay empiric antibiotic therapy. Antibiotic exposure prior to biopsy does not negatively impact pathogen recovery, though longer antibiotic use can decrease yield of culture. The importance of diagnostic aspiration is more in newborns and in the immunocompromised where the etiology is more diverse and drug resistant.

Empiric antimicrobial therapy should always be parenteral to begin with (Table 1).

TABLE 1: Empiric antimicrobial therapy for acute hematogenous osteomyelitis/septic arthritis.

Age	*Antibiotics (intravenous)*
Infants 0–2 months	Cloxacillin/Cefazolin* + Cefotaxime**
Children 2 months to 5 years	Cloxacillin/Cefazolin* + Ceftriaxone
Children >5 years	Cloxacillin* or Cefazolin*

*If there is concern for MRSA (local rates of MRSA >10%), anti-MRSA drug should also be added to the regime. Crude data from India suggests prevalence rates of MRSA of 20–40% in bone and joint infections. By these criteria, anti-MRSA drug may be needed in all patients. However, rates vary from center to center. So the decision to add anti-MRSA depends largely on previous microbial etiology at the center, degree of sickness, and toxicity. In stable patients, anti-MRSA drug may be withheld till cultures are available or response to therapy seen.

**In newborns who are sick or have prior history of infection with drug resistant gram-negative bacteria cefotaxime may be replaced with beta lactam (BL)-beta-lactamase inhibitor (BLI) combinations including piperacillin tazobactam/ cefoperazone sulbactam or carbapenems with or without aminoglycosides.

Definite Antimicrobial Therapy

After initial empiric therapy, the antibiotics should be tailored based on the biopsy/aspirate/blood culture, and sensitivity.

Methicillin-susceptible *S. aureus* (MSSA) can be successfully treated with cloxacillin or cefazolin. Ceftriaxone is also very good for bone and joint infections and can be given as once a day therapy on an outpatient basis after initial therapy with cloxacillin/cefazolin in hospital. However, if MSSA bacteremia is present cloxacillin/cefazolin should be continued for 2 weeks and step down to ceftriaxone avoided. If there is beta lactam allergy daptomycin can be used. The glycopeptides (vancomycin/teicoplanin) are inferior to beta lactams in treatment of MSSA. The oral options for therapy of MSSA include cephalexin (drug of choice), cloxacillin, cotrimoxazole or clindamycin.

In the case of MRSA, several options for therapy are available. Options for initial parenteral therapy include vancomycin, teicoplanin, daptomycin, linezolid, clindamycin, and cotrimoxazole. Options for oral switch include clindamycin, cotrimoxazole, and linezolid. Though vancomycin is the gold standard, need for frequent dosing, infusion-related side effects and nephrotoxicity are limiting factors. Also vancomycin levels in bone are less than optimal. Oral switch over to drug from another class is needed. Teicoplanin is an attractive option since it is concentrated well in the bone, can be given once a day, has less infusion-related toxicity/nephrotoxicity, and can also be given as an outpatient. However, higher doses may need to be used. MRSA infections can also be successfully treated with daptomycin, a drug which may be used if there is nephrotoxicity precluding the use of vancomycin or if once daily administration as outpatient is desired. Clindamycin is an appropriate antibiotic if susceptible because of its excellent bone penetration. It can be easily switched over from IV to oral therapy. Strains that are erythromycin-resistant and clindamycin-susceptible should be evaluated by the "D test" to determine the presence of inducible macrolide-lincosamide-streptrogramin B ($MLS_{B)}$ resistance. If present, clindamycin should be avoided. Cotrimoxazole can also be used successfully to treat MRSA bone and joint infections if susceptible; it achieves good levels in the bone and oral switch option is available. Linezolid is another drug that can be used for treatment of MRSA bone and joint infections and allows switch over to oral therapy. However, myelosuppression and optic and peripheral neuropathies are known side effects associated with prolonged linezolid use of more than 3 weeks which can limit use of linezolid. It is better to reserve use of linezolid if other options are available. If there is concomitant MRSA bacteremia with osteomyelitis, options for initial therapy include vancomycin and daptomycin and possibly teicoplanin. Other MRSA drugs discussed earlier cannot be used since they are not ideal for bacteremia. There is some data to suggest that adding rifampicin to the background regime for MRSA osteomyelitis improves the cure rates and reduces risk of relapse.

Since *S. aureus* is by far the most common cause acute hematogenous bone and joint infections, we have dealt with the treatment of MSSA and MRSA in some detail. Table 2 for doses. If the culture grows another micro-organism, the antibiotic therapy should be tailored according to its susceptibility pattern.

Changing Parenteral to Oral Antimicrobial Therapy

If staphylococcal bacteremia is demonstrated then parenteral therapy has to continue for 14 days. In other cases, shorter duration of parenteral therapy may be used.

TABLE 2: Dosages of commonly used antibiotics in bone and joint infections.

Antibiotic	*Dose*	*Max. dose/day*	*Route*
Cloxacillin	100–200 mg/kg/day ÷ Q 6 h	12,000 mg	IV/oral
Cefazolin	50–150 mg/kg/day ÷ Q 8 h	6,000 mg	IV
Ceftriaxone	50–100 mg/kg/day ÷ Q 12/24 h	4,000 mg	IV
Cefotaxime	150 mg/kg/day ÷ Q 8 h	8,000 mg	IV
Vancomycin	45 mg/kg/day ÷ Q 8 h	4,000 mg	IV
Teicoplanin	10–12 mg/kg/day Q 24 h	800 mg	IV/IM
Daptomycin	6–8 mg/kg/day Q 24 h	350 mg	IV
Clindamycin	30–40 mg/kg/day ÷ Q 8 h	1,800 mg	IV/oral
Co-trimoxazole (TMP)	10–12 mg/kg/day ÷ Q 8 h	480 mg	IV/oral
Cephalexin	100–150 mg/kg/day ÷ Q 6 h	6,000 mg	Oral
Linezolid	<12 years 30 mg/kg/day ÷ Q 8 h >12 years 600 mg twice daily	1,200 mg	IV/oral
Rifampicin	10–20 mg/kg/day Q 12–24 hourly	900 mg	Oral

Evidence-based data on the appropriate time to switch parenteral to oral therapy are limited and there are no defined criteria established to enable this switch. Shorter duration of parenteral therapy of less than 7 days is associated with similar cure rates compared with those who had parenteral therapy more than 7 days (95.2% vs. 98.8%) based on a meta-analysis on children between 3 months and 16 years with acute hematogenous osteomyelitis. The decision to switch to oral therapy is based on the availability of an appropriate oral antibiotic, the ability of the child to take medication orally, and reliability of the parent/caregiver to administer the oral antibiotic. The switch to oral therapy can be made when the child becomes afebrile, the symptoms and signs are resolving and the C-reactive protein (CRP) is returning to normal. Weekly monitoring of CRP and erythrocyte sedimentation rate (ESR) can be used to assess response to therapy. Typically CRP returns to baseline in about a week of effective therapy and can be used as a marker for transition from parenteral to oral therapy. Infants less than 3 months of age are best treated with parenteral therapy for the total duration of antibiotic therapy.

Duration of Antimicrobial Therapy

Duration of antimicrobial therapy depends on the presence of underlying risk factors, extent of infection, clinical response, and normalization of CRP and ESR. Acute hematogenous osteomyelitis can be treated with 4–6 weeks of total antimicrobial therapy if there is good clinical response and normalization of the CRP and ESR. In MRSA osteomyelitis, treatment for longer duration up to 8–12 weeks is recommended. Candida osteomyelitis needs treatment for up to 6 months.

If there are X-ray changes seen at the time of initiation of appropriate antibiotics, the osteomyelitis is subacute or chronic and the duration of therapy will have to be longer based on clinical response and normalization of inflammatory markers. The duration of antibiotic therapy in chronic osteomyelitis may have to be extended for up to 3–6 months due to biofilm formation. Surgical debridement and removal of implant/foreign body may be necessary to augment antibiotic therapy in chronic osteomyelitis.

In infants and children with uncomplicated septic arthritis, the treatment duration is dependent on the clinical response to therapy and the suspected organism. *S. pneumoniae*, Hib, *K. kingae* and *N. gonorrhoea*e are treated with appropriate antibiotics for 2–3 weeks. Infections with *S. aureus* and Gram-negative organisms are treated longer for 3–4 weeks. If there is associated osteomyelitis (complicated septic arthritis), the duration of antibiotics would be as for osteomyelitis. In resource-limited settings, associated osteomyelitis can be ruled out by performing an X-ray of the affected joint to look for bony changes consistent with osteomyelitis at the end of 2–3 weeks of therapy.

PROGNOSIS

Long-term sequelae are uncommon in those treated appropriately for acute osteomyelitis. Recurrence of infection can occur in about 5% and chronic osteomyelitis in less than 5%, mostly occurring in those with contiguous spread of osteomyelitis. The proportion of neonates with osteomyelitis developing sequelae ranges from 6% to 50% and include permanent effects such as disturbance in bone growth, limb length discrepancies, arthritis, abnormal gait, and pathological fractures. Complications following osteomyelitis are related to delayed diagnosis (>5 days), short duration of therapy, young age at time of illness, concurrent septic arthritis pyomyositis or abscess, location (hip 40%, ankle 33%, and knee 10%) and the infecting organism being MRSA, *S. pneumonia* or bearing the PVL toxin.

Complications following pyogenic arthritis are reported in 10–25% of all cases and include abnormal bone growth, limp, unstable articulation of the affected joint, and decreased range of motion. Risk factors for sequelae are similar to those for acute osteomyelitis. Adjacent bone involvement with septic arthritis is associated with more sequelae.

RECOMMENDED READING

1. Brady RA, Leid JG, Calhoun JH, et al. Osteomyelitis and the role of biofilms in chronic infection. FEMS Immunol Med Microbiol. 2008;52(1):13-22.
2. Chen C-J, Chiu C-H, Lin T-Y, et al. Experience with linezolid therapy in children with osteoarticular infections. Pediatr Infect Dis J. 2007;26(11):985-8.
3. Dartnell J, Ramachandran M, Katchburian M. Haematogenous acute and subacute paediatric osteomyelitis: A systematic review of the literature. J Bone Joint Surg Br. 2012;94(5):584-95.
4. Gutierrez K. Bone and joint infections in children. Pediatr Clin North Am. 2005;52(3):779-94.
5. Harik NS, Smeltzer MS. Management of acute hematogenous osteomyelitis in children. Expert Rev Anti Infect Ther. 2010;8(2):175-81.
6. Howard A, Wilson M. Septic arthritis in children. BMJ. 2010;341:c4407.

7. Iliadis AD, Ramachandran M. Paediatric bone and joint infection. EFORT Open Rev. 2017;2(1):7-12.
8. Le Saux N, Howard A, Barrowman NJ, et al. Shorter courses of parenteral antibiotic therapy do not appear to influence response rates for children with acute hematogenous osteomyelitis: A systematic review. BMC Infect Dis. 2002;2:16.
9. Liu C, Bayer A, Cosgrove SE, et al. Infectious Diseases Society of America. Clinical practice guidelines by the infectious diseases society of America for the treatment of methicillin-resistant Staphylococ*cus aureus* infections in adults and children. Clin Infect Dis. 2011;52(3):e18-55.
10. Marschall J, Bhavan KP, Olsen MA, et al. The impact of prebiopsy antibiotics on pathogen recovery in hematogenous vertebral osteomyelitis. Clin Infect Dis Off Publ Infect Dis Soc Am. 20111;52(7):867-72.
11. Messina AF, Namtu K, Guild M, et al. Trimethoprim-sulfamethoxazole therapy for children with acute osteomyelitis. Pediatr Infect Dis J. 2011;30(12):1019-21.
12. Montgomery CO, Siegel E, Blasier RD, et al. Concurrent septic arthritis and osteomyelitis in children. J Pediatr Orthop. 2013;33:464.
13. Pappas PG, Kauffman CA, Andes DR, et al. Clinical practice guideline for the management of candidiasis: 2016 update by the Infectious Diseases Society of America. Clin Infect Dis. 2016;62(4): 409-17.
14. Pääkkönen M. Septic arthritis in children: Diagnosis and treatment. Pediatr Health Med Ther. 2017;8:65-8.
15. Steward CD, Raney PM, Morrell AK, et al. Testing for induction of clindamycin resistance in erythromycin-resistant isolates of *Staphylococcus aureus*. J Clin Microbiol. 2005;43:1716-21.
16. Syrogiannopoulos GA, Nelson JD. Duration of antimicrobial therapy for acute suppurative osteoarticular infections. Lancet Lond Engl. 1988;1(8575-6):37-40.
17. Yagupsky P, Porsch E, St Geme JW. *Kingella kingae*: An emerging pathogen in young children. *Pediatrics.* 2011;127(3):557-65.
18. Yeo A, Ramachandran M. Acute haematogenous osteomyelitis in children. BMJ. 2014;348:g66.
19. Zhorne DJ, Altobelli ME, Cruz AT. Impact of antibiotic pretreatment on bone biopsy yield for children with acute hematogenous osteomyelitis. Hosp Pediatr. 2015;5(6):337-41.

Antimicrobial Therapy in Central Nervous System Infections

26
Chapter

Ayesha J Sunavala, Vrajesh Udani

BACTERIAL MENINGITIS

Introduction

Bacterial meningitis remains an important cause of childhood morbidity and mortality in the developing world. The etiology of bacterial meningitis is unique to the age of the child and is somewhat different in developing versus developed countries. The three most common pathogens, *Haemophilus influenzae, Streptococcus pneumoniae, and Neisseria meningitidis* account for more than 80% of cases. With the introduction of the *Haemophilus influenzae* type b (Hib) and pneumococcal conjugate vaccines in the infant immunization schedule in the Western world, the incidence of bacterial meningitis declined in all age groups except children younger than 2 months. The median age shifted from less than 5 years to 42 years. Hib and pneumococcal vaccines have been recently introduced as part of the Universal Immunization Program of India, and hence the total impact of these vaccines on disease burden in our population has not been established as yet. However, a prospective study from CMC, Vellore, found a significant decline in the annual mean number of culture-confirmed Hib meningitis cases (10.7 prior to Hib vaccine introduction, falling to 3.8 cases following introduction) after introduction of the vaccine.

The mortality rate of untreated bacterial meningitis approaches 100%. Even with optimal therapy, significant morbidity with neurological sequelae are common among survivors and thus timely and rational use of empiric antimicrobials as well as prompt diagnosis of the specific causative agent is essential to optimize management. Finally, the emergence of resistant *Streptococcus pneumoniae* isolates from various parts of the country warrant new empiric strategies for the management of bacterial meningitis.

This chapter discusses community-acquired bacterial meningitis, see chapter 30 for nosocomial meningitis.

Etiology

Neonatal Age (<4 weeks)

The etiological spectrum responsible for neonatal meningitis in developing countries differs from that in developed countries, probably reflecting differences in bacterial colonization of the maternal tract, genetic differences in immune response and possibly differences in facilities for pathogen isolation and reporting.

Neonatal meningitis is usually classified as early onset (<7 days), which is mainly caused by bacteria acquired vertically from maternal vaginal flora or the delivery room while late onset sepsis is due to nosocomial pathogens. Group B streptococci (GBS), enterobacteriaceae, and *Listeria monocytogenes* have been found to be the most commonly detected organisms in early onset neonatal sepsis and meningitis from the developed world. Although, there is relative paucity of Indian data, a recent study on neonatal meningitis from Northeast India found that *Enterococcus, E. coli,* GBS, *Globicatella* spp., *Sneathia* spp. all known vaginal colonizers were isolated from neonates who were born through vaginal delivery and had an early onset of symptoms. The National neonatal perinatal database published in 2005 from multiple tertiary centers suggests that Gram-negative organisms like *E. coli* and *Klebsiella* are the most common pathogens in early/late onset sepsis. A recent study from Delhi which included both neonates born at home or at hospital revealed that Gram-negative organisms including *Klebsiella, E. coli,* and *Acinetobacter* were the most common pathogens causing neonatal sepsis and organisms causing late onset and early onset sepsis were not different. Additionally, these pathogens had very high rates of cephalosporin and carbapenem resistance (40–80%). Candida was isolated in 25% of the patients and also in babies who weighed more than 1,500 g and who were born at term. Candida in neonates has very high rates of tropism to the brain and hence is an important cause of late onset meningitis in neonates with neonatal intensive care unit (NICU) stay. GBS is found to be an infrequent cause of neonatal sepsis in India; however, the true incidence may be underestimated. One must be aware of the possibility of HSV as a cause of neonatal meningitis and investigate for it accordingly.

Infants and Older Children

In children older than 4 weeks, *S. pneumoniae, H. influenzae b,* and *N meningitidis* are the most common etiologic agents. In a hospital-based surveillance study from 10 hospitals from India conducted between 2012 and 2013, of 257 cases of microbiologically confirmed meningitis among 3,104 cases of clinically suspected meningitis in children below 5 years, 83% were due to *Pneumococcus,* 14.4% due to *H. influenzae* and only 2.7% were due to meningococci.

In a systematic review by Singh et al. which included seven studies published from 2009 to 2016 in children below 5 years the incidence of penicillin resistance was 10% and cefotaxime resistance was 4%. In the Alliance for Surveillance of Invasive Pneumococcal Serotypes (ASIP) study in children below 5 years which included 361 isolates, the penicillin resistance was 8% and no cephalosporin resistance was reported.

However, there is increase in rates of penicillin and cephalosporin resistance in India. In a recent study from CMC, Vellore, a total of 830 invasive pneumococcal isolates were investigated, of which 37.5% of the isolates were in children aged less than 5 years, 12.8% in children aged 5–16 years, and 49.7% of the isolates were from those 16 years of age and older. About 20.1% (167) of the isolates were from meningeal infection. Of the 167 cerebrospinal fluid (CSF) isolates, 43.7%, and 14.9% were nonsusceptible to penicillin and cefotaxime, respectively. Of the 25 isolates that were resistant to cephalosporins, 8 were fully resistant [minimum inhibitory concentration (MIC) $\geq$ 4] and 17 were intermediately resistant (MIC 2). Penicillin resistance in pneumococcal meningeal isolates has increased from less than 10% in 2008 to over 40% by 2016 and cephalosporin resistance from 4.7% in 2008 to 28.5 % in 2016.

Immunocompromised

Here the etiology is diverse and depends on the type of immuncompromise. Pathogens include listeria, resistant Gram-negative, *Nocardia,* tuberculosis, *Cryptococcus, Candida,* dematiaceous fungi, and molds.

Principles of Therapy

Avoidance of Delay

Community-acquired meningitis is a medical emergency of catastrophic consequences; hence, appropriate empiric antibiotic therapy should be initiated as soon as possible after the diagnosis is considered likely. A Danish study which assessed outcome in community-acquired bacterial meningitis found a 10% increase of in-hospital mortality and risk for unfavorable outcomes at discharge with each hour of delay of antibiotics for the first 6 hours of admission.

It is recommended that appropriate empiric antibiotic therapy should be initiated as soon as lumbar puncture (LP) is performed. However, in patients in whom LP is delayed or a computerized tomography (CT) scan is performed, there may be a significant interval between establishing the diagnosis of bacterial meningitis and initiating appropriate therapy. In these patients, blood samples must be obtained for culture and appropriate antimicrobial and adjunctive therapy given prior to LP or before the patient is sent for CT scan.

Although the administration of antimicrobial therapy before LP may affect the yield of CSF Gram stain and culture, pathogens other than *Meningococcus* usually can be identified in the CSF up to several hours after the administration of antibiotics and more so now with use of multiplex polymerase chain reaction (PCR) in CSF for etiologic diagnosis.

Antibiotic Regimen

Bactericidal agents: The CSF is a site of impaired humoral immunity; hence, antibiotics must achieve a bactericidal effect within CSF to result in optimal microbiologic cure.

Drug entry into CSF: Normally, the blood–brain barrier blocks macromolecule entry into the CSF, with small, lipophilic molecules penetrating most easily. Most drugs reach peak concentrations in the CSF that are only 10–20% of peak concentrations in the serum. However, in meningitis, the peak concentration of several drugs in CSF increases with inflammation of the blood–brain barrier. This was illustrated in one study that sequentially monitored CSF and serum penicillin levels in children with bacterial meningitis. The mean CSF/serum ratio 2 hours after administration of the same intravenous dose of penicillin was 42% on the first day of therapy but fell to less than 10% on the 10th day, when the inflammatory changes had subsided. Owing to the general limitation in antibiotic penetration into the CSF, drugs must be administered intravenously to increase the bioavailability. Administration of antibiotics directly in the CSF is an attractive option to achieve good local levels. However, based on a recent Cochrane review, the use of intraventricular antimicrobial agents is not recommended routinely in neonates or infants as it resulted in a three-fold increased risk of mortality when compared to standard therapy. However, the use of intraventricular or intrathecal antibiotics can be considered in the treatment of healthcare-associated meningitis associated with multidrug-resistant pathogens.

Optimizing PK/PD: Higher antimicrobial doses at appropriate dosing intervals have been recommended based on pharmacokinetic studies to optimize outcomes in bacterial meningitis.

Specific Classes of Antimicrobial Agents

Penicillins

Ampicillin either alone or with chloramphenicol in postneonatal meningitis and with an aminoglycoside in neonatal meningitis were the usual first-line empiric antibacterial agents used in the 1970s and 1980s. However, recent Indian studies have revealed 35–44% penicillin resistance among *S. pneumoniae* isolates and up to 80% ampicillin resistance for *H. influenzae* isolates. Similarly Gram-negative organisms in neonatal meningitis are routinely resistant to ampicillin, with a recent study on neonatal meningitis showing 100% resistance. These rates preclude the use of the penicillin or ampicillin as empiric agents in bacterial meningitis both in the neonatal period and beyond. However, ampicillin in combination with gentamicin is the drug of choice for meningitis due to *Listeria* and susceptible enterococci.

Chloramphenicol

This is an excellent drug for meningitis as it has excellent central nervous system (CNS) penetration and achieves high concentrations in the CNS making it very useful when long-term treatment is sometimes necessary in complicated meningitis (when IV access maybe a problem). Although chloramphenicol is a bacteriostatic drug for most enteric Gram-negative rods; it is usually bactericidal for *H. influenzae, Neisseria meningitidis,* and *Streptococcus pneumoniae* and has been used extensively and successfully to treat meningitis caused by these organisms especially in the meningococcal belt of Africa. However, resistance rates have soared with *H. influenzae* being resistant in up to 38–60% of cases. It should now be considered only when no other options are available.

Aminoglycosides

Cerebrospinal fluid penetration of aminoglycosides is an issue but these have been found useful in management of neonatal meningitis where Gram-negative pathogens are common. They may also be used for intrathecal/intraventricular administration.

Cephalosporins

The treatment of bacterial meningitis has been revolutionized by the availability of the third-generation cephalosporins. They are usually highly effective against community-acquired agents like *H. influenzae, S. pneumoniae* and *N. meningitidis*. Cefotaxime and ceftriaxone are very effective in meningitis caused by susceptible strains of aerobic Gram-negative bacilli (e.g. *Escherichia coli* or *Klebsiella* species). Ceftazidime has also shown efficacy in several studies of patients with *Pseudomonas* meningitis. The fourth-generation cephalosporin, cefepime, has been shown to be safe and therapeutically equivalent to cefotaxime in the treatment of bacterial meningitis in infants and children.

However, emerging resistance in pneumococci to cephalosporins as discussed earlier is compromising their use as empiric monotherapy for bacterial meningitis. Increasing extended-spectrum beta-lactamases (ESBL) rates among enterobacteriaceae and Gram-negative pathogens in hospital setting is making third-generation cephalosporins redundant in management of healthcare-associated meningitis and compromising their efficacy in neonatal meningitis. The organisms *Serratia* spp., *Providencia* spp., indole-positive *Proteus, Citrobacter* spp. and *Enterobacter* spp. (SPICE) some of which cause serious community-acquired neonatal meningitis exhibit stable derepression of the chromosomal beta-lactamase AmpC. Even if these organisms test susceptible in vitro, the use of a third-generation cephalosporin as a single agent for treatment of serious infections due to these bacteria can lead to the emergence of resistance during therapy and is thus not recommended.

Vancomycin

Vancomycin has proven useful in the therapy of bacterial meningitis caused by penicillin-resistant pneumococci. Due to poor CSF penetration, vancomycin should always be combined with a third-generation cephalosporin even in patients with meningitis caused by penicillin- and cephalosporin-resistant strains. Vancomycin has a role in late onset neonatal meningitis, postneurosurgery and postshunt meningitis caused by methicillin-resistant *Staphylococcus aureus* (MRSA) and methicillin-resistant *Staphylococcus epidermis* (MRSE). When used for the treatment of bacterial meningitis, vancomycin should be administered to maintain serum vancomycin through concentrations of approximately 15–20 mg/mL. Intrathecal administration of vancomycin may be considered in patients who are not responding to parenteral administration.

Rifampin

This drug has good CSF penetration and in vitro activity against many meningeal pathogens. However, when used alone, resistance rapidly develops; hence, rifampin must be used in combination with a third-generation cephalosporin, with or without vancomycin, in patients with pneumococcal meningitis caused by highly cephalosporin-resistant strains. Addition of rifampicin should be considered if cephalosporin MIC more than 4 μg/mL, if the child's condition is worsening after 48 hours of vancomycin + ceftriaxone, if dexamethasone has been given or if repeat LP shows presence of bacteria.

Rifampin should also be combined with vancomycin in patients with CSF shunt infections caused by staphylococci, especially in cases in which the shunt cannot be removed.

Carbapenems

Meropenem which has a broad range of in vitro activity and less seizure proclivity than imipenem, has been studied in both children and adults with bacterial meningitis. In these studies, meropenem has been shown to have clinical and microbiologic outcomes similar to those of cefotaxime or ceftriaxone and can be recommended as an alternative to these agents for treatment of bacterial meningitis. Meropenem has also been used successfully in meningitis caused by Gram-negative isolates that are resistant to standard therapy a commonly encountered situation in neonatal meningitis and healthcare-associated meningitis. In a recent study 20 cefotaxime-resistant *S. pneumoniae* isolates, 4 were intermediate and 13 were resistant to meropenem, suggesting that meropenem may not be a useful alternative agent for treatment of pneumococcal isolates that are resistant to penicillin and cephalosporins.

Fluoroquinolones

These agents have been considered useful for treating Gram-negative meningitis in the newborn as they have good penetration into CSF and cerebral tissues. It is suggested that fluoroquinolones may reduce the chances of cerebral abscess formation in neonates and immunocompromised hosts. The CSF penetration of the newer fluoroquinolones is better than the older drugs. Empiric use of this group of drugs however, is discouraged due to high gram-negative resistance rates in India. However, they can be considered in treatment of Gram-negative meningitis if susceptibility is demonstrated or if there is serious allergy to the beta-lactams. Moxifloxacin is the preferred drug due to its better CNS penetration.

Polymyxins

The burgeoning rates of carbapenem-resistant Gram-negative isolates have forced us to explore this group of drugs for healthcare-associated infections including meningitis and ventriculitis. CSF penetration is known to be poor and studies reveal CSF levels barely above the MIC for many nosocomial isolates in patients with meningitis thus prompting additional intrathecal or intraventricular administration. In a systemic review on the use of intrathecal or intraventricular polymyxins for meningitis in adults and children, success rates of 80% were noted in 30 children. Although dose-dependent neurotoxicity was not uncommon, irreversible toxicity was not reported in any study.

Empiric Treatment in Patients with Suspected Bacterial Meningitis (Table 1)

Neonates

In early onset meningitis, empiric therapy should necessarily cover community-acquired agents from the maternal flora like *E. coli* and *Klebsiella*. Group B streptococci and *Listeria monocytogenes* have not been commonly reported from Indian studies but should be considered while fashioning empiric treatment.

For both early onset neonatal meningitis and for community-acquired late onset meningitis in an antibiotic naïve patient where Gram-negative organisms are the predominant

TABLE 1: Empiric treatment options for bacterial meningitis.

Age	*Possible etiology*	*Empiric antibiotic*
Neonates (early onset <7 days)/ community-acquired late onset	*E. coli*, *Klebsiella* spp. GBS *Listeria monocytogenes* HSV	Cefotaxime + aminoglycoside ± ampicillin *or* Meropenem
Late onset nosocomial sepsis	MDR/XDR Gram-negatives MRSA/MRSE *Candida*	Meropenem with/without vancomycin Add colistin if unit has high incidence of carbapenem resistance and especially if baby in septic shock
Children	*S. pneumoniae*, *H. influenzae*, *N. meningitidis*	Cefotaxime or ceftriaxone plus vancomycin
Nosocomial/device associated	*S. aureus*, CONS, MDR/XDR gram-negative pathogens,	Meropenem plus vancomycin (consider intrathecal administration)
Immunosuppressed child	*S. pneumoniae*, *H. influenzae*, *N. meningitidis* *S. aureus*, CONS, DR Gram-negative pathogens *plus* Opportunistic pathogens (*Listeria*, *Nocardia*, TB *Rhodococcus*, *Candida* spp., molds, cryptococci)	Meropenem plus vancomycin (Empiric treatment difficult: Identification of causative organism critical)

(CONS: coagulase-negative staphylococci; GBS: group B streptococci; HSV: herpes simplex virus; MDR: multidrug-resistant; MRSA: methicillin-resistant *Staphylococcus aureus*; MRSE: methicillin-resistant *Staphylococcus epidermidis*; XDR: extensively drug-resistant)

etiology, empiric therapy should include cefotaxime in combination with an aminoglycoside. Ceftriaxone should be avoided as it causes sludging of bile and may increase the risk of bilirubin encephalopathy in high-risk newborns. In situations of suspected *Listeria monocytogenes,* additional ampicillin is recommended as these organisms are intrinsically resistant to cephalosporins. However, the rising prevalence of ESBL production even in early onset neonatal sepsis/community-acquired infections in neonates in various recent studies is likely to make this regime poorly efficacious. Hence, one may elect to use carbapenems as empiric therapy in this setting if local experience suggests so.

For nosocomially-acquired neonatal meningitis empiric therapy must be guided by the local epidemiology and antibiogram of the neonatal center and usually includes meropenem. Vancomycin should be added empirically is MRSA/MRSE rates in the unit is high.

Infants and Children

Initial antibiotic selection should provide coverage for all three common pathogens: *S pneumoniae, N. meningitidis,* and *H. influenzae.*

Till sometime ago empiric therapy with ceftriaxone/cefotaxime was considered adequate for bacterial meningitis in this age group. This practice has since changed in countries with an evolving pneumococcal resistance to the third-generation cephalosporins. It is now recommended by the American Academy of Pediatrics and Infectious Disease Society of America to use a combination of ceftriaxone and vancomycin in suspected bacterial meningitis. With the increasing trend of pneumococcal resistance reported from recent Indian studies, it seems reasonable to follow the above recommendations for empiric therapy pending culture results.

Modification of Therapy

Therapy should be modified on basis of culture results. If pneumococci are isolated and are penicillin/cephalosporin susceptible vancomycin should be stopped. If the organism is highly drug resistant especially to carbapenems one may use intrathecal/intraventricular antibiotics. A recent Cochrane review on the use of intraventricular antibiotics in neonatal meningitis concluded that there is no place for this practice at the present time as the only randomized controlled trial showed a 3-fold increase in mortality when this procedure was adopted. However in situations where neonatal meningitis is caused by unusual pathogens like *Elizabethkingia meningoseptica* or carbapenem-resistant Gram-negative isolates intraventricular antibiotics may be considered. Table 2 lists the dosages of commonly used drugs in bacterial meningitis.

Duration of Therapy

The duration of antimicrobial therapy should be based upon the causative organism and the clinical course. There is limited evidence from high quality studies to guide the duration of treatment for bacterial meningitis. If the cultures are negative treatment for 2 weeks is recommended. The recommended durations of therapy for uncomplicated meningitis caused by the following organisms are:

- *S. pneumoniae*—10–14 days
- *N. meningitidis*—5–7 days
- *H. influenzae* type b (Hib) - 7–10 days
- *L. monocytogenes*—14–21 days

TABLE 2: Dosage of antimicrobial agents in infants and children.

Agent	*Total daily dose (dosing interval in hours)*
Amikacin	20–30 mg/kg (8)
Ampicillin	300 mg/kg (6)
Cefipime	150 mg/kg (8)
Cefotaxime	200 mg/kg (6–8)
Ceftazidime	150 mg/kg (8)
Ceftriaxone	100 mg/kg (12)
Chloramphenicol	75–100 mg /kg (6)
Gentamicin	7.5 mg/kg (8)
Meropenem	120 mg/kg (8)
Oxacillin	200 mg/kg (6)
Rifampicin	10–20 mg/kg (12–24)
Vancomycin	60 mg/kg (6)

- *S. aureus*—at least 2 weeks
- Gram-negative bacilli: 3 weeks or a minimum of 2 weeks beyond the first sterile CSF culture, whichever is longer.

In neonatal meningitis, treatment should be continued for 3 weeks after the last negative culture and even longer for up to 6-8 weeks if there is ventriculitis.

For children with negative CSF cultures at 48-72 hours, further course of antimicrobials depends upon:

- Discontinue antimicrobials if normal CSF profile, negative blood and CSF culture.
- For those who have a CSF pleocytosis and positive blood culture, but negative CSF culture, treat for meningitis caused by the organism isolated from the blood culture (i.e. management is the same as if the CSF culture was positive for the same organism).
- For those who have a CSF pleocytosis, negative blood culture, and negative CSF culture, it is recommended to individualize the duration of antimicrobial therapy based on clinical parameters.

Many children in our scenario are diagnosed late, partly treated or already have complications like subdural empyema necessitating much longer durations. Often this would need the duration of therapy to be individualized on the basis of the patient's clinical response. Also in case of a significant subdural empyema surgical drainage often with large craniotomies would be necessary to ensure an optimal result.

Role of Adjunctive Dexamethasone Therapy in Patients with Bacterial Meningitis

At present, there are insufficient data to make a recommendation on the use of adjunctive dexamethasone in neonates with bacterial meningitis. A small, randomized trial that did not have a placebo arm evaluated the use of dexamethasone in reducing the risk of neurologic sequelae in neonatal meningitis. As per this study, the administration of dexamethasone did not significantly affect mortality or neurologic outcome at 2 years of age. Thus dexamethasone therapy is not currently recommended in neonatal meningitis.

A recently concluded Cochrane review on adjunctive steroids in bacterial meningitis included 16 trials from high-income countries and 9 from low-income countries with 4,121 participants (2,511 children and 1,517 adults; 93 mixed population). The overall results showed no overall impact on mortality, but reduced risk of severe hearing loss, any hearing loss and neurologic sequelae. Sub-group analysis showed mild reduction in mortality in *Pneumococcus* [risk ratio (RR) 0.84 95%; confidence interval (CI) 0.72–0.98], but no mortality benefit in meningitis due to Hib or *Meningococcus*. There was reduction in hearing loss due to Hib disease in children but not in non-Hib meningitis. Furthermore corticosteroids showed no impact at all in trials in low-income countries. No significant adverse effects of steroids were noted in either low/high-income countries. An earlier RCT had actually shown adverse outcome with use of steroids in African children with bacterial meningitis.

It is therefore clear that the benefit of steroids is controversial in children with bacterial meningitis. Other arguements against using steroids are reduction in the incidence of Hib meningitis due to vaccination (which is the main benefactor from steroids), prior use of antibiotics in many children with meningitis, and the inability to determine the etiology of meningitis at the time of presentation (multiplex PCR is not available in most settings). Furthermore with increase in incidence of cephalosporin-resistant pneumococcal meningitis and need to use vancomycin as companion therapy, the penetration of vancomycin in CSF may be hampered by use of dexamethasone. In fact some experts suggest that if dexamethasone is administered, rifampicin should be added to the empiric regimen of vancomycin and ceftriaxone/cefotaxime. Other potential adverse effects of steroids include masking of clinical signs and symptoms thus interfering with the ability to assess true clinical response to therapy and gastrointestinal bleeding (in approximately 1–2% of children).

In summary, the use of dexamethasone in children with meningitis other than Hib, or in whom bacterial meningitis is suspected but the etiology unknown, must be individualized after careful analysis of the potential risks and benefits. If they are at all used, dexamethasone should be initiated 10–20 minutes prior to, or at least concomitant with, the first antimicrobial dose, at 0.15 mg/kg every 6 hours for 48–96 hours. It is thought to be of no likely benefit if given more than 1 hour later.

Adjuvant Glycerol in Childhood Bacterial Meningitis

Glycerol is a hyperosmolar osmotic diuretic that has been used in neurosurgery, neurology, and ophthalmology to reduce raised tissue pressure. It appears an attractive adjunctive measure as it may reduce meningeal inflammation by scavenging free oxygen radicals and is safe, easily available, and inexpensive.

It is administered as 1.5 g/kg (max 25 g) four times daily for the 1st 48 hours only. However, a 2018 meta-analysis of various trials on glycerol in patients with bacterial meningitis concluded that the use of adjunctive glycerol may reduce the risk of deafness and neurologic disability but has no effect on mortality. These studies were fraught with several limitations including lack of long-term follow-up for subtle neurologic sequelae, variations in population and environment, and the use of different methods to assess hearing. Hence, additional studies are necessary before glycerol therapy can be routinely recommended for bacterial meningitis in children.

BRAIN ABSCESS

Brain abscesses are most common in children between 4 years and 8 years. Causes of brain abscess include embolization due to congenital heart disease with right-to-left shunts, meningitis (especially neonatal), ear and mastoid infections, soft-tissue infection of face and scalp, orbital cellulitis and sinusitis (mostly in frontal lobe), dental infections, penetrating head injuries, postneurosurgical procedures, immunodeficiency states, and rarely as a result of shunt infections.

The etiology determines the microbiology. The microbiologic causes are listed in Table 3. At least two sets of blood cultures should be sent prior to initiating therapy. Diagnostic aspiration is very crucial in the immunocompromised where the etiology is very diverse. All efforts must be made to aspirate the abscess and obtain material for Gram stain, aerobic/anaerobic culture and if indicated mycobacterial and fungal culture. Exceptions are multiple abscesses, poor surgical risk, positive blood culture, or difficult location.

Empiric therapy prior to obtaining culture results or if cultures are negative or not possible depends on the setting and is discussed in Table 3. Therapy is altered once cultures are available. Patients with cerebritis, multiple or small abscess less than 3 cm, as well as abscesses in inaccessible areas of the brain may be treated with medical therapy alone. Clearly surgical drainage by repeated aspiration or excision is an important part of management of large abscesses especially if these are chronic and thick walled or is causing life-threatening mass

TABLE 3: Etiology and empiric therapy for brain abscess.

Predisposing factor	*Likely etiology*	*Empiric therapy*
Penetrating head injury	*S. aureus*, *Clostridium* species	Cefotaxime/ceftriaxone and vancomycin
Postneurosurgery	*S. aureus*, CONS, resistant gram-negative bacilli	Meropenem and vancomycin
Hematogenous spread cyanotic congenital heart disease/lung infections/endocarditis	Aerobic/microaerophilic/ anaerobic streptococci, *S. aureus*	Cefriaxone and metronidazole with/without vancomycin
Continuous spread from otitis media/mastoiditis/sinusitis/dental infection	Aerobic, microaerophilic, anaerobic streptococci, Anaerobic gram-negative bacilli (*Fusobacterium, Prevotella, Porphyromonas*), *S. aureus, Pseudomonas*	Ceftriaxone/cefepime and metronidazole
Neonates	Citrobacter/Enterobacteriaceae, Candida	Meropenem
HIV	*Mycobacterium TB, Nocardia, Toxoplasma, Cryptococcus, Listeria*	No empiric therapy
Immunocompromised	*Nocardia, Mycobacterium, Toxoplasma, Mucorales, Aspergillus, Listeria, Cryptococcus, Candida.*	

(CONS: coagulase-negative staphylococci)

effect and increased intracranial pressure (ICP). Duration of therapy is 4–12 weeks if abscess is drained/excised. If abscess not drained then longer duration may be required till radiological resolution (4 months till 1 year).

CEREBROSPINAL FLUID SHUNT INFECTIONS

Introduction and Microbial Etiology

The rate of internalized CSF shunt infection in most studies has ranged from approximately 5%–15%. The highest rates are reported in young infants. Most infections are a result of intraoperative contamination of the surgical wound by skin flora. Accordingly coagulase-negative staphylococci are isolated in more than half of the cases. *Staphylococcus aureus* is isolated in approximately 20% and Gram-negative bacilli in 15%. A fastidious pathogen is *Cutibacterium acnes* (formerly *Propionibacterium acnes*). Four distinct clinical syndromes have been described: Colonization of the shunt, infection associated with wound infection, distal infection with peritonitis, and infection associated with meningitis. The most common type of infection is "colonization" of the shunt with symptoms occurring few months after the surgical procedure. Wound infection presents with obvious infection or dehiscence along the shunt tract and most often occurs within days to weeks of the surgical procedure. Whereas, CONS, *Cutibacterium acnes,* and *S. aureus* are the most common organisms associated with colonization and wound infection respectively, Gram-negative enteric bacilli are predominantly isolated from distal infection of the VP shunt with peritonitis.

Treatment

The most crucial aspect of treating a shunt infection is removal of the shunt. Both the distal and proximal end of the shunt should be sent for culture. The laboratory should be asked to process and incubate to detect *Propionibacterium acnes*. A temporary external ventricular drain should be placed. Empiric antibiotic therapy usually includes ceftriaxone with vancomycin or meropenem with vancomycin depending on local susceptibility patterns, severity of illness, and timing of infection since placement of shunt. Cultures should be repeated to document culture negativity. The duration of antibiotics and timing of the placement of the new shunt depends on the causative organism and is discussed in Table 4.

In some situations when the shunt cannot be removed, combination of systemic antimicrobial therapy and local intraventricular antibiotics may be administered (see chapter 30 for doses) to salvage the shunt. A recent systematic review sponsored by the American Association of Neurological Surgeons/Congress of Neurological Surgeons noted insufficient evidence for

TABLE 4: Timing of reimplantation of shunt depending on causative organism.

Etiology	*Timing of shunt reimplantation*
CONS, P. acnes with no CSF abnormalities	48 hours after repeat CSF cultures are negative
CONS, P. acnes with CSF abnormalities	7 days if repeat CSF cultures are negative. If repeat cultures are positive then 7–10 days after the last negative culture
Gram-negative bacilli and *S. aureus*	10 days after repeat CSF cultures are negative

(CONS: coagulase-negative staphylococci; CSF: cerebrospinal fluid)

intraventricular antibiotics to recommend their use in pediatric shunt infections. However, smaller case series have described quick sterilization of the CSF, low relapse rates, and survival in children who received intraventricular antibiotics for CSF shunt infection. If conservative therapy fails then the shunt will have to be removed.

Important strategies to prevent infections related to shunts and external ventricular drains includes using antibiotic impregnated shunts/drains, using appropriate perioperative prophylaxis for shunts and placement of external ventricular drains and using strict asepsis at the time of insertion. Fixed interval change of external ventricular drains (EVDs) and continuing antibiotics for the whole duration of the drain is however not recommended.

RECOMMENDED READING

1. American Academy of Pediatrics. Pneumococcal infections. In: Kimberlin DW, Brady MT, Jackson MA, Long SS (Eds). Red Book: 2015 Report of the Committee on Infectious Diseases, 30th edition. Elk Grove Village, IL: American Academy of Pediatrics; 2015. p. 626.
2. Arnell K, Enblad P, Wester T, et al. Treatment of cerebrospinal fluid shunt infections in children using systemic and intraventricular antibiotic therapy in combination with externalization of the ventricular catheter: Efficacy in 34 consecutively treated infections. J Neurosurg. 2007;107(3):213-7.
3. Baddour LM, Flynn PM, Fekete T et al. Infections of cerebrospinal fluid shunts and other devices. Uptodate 2017.
4. Bodilsen J, Dalager-Pedersen M, Schønheyder HC, et al. Time to antibiotic therapy and outcome in bacterial meningitis: a Danish population-based cohort study. BMC Infect Dis. 2016;16:392.
5. Brouwer MC, McIntyre P, Prasad K, et al. Corticosteroids for acute bacterial meningitis. Cochrane Database Syst Rev. 2015;12(9):CD004405.
6. Buckingham SC, Davis Y, English BK. Pneumococcal susceptibility to meropenem in a mid-South children's hospital. South Med J. 2002;95:1293-6.
7. Devi U, Bora R, Malik V, et al. Bacterial aetiology of neonatal meningitis: A study from North-East India. Indian J Med Res. 2017;145(1):138-43.
8. Edwards MS, Baker CJ. Bacterial meningitis in the neonate: Clinical features and diagnosis. Up to date May 2018.
9. Jajoo M, Manchanda V, Chaurasia S, et al. Investigators of the Delhi Neonatal Infection Study (DeNIS) collaboration, New Delhi, India. Alarming rates of antimicrobial resistance and fungal sepsis in outborn neonates in North India. PLoS One. 2018;13(6):e0180705.
10. Jayaraman Y, Veeraraghavan B, ChethrapillyPurushothaman GK, et al. Hospital Based Sentinel Surveillance of Bacterial Mening*itis (HBSSBM) Network T*eam. Burden of bacterial meningitis in India: Preliminary data from a hospital based sentinel surveillance network. PLoS One. 2018;13(5):e0197198.
11. Kanegaye JT, Soliemanzadeh P, Bradley JS. Lumbar puncture in pediatric bacterial meningitis: Defining the time interval for recovery of cerebrospinal fluid pathogens after parenteral antibiotic pretreatment. Pediatrics. 2001;108(5):1169.
12. Kaplan SL. Bacterial meningitis in children older than one month: treatment and prognosis. Uptodate 2018.
13. Kuruvilla KA, Thomas N, Jesudasan MV, et al. Neonatal group B Streptococcal bacteraemia in India: Ten years' experience. Acta Paediatr. 1999;88:1031-2.
14. National Neonatal Perinatal Database: Report 2002-2003 ICMR, New Delhi Publications 2005; 45-57.
15. Peltola H, Anttila M, Renkonen OV. Randomised comparison of chloramphenicol, ampicillin, cefotaxime, and ceftriaxone for childhood bacterial meningitis. Finnish Study Group. Lancet. 1989;1(8650):1281-7.
16. Ramchandran P, Fitzwater SP, Aneja S, et al. Prospective multi-centre sentinel surveillance for Haemophilus influenzae type b & other bacterial meningitis in Indian children. Indian J Med Res. 2013;137:712-20.

17. Ricard JD, Wolff M, Lacherade JC, et al. Levels of vancomycin in cerebrospinal fluid of adult patients receiving adjunctive corticosteroids to treat pneumococcal meningitis: A prospective multicenter observational study. Clin Infect Dis. 2007;44(2):250.
18. Saez-Llorens X, O'Ryan M. Cefepime in the empiric treatment of meningitis in children. Pediatr Infect Dis J. 2001;20:356-61.
19. Shah SS, Ohlsson A, Shah VS. Intraventricular antibiotics for bacterial meningitis in neonates. Cochrane Database Syst Rev. 2012;7:CD004496.
20. Singh J, Sundaresan S, Manoharan A, et al. Serotype distribution and antimicrobial susceptibility pattern in children ≤5 years with invasive pneumococcal disease in India: a systematic review. Vaccine. 2017;35(35 Pt B):4501-9.
21. Southwick FS. Treatment and prognosis of bacterial brain abscess. Uptodate 2017.
22. Thigpen MC, Whitney CG, Messionier NE, et al. Bacterial meningitis in the United States, 1998-2007. Emerging Infections Programs Network. N Engl J Med. 2011;364(21):2016.
23. Tunkel AR, Hartman BJ, Sheldon L, et al. IDSA practice guidelines for the management of bacterial meningitis. CID. 2004:39;1267-84.
24. Tunkel AR, Hasbun R, Bhimraj A. 2017 Infectious Diseases Society of America's clinical practice guidelines for healthcare-associated ventriculitis and meningitis. CID. 2017;64(6):e34-e65.
25. Velissariou IM. The use of fluoroquinolones in children: recent advances. Expert Rev Anti Infect Ther. 2006;4(5):853-60.
26. Verghese VP, Veeraraghavan B, Jayaraman R, et al. Increasing incidence of penicillin- and cefotaxime-resistant *Streptococcus pneumoniae* causing meningitis in India: time for revision of treatment guidelines? Indian J Med Microbiol. 2017;35(2):228-36.
27. Wall EC, Ajdukiewicz KM, Bergman H, et al. Osmotic therapies added to antibiotics for acute bacterial meningitis. Cochrane Database Syst Rev. 2018;2:CD008806.

Antimicrobial Therapy in Infective Endocarditis

27

Chapter

Neha Gupta, Soni Chawla, Ranjit Sah

INTRODUCTION

Infective endocarditis (IE) is microbial infection of the endothelial surfaces of the heart or iatrogenic foreign bodies like prosthetic valves and other intracardiac devices. IE is one of the most intriguing syndromes to diagnose and treat in the landscape of infectious diseases. Early detection and appropriate management of IE with appropriate antibiotics and surgery has implications on healthcare costs, length of hospital stay, mortality, and antimicrobial resistance.

Infective endocarditis appears to be changing globally. There is a change in spectrum and antimicrobial susceptibility of organisms causing IE along with changes in the disease characteristics, treatment, and outcome. Increasing antibiotic resistance may have implications for empiric therapy of culture-negative IE. Nosocomial IE due to multidrug-resistant organisms is on the rise; infection control measures need to be emphasized for preventing nosocomial IE.

EPIDEMIOLOGY

Recently, there has been substantial change in epidemiology of IE. In India, IE is becoming increasingly common in older age group (> 40 years) with no previously known valve disease as compared to younger patients (with mean age 25 years) with underlying valvular heart disease. This is comparable to the data reported by developed countries. In children, the common risk factors include congenital heart disease (CHD) including ventricular septal defect (VSD), cyanotic CHD including shunts, and rheumatic heart disease (RHD).

The most common pathogens causing IE in adults are the Gram-positive cocci including viridians group streptococci, *Staphylococcus aureus* and the enterococci. Overall, prevalence of methicillin-resistant *S. aureus* (MRSA) is less than 10% in the various studies reported. A summary of recent studies relating to etiology of IE in adults in India is summarized in Table 1.

The common causes of endocarditis in children are viridans group streptococci (VGS) and staphylococci. Enterococcal endocarditis is less common in children as compared to adults. There are no large series pertaining to childhood IE from India. However, there is a large series from the United States national inpatient sample database from 2000 to 2010 of IE in children aged less than or equal to 19 years old. An estimated 3,840 children had a discharge diagnosis of IE. The overall incidence was 0.43 per 100,000 children. The incidence was stable over the study period (P = 0.4 for trend). The majority of patients 56.2% were more than or equal to 11 years old and 15.4% were less than or equal to 1 year. Underlying cardiac conditions were present in 53.5% of patients. Overall 30.2% of cases were culture negative. Among those with identified pathogens, *Staphylococcus* species were most common (43.1%) followed by *Streptococcus*

TABLE 1: Microbiologic profile of infective endocarditis in adults.

Study	*Culture positive cases (%)*	*Etiology*
Soman et al. (2018)	53 cases with culture positive endocarditis	VGS (32%), Enterococci (20%), NTM (16%), MSSA (7%), *Candida* (5%), *Aspergillus* (2%),
Gupta et al. (2015)	69% (22/32)	VGS (16%), Enterococci (16%), MSSA (9%), MRSA (6%), *Pseudomonas* (3%), *Klebsiella pneumoniae* (3%), *Scedosporium* (3%), *Candida* (6%), *Brucella* (3%)
Subhramanian et al. (2010)	22.3% (27/121)	VGS (55.5%), *Staphylococcus* species—4 (14.8%) cases. Other species such as *Pseudomonas* species (2/27, 7.4%), *Corynebacterium diphtheriae* (1/27, 3.7%); *Acinetobacter baumannii* complex (1/27, 3.7%), *Salmonella enterica serovar* typhi (1/27, 3.7%), *Granulicatella adiacens* (1/27, 3.7%)

(MRSA: methicillin-resistant *S. aureus*; MSSA: methicillin-sensitive *Staphylococcus aureus*; NTM: nontuberculous mycobacteria; VGS: viridans group streptococci)

species (39.5%). Viridans *Streptococcus* group was most common in those with underlying heart disease (32.7%) and *S. aureus* was most common in those without heart disease (46.9%). Among culture-positive patients, there was a decline in proportion of staphylococcal IE (P = 0.03) and an increase in proportion of streptococcal IE (P = 0.04). Overall mortality was 2.8%. Patients with staphylococcal IE had longer median length of stay (12 vs. 9 days; P < 0.01) and the highest mortality (4.7%).

ANTIMICROBIAL THERAPY FOR INFECTIVE ENDOCARDITIS

Principles

Management of IE is challenging. This is perhaps because:
- The vegetation is avascular. This results in decrease penetration of antibiotic within the vegetation.
- The bacteria are largely nongrowing, metabolically inactive.
- The local host defenses are deficient. Thus, the bacteria are less easily killed by antibiotics.

Thus, it is difficult to eradicate bacteria from the avascular vegetation. Therefore, therapy must be *bactericidal, parenteral, and prolonged.* Antibiotics are generally given parenteral to achieve serum concentrations that, through passive diffusion, lead to effective concentrations in the depths of the vegetation. For β-lactams, as it is the time more than minimum inhibitory concentration (T > MIC) which determines pharmacokinetic-pharmacodynamic (PKPD) parameter more frequent dosing of β-lactam antibiotics are desirable for cure of IE.

Empirical Therapy

Treatment of IE should be started promptly. In sick patients, three sets of blood cultures (one aerobic and one anaerobic) should be drawn at 30 minutes interval before initiation of antibiotics. If the patient is stable then, three sets of cultures should be drawn over 24 hours and if the culture remain negative on day 2, then two to three additional sets can be obtained before initiating antimicrobials. The laboratory should be asked to use special techniques and media to help isolate fastidious organisms such as nutritionally variant streptococci.

The initial choice of empirical treatment depends on which is the likely organism and its likely susceptibility for IE. To arrive at this, a detailed history regarding the onset, duration, and progression of symptoms, predisposing conditions and nosocomial procedures including surgery and valve replacement, history of skin and soft tissue infection (as abscesses), history of urinary tract infection (UTI) or constipation or any genitourinary or gastrointestinal procedures, and prior antibiotic therapy needs to be sought. For children with congenital heart disease, VGS are the most common cause. For patients with indwelling catheters and history of cardiac surgery or prosthetic valve replacement, staphylococci [*S. aureus*/CONS (coagulase-negative staphylococci)] are the most common. Gram-negative bacilli are less common causes of endocarditis because they cannot adhere well to the valvular material with the exception of *Pseudomonas aeruginosa*. Fungal/*Candida* endocarditis is becoming increasingly common in this setting. In newborns, common causes of endocarditis include CONS, *S. aureus,* and *Candida*. Acutely developing endocarditis is more likely to be due to *S. aureus* whereas subacute endocarditis is more likely to be due to CONS/VGS.

Empiric therapy should be started promptly after collecting cultures in sick patients but can be withheld for 48 hours in stable patients till more cultures are collected. Empirical antibiotic therapy is summarized in Table 2 and is based on the principles discussed above.

TABLE 2: Empirical antibiotic therapy for infective endocarditis (IE) (pending blood culture results or when cultures are negative).

	Etiologies (usual)	*Suggested regimens (Primary)*	*Adjunct diagnostic or therapeutic measures or comments*
Native valve endocarditis (no risk factors like indwelling catheters/ surgery/procedures) or late onset prosthetic valve endocarditis (> 1 year)	VGS, *Staphylococcus aureus*, CONS, *Streptococcus gallolyticus,* NVS, enterococci	Ampicillin-sulbactam 3g q6h (Ampicillin—150 mg/ kg/day or sulbactam 50 mg/kg/day) in four divided doses *or* Ceftriaxone 2 g IV q24h Pediatric dose: 80–100 mg/kg/day) in two divided doses *and* Gentamicin 1 mg/kg q8h or 3 mg/kg single dose	Ampicillin sulbactam and gentamicin covers VGS, NVS, MSSA, methicillin-susceptible CONS, enterococci and HACEK group of organisms but not MRSA Combination of ceftriaxone with gentamicin does not cover *Enterococcus* which is not a common cause of infective endocarditis in children
Early prosthetic valve endocarditis (< 1 year)/ recent cardiac surgery/ indwelling catheters/ nosocomial endocarditis	MSSA, MRSA, MR CONS, gram-negative bacilli	Meropenem 60 mg/kg/ day in three divided doses *and* Vancomycin (30–60 mg/ kg/24 hours IV given 6–8 hourly) *and* Rifampicin 300–600 mg q12H po/IV (if prosthetic material present)	Meropenem is for patients with endocarditis very soon after surgery/ with indwelling catheters and especially if there is high prevalence of gram-negative infections in the unit Daptomycin can be used instead of vancomycin if nephrotoxicity

(CONS: coagulase-negative *staphylococci;* HACEK: *Haemophilus* species, *Aggregatibacter* species, *Cardiobacterium hominis, Eikenella corrodens,* and *Kingella* species; IV: intravenous; MR: methicillin resistant; MRSA: methicillin-resistant *Staphylococcus aureus;* MSSA: methicillin-sensitive *Staphylococcus aureus; NVS: nutritionally variant streptococci; PO: per os; VGS:* viridans group streptococci)

DEFINITIVE ANTIMICROBIAL TREATMENT FOR INFECTIVE ENDOCARDITIS

Once cultures are positive, therapy should be optimized as per the organism and drug susceptibility. Blood cultures should be repeated every 2–3 days till negative and the duration of therapy is time after the cultures turn negative. If the patient has been operated then the vegetation should be sent for culture. If the vegetation is negative, duration is from the time treatment was started and if positive, it is from the time of the surgical intervention.

Infective Endocarditis due to Viridans Group of Streptococci, *Streptococcus Gallolyticus* (Formerly Known as *S. Bovis*), *Abiotrophia Defectiva*, and *Granulicatella Species*

Viridans group of streptococci are common pathogenic agents in community-acquired neovascularization elsewhere (NVE) in patients. There are no disc diffusion criteria for VGS and susceptibility should be reported as per penicillin MIC by E-test (epsilometer test) as per Clinical and Laboratory Standards Institute (CLSI). A higher MIC indicates a higher resistance and a bactericidal antibiotic combination for longer duration with addition to gentamicin to the regimen is advised. Gentamicin is administered as a single daily dose in susceptible and relatively resistant VGS IE to achieve maximum concentration above MIC, to decrease nephrotoxicity, for postantibiotic effect (PAE), and postantibiotic leukocyte enhancement. Antibiotic therapy for VGS IE is summarized in Table 3.

TABLE 3: Antibiotic therapy for native valve infective endocarditis (IE) due to viridans group streptococci (VGS) and group D streptococci.

Regimen	*Highly penicillin-susceptible VGS and Streptococcus gallolyticus (bovis) (MIC ≤0.12* µg/mL)	*Relatively resistant VGS (MIC > 0.12–0.5 µg/mL)*	*VGS isolates with a penicillin MIC ≥ 0.5 µg/mL and Abiotrophia and Granulicatella spp. (nutritionally variant streptococci)*
Preferred	Aqueous crystalline penicillin G (CP) sodium 20–40,00,000 units/kg/day IV 4 hourly *Or* 12–18 million U/24 h IV in 4–6 divided doses or continuously if possible	Aqueous crystalline penicillin G (CP) sodium Plus Gentamicin	Aqueous crystalline penicillin G (CP) sodium Plus Gentamicin
Alternative	Ampicillin 200 mg/kg/day in 6 divided doses (Maximum dose—2 g IV in q4h) *Or* Ceftriaxone 50–100 (60 mg/kg/day) in two divided doses (Maximum dose–2 g IV q24h) For penicillin allergy—vancomycin for 4 weeks is an alternative	Ampicillin or ceftriaxone Plus Gentamicin For penicillin allergy—vancomycin for 4 weeks is an alternative	Ampicillin or ceftriaxone (not for NVS) Plus Gentamicin For penicillin allergy—vancomycin for 4 weeks is an alternative

Contd...

Contd...

Regimen	*Highly penicillin-susceptible VGS and Streptococcus gallolyticus (bovis) (MIC ≤ 0.12* μg/mL)	*Relatively resistant VGS (MIC > 0.12–0.5 μg/mL)*	*VGS isolates with a penicillin MIC ≥ 0.5 μg/mL and Abiotrophia and Granulicatella spp. (nutritionally variant streptococci)*
Duration of antibiotic therapy	If only β-lactam is used—then, 4 weeks But if combination of β-lactam with gentamicin (3 mg/kg/day) is used—then, 2 weeks is sufficient except in with known cardiac or extracardiac abscess	β-lactam for 4 weeks and gentamicin for 2 weeks	β-lactam and gentamicin for 6 weeks
Prosthetic valve endocarditis	CP/ampicillin/ceftriaxone for 6 weeks with/without gentamicin for 2 weeks Penicillin allergic—vancomycin for 6 weeks	CP/ampicillin/ceftriaxone for 6 weeks and gentamicin as single dose for 6 weeks Penicillin allergic—vancomycin for 6 weeks	

(MIC: minimum inhibitory concentration; NVS: nutritionally variant streptococci)

Staphylococcal Infective Endocarditis

Infective endocarditis may be caused by staphylococci that are coagulase positive (*S. aureus*) or coagulase negative (*S. epidermidis, S. lugdunensis,* and various other species). A single blood culture positive with *S. aureus* should be considered significant and IE should be ruled out in case of persistent fever or bacteremia or prosthesis. Oxacillin/cefoxitin susceptible *S. aureus* is methicillin-sensitive *S. aureus* (MSSA) whereas oxacillin/cefoxitin resistant *S. aureus* is MRSA.

On the contrary, *S. haemolyticus,* CONS, is a common skin colonizer and blood culture contaminant. It is considered significant only when multiple blood cultures are positive especially in the presence of a prosthesis. Gentamicin should not be used for treatment of NVE caused by MSSA or MRSA. Clindamycin is not recommended as a result of an increased IE relapse rate (Table 4).

TABLE 4: Antibiotic therapy for infective endocarditis (IE) due to staphylococci (doses in Table 2).

Native valve MSSA IE	Cloxacillin/flucloxacillin in 6 divided doses or Cefazolin in 3 divided doses Duration 6 weeks (uncomplicated right-sided endocarditis 2 weeks) Daptomycin in penicillin allergic patients
Prosthetic valve MSSA IE	Cloxacillin or flucloxacillin with Rifampicin pediatric 15 mg/kg/day (maximum dose 900 mg) in 3 divided doses, for 6 weeks with Gentamicin 1 mg/kg TDS for 2 weeks Daptomycin in penicillin allergic patients
Native valve MRSA IE	Vancomycin or daptomycin for 6 weeks
Prosthetic valve MRSA IE	Vancomycin or daptomycin for 6 weeks with rifampicin for 6 weeks with gentamicin 1 mg/kg TDS for 2 weeks

(MRSA: methicillin-resistant *Staphylococcus aureus; MSSA: methicillin-sensitive Staphylococcus aureus;* TDS: thrice a day)

TABLE 5: Antibiotic therapy for infective endocarditis due to *Enterococcus spp.*

	Ampicillin sensitive (MIC ≤ 4 mg/L) and non-HLAR (MIC ≤ 128 mg/L)	*Ampicillin resistant (β-lactamase producing) and non-HLAR*	*Ampicillin resistant (β-lactamase producing) and HLAR/risk of nephrotoxicity*	*Ampicillin resistant (aPBP) and HLAR*
Regimen	Ampicillin with gentamicin	Ampi-sulbactam with gentamicin	Ampi-sulbactam with ceftriaxone	Vancomycin with gentamicin or if risk of nephrotoxicity daptomycin
*Duration**	4–6 weeks	4–6 weeks	6 weeks	6 weeks

(non-HLAR: non-high-level aminoglycoside resistant)

Ampicillin: 200 mg/kg/day in 6 divided doses (maximum dose—2 g IV in q4h). Native valve: 4-week therapy recommended for patients with symptoms of illness less than 3 months; 6-week therapy recommended for native valve symptoms more than 3 months and for patients with prosthetic valve or prosthetic material. Recommended for patients with creatinine clearance more than 50 mL/minute

Ampi-sulbactam with gentamicin: (Ampicillin—150 mg/kg/day and sulbactam 50 mg/kg/day) in 4 divided doses and gentamicin 3 mg/kg/24 hours IV or IM in 3 equally divided doses

Ampi-sulbactam with ceftriaxone: (Ampicillin—150 mg/kg/day with sulbactam 50 mg/kg/day)

Vancomycin with gentamicin: Vancomycin 30 mg/kg/24 hours IV in 2 equally divided doses and gentamicin 3 mg/kg/24 hours IV or IM in 3 equally divided doses

Daptomycin: 8–10 mg/kg/day

Enterococcal Endocarditis

Enterococci IE is increasingly becoming common. Antibiotic therapy is summarized in Table 5.

Haemophilus Species, *Aggregatibacter* Species, *Cardiobacterium Hominis, Eikenella Corrodens,* and *Kingella* Species Endocarditis

Treatment should be with a β-lactamase-stable cephalosporin or amoxicillin if the isolate is susceptible. Gentamicin should only be added for the first 2 weeks of therapy. Ciprofloxacin can be considered an alternative agent. NVE should receive 4 weeks and prosthetic valve endocarditis (PVE) 6 weeks of treatment.

Fungal Endocarditis

Candida is emerging as an important cause of nosocomial endocarditis in neonates, children, and adults. The management of IE due to *Candida* is complex and includes antifungal therapy and surgery. The choice of antifungal therapy depends on susceptibility. The preferred regime is liposomal amphotericin B with flucytosine for at least 6 weeks. Alternative option is to use double dose echinocandins for the same period. Fungal endocarditis was earlier considered an absolute indication for surgery. However, a recent retrospective observational cohort study did not find any difference in the outcome of patients treated with surgery and antifungal therapy as compared to those treated with antifungal therapy. With this, one may defer or avoid surgery in patients who are at high risk for complications or mortality due to cardiac surgery. The new Infectious Diseases Society of America (IDSA) guidelines also recommend maintenance oral therapy with azoles for life in all cases of fungal endocarditis (whether treated medically/surgically) due to high risk of recurrence. This may not always be practically possible due to compliance issues, adverse events, and especially if the isolate is fluconazole resistant.

Culture Negative Infective Endocarditis

Studies show that 30–50% of all endocarditis may be culture negative. This may be due to inadequate microbiologic techniques, fastidious organisms, or administration of antibiotics before collection of the cultures. Therapy of culture negative endocarditis is challenging. An epidemiologic risk assessment should be done to try and determine the most likely cause. The regime is same as that recommended for empiric therapy in Table 2.

SURGERY IN INFECTIVE ENDOCARDITIS

Decisions on surgical intervention are complex and depend on many clinical and prognostic factors that vary among patients, including infecting organism, vegetation size, presence of perivalvular infection, presence of embolism or heart failure, age, noncardiac comorbidities, and available surgical expertise. There is a paucity of evidence available to define the optimal timing of valve surgery. Literature suggests early surgery is associated with improved clinical outcomes in IE (Table 6).

CONCLUSION

Infective endocarditis is a complex illness and should be managed by a multispecialty team with expertise in cardiology, imaging, cardiothoracic surgery, and infectious diseases.

TABLE 6: Indication for surgery in patient with associated condition.

Indication for surgery	*Timing*
Heart failure	
Aortic/mitral IE with severe regurgitation/valve obstruction causing pulmonary edema or cardiogenic shock	Emergency
Aortic/mitral IE with fistula into cardiac chamber or pericardium causing refractory pulmonary edema or shock	Emergency
Aortic/mitral IE with severe acute regurgitation or valve obstruction and persisting heart failure (HF) or echocardiographic signs of poor hemodynamic tolerance	Urgent
Aortic/mitral IE with severe regurgitation and no HF	Elective
Uncontrolled infection	
Locally uncontrolled infection (abscess/aneurysm/fistula/enlarging vegetation)	Urgent
Persisting fever and positive blood culture > 7–10 days	Urgent
Infection caused by fungi or multiresistant organism	Urgent
Prevention of embolism	
Aortic/mitral IE with large vegetation (> 10 mm) following episode of embolism despite appropriate antibiotic therapy	Urgent
Aortic/mitral IE with large vegetation (> 10 mm) and predictor of complicated course	Urgent
Isolated very large vegetation (> 15 mm)	Urgent

(IE: infective endocarditis)

RECOMMENDED READING

1. Agarwal R, Bahl VK, Malaviya AN. Changing spectrum of clinical and laboratory profile of infective endocarditis. J Assoc Physicians India. 1992;40:721-3.
2. Baddour LM, Wilson WR, Bayer AS, et al. Infective endocarditis in adults: diagnosis, antimicrobial therapy, and management of complications. Circulation. 2015;132:1-53.
3. Baltimore RS, Gewitz M, Baddour LM, et al. American Heart Association Rheumatic Fever, Endocarditis, and Kawasaki Disease Committee of the Council of Cardiovascular Disease in the Young and the Council on Cardiovascular and Stroke Nursing. Infective Endocarditis in Childhood: 2015 Update: A scientific statement from the American Heart Association. Circulation. 2015;132(15):1487-515.
4. Fowler VG, Scheld WM, Bayer AS. Chapter 82: Endocarditis and intravascular infections. In: Mandell GL, Bennett JE, Dolin R (Eds). Principles and Practice of Infectious Diseases, 8th edition. Philadelphia, PA: Elsevier Churchill Livingstone; 2015. pp. 990-1028.
5. Garg N, Kandpal B, Tewari S, et al. Characteristics of infective endocarditis in a developing country-clinical profile and outcome in 192 Indian patients, 1992-2001. Int J Cardiol. 2005;15:98:253-60.
6. Gavaldà J, Torres C, Tenorio C, et al. Efficacy of ampicillin plus ceftriaxone in treatment of experimental endocarditis due to Enterococcus faecalis strains highly resistant to aminoglycosides. Antimicrob Agents Chemother. 1999;43:639-46.
7. Gould FK, Denning DW, Elliott TS, et al. Guidelines for the diagnosis and antibiotic treatment of endocarditis in adults: a report of the working party of the British Society for antimicrobial chemotherapy. J Antimicrob Chemother. 2012;67:269-89.
8. Gupta N, Khurana P, Tomar M, et al. Brucella endocarditis-one of the many faces of Brucellosis. Haryana Medical Journal. 2018:41;53-128.
9. Gupta S, Sakhuja A, McGrath E, et al. Trends, microbiology, and outcomes of infective endocarditis in children during 2000-2010 in the United States. Congenit Heart Dis. 2017;12(2):196-201.
10. Habib G, Lancellotti P, Antunes MJ, et al. 2015 ESC guidelines for the management of infective endocarditis. Eur Heart J. 2015;36(44):1-54.
11. Kang DH, Kim YJ, Kim SH, et al. Early surgery versus conventional treatment for infective endocarditis. N Engl J Med. 2012;366:2466-73.
12. Palraj R, Knoll BM, Baddor LM, et al. Chapter 83: Prosthetic valve endocarditis. In: Mandell GL, Bennett JE, Dolin R (Eds). Principles and Practice of Infectious Diseases, 8th edition. Philadelphia, PA: Elsevier Churchill Livingstone; 2015. pp. 1029-40.
13. Pappas PG, Kauffman CA, Andes DR, et al. Clinical Practice Guideline for the Management of Candidiasis: 2016 Update by the Infectious Diseases Society of America. Clin Infect Dis. 2016;62(4): 409-17.
14. Soman R, Gupta N, Shetty A, et al. Implications for diagnosis and treatment of infective endocarditis: Eight year experience of an infectious diseases team in a private tertiary care centre. J Assoc Physicians India. 2018;66:22-5.
15. Soman R, Gupta N, Shetty A, et al. Stent-related NTM endocarditis. J Assoc Physicians India. 2015;63(1):18-21.

Antimicrobial Therapy in Neonatal Sepsis

28
Chapter

Umesh Vaidya, Deepak Karpe, Shilpa Kalane, Gaurav Patwardhan

INTRODUCTION

Management of neonatal sepsis constitutes the major clinical workload of all neonatal units, in view of its prevalence and high mortality and morbidity. The clinician faces challenges in the diagnosis of sepsis, indications and choice of antimicrobials, and duration of treatment. Considerable variations in recommendations, wide choice of drugs, nonavailability of standard bacteriology/reliable sepsis screen markers, and variable local antibiotic resistance patterns lead to indiscriminate and inconsistent use of antimicrobials. The morbid "sepsis phobia" in clinicians leads to anxiety and overtreatment of "precious" babies. The overanxious clinician would attribute any neonatal symptom to sepsis and antibiotics are initiated on the slightest pretext. No wonder, India is facing an enormous and growing problem of antibiotic use and abuse in newborn care. Experts have expressed a lot of concern regarding antibiotic abuse and increasing resistance and the need to bring in rationality in practice guidelines. The present article provides standard recommendations for rational antimicrobial use in neonatal infections.

CURRENT SCENARIO IN INDIA

The National Neonatal Perinatal Database (NNPD) Report 2002–2003 reveals an incidence of neonatal systemic infection of 3% in intramural and 39.7% in extramural births. Septicemia contributes to 18.6% and 39% mortality in the two groups, respectively. In hospital settings, 12.9% of intramural babies and 84.2% extramural babies received antibiotic therapy. In babies diagnosed with systemic infection, only one-third grew organisms in blood culture (proven sepsis); the remaining were clinical sepsis (probable sepsis). The common organisms causing neonatal septicemia were not remarkably different in the intramural and extramural babies. *Klebsiella* (27%), *Staphylococcus aureus* (15%), *Escherichia coli* (12%), and *Pseudomonas* (13%) were the common isolated organisms. Group B *Streptococcus* (GBS) did not figure in the list of isolates.

In a large community-based study carried across 223 villages in Odisha between 2002 and 2005 but published recently in 2017, Panigrahi P et al. reported incidence of culture confirmed sepsis in neonates less than 60 days to be 6.7/1,000 births (84 isolates) with 51% Gram-negative organisms (*Klebsiella* predominating) and 26% gram-positive organisms (most common *S. aureus*). A very high level of resistance to penicillin and ampicillin, moderate resistance to cephalosporins (50%), and extremely low resistance to gentamicin and amikacin was observed.

In another community-based study from South Asia, conducted in Bangladesh, Pakistan, and India (two sites Vellore and Odisha), community healthcare workers visited newborns regularly till the age of 60 days and investigated sepsis-like episodes with blood cultures and molecular studies in blood and respiratory infections. The incidence of possible serious bacterial infections was 95.4/1,000 live births. Etiology could be established in 28% of the cases of which 16% were bacterial and 12% viral. The most common pathogens (as % of all episodes) were RSV (6.5%), *Ureaplasma* (2.8%), *Klebsiella* (1.5%), *E. coli* (1%), Enterovirus/Rhinovirus (1%), *Salmonella* (1%), *Streptococcus pneumoniae* (1%), GBS (1%), and *S. aureus* (1%). The susceptibility of bacterial isolates was fair with 51% being susceptible to ampicillin/penicillin and 75% to gentamicin. 46% of deaths in neonates were due to possible serious bacterial infection (92% bacterial, *E. coli* the most common followed by *Ureaplasma*).

In sharp contrast to the above study, a recently published hospital-based study by the Delhi Neonatal Infection Study (DeNIS) collaboration in *inborn* neonates at three big hospitals, the overall incidence of sepsis was 14·3% of which culture-positive sepsis was 62%. Nearly two-thirds of total episodes occurred at or before 72 hours of life (early onset). 64% of the isolates were Gram-negative organisms (*Acinetobacter* species 22%, *Klebsiella* species 17%, and *E. coli* 14%). The pathogen mix in early-onset sepsis did not differ from that of late-onset sepsis. High rates of multidrug resistance/carbapenem resistance were observed in 40–80% of Gram-negative isolates. Methicillin resistance prevailed in 61% of coagulase-negative staphylococci (CONS) and 38% of *S. aureus* isolates.

In another study by the same group in another hospital in New Delhi which included 2,588 neonates between 2011 and 2015 both outborn and inborn as well as some who were delivered at home, high rates of sepsis were noted [54.7% culture negative sepsis (case fatality rate—CFR 11%), and 13.1% culture positive sepsis (CFR 23.4%)]. A total of 401 pathogens were isolated of which the predominant were *Klebsiella* 12.5% and *Acinetobacter* 11.5%. multidrug-resistant (MDR) and carbapenem resistance was seen in up to 80%. *Candida* was isolated in 22.7% (previously hospitalized babies) but more than three-fourths were babies born at 32 weeks above the weight of 1,500 g.

In our institute, sepsis surveillance (2016–2017) revealed Gram-negative organisms in 70.1% of cases, with *Klebsiella* (47.7%), *Acinetobacter baumannii* (13.6%), and *E. coli* (2.3%) being the common microbes. CONS was the major Gram-positive organism isolated (10.2%) and *S. aureus* had an incidence of 6.8%. Most Gram-negative isolates were sensitive to colistin and amikacin. Resistance to meropenem was very high in the 2015–2016 surveillance after which it was omitted from our formulary leading to re-emergence of better sensitivity profile *(unpublished data)*.

Hence to summarize, the predominant cause of neonatal sepsis in India is Gram-negative (*Klebsiella, E. coli, Acinetobacter*) followed by *S. aureus*. The rates of drug resistance are variable, moderate in community-based studies, and very high in hospital-based studies (even in babies born at home and then admitted directly to the study hospital).

DEFINITION AND DIAGNOSIS OF NEONATAL SEPSIS

Use of standard definitions in reporting neonatal sepsis facilitates proper recording of data and policy making. The following definitions are acceptable and as per standard nomenclature.

Culture Positive/Proven Sepsis

In an infant having clinical picture suggestive of septicemia, pneumonia, or meningitis, the presence of either of the following:

- Isolation of pathogens from blood or cerebrospinal fluid (CSF) or urine or abscess (es)
- Pathological evidence of sepsis on autopsy.

Culture Negative/Probable Sepsis

In an infant having clinical picture suggestive of septicemia, the presence of any one of the following criteria is enough for assigning probable diagnosis of sepsis:

- Existence of predisposing factors: Maternal fever or foul smelling liquor or prolonged rupture of membranes (>24 hours) or gastric polymorphs (>5 per high power field).
- Positive septic screen (two of the four parameters) (1) TLC less than 5,000/mm and band to total polymorph ratio of more than 0.2 (both essential), (2) absolute neutrophil count less than 1,800/cu mm, (3) C-reactive protein (CRP) more than 1 mg/dL, and (4) micro-ESR (erythrocyte sedimentation rate) more than 10 mm 1st hour.
- Radiological evidence of pneumonia.

Early onset sepsis (EOS) is occurrence of sepsis within first 72 hours of life, whereas late onset sepsis (LOS) in occurrence beyond 72 hours of life.

It is mandatory to send blood cultures in neonatal sepsis. Due to high levels of bacteremia, even 0.5–1 mL of blood is sufficient. It is ideal to send a set of cultures (one aerobic and one anaerobic) since the sensitivity is higher and it helps differentiation between contamination and infection (particularly important for CONS). If there is a central line, one set should be sent from the central line and one from the peripheral venipuncture.

APPROACH TO NEONATE WITH SUSPECTED SEPSIS

"Suspected sepsis" is one of the most common diagnoses made in the neonatal intensive care unit (NICU). However, the signs of sepsis are nonspecific, and inflammatory syndromes of noninfectious origin mimic those of neonatal sepsis. As discussed above, all the available diagnostic techniques have their own set of limitations and thus the question of when to start antibiotics is one of the most contentious issues in neonatology.

Early Onset Sepsis

There is scarcity of data and studies evaluating various strategies for management of suspected EOS in preterm neonates especially those who are below 35 weeks gestation after the implementation of intrapartum antibiotic prophylaxis. Traditional approach has been based on presence of various maternal risk factors. These risk factors identified in various studies are presence of chorioamnionitis, prolonged rupture of membranes for more than 18 hours, foul smelling liquor, maternal pyrexia, GBS colonization of maternal genital tract, history of previous sibling with invasive GBS disease, unclean or multiple per vaginal examination, meconium stained amniotic fluid, and low APGAR scores.

There are various predictor scores available, one of which was developed by Singh M et al. This has four independent risk factors each having a score of 2 and two dependent risk factors each with a score of 1. The independent risk factors in this score were foul smelling liquor, maternal pyrexia (≥38°C), unclean vaginal examination, and birth asphyxia. The dependent factors were premature rupture of membranes (PROM) more than or equal to 18 hours and prolonged labor. A score of 4 or more was predictive of EOS in neonates with birth weight of more than 2,500 g and a score of even 1 was predictive of EOS in low birth weight babies as preterm infants (<34 weeks' gestation or <1,500 g) are at significantly increased risk for EOS. Additional data are needed to ascertain the independent roles of maternal risk factors (including chorioamnionitis), clinical signs of illness, and laboratory findings in guiding empiric antibiotic therapy. Until such data are available, it is reasonable to continue to stratify risk based on those traditional risk factors. Because most preterm infants have clinical signs of illness, most will qualify for empiric treatment. Preterm infants who appear well and have minimal or no risk factors (e.g. no chorioamnionitis, preterm premature rupture of membranes, or GBS colonization with inadequate intrapartum prophylaxis) may be candidates for close monitoring and serial laboratory evaluation.

Among asymptomatic late-preterm and term infants with risk factors as defined by the Centers for Disease Control and Prevention (CDC) (including but not limited to clinical chorioamnionitis), the risk of EOS is extremely low. In infants more than 34 weeks of gestational age, there have been attempts to decrease the use of empirical antibiotic therapy. Investigators in Boston and Northern California have taken the lead in implementing a change in practice. Recognizing the potential inconsistency in making the diagnosis of chorioamnionitis, they have chosen to rely upon maternal fever alone as a surrogate for the risk associated with chorioamnionitis. Using data from more than 600,000 infants more than or equal to 34 weeks' gestation at birth, they developed a model for EOS risk prediction based on maternal factors (gestational age, GBS colonization, duration of ruptured membranes, highest intrapartum temperature, and nature and duration of intrapartum antibiotics), and then combined that model with findings from examination of the infants to stratify subgroups according to EOS attack rates. Based on the maternal factors, the neonates are classified into three groups according to EOS risk at birth (<0.65, 0.65–1.54 or ≥1.54 per 1,000 births). These neonates were further classified as treat empirically (4.1% of all live births, 60.8% of all EOS cases, sepsis incidence of 8.4/1,000 live births), observe and evaluate (11.1% of births, 23.4% of cases, 1.2/1,000), and continued observation (84.8% of births, 15.7% of cases, incidence 0.11/1,000) based on clinical examination findings. They concluded that it is possible to combine objective maternal data with evolving objective neonatal clinical findings to define more efficient strategies for the evaluation and treatment of EOS in term and late preterm infants and judicious application of their protocol could result in decreased antibiotic treatment in 80,000–240,000 US newborns. Based on this strategy, they have devised a predictive score for EOS which is available for free access at *https://neonatalsepsiscalculator.kaiserpermanente.org/*.

To summarize, the approach to a baby with suspected EOS depends on the gestation, maternal risk factors, and clinical appearance. Flowchart 1 gives an algorithm of management of suspected EOS.

Late Onset Sepsis

The organisms causing hospital-acquired infections are invariably resistant to first-line antibiotics. Most of the cases are by Gram-negative organisms in India. Gram-negative septicemia is generally more severe and is associated with acute deterioration and septic shock. CONS and fungal sepsis are more indolent. Biomarkers for sepsis such as CRP, immature to total leukocyte ratio, and absolute neutrophil count have a better sensitivity and specificity in LOS as compared to EOS.

Flowchart 2 shows a simple approach to a neonate with suspected LOS. As the signs of sepsis in a neonate are variable and diverse, clinical experience and close observation are essential for diagnosis. Both overdiagnosis and complacency can be detrimental and objective evaluation rather than "personal anxiety" should be used in diagnosis. If the clinical condition of the baby

Flowchart 1: Management of suspected early onset sepsis (EOS).

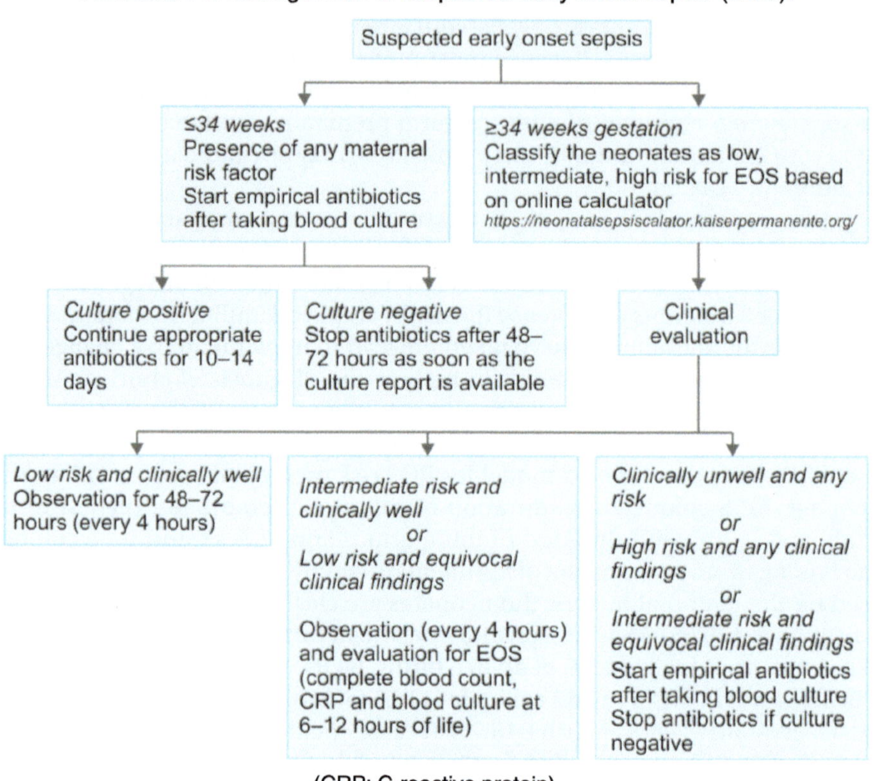

(CRP: C-reactive protein)

is stable, one should wait for results of the sepsis screen before initiation of antibiotic therapy. Appropriate clinical stabilization may be done while awaiting results. However, if there is reasonable clinical ground for suspicion of sepsis of rapid deterioration in general condition, early antibiotic therapy is mandatory. A lumbar puncture is recommended in all neonates with suspected sepsis prior to or along with initiation of antibiotic therapy.

WHICH ANTIBIOTIC TO USE FOR EMPIRIC THERAPY?

Universal recommendation for empiric therapy cannot be made as considerable variations occur in bacteriological patterns across units. Most of the recommendations for empirical therapy are dated and are based on the most common organisms isolated which used to be GBS causing EOS and CONS, *S. aureus,* and *Candida* causing LOS. Thus, the recommendations are for penicillin/ semisynthetic penicillin or cephalosporin with an aminoglycoside. As discussed earlier, penicillin/ semisynthetic penicillin and now even cephalosporins have widespread resistance in most available surveillance data, although aminoglycosides continue to be very useful first-line drugs. As most cases of both early and LOS are due to Gram-negative organisms, the recommendations for empirical therapy continue to include an aminoglycoside. However, aminoglycosides cannot be used alone and need a beta lactam. The choice of the beta lactam is variable and depends on the likelihood of resistance and may include either cefotaxime or piperacillin-tazobactam or a

Flowchart 2: Approach to a neonate with suspected late onset sepsis.

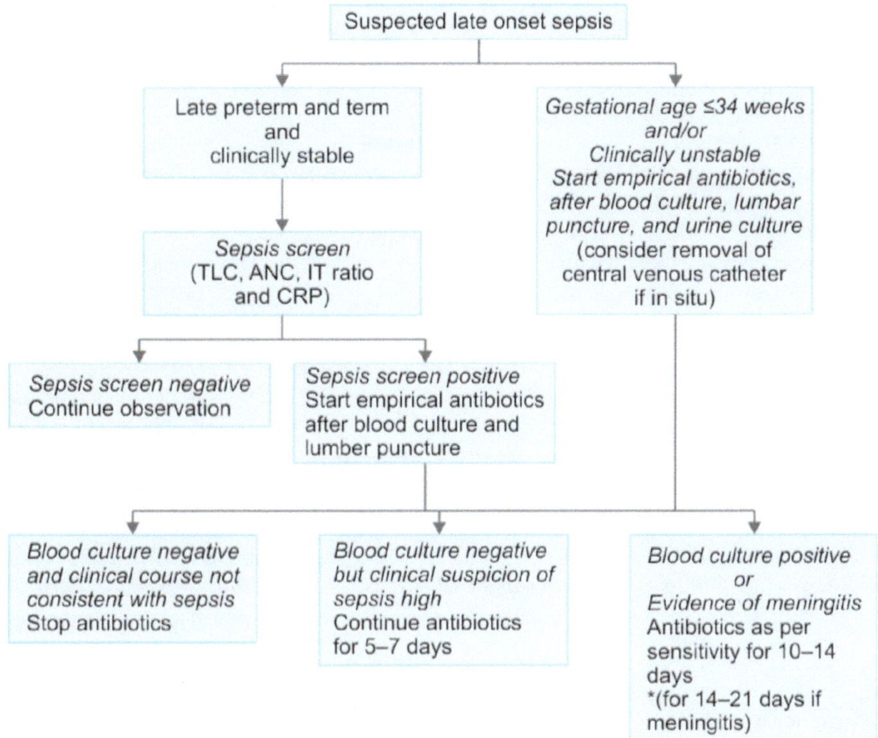

(ANC: absolute neutrophil count; CRP: C-reactive protein; IT ratio: immature neutrophils to total neutrophil count ratio; TLC: total leukocyte count)

carbapenem. Thus, the best policy can only be framed and implemented with regular bacteriological surveillance and data on sensitivity patterns. Hospitals need to form an antibiotic stewardship committee consisting of microbiologists, clinicians, nurses, and members of administration, to carry out surveillance and forming antibiotic policy that is best suited to respective units. All newer antibiotics should be periodically evaluated and use should be regulated.

The antibiotic policy practiced in NICUs in most corporate hospitals is shown in Tables 1 and 2. It is needless to state that certain alterations from the basic policy may be necessary in individual situations. The antibiotic policy needs to be reviewed for its suitability over a period of time.

MODIFICATION OF THERAPY

This is dependent on the clinical course and reports of culture susceptibility. If cultures are positive, therapy should be optimized. If cultures and negative then antibiotics can be stopped if sepsis is unlikely (*see* Flowcharts 1 and 2). If cultures are negative and the baby is deteriorating, cultures should be repeated and therapy escalated as per the unit protocol. The doses of commonly used antibiotics in neonatal sepsis is listed in Table 2.

TABLE 1: Empiric antibiotic policy for neonatal sepsis.

	Indication	*Antibiotics*	*Comments*
First line	Risk of sepsis (premature rupture of membranes, maternal fever, foul smelling liquor)	Third-generation cephalosporin + gentamicin	
Second line	Nosocomial/outborn referral with no previous antibiotic use	Piperacillin tazobactam/ meropenem With amikacin	Vancomycin if *Staphylococcus* suspected
Third line	Nosocomial infection with prior extreme antibiotic use Outborn referral of neonate who is very sick and shows rapid deterioration along with extreme prior antibiotic use	Colistin + Meropenem	Choice may vary based on previous antibiotic use and local susceptibility patterns Vancomycin if MRSA/ MRSE rates high Antifungals (fluconazole/ amphotericin B if indicated)

(MRSA: Methicillin-resistant *Staphylococcus aureus*; MRSE: methicillin-resistant *Staphylococcus epidermidis*)

TABLE 2: Drug doses (mg/kg) of commonly used antibiotics in neonates.

Drug	*Route*	*Birth weight <2,000 g*		*Birth weight >2,000 g*	
		0–7 days	*>7 days*	*0–7 days*	*>7 days*
Amikacin	IV, IM	7.5q 12 h	7.5q 8 h	7.5q 12 h	7.5q 8 h
Ampicillin, Doses for meningitis	IV IV, IM	25q 12 h 50q 12 h	75q 8 h 50q 8 h	75q 8 h 50q 8 h	100q 6 h 75q 6 h
Cefotaxime	IM, IV	50q 12 h	50q 12 h	50q 8 h	50q 6 h
Ceftazidime	IM, IV	50q 12 h	50q 8 h	50q 8 h	50q 8 h
Ceftriaxone	IM, IV	50q 24 h	50q 24 h	50q 24 h	75q 24 h
Ceftizoxime	IV, IM	50q 12 h	50q 12 h	50q 12 h	50q 12 h
Colistin	IV	Loading dose of 150,000 IU and then the same dose in 2–3 divided doses			
Gentamicin	IV, IM	4q 48 h	4q 24 h	4q 36 h	4q 24 h
Levofloxacin	IV	10q 12 h	10q 12 h	10q 12 h	10q 12 h
Meropenem Dose for meningitis	IV, IM	20q 12 h 40q 12 h	20q 8 h 40q 12 h	20q 12 h 40q 12 h	20q 8 h 40q 12 h
Penicillin G*	IV, IM	25,000 U q 12 h 75,000–100,000 U q 12 h	25,000 U q 8 h 75,000–100,000 U q 8 h	25,000 U q 8 h 75,000–100,000 U q 8 h	25,000 U q 6 h 75,000–100,000 U q 6 h
Piperacillin tazobactam (dosed for piperacillin)	IV, IM	75q 12 h	75q 8 h	75q 8 h	75q 6 h
Vancomycin	IV	15 mg q 18 h	15 mg q 12 h	15 mg q 12 h	15 mg q 8 h
Linezolid	IV	10 mg q 12 h	10 mg q 8h	10 mg q 8 h	10 mg q 8 h

*All doses except penicillin G are expressed in mg/kg
(IM: intramuscular; IV: intravenous)

MANAGEMENT OF SPECIFIC INFECTIONS IN NEONATES

Neonatal Meningitis

Antibiotic therapy should achieve adequate drug levels to sterilize the CSF. Antibiotics, which have a good CSF penetration, should be chosen. Until a definitive diagnosis has been made, a combination of a third-generation cephalosporin and an aminoglycoside should be started intravenously immediately after the cultures have been drawn. Third-generation cephalosporins are recommended because of good CSF penetration and safety profile. Aminoglycosides have poor CSF penetration and should not be used as sole agents for therapy of meningitis. Controlled trials have failed to show any benefit of intraventricular or intrathecal therapy over systemic therapy. For nosocomially acquired meningitis or meningitis after previous antibiotic use, a carbapenem (meropenem) with/without an aminoglycoside may be indicated.

Once a specific pathogen has been isolated and its susceptibilities identified, the best drug or combination of drugs should be employed. Benzyl penicillin/ampicillin is the drug of choice for GBS infection. A combination of ampicillin and gentamicin, which have synergistic action, is preferred in infections with *Listeria* and *Enterococci*. In most hospital-acquired cases of meningitis, usually carbapenems with or without colistin may be required owing to the high prevalence of resistance in Gram-negative organisms.

A CSF examination should be repeated 48 hours after initiation of antibiotics to document improvement. With appropriate antibiotic therapy, the CSF becomes sterile very quickly. Pleocytosis and alteration of CSF chemistry may continue for some weeks making later CSF results difficult to interpret. Antimicrobial therapy should be continued for a minimum of 14 days for Gram-positive organisms (4 weeks for *S. aureus*) and 21 days for Gram-negative organisms.

Neonatal Pneumonia

Pneumonia in neonates may be acquired in utero (congenital), during birth, or nosocomially. Congenital pneumonia may be caused by TORCH (Toxoplasmosis, Other (syphilis, varicella-zoster, parvovirus B19), Rubella, Cytomegalovirus (CMV), and Herpes infections) group of organisms, *Listeria,* or secondary to chorioamnionitis. Pneumonia acquired during passage through the maternal genital tract may be due to GBS, *E. coli, Klebsiella* species, *Mycoplasma hominis, Ureaplasma urealyticum,* and *Chlamydia trachomatis.* In nosocomial pneumonia, common organisms involved are *S. aureus, S. epidermidis, E. coli, Klebsiella,* and *P. aeruginosa.*

For early onset pneumonia, therapy should be with ampicillin/penicillin or third-generation cephalosporin/beta lactam-beta lactamase inhibitor combination and an aminoglycoside. The choice depends on the setting and local resistance patterns. For nosocomial pneumonia, choice depends on the prevalent microbial flora in NICU and their sensitivity. Azithromycin or erythromycin is the drug of choice for suspected infections due to atypical pathogens. There is no consensus regarding duration of therapy but shorter courses may be as effective as prolonged courses.

Urinary Tract Infection

The most frequent infecting organism is *E. coli,* but *Klebsiella* species and *Enterococci* can also cause urinary tract infection (UTI). In very preterm LBW babies and who have received long courses of antibiotics, *Candida albicans* is an important etiological agent.

Empirical therapy with a broad-spectrum cephalosporin and gentamicin may be started but antibiotics must be changed according to urine culture reports. Treatment duration in absence of a positive blood or CSF culture is 10–14 days. It is recommended that infants with UTI undergo renal ultrasound and vesicourethrocystogram imaging to identify any underlying anatomic or functional abnormalities (reflux) that may have contributed to the development of the UTI. Infants should receive UTI prophylaxis with amoxicillin (10-20 mg/kg once a day) after completing UTI treatment until imaging studies are performed.

Osteomyelitis and Septic Arthritis

The most common organism causing osteomyelitis and septic arthritis is *S. aureus*. Group B streptococci; *Klebsiella,* and *E. coli* are also prominent. *S. epidermidis* and *C. albicans* are emerging as important etiological agents in extremely preterm infants.

All efforts should be made to obtain material for culture and sensitivity. In patients with community-acquired infection, third-generation cephalosporin with cloxacillin should be started until culture and sensitivity results are available. In patients with history of prolonged NICU stay, treatment depends on local flora and should include an antifungal. Therapy should be continued for at least 6 weeks.

Neonatal Tetanus

Treatment of neonatal tetanus consists of the administration of human tetanus immunoglobulin (Ig) (500 units) and crystalline penicillin (50,000 units/kg/day) for 10–14 days as well as supportive care with mechanical ventilation, sedatives, and muscle relaxants.

DURATION OF ANTIBIOTIC THERAPY

Standard recommendations for duration of antibiotic treatment are shown in Table 3. Recent evidence suggests that it is rational and safe to stop antibiotics after 48–72 hours, if sepsis screen and blood culture are negative. The decision should include consideration of the clinical course as well as the risks associated with longer courses of antimicrobial agents. In a retrospective study by Cordero and Ayers, the average duration of treatment in 695 infants (<1,000 g) with negative blood cultures was 5 ± 3 days. Cotten et al. have suggested an association with prolonged

TABLE 3: Duration of antibiotic therapy.

Condition/diagnosis	*Duration*
Bone/joint infection	4–6 weeks
Meningitis • Gram-positive organisms (except *Staphylococcus aureus*) • *S. aureus* • Gram-negative organisms	 14 days 28 days 21 days
Pneumonia (culture negative)	7–10 days
Urinary tract infection	10–14 days
Culture positive sepsis (no meningitis)	14 days
Clinical sepsis (based on clinical suspicion and/or septic screen positivity	7–10 days

administration of antimicrobial agents (>5 days) in infants with suspected early-onset sepsis (and negative blood cultures) with death and necrotizing enterocolitis (NEC). Two recent papers also support this association. Unwarranted prolonged use of antibiotics increases the risk of emergence of resistant strains.

There is also controversy regarding duration of therapy in those with proven sepsis. Recent data shows shorter courses of antibiotics to be as effective as traditional long courses. One trial comparing 10 versus 14 days of therapy found that there was no difference in treatment failure if the neonate was asymptomatic and with normal CRP at the 7th day, but the 10-day group had significantly shorter hospitalizations. Another trial testing 7 days versus 14 days of therapy, in asymptomatic newborns at day 7, found a nonsignificant trend toward greater treatment failure in the short course arm. Both of these trials had small sample sizes and were performed in neonates with a gestational age more than 32 weeks and birth weight more than 1,500 g. The length of optimal duration might also depend on the pathogen. In *S. aureus* infection, a short course of antibiotic (7 versus 14 days) is significantly associated with higher treatment failures. Conversely, treatments of only 3 days have been effective in CONS sepsis. Until more data is available, the traditional duration of therapy is recommended which is shown in Table 3.

FUNGAL SEPSIS

As discussed earlier, fungi are assuming an important role in nosocomial sepsis especially in extremely low-birth weight and very low-birth weight infants who have prolonged NICU stay and who have received antibiotics. Receipt of total parenteral nutrition (TPN) especially intralipids and presence of central lines and gut surgery are other important risk factors. Empirical antifungal therapy should be initiated appropriately in babies with these risk factors and clinical features of sepsis. Thrombocytopenia and indolent course may be a pointer. Blood cultures are positive only in 50% of instances. The choice of empirical therapy depends on whether the baby has received fluconazole in the past and the prevalence of azole resistant *Candida* in the unit. Choices include fluconazole at the rate of loading at 25 mg/kg and then 12 mg/kg/day or amphotericin B. Recent guidelines from the Infectious Diseases Society of America (IDSA) prefer the use of conventional amphotericin B for neonatal candidiasis as opposed to liposomal amphotericin B owing to high incidence of renal involvement in neonates where the liposomal amphotericin B is ineffective. Echinocandins are not the preferred drugs since there is lack of data and poor penetration of brain and kidneys which are commonly involved in neonatal candidiasis. The duration of therapy for systemic fungal infection is 3 weeks after blood cultures are negative. Ophthalmic examination should be done to rule out endophthalmitis. CSF should be done to rule out meningeal involvement. If CNS involvement is present, treatment is required for several weeks till all clinical, CSF, and radiologic abnormalities have resolved.

ANTIMICROBIAL PROPHYLAXIS

There is no role for prophylactic antibacterial therapy in neonates. Prophylactic treatment has been studied in neonates with central venous catheters, invasive ventilation, meconium aspiration, and NEC and none of the studies have found significant benefit considering the risk of development of antimicrobial resistance.

Antifungal prophylaxis has some role especially in extremely low-birth weight neonates. Antifungal prophylaxis appears to be effective in reducing the incidence of *Candida* colonization and invasive *Candida* infections in the NICU. Both nystatin and fluconazole have been studied;

however, most of the literature has evaluated fluconazole beginning soon after birth and continuing for the first 4–6 weeks of life. A recent meta-analysis reported reduction in invasive candidiasis in neonates receiving fluconazole with no impact on resistance. Current guidelines from the IDSA recommend intravenous (IV) or oral fluconazole, 3–6 mg/kg twice weekly for 6 weeks in neonates with birth weights less than 1,000 g in nurseries with high rates (>10%) of invasive candidiasis.

ADJUNCTIVE THERAPY IN NEONATAL SEPSIS (TABLE 4)

Few immunologic interventions to treat or prevent neonatal sepsis have been reliably evaluated in randomized controlled trials (RCTs), because of inadequate sample sizes. Promising or possible therapeutic interventions in severe or Gram-negative sepsis include exchange transfusions, pentoxifylline, and IgM-enriched intravenous immunoglobulin (IVIG). Promising or possible prophylactic interventions include lactoferrin, with or without a probiotic; selenium; early curtailment of antibiotics after sterile cultures; and earlier initiation of breast milk (colostrum) in high-risk preterm infants. Current probiotic products are safe and effective in substantially reducing all-cause mortality and NEC, with no increase in sepsis.

TABLE 4: Adjunctive therapy in neonatal sepsis.

Intervention	*Outcomes and conclusions*
Granulocyte transfusion	No difference shown in mortality or sepsis: more RCTs needed
G-CSF or GM-CSF	No difference shown in mortality or sepsis: more RCTs needed GM-CSF improves survival in sepsis with neutropenia
Activated protein C	Not recommended
Exchange transfusion	Improves survival in Gram-negative sepsis
Pentoxifylline	Improves survival in proved sepsis, more RCTs needed
Reduce oxidative stress: Selenium	Insufficient evidence
Melatonin	Insufficient evidence
Glutamine	No difference shown in mortality or sepsis or disability free survival: More RCTs not a high priority
Lactoferrin	Reduce late-onset sepsis, RCTs needed to evaluate effects on disability-free survival
Probiotic	Reduce all-cause mortality and NEC
Prebiotics	Insufficient evidence
Broad-spectrum peripartum antibiotics	Broad-spectrum antenatal antibiotics increase NEC, functional impairment, and cerebral palsy at 7 years Prolonged postnatal antibiotic therapy after sterile cultures is associated with increased risk of death and NEC. RCTs needed to evaluate effect of early curtailment of antibiotics after sterile cultures on disability-free survival
IVIG	No role
Breast milk	Reduces sepsis

(G-CSF: granulocyte-colony stimulating factor; GM-CSF: granulocyte/macrophage-colony stimulating factor; IVIG: intravenous immunoglobulin; NEC: necrotizing enterocolitis; RCT: randomized controlled trial)

GOLDEN RULES FOR RATIONAL USE OF ANTIBIOTICS IN NEONATES

- Enforce strict measures to prevent nosocomial infection. Relook at hand washing practices, disinfection protocols, procedure asepsis, minimum invasion, equipment sharing, nurse patient ratio, isolation policy, and training (Box 1).
- Form Neonatal Infection Review Group and monitor bacteriological patterns and sensitivity on a monthly basis. Such group should include microbiology personnel, nurse, residents along with neonatologist.
- Improve laboratory capabilities in bacteriology and sepsis screen makers sufficiently, so that antibiotics can be stopped with confidence if sepsis work up is negative. Prolonged, unwarranted use of antibiotics does not prevent, but in fact causes antibiotic resistance.
- Formulate antibiotic policy using bacteriology surveillance data. Use antibiotics with low resistance potential like amikacin, piperacillin, quinolones, and cefepime.
- Restrict use of antibiotics with high resistance potential such as ceftazidime and meropenem.
- Always perform sepsis screen/blood culture before starting antibiotics.
- Never treat colonization such as positive endotracheal tube (ETT) culture/catheter tip culture unless strong clinical/systemic infection.
- Do not start prophylactic antibiotics just because of central catheter, chest drain, surgery, etc. Such procedures are expected to be done in an aseptic manner.
- Follow standard recommendations on dose and duration of antibiotic treatment in proven sepsis.
- Avoid indiscriminate use of newer antibiotics in clinical practice unless appropriately studied for sensitivity pattern.

BOX 1: Potential better practices for preventing nosocomial infection.

Hand washing
- Meticulous attention to hand washing, with regular monitoring and surveillance of hand washing practice and reporting of compliance

Nutrition
- No alteration of hyperalimentation solutions after preparation
- Initiation of enteral feedings as early as possible
- Reduced exposure to IV lipids and hyperalimentation
- Promotion of the use of human milk, ensuring proper collection and storage

Skin care
- Initiation of a skin care protocol for all neonates weighing <1,000 g, the goals of which are to promote skin maturation and to prevent skin breakdown
- Reduced laboratory testing that requires venipuncture or heel stick
- Development of a systematic approach to IV therapy that reduces the frequency and number of skin punctures for placement of an IV catheter

Respiratory care
- Minimization of intubation days
- Minimization of the interruption of the ventilator-endotracheal tube circuit

Vascular access
- Minimization of the use of central lines, and when used, minimization of the frequency of daily entries and the duration of use
- Prospective placement of central lines when IV therapy will be of long duration
- Establishment of sound policies and procedures for line care and access and regular monitoring of compliance

RECOMMENDED READING

1. Benitz WE, Wynn JL, Polin RA. Reappraisal of guidelines for management of neonates with suspected early-onset sepsis. J Pediatr. 2015;166(4):1070-4.
2. Cantoni L, Ronfani L, Da Riol R, et al. Perinatal Study Group of the Region Friuli-Venezia Giulia. Physical examination instead of laboratory tests for most infants born to mothers colonized with group B *Streptococcus*: support for the Centers for Disease Control and Prevention's 2010 recommendations. J Pediatr. 2013;163:568-73.
3. Chowdhary G, Dutta S, Narang A. Randomized controlled trial of 7-day vs. 14-day antibiotics for neonatal sepsis. J Trop Pediatr. 2006;52:427-32.
4. Cordero L, Ayers LW. Duration of empiric antibiotics for suspected early-onset sepsis in extremely low birth weight infants. Infect Control Hosp Epidemiol. 2003;24:662-6.
5. Cotten CM, Taylor S, Stoll B, et al. NICHD Neonatal Research Network. Prolonged duration of initial empirical antibiotic treatment is associated with increased rates of necrotizing enterocolitis and death for extremely low birth weight infants. Pediatrics. 2009;123:58-66.
6. Escobar G, Zukin T, Usatia NI, et al. Early discontinuation of antibiotic treatment in newborns admitted to rule out sepsis, a decision rule. Pediatr Infect Dis J. 1994;13:860-6.
7. Escobar GJ, Puopolo KM, Wi S, et al. Stratification of risk of early-onset sepsis in newborns ≥ 34 weeks' gestation. Pediatrics. 2014;133:30-6.
8. Flidel-Rimon O, Galstyan S, Juster-Reicher A, et al. Limitations of the risk factor based approach in early neonatal sepsis evaluations. Acta Paediatr. 2012;101:e540-4.
9. Gathwala G, Sindwani A, Singh J, et al. Ten days vs. 14 days antibiotic therapy in culture-proven neonatal sepsis. J Trop Pediatr. 2010;56:433-5.
10. Hashavya S, Benenson S, Ergaz-Shaltiel Z, et al. The use of blood counts and blood cultures to screen neonates born to partially treated group B *Streptococcus*-carrier mothers for early-onset sepsis: is it justified? Pediatr Infect Dis J. 2011;30:840-3.
11. Hemels MA, van den Hoogen A, Verboon-Maciolek MA, et al. Shortening the antibiotic course for the treatment of neonatal coagulase-negative staphylococcal sepsis: fine with three days? Neonatology. 2012;101:101-5.
12. Investigators of the Delhi Neonatal Infection Study (DeNIS) collaboration. Characterisation and antimicrobial resistance of sepsis pathogens in neonates born in tertiary care centres in Delhi, India: a cohort study. Lancet Glob Health. 2016;4(10):e752-60.
13. Isaacs D, Wilkimson AR, Moxon ER. Duration of antibiotic courses for neonates. Arch Dis Childhood. 1987;62:727-44.
14. Isacs D. Neonatal sepsis: the antibiotic crisis. Indian Pediatr. 2005;42:9-13.
15. Jackson GL, Rawiki P, Sendelbach D, et al. Hospital course and short-term outcomes of term and late preterm neonates following exposure to prolonged rupture of membranes and/or chorioamnionitis. Pediatr Infect Dis J. 2012;31:89-90.
16. Jajoo M, Manchanda V, Chaurasia S, et al. Investigators of the Delhi Neonatal Infection Study (DeNIS) collaboration, New Delhi, India. Alarming rates of antimicrobial resistance and fungal sepsis in outborn neonates in North India. PLoS One. 2018;13(6):e0180705.
17. Kuppala VS, Meinzen-Derr J, Morrow AL, et al. Prolonged initial empirical antibiotic treatment is associated with adverse outcomes in premature infants. J Pediatr. 2011;159:720-5.
18. Mordi T, Isaacs D, Dutta S, et al. Adjuncive immunological interventions in neonatal sepsis. Clin Perinatol. 2010;37:481-99.
19. National Neonatal Perinatal Database: Report 2002-2003. ICMR, New Delhi Publications; 2005. pp. 45-57.
20. Ottolini MC, Lundgren K, Mirkinson LJ, et al. Utility of complete blood count and blood culture screening to diagnose neonatal sepsis in the asymptomatic at risk newborn. Pediatr Infect Dis J. 2003;22:430-4.

21. Panigrahi P, Chandel DS, Hansen NI, et al. Neonatal sepsis in rural India: timing, microbiology and antibiotic resistance in a population-based prospective study in the community setting. J Perinatol. 2017;37(8):911-21.
22. Pappas PG, Kauffman CA, Andes DR, et al. Executive summary: Clinical Practice Guideline for the Management of Candidiasis: 2016 Update by the Infectious Diseases Society of America. Clin Infect Dis. 2016;4:409-17.
23. Paul VK, Agarwal R. Neonatal sepsis. NNF Manual of Neonatal Care, 1st edition. Prism Books Pvt Ltd; 2014. pp. 121-34.
24. Polin RA, Saiman L. Nosocomial infections in the neonatal intensive care unit. Neoreviews. 2003;4:e81
25. Puopolo KM, Draper D, Wi S, et al. Estimating the probability of neonatal early-onset infection on the basis of maternal risk factors. Pediatrics. 2011;128:e1155-63.
26. Saha SK, Schrag SJ, El Arifeen S, et al. Causes and incidence of community-acquired serious infections among young children in south Asia (ANISA): an observational cohort study. Lancet. 2018;392(10142):145-59.
27. Singh M1, Narang A, Bhakoo ON. Predictive perinatal score in the diagnosis of neonatal sepsis. J Trop Pediatr. 1994;40(6):365-8.
28. Volpe JJ. Neonatal meningitis. In: Volpe JJ (Ed). Neurology of the Newborn, 3rd edition. Philadelphia: WB Saunders; 1995. pp. 730-68.
29. Wamg EE, Ohlsson A, Kelner JD. Association of Ureaplasma urealyticum colonisation with CLD of prematurity: result of a meta analysis. J Pediatr. 1995;127:640-4.

Antimicrobial Therapy in Septic Shock

29
Chapter

Soonu Udani, Ambreen A Pandrowala

INTRODUCTION

Sepsis is a clinical syndrome complicating severe infection that is characterized by systemic inflammation, immune dysregulation, microcirculatory derangements, and end-organ dysfunction. Septic shock refers to sepsis with cardiovascular dysfunction (i.e. need for vasoactive drug administration to maintain perfusion) despite fluid resuscitation. Severe sepsis and septic shock are characterized by dysfunction of two or more organ systems and cardiovascular dysfunction.

Shock is a life-threatening condition of circulatory failure that most commonly presents with hypotension. It can also have other vital sign changes with elevated serum lactate levels. The effects of shock are initially reversible but can rapidly become irreversible, resulting in multiorgan failure (MOF) and death. Thus, when a patient presents with undifferentiated hypotension and/or is suspected of having shock, it is important that the clinician rapidly identify the etiology so that appropriate therapy can be administered to prevent MOF and death.

Prompt identification of shock, rapid resuscitation, and antibiotic therapy as closely targeted to the cause, form the first-line of the management bundle.

MICROBIAL ETIOLOGY OF SEPTIC SHOCK

The microbial etiology of septic shock depends on the age, whether infection is community or hospital acquired and the underlying immune status of the individual.

In community-acquired infections (CAIs), the usual source of infection is most commonly pneumonia followed by intra-abdominal and urinary tract infections (UTIs). The most common pathogens here are *Streptococcus pneumoniae, Staphylococcus aureus, Escherichia coli,* and *Klebsiella pneumoniae.* During recent years with alarming rise in multidrug resistance it is not uncommon for sepsis due to community-acquired bacteria to be multidrug resistant. In nosocomial infections, the usual causes are multidrug resistant Gram-negative pathogens including *E. coli, K. pneumoniae, Acinetobacter,* and *Pseudomonas*. Methicillin-resistant *S. aureus* (MRSA) and *Candida* also account for some infections. In neonates, the usual pathogens are again enteric Gram-negative pathogens including *E. coli* and *Klebsiella* as well as *S. aureus.* Certain host conditions predispose to fungal or unusual infections, e.g. neutropenia, primary immunodeficiency, etc.

In a study from Kochi, India in children with severe sepsis and septic shock, the predominant isolates were *E. coli* (30.4%), *K. pneumoniae* (20.3%), and *S. aureus* (8.9%). In patients with severe sepsis, the main isolate from blood specimens was *E. coli* (21/65, 32.3%) followed by *K. pneumoniae* (11/65, 16.9%). A point prevalence study to determine the global epidemiology of pediatric sepsis [the SPROUT (Sepsis Prevalence, Outcomes, and Therapies) study] recruited 6,925 patients from 128 pediatric intensive care units (PICUs) in 26 countries (two sites from India). In the Indian sites, the prevalence of severe sepsis was 8.2%; median age was 3 years; the respiratory tract was the most common site; and 65% of all cases were culture positive. Gram-positive and Gram-negative pathogens contributed to a quarter each of severe sepsis while fungi were isolated in 13%. *S. aureus was the most common pathogen. The mortality rate was 25%.* Recent couple of large studies in neonatal sepsis from Delhi, India in both inborn and outborn babies has shown a predominance of Gram-negative pathogens with very high rates of multidrug and carbapenem resistance.

FIRST HOUR BUNDLE FOR SEPTIC SHOCK

The "bundle" approach to septic shock has been advocated by several consensus groups. The outcome improves with a team approach and a fixed time frame with goals at every stage. Quick and often empirical treatment of the infection, which is often unknown, is an important intervention, as most other interventions are purely supportive (Box 1).

Unless the organism and sensitivity are known, broad-spectrum intravenous (IV) antibiotic therapy should begin in 1 hour of arrival/presentation, preferably after obtaining appropriate blood or other site cultures. The regimen should cover all likely pathogens since there is little margin for error in critically ill patients.

Two large bore IV sites need to be obtained for adequate delivery of fluids and antibiotics in the appropriate time frame of the 1st hour. Antibiotics should *not be withheld if lumbar puncture cannot be performed. Neither should a delay occur because blood or other cultures cannot be collected.*

The rationale for the 1-hour target for antimicrobial administration comes from observational studies that show poor outcomes with delays in antibiotic therapy. In one pediatric series of 130 patients with severe sepsis or septic shock, delays greater than 3 hours were associated with significantly increased mortality [odds ratio (OR) 4.0 (95% confidence interval 1.3–12.1)]. In another prospective observational study, mortality from septic shock was 1% among children who met goals for timely administration of fluids within 1 hour and antibiotics within 3 hours versus 4% for those who did not. Each hour delay in antibiotic administration has been associated with an approximately 8% increase in mortality in adults.

BOX 1: First hour bundle.

In the 1st hour of resuscitation, the goals are to restore or maintain:
- Airway, oxygenation, and ventilation
- Circulation
- Threshold heart rate (i.e. heart rate that is neither too low nor too high to ensure adequate cardiac output)

After identification of severe sepsis or septic shock, this approach emphasizes the following actions:
- Obtain vascular access [IV or intraosseous (IO)] within 5 minutes
- Start appropriate fluid resuscitation within 30 minutes
- Begin broad-spectrum antibiotics within 60 minutes
- For patients with fluid-refractory shock, initiate peripheral or central inotropic infusion within 60 minutes

The feasibility of a 1-hour target has not been tested outside of tertiary care pediatric institutions.

EMPIRIC REGIMENS

The regimen chosen should consider various factors (Box 2 and Tables 1 and 2). A distinction between CAIs and hospital-acquired infections (HAIs) is very important.

Equally important to remember is that virulence should not be confused or equated with resistance. An exquisitely sensitive Streptococcal infection can be extremely virulent and antibiotic therapy will remain the same. Similarly, an indolent *Acinetobacter infection is likely to be highly resistant.*

DOSING OF ANTIMICROBIAL DRUGS

In patients with severe sepsis, the highest recommended doses should be used as per recommended dosing interval. Attention should be paid to pharmacokinetic and pharmacodynamic parameters. Loading doses are needed for antibiotics such as colistin, polymyxin, tigecycline, and vancomycin. Antibiotics which have time dependent action like beta-lactams can be given as prolonged infusions over 3–4 hours to treat resistant infections. For beta-lactam-beta-lactamase inhibitor (BL-BLI) combinations, dosing should be on the basis

BOX 2: Issues to consider for empiric choice.

- Age
- Likely site of the infection
- Likely pathogen and likely resistance (Table 1)
- Level of immunocompetence
- Host comorbidities
- Previous antibiotic administration
- Antibiotic spectrum and need for combination therapy
- Antibiotic activity: Bactericidal/bacteriostatic
- Site of infection and achievable antibiotic concentration
- Dosage and pharmacodynamic principles

TABLE 1: Patient risk stratification (RS) for assessment of likelihood of drug resistance.

Type 1 *Risk of drug resistant pathogens low*	*Type 2* *Risk of drug resistant pathogens moderate*	*Type 3* *Risk of multidrug resistant pathogens very high*
Meeting *all* below mentioned criteria • No contact with hospital in last 90 days • No antibiotics in last 90 days • No comorbid conditions	Meeting *any one* of below mentioned criteria • Contact with hospital in last 90 days *without* invasive procedure/devices • Antibiotic therapy (oral/parenteral) in last 90 days • Patient with two or less comorbidities	Meeting *any one* of below mentioned criteria • Hospitalization in last 90 days with invasive procedure/devices • *More than* two antibiotics (oral/parenteral) in last 90 days • Greater than two comorbidities (e.g. DM, HT, CLD immunodeficiency)

(CLD: chronic liver disease; DM: diabetes mellitus; HT: hypertension)

TABLE 2: Empiric regimens for severe sepsis/septic shock.

Type of setting	*Likely pathogens*	*Choice of drug*	*Comments*
Community-acquired infections with normal immune status			
No clinical focus	• *Streptococcus pneumoniae* • *Escherichia coli* • *Klebsiella pneumoniae*	Ceftriaxone + aminoglycoside	Add doxycycline in *Rickettsia* endemic areas, artesunate if malaria a possibility
Respiratory focus	• *S. pneumoniae* • *Staphylococcus aureus* • *Mycoplasma* • Viruses	Co-amoxiclav/ ceftriaxone	• Add macrolide in children above 5 years or if suspected mycoplasma • Add anti-MRSA cover if features of staphylococcal infection • Add oseltamivir if flu suspected
Genitourinary source	• *E. coli* • *K. pneumoniae* • (ESBL common)	Ceftriaxone with aminoglycoside OR BL-BLI combination (RS2)	Carbapenems if history of previous ESBL or multiple antibiotics (RS3)
Intra-abdominal source	• *E. coli* (ESBL common) • Anaerobes	BL-BLI combinations	Carbapenems if source control not possible immediately
Skin and soft tissue	• *S. pyogenes* • *S. aureus*	Ceftriaxone and clindamycin	Add anti-MRSA cover if purulent SSTI
Bone and Joint	• *S. aureus* including • MRSA	Cefazolin and vancomycin	Daptomycin can be used as monotherapy
Nosocomial infections (depends on local patterns, also see chapter 30)*			
No obvious source/ CLABSI/VAP/ SSI	• MDR/XDR Gram-negatives • MRSA • *Candida*	BL-BLI/carbapenems with or without aminoglycoside	• Add MRSA cover if high incidence of MRSA in the unit • Add colistin/polymyxin if high incidence of carbapenem resistance in the unit • Add antifungal (azole/ echinocandin/amphotericin B if risk factors for candida)
Immunocompromised host (neutropenia, steroids, HIV) (see chapter 31)			
No obvious focus	• *Listeria* • Resistant Gram-negatives • MRSA • *Candida*	BL-BLI/carbapenems with or without aminoglycoside	• Add other drugs depending on the type of immunocompromise • Microbial etiology important
Neonates (see chapter 28)			
	Gram-negative (high prevalence of resistance), MRSA, *Candida* HSV, enterovirus	Cefotaxime/BL-BLI and gentamicin/ amikacin *or* meropenem	• BL-BLI/meropenem preferred in newborns with history of possible exposure to resistant pathogens and in very sick neonates • Ampicillin to be added if *Listeria* suspected

Contd...

Contd...

			• Add polymyxins if nosocomial and high rates of carbapenem resistance • Antifungals if risk factors for *Candida* (no previous prophylaxis) • Investigate for HSV if cultures negative

(*BL-BLI: beta-lactam–beta-lactamase* inhibitor; CLABSI: central-line associated bloodstream infection; ESBL: extended-spectrum beta-lactamase; HIV: human immunodeficiency virus; HSV: herpes simplex virus; MDR: multidrug-resistance; MRSA: Methicillin-resistant *S. aureus*; NICU: neonatal intensive care unit; SICU: surgical intensive care unit; SSI: surgical site infection; SSTI: skin and soft tissue infection; VAP: ventilator-associated pneumonia; XDR: extensively drug-resistant)

of the parent beta lactam and not the whole combination. Since patients with severe sepsis are on several other drugs, the prescription should be checked for any drug interactions. Renal function should be monitored and doses of antibiotics adjusted, if needed. The first dose in a patient with impairment of renal function is always the full dose.

MODIFICATION OF FURTHER ANTIBIOTIC THERAPY

The empirical antibiotic therapy should be reviewed at 24–48 hours. If a diagnosis of a nonbacterial infection is made, antibiotics can be stopped. If cultures are positive, then therapy should be optimized as per cultures. The culture and susceptibility reports should be interpreted carefully and attention given to minimum inhibitory concentration (MIC) data if available. If cultures are negative, but patient is improving then the same antibiotics may be continued. If cultures are negative and the child is not improving or worsening, upgradation of antibiotics can be considered. Before upgrading antibiotics, fresh cultures should be sent and other causes of poor response should be considered. These include nondrainage of pus, nonremoval of an infected central venous catheter, or a different pathogen, which will not respond to the current antimicrobial regimen (e.g. rickettsial infections and atypical organisms will not respond to beta-lactams).

SOURCE CONTROL

The nature and site of infection will affect duration of therapy. Infectious foci suspected to cause septic shock should be controlled as soon as possible following successful initial resuscitation. Observational studies have shown better survival if source control is achieved in 6–12 hours especially for intra-abdominal focus of infection. The risks and benefits must be weighed when selecting the specific intervention as source control intervention can cause complications, e.g. bleeding, fistulas, etc.

Both short- and long-term intravascular catheters can be the source of sepsis. Long-term catheters should be removed from patients with severe sepsis and bloodstream infection that continues despite 12 hours of antimicrobial therapy to which the infecting microbes are susceptible, or infections due to *S. aureus*, fungi, or mycobacteria. Short-term catheters should be removed once another site for vascular access is obtained if suspected to be the source.

BOX 3: Bedside approach to de-escalation

- Every patient on antibiotics should have the need for this considered and formally documented every day
- No later than day 3, a full assessment of investigation, results, and clinical progress should be performed, and a positive decision should be captured to:
  - Stop the treatment (no infection is present)
  - Narrow the spectrum of the therapy
  - Reduce the number of antibiotics being used, for example, there is redundancy in the therapy or such clinical progress that multiple agents active against the same pathogen(s) are not necessary
  - Not to de-escalate with the specific reason for not de-escalating documented
- Every day thereafter a decision to stop, change, or continue the therapy should be made against specific reasons

ESCALATION AND DE-ESCALATION

Management of sepsis requires rapid adequate therapy with broad-spectrum antibiotics. Antibiotic stewardship and restriction of antibiotic use is an important strategy to reduce development of bacterial resistance and cost but it is not the appropriate one for initial therapy of sepsis [Surviving Sepsis Campaign (SSC)]. The concept of "hit hard, hit early" should be followed by focused de-escalation.

The definition of antimicrobial de-escalation is that it is a mechanism whereby the provision of effective initial antibiotic treatment, particularly in cases of severe sepsis, is achieved while avoiding unnecessary antibiotic use that would promote the development of resistance (Box 3).

DURATION OF ANTIBIOTIC THERAPY

Duration of antibiotic therapy depends on the microbial etiology and site of infection. In neonates, culture negative sepsis needs to be treated for 7 days, culture positive sepsis for 2 weeks, and meningitis for 3 weeks. In older children, most infections can be adequately treated in 10–14 days; staphylococcal infections, bone and joint infections, and endocarditis need longer treatment for 4–6 weeks. There has been a trend toward reducing the duration of antibiotics for most infections. Uncomplicated community-acquired pneumonia can be adequately treated with 5–7 days therapy. Primary bacterial peritonitis, acute cholecystitis, and appendicitis may be treated for as short as 5 days. The PROcalcitonin to Reduce Antibiotic Treatments in Acutely ill patients (PRORATA) trial and Stop Antibiotics on Procalcitonin Guidance Study (SAPS), two large multicenter randomized trials in patients with sepsis, have demonstrated that procalcitonin levels could be used as a marker for stopping antibiotics once the patient stabilizes.

WHAT SHOULD BE AVOIDED IN MANAGEMENT OF SEPSIS?

- Treating noninfectious or nonbacterial syndrome
- Treating colonization or contamination
- Treating longer than necessary
- Failing to make adjustments in a timely manner
- Prescribing an antibiotic with spectrum of activity not indicated.

OTHER MEASURES

- *Immunoglobulin use*: There have been three Cochrane reviews till date, the latest one showing no survival benefit. There are no plasma immunoglobulin G (IgG) levels cutoffs for septic patients for which intravenous immunoglobulin (IVIG) substitution could be recommended.
- Granulocyte-colony stimulating factor (GCSF/G-CSF) and granulocyte-macrophage colony-stimulating factor (GM-CSF) have shown promise in the treatment of infection in non-neutropenic hosts in many animal models. GM-CSF is produced by monocytes-macrophages, T and B cells, mast cells, fibroblasts, and epithelial cells at low level during steady state which is significantly increased during inflammatory conditions. Use of GM-CSF in sepsis studies are characterized by a small number of patients and high heterogeneity of diagnosis and clinical presentation. Till date, clinical trials have not shown any benefit of GM-CSF treatment during sepsis. GCSF not only causes neutrophil proliferation but also enhances neutrophil production of cytokines. Bo et al. conducted a meta-analysis on impact of GCSF in sepsis. They showed no survival benefit or a significant rate of adverse effects.

CONCLUSION

Sepsis is one of the oldest and elusive problems in medicine. With increased understanding of pathogen and host response along with advances in intensive care, outcome has improved significantly. In addition, quality improvement bundles for sepsis care have reduced mortality when compliance is high. The emerging multidrug resistance is in not only Gram-positive and Gram-negative bacteria but also in fungal pathogens, e.g. *Candida auris* will pose a challenge in management of these patients.

RECOMMENDED READING

1. Alejandria MM, Lansang MA, Dans LF, et al. Intravenous immunoglobulin for treating sepsis, severe sepsis and septic shock. Cochrane Database Syst Rev. 2013;9:CD001090.
2. Angus DC, van der Poll T. Severe sepsis and septic shock. N Engl J Med. 2013;369:840-51.
3. Azuhata T, Kinoshita K, Kawano D, et al. Time from admission to initiation of surgery for source control is a critical determinant of survival in patients with gastrointestinal perforation with associated septic shock. Crit Care. 2014;18(3):R87.
4. Babu M, Menon VP, Devi U. Prevalence of antimicrobial resistant pathogens in severe sepsis and septic shock patients. J Young Pharm. 2018;10(3):358-61.
5. Bo L, Wang F, Zhu J, et al. Granulocyte-colony stimulating factor (G-CSF) and granulocyte-macrophage colony stimulating factor (GM-CSF) for sepsis: a meta-analysis. Crit Care. 2011;15(1):R58.
6. Davis AL, Carcillo JA, Aneja RK, et al. American College of Critical Care Medicine Clinical Practice Parameters for Hemodynamic Support of Pediatric and Neonatal Septic Shock. Crit Care Med. 2017;45(6):1061-92.
7. Jajoo M, Manchanda V, Chaurasia S, et al. Investigators of the Delhi Neonatal Infection Study (DeNIS) collaboration, New Delhi, India. Alarming rates of antimicrobial resistance and fungal sepsis in outborn neonates in North India. PLoS One. 2018;13(6):e0180705.
8. Lane RD, Funai T, Reeder R, et al. High reliability pediatric septic shock quality improvement initiative and decreasing mortality. Pediatrics. 2016;138(4):e20154153.
9. Manian FA. IDSA guidelines for the diagnosis and management of intravascular catheter-related bloodstream infection. Clin Infect Dis. 2009;49:1770-1.
10. Masterton RG. Antibiotic de-escalation. Crit Care Clin. 2011;27(1):149-62.

11. Paul R, Melendez E, Stack A, et al. Improving adherence to PALS septic shock guidelines. Pediatrics. 2014;133(5):e1358.
12. Rhee C. Using procalcitonin to guide antibiotic therapy. Open Forum Infect Dis. 2017;4(1):ofw249.
13. Shankar-Hari M, Culshaw N, Post B, et al. Endogenous IgG hypogammaglobulinaemia in critically ill adults with sepsis: systematic review and meta-analysis. Intensive Care Med. 2015;41(8):1393-401.
14. Weiss SL, Fitzgerald JC, Balamuth F, et al. Delayed antimicrobial therapy increases mortality and organ dysfunction duration in pediatric sepsis. Crit Care Med. 2014;42(11):2409-17.
15. Weiss SL, Fitzgerald JC, Pappachan J, et al. Sepsis Prevalence, Outcomes, and Therapies (SPROUT) Study Investigators and Pediatric Acute Lung Injury and Sepsis Investigators (PALISI) Network. Global epidemiology of pediatric severe sepsis: the sepsis prevalence, outcomes, and therapies study. Am J Respir Crit Care Med. 2015;191:1147-57.

Antimicrobial Therapy of Healthcare-associated Infections

30
Chapter

Tanu Singhal

INTRODUCTION

Nosocomial infections (NIs) now better termed as healthcare-associated infections (HAIs) are those that occur as a consequence of medical care and may arise during or following hospitalization. The vast majority of HAI in children are viral respiratory tract infections including influenza, gastrointestinal infections, and various exanthematous illnesses. These often result from exposure in crowded outpatient clinics. However, the classical HAI arising as a consequence of invasive devices and procedures include bloodstream infections (BSIs) (most common), pneumonia, urinary tract infections (UTIs), and surgical site infections (SSIs). These occur predominantly in the pediatric and neonatal intensive care unit (ICU). The incidence, type of infections, causative organisms, susceptibility profile vary tremendously between hospitals due to differences in infection control policies, microbial flora, antimicrobial use, patient profile, and other factors. NIs are responsible for considerable morbidity, mortality, expense, increased length of stay, antibiotic use, and antibiotic resistance.

ETIOLOGY AND ANTIMICROBIAL RESISTANCE PATTERN OF NOSOCOMIAL INFECTIONS IN INDIA

The most common etiologic agents for NIs in India in both adult and pediatric ICUs (PICUs) are gram-negative pathogens including *Klebsiella*, *Escherichia coli*, *Pseudomonas*, *Acinetobacter*, and *Enterobacter*. These are followed by Gram-positive organisms including *Staphylococcus aureus*, *Staphylococcus epidermidis*, and enterococci. There is an increasing incidence of invasive candida infections in critically sick children. Most of the nosocomial pathogens are multidrug-resistant. Foremost is drug resistance in Gram-negative pathogens with 80% of nosocomial *E. coli* and *Klebsiella* infections being resistant to third-generation cephalosporins by virtue of production of extended-spectrum beta-lactamases (ESBL). The emergence of AmpC-mediated resistance, traditionally found in *Pseudomonas*, *Enterobacter*, *Serratia*, and *Citrobacter* but now even in other Gram-negative bacilli, has made third-generation cephalosporins and beta-lactam-beta-lactamase inhibitor combinations ineffectual. The fall out of ESBL and AmpC-mediated resistance has been excessive use of carbapenems in the ICU. This has led to emergence of carbapenem resistance with nearly 50% of Gram-negative isolates in certain ICUs exhibiting carbapenem resistance. This has lead to increased use of the polymyxins with consequent emergence of colistin resistance. While most nosocomial *S. aureus* are methicillin-resistant, vancomycin-resistant *S. aureus*/enterococci are not a major problem in India unlike the West. Similarly, seen over time with increasing use of fluconazole, is increasing fluconazole resistance. However, one must remember that there are significant differences between ICUs in terms of microbial etiology and antimicrobial susceptibility and the same must be considered while designing empiric therapy regimens.

GENERAL PRINCIPLES OF TREATMENT

Distinguishing Infectious from Noninfectious causes of Fever

The usual setting when a NI is suspected is when a hospitalized patient develops fever. However, fever can also result from noninfectious causes such as postoperative atelectasis, drug fever, thrombophlebitis, transfusions, deep venous thrombosis, central fever, etc. Similarly leukocytosis may not always be due to an infection; noninfectious causes of leukocytosis include stress, bleeding, atelectasis, and steroids.

Determining the Site of Infection

Once, major noninfectious causes are excluded a thorough clinical assessment should be to determine the site of infection. Common sites are BSIs especially in patients who have central lines, sinusitis/tracheobronchitis/pneumonia in patients on invasive ventilation, UTIs in those who have indwelling urinary catheters, and SSIs in postsurgical patients. Central nervous system (CNS) infections and intra-abdominal sepsis should be also considered in children with predisposing procedures/interventions at these sites. *Clostridium difficile* is less common in children as compared to adults. Occult sites of infection include sinusitis, osteomyelitis, and septic arthritis. Eliciting symptoms referable to a particular system is often difficult in very sick children, but should be done whenever possible. A head to toe assessment should be done with careful inspection of the central line exit site, respiratory system, nature of tracheal secretions, abdomen, bones, joints, examination of neck stiffness and surgical sites, and the skin. It is important to disrobe and examine the entire skin as these might show areas of cellulites, eschars, and pustules which often indicate bacteremia/fungemia.

Appropriate Investigations

The initial investigations include a complete blood count and peripheral smear evaluation with acute phase reactants such as C-reactive protein (CRP)/procalcitonin (PCT). At least one set (one aerobic and one anaerobic) and preferably two set of cultures should be sent. If there is a central catheter then one culture should be sent from the catheter lumen and the other from peripheral venipuncture. The total volume of blood collected should be around 1% of the circulating blood volume. Fungal cultures should be sent if candida is suspected. In children with indwelling urinary catheter a routine urine analysis and culture should be sent. Results of these investigations should be interpreted carefully as some degree of pyuria and significant bacteriuria (colony count of more than 10^5/mL) may be seen in any catheterized patient. For suspected ventilator-associated pneumonia (VAP), cultures of the respiratory secretions (quantitative endotracheal aspirates, bronchoalveolar lavage, and protected specimen brush) should be sent. Cultures should also be sent from other suspected sites of infection such surgical sites, cerebrospinal fluid (CSF), abscesses, etc. Care should be taken to send deep samples; skin swabs and cultures from drains may just indicate colonization. Imaging also assists in diagnosis. Basic imaging includes chest X-ray (CXR) and ultrasonography (USG) abdomen. In some patients computerized scans of the thorax and abdomen may be needed for diagnosis.

Distinguishing Infection from Colonization in the Nosocomial Setting

An important issue in managing NIs is to differentiate infection from colonization. In ICUs, cultures are sent from nonsterile sites such as endotracheal tubes, central lines, urinary catheters, and drains will always grow microbes as these sites are inevitably colonized. Careful interpretation of the results of such cultures in light of the clinical setting is needed to differentiate colonization from true infection. It is important that these colonizations are not treated with antibiotics as it will lead to selection of resistant organisms.

OVERVIEW OF THERAPY

Empirical Therapy

Various factors determine the empiric choice of antibiotics and include:

- *Local epidemiologic data*: Knowledge of common microbial pathogens and their resistance profile in a particular ICU helps in making empirical choice of antibiotics till cultures are available.
- *Previous antibiotic usage*: This again helps in predicting the likely resistance profile of the microbe till culture results are available. Additionally, it helps in guessing what pathogens have not been appropriately covered till now.
- *Severity of infection*: This is perhaps the most important factor. For a patient who is in septic shock, broad spectrum and high end antimicrobial agent should be chosen based with the least likelihood of failure (de-escalation strategy). On the other hand, if the infection is nonsevere, treatment may be initiated with a lower antimicrobial and upgraded if nonresponse (escalation strategy).
- *Associated comorbidities*: These are important considerations. For instance if there is associated renal compromise, nephrotoxic drugs should be avoided or used with caution.
- *Site of the infection*: In the presence of a CNS infection, a drug with good CSF penetration must be used.

Though the empiric choice is governed by above mentioned factors, given the fact that most NIs in the Indian health care setting are due to ESBL producing Gram-negative organisms, the initial choice is either a beta-lactam-beta-lactamase inhibitor combination (piperacillin tazobactam/cefoperazone-sulbactam/cefepime-tazobactam) or a carbapenem (meropenem/imipenem) with or without an aminoglycoside. Addition of polymyxin B/colistin is indicated in a setting of high carbapenem resistance. A methicillin-resistant *S. aureus* (MRSA) cover (vancomycin/teicoplanin) is indicated in those units where incidence of MRSA is high. Antifungals should be considered in those cases with high risk for invasive candidiasis. Table 1 lists the empiric approach to management of NI at the author's institution where Gram-negative pathogens are implicated in 80% of infections, Gram-positive in 10%, and candida in 10%. The ESBL prevalence is more than 80% and carbapenem resistance in BSIs is 50% and VAP is 80%.

TABLE 1: Empiric antibiotic choices for healthcare-associated infections at the author's institution (Kokilaben Dhirubhai Ambani Hospital, Mumbai).

Suspected site	*Likely organisms*	*Stable patient/no prior antibiotic exposure*	*Patient in septic shock/ already received first-line agents*
Bloodstream infection	*Klebsiella, E. coli, Pseudomonas, Acinetobacter*	Piperacillin tazobactam/ cefoperazone sulbactam/ meropenem/imipenem with or without amikacin	Colistin/polymyxin B with meropenem/imipenem with/without high dose tigecycline with/without fluconazole/echinocandin
Ventilator-associated pneumonia	*Acinetobacter, Pseudomonas, Klebsiella, E. coli*	Piperacillin tazobactam/ cefoperazone sulbactam/ imipenem/meropenem	Colistin/polymyxin B with tigecycline
Urinary tract infection	*E. coli, Klebsiella, Pseudomonas*	Fosfomycin/amikacin/wait for cultures	Colistin
Surgical site infection	*E. coli, Klebsiella, Acinetobacter/ Pseudomonas/S. aureus*	Piperacillin tazobactam/ cefoperazone sulbactam with or without vancomycin/linezolid	Colistin/polymyxin B with carbapenem with/without vancomycin/linezolid
Meningitis	*E. coli, Klebsiella, Acinetobacter, Pseudomonas*	High dose meropenem	Colistin/polymyxin B and meropenem

Source Control

Adequate source control is paramount. This may involve removal of infected lines/catheters, drainage of pus/collections. In very sick patients who are not candidates for surgical drainage, radiologically-guided drains/pigtails can be inserted. The role of source control is even more important in today's age of multidrug-resistant infections.

Dosing of Antibiotics

Adequate attention is needed towards administration of appropriate doses. Loading dose is indicated for antibiotics such as polymyxin B/colistin/vancomycin/fluconazole/echinocandins. Higher doses are indicated for serious infections. Time-dependent antibiotics such as beta-lactams should be dosed frequently to maintain serum levels continuously above the minimum inhibitory concentration (MIC). Recent data supports administration of beta-lactams by continuous infusion in infections with organisms with high MICs. On the other hand, concentration-dependent antibiotics such as aminoglycosides may be effectively dosed once a day. Antibiotic doses should be adjusted for renal and hepatic dysfunction. However, even in patients with renal failure the first dose should be the full dose.

Definitive therapy, De-escalation, and Escalation

Once culture reports are available therapy should be optimized to the most appropriate antibiotic for that pathogen. Every effort should be made to de-escalate to a more narrow spectrum drug if possible and drop antibiotics which are no longer indicated. De-escalation is difficult with negative cultures but can still include stopping the MRSA cover if no Gram-positive pathogen has been isolated. In patients who are not improving with the empiric regime, other causes of nonresponse such as noninfectious causes, poor source control should be addressed before escalation of antibiotics.

Duration of Therapy

This depends on the site/severity of infection and underlying pathogen. Emerging data supports the use of reduced duration antibiotic therapy (usually 7 days) for most NIs (exception *S. aureus*, invasive candidiasis, and necrotizing pneumonias). Shortening therapy helps in reducing the risk of selection of resistant pathogens apart from reducing costs.

CATHETER-ASSOCIATED BLOODSTREAM INFECTIONS

Confirmation of the diagnosis of a catheter-related BSI involves isolation of the same organism with the same antibiogram from simultaneous cultures obtained through peripheral venipuncture and the catheter lumen. A differential time to positivity (DTP) of more than 120 minutes (central line culture 120 minutes before the peripheral puncture) indicates the catheter as a source of infection. A positive catheter/catheter tip culture alone has poor positive predictive value for catheter-associated bloodstream infection (CLABSI) as it may just indicate colonization; but high negative predictive value (90%). However, in certain situations where the peripheral culture cannot be sent or is negative and there is no other identifiable focus of infection, consideration may have to be given to the central line culture.

Management of BSI is determined by several factors including the severity of the infection, the type of catheter, whether or not local infection is present, the etiologic agent as well as the certainty of diagnosis.

The central line should be removed after (sending cultures) if the patient with a suspected BSI is in septic shock or has local exit site infection of if there is evidence of metastatic infection such as endocarditis/osteomyelitis. The central line may be retained if the patient is hemodynamically stable and if it is a precious catheter (implanted catheter/port). The choice of empiric therapy depends on factors discussed earlier and usually includes a beta-lactam-beta-lactamase combination/carbapenems with or without aminoglycosides. Polymyxins/anti-MRSA drugs may have to be used empirically in units where prevalence of carbapenem-resistant bugs or MRSA is high. Empirical antifungals should be added if risk factors for invasive candidiasis are present such as prolonged ICU stay, antibiotic use, mechanical ventilation, gut surgery, renal failure, total parenteral nutrition including intralipids, use of corticosteroids and other immunocompromised states, renal failure, and extreme prematurity. Other pointers to candidemia as a cause of sepsis include isolation of candida from multiple nonsterile sites, nonresponse to appropriately chosen antibacterials and sepsis with low PCT levels. The choice of antifungal depends on previous azole exposure, the azole susceptibility of candida species isolated in the unit, and the severity of infection and associated comorbidities and may include fluconazole, amphotericin B or echinocandins.

Subsequent therapy depends on the culture reports. Cultures may be negative in 50% of BSIs. In culture negative cases, an alternative focus should be searched for and antimicrobials stopped/modified/escalated depending on the diagnosis and clinical response. If cultures are positive then therapy should be optimized for that particular pathogen. If coagulase negative *Staphylococcus* has been isolated the catheter can be safely retained and appropriate antimicrobials administered for 7–10 days. If Gram-negative bacteria are isolated then therapy needs to be continued for 7–10 days. For Gram-negative infections tunneled and implanted catheters can be retained but a percutaneous central venous catheter (CVC) should be removed. If *S. aureus* is the culprit than the catheter should be removed, an echocardiography (ECHO) done to rule out endocarditis and a watch kept for complications like abscesses and osteomyelitis. Blood cultures should be repeated after 3–4 days to document negativity. Duration of therapy is 2 weeks for uncomplicated cases and 4–6 weeks for complications. If candida has been isolated then the catheter should be removed, blood cultures repeated every 48–72 hours, and appropriate antifungals administered for 2 weeks after the last negative blood culture. A dilated retinal examination is indicated before completion of therapy to rule out endophthalmitis.

In selected cases of CLABSI where catheter removal is indicated but cannot be done due to logistic/access issues antibiotic lock therapy with an appropriate antimicrobial can be done to salvage the catheter.

VENTILATOR-ASSOCIATED PNEUMONIA

Ventilator-associated pneumonia is the second commonest hospital-associated infection in critically ill children and neonates and develops in 3–10% of PICU patients (as against 15–30% in adults). The diagnosis of VAP is challenging since many noninfectious conditions such as atelectasis, pulmonary edema, pulmonary embolism mimic VAP, and isolation of microorganisms from the tracheobronchial tree may just represent colonization. In most instances, diagnosis of VAP is established by a combination of clinical (fever, purulent/increased secretions, leukocytosis/leukopenia, new auscultatory findings, and worsening gas exchange), radiologic (new infiltrates) and microbiologic (isolation of a significant colony count of microorganism from endotracheal aspirate/bronchoalveolar lavage/protected specimen brush).

The etiology of VAP in children is generally independent of the duration of ventilation (unlike adults). Most studies from India in both adults and children have incriminated multidrug-resistant Gram-negative pathogens including *Acinetobacter*, *Pseudomonas*, *Klebsiella*, *E. coli*, and *Enterobacter* as causative agents; Gram-positive organisms have been infrequently reported. Candida species are almost never the cause of VAP and their isolation from tracheal secretions reflects colonization rather than true infection.

Empiric therapy is governed by factors discussed previously as well as the pulmonary penetration of in view of the etiologic and resistance profile in Indian ICUs, initial therapy with beta-lactam-beta-lactamase inhibitor combination (piperacillin tazobactam/cefoperazone sulbactam) or carbapenems with or without an aminoglycoside maybe chosen. In some units where carbapenem resistance is high, empirical use of colistin in very sick patients is sometimes necessary. A MRSA cover should be given if the MRSA rates in the ICU (>20%) are high or if the Gram stain of endotracheal aspirate shows Gram-positive cocci; there is some data to suggest that linezolid may be superior to vancomycin for pneumonia. There is no data to support routine use of inhalational antibiotics in VAP.

Therapy should be modified and de-escalated as per culture results to narrower spectrum drugs or even a single drug. If cultures are sterile and the patient had not received antibiotics in 48–72 hours preceding cultures, antimicrobials should be stopped. Treatment for 8 days has been shown to be as effective as 15 days; longer therapy for 14–21 days is recommended for multilobular involvement, cavitation, and necrotizing pneumonias and should be considered for infection with *Pseudomonas aeruginosa* and *Acinetobacter*.

CATHETER-ASSOCIATED URINARY TRACT INFECTIONS

Catheter-associated urinary tract infection (CAUTI) is an uncommon NI in children unlike adults. The etiology of CAUTIs is usually multidrug-resistant Gram-negative bacilli including *E. coli, Klebsiella,* and *Pseudomonas.* The diagnosis of nosocomial UTI in is complicated by the fact that critically sick children and those with catheters do not manifest/cannot report symptoms such as urgency, frequency, dysuria, abdominal pain, and tenderness. A urine culture with a significant colony count may be due to catheter colonization. Pyuria may be due to catheter-related cystitis. Hence, the diagnosis of CAUTI should be done carefully to prevent treating asymptomatic bacteriuria or cystitis. Urine for culture in catheterized patients should be obtained from the aspiration port and not from the collection bag.

Empirical therapy for nosocomial UTI should be based on local epidemiology of the ICU, prior antibiotic therapy as well as reports of the Gram stain [if Gram-positive cocci are seen then cover for coagulase negative staphylococci (CoNS)/*Enterococcus* may be needed]. Usual empiric choices include beta-lactam-beta-lactamase inhibitor combinations such as piperacillin tazobactam/cefoperazone sulbactam/carbapenems/aminoglycosides. Therapy should be tailored once reports of susceptibility are available. It is not uncommon to isolate carbapenem-resistant Gram-negative bacteria in CAUTI. After excluding colonization, these infections may need treatment with colistin (polymyxin B does not penetrate the urine), aminoglycosides/fosfomycin.

It is very common to isolate candida in patients suspected to have CAUTI. In most instances, this represents colonization since most of these children have indwelling catheters and are on broad spectrum antibiotics. There is no reliable cutoff to differentiate candida colonization from true infection. Most cases of candiduria resolve with catheter removal and stopping antibiotics. Asymptomatic candiduria should be treated only in severely neutropenic or in those undergoing urologic manipulation. In preterm/very low birth weight neonates, candiduria indicates invasive candidiasis and should be treated aggressively. Isolation of candida from urine or from other nonsterile sites should be evaluated for underlying candidemia by appropriate tests. Patients with symptomatic candida UTIs (where no other cause for fever/urinary symptoms apart from candiduria is found) should be treated. Fluconazole (3–6 mg/kg/day) achieves excellent urinary levels and is the drug of choice if the candida is susceptible. Treatment of fluconazole resistant candida UTI is challenging since drugs like liposomal amphotericin B, voriconazole, and echinocandins do not achieve good urinary levels. Here amphotericin B deoxycholate may have to be used.

SURGICAL SITE INFECTIONS

The incidence of SSIs is largely determined by the wound class; rates being lowest (1–2%) for clean wounds. Nearly half of all SSI in the Indian setting are caused by Gram-negative bacilli including *Klebsiella, Pseudomonas, Acinetobacter,* and *E. coli.* The other half is due to Gram-positive cocci of which *S. aureus* is the commonest followed by coagulase negative *Staphylococcus.* Candida and anaerobes account for some infections. The usual features of SSI are pain, redness, induration, and discharge from the wound occurring within 30 days of surgery. SSI may be classified as superficial site infections (skin or subcutaneous tissues), deep incisional SSI (muscle and fascia), and organ/space infections. Pus aspirate/tissue cultures should be sent to guide therapy; superficial swabs may not always be representative.

Some infections may resolve with topical antibiotic therapy (mupirocin, fusidic acid, and povidone iodine) but others need systemic antimicrobial therapy. Choice of empiric therapy depends on severity of infection/local epidemiology. Mild infections can be treated on an outpatient basis with oral cephalexin/cefuroxime/co-amoxiclav pending culture results. For serious infections, piperacillin-tazobactam/carbapenems with an anti-MRSA cover such as vancomycin/teicoplanin/linezolid may be required. Source control is crucial including drainage of fluid collections, debridement of devitalized tissue, relief of tension, and pressure in the affected area and removal of foreign bodies (e.g. shunt in shunt infections). Antibiotic therapy should be modified and de-escalated as per culture results. Treatment duration varies from 7–14 days.

HEALTHCARE/NOSOCOMIAL MENINGITIS/VENTRICULITIS

Healthcare-associated meningitis/ventriculitis is seen in patients undergoing neurosurgeries, head trauma, external ventricular drainage, lumbar punctures, etc. Diagnosis is a challenge since sensorial obtundation (a cardinal symptom of meningitis) may be due to the underlying disease/surgery. The CSF may be abnormal due to pre-existing bleed/surgery induced chemical meningitis. The patients are frequently on antibiotics and hence microbial isolation rates are low. CSF examination including lactate estimation and contrast magnetic resonance imaging (MRI) are the recommended investigations. The etiology depends on local epidemiology, but commonly includes multidrug/extremely drug-resistant Gram-negative pathogens including *Acinetobacter, Pseudomonas, Klebsiella,* and S. *aureus*/*epidermidis*.

Empirical therapy depends on local flora, but usually includes high dose meropenem with vancomycin. Therapy should be modified based on culture reports. Surgical drainage of pus and removal of hardware may be needed. For carbapenem-resistant pathogens, intraventricular/intrathecal therapy with colistin/polymyxin B/aminoglycosides is indicated. The drugs are best administered through injection of Ommaya reservoir, but may sometimes have to be given through external ventricular derivation (EVD)/lumbar punctures. Doses of drugs that can be administered in the CSF are listed in Table 2. The duration of therapy varies depending on the causative organism but is generally 2–3 weeks.

TABLE 2: Doses of drugs to be given by intrathecal/intraventricular route.

Drug	*Dose*
Vancomycin	5–20 mg
Teicoplanin	5–40 mg
Amikacin	5–50 mg
Gentamicin	1–8 mg
Colistin	10–20 mg
Polymyxin B	50,000 units
Daptomycin	2–5 mg
Tobramycin	5–20 mg

CLOSTRIDIUM DIFFICILE INFECTION

This is discussed in chapter 17.

CONCLUSION

The incidence of NI is on the rise due to advancements in intensive care, neonatal care, cancer therapy, human immunodeficiency virus (HIV), and transplant. The frequency, type, etiology, and susceptibility of NI vary with each unit and is a reflection of the infection control practices and antimicrobial use. Therapy of NI is getting more and more difficult and expensive with evolving drug resistance and exhaustion of antibiotic options; the latest in the list is carbapenem resistance. In this scenario an active infection control program and an antimicrobial stewardship program is needed to address the problem of NI.

RECOMMENDED READING

1. Alagesan M, Gopalakrishnan R, Panchatcharam SN, et al. A decade of change in susceptibility patterns of Gram-negative blood culture isolates: a single center study. Germs. 2015;5(3):65-77.
2. Alfouzan WA, Dhar R. Candiduria: evidence-based approach to management, are we there yet? J Mycol Med. 2017;27(3):293-302.
3. Balasubramanian P, Tullu MS. Study of ventilator-associated pneumonia in a pediatric intensive care unit. Indian J Pediatr. 2014;81:1182-6.
4. Chakrabarti A, Sood P, Rudramurthy SM, et al. Incidence, characteristics and outcome of ICU-acquired candidemia in India. Intensive Care Med. 2015;41(2):285-95.
5. Chastre J. Antimicrobial treatment of hospital-acquired pneumonia. Infect Dis Clin N Am. 2003;17: 727-37.
6. Datta S, Wattal C, Goel N, et al. A ten year analysis of multi-drug resistant blood stream infections caused by *Escherichia coli & Klebsiella pneumoniae* in a tertiary care hospital. Indian J Med Res. 2012;135(6):907-12.
7. Garner JS, Jarvis WR, Emori TG, et al. CDC Definitions for NI, 1988. Am J Infect Control. 1988;16:128-40.
8. Huskins WC, Goldmann DA. Nosocomial infections. In: Feigin RD, Cherry JD (Eds). Textbook of pediatric infectious diseases. 4th edition. Philadelphia: WB Saunders Company; 1998. pp. 2545-85.
9. Kalil AC, Metersky ML, Klompas M, et al. Management of adults with hospital-acquired and ventilator-associated pneumonia: 2016 Clinical Practice Guidelines by the Infectious Diseases Society of America and the American Thoracic Society. Clin Infect Dis. 2016;63(5):e61-111.
10. Lodha R, Natchu UC, Nanda M, et al. Nosocomial infections in pediatric intensive care units. Indian J Pediatr. 2001;68:1063-70.
11. Mermel LA, Allon M, Bouza E, et al. Clinical practice guidelines for the diagnosis and management of intravascular catheter-related infection: 2009 Update by the Infectious Diseases Society of America. Clin Infect Dis. 2009;49(1):1-45.
12. Shah S, Singhal T, Naik R. A 4-year prospective study to determine the incidence and microbial etiology of surgical site infections at a private tertiary care hospital in Mumbai, India. Am J Infect Control. 2015;43:59-62.
13. Shah S, Singhal T, Naik R. High incidence of antimicrobial resistance in gram negative pathogens causing central line associated blood stream infections in the adult intensive care unit of a tertiary care hospital in Mumbai, India. Philadelphia, PA, USA: Program and abstracts of the 52nd Annual Meeting of the Infectious Diseases Society of America; 2014.
14. Tunkel AR, Hasbun R, Bhimraj A, et al. 2017 Infectious Diseases Society of America's Clinical Practice Guidelines for Healthcare-Associated Ventriculitis and Meningitis. Clin Infect Dis. 2017.

Antimicrobial Therapy in Febrile Neutropenia

31
Chapter

Nitin Shah, MR Lokeshwar

INTRODUCTION

The survival of childhood cancer patients has significantly improved in the last two to three decades due to availability of better chemotherapeutic protocols, improved supportive care including blood components, and effective antimicrobial therapy. The current treatment protocols are very intense which frequently expose the patients to episodes of severe neutropenia during which the patient is at risk of developing potentially fatal invasive infections. In fact, the causation of cancer mortality has shifted from one due to bleeding in past to one due to infections currently. Though better understanding and timely management of infections have reduced mortality in cancer patients, it still is a leading cause of morbidity and mortality. Availability of colony stimulating factors, though shortening the duration of neutropenia, has not reduced the mortality rates due to infections.

Besides malignancies, other situations where one faces a patient with febrile neutropenia include neonate with sepsis, bone marrow failure syndromes, hematopoietic stem cell transplant recipients, HIV infection, organ transplant recipients, congenital neutropenia, drug-induced neutropenia, and though rare in pediatric patients, pre-leukemic conditions like myelodysplastic syndrome.

Like in many other clinical challenges, there is no substitute to a systematic approach to a child who has febrile neutropenia.

DEFINITIONS

Fever is defined as a single oral temperature record of more than or equal to 38.3°C (101°F) or a temperature of more than or equal to 38°C (100.4°F) for more than or equal to 1 hour. Neutropenia is defined as absolute neutrophil count (ANC) less than 500 cells/mm^3 or a count of less than 1,000 cells/mm^3 with predicted fall to less than 500 cells/mm^3 in next few days.

GENERAL CONSIDERATIONS

Though there are many other causes of fever in a setting of neutropenia, occult or overt infections account for 50% of these episodes, 85% of which are bacterial in origin, 50% of them are bacteremic at onset, 80% of them originate from patient's own flora, and 50% of the times the patient is colonized while in hospital. The other causes of fever in a neutropenic patient include blood products, drugs, malignant process itself especially before remission is achieved, thrombophlebitis, etc. A sick looking patient with chills and hypotension is always likely to have sepsis.

The incidence of infection is inversely proportional to the neutrophil count and duration of neutropenia. The chances of infection are 14% when the ANC is 500–1,000 as compared to 24–60% when it is less than 100 cells/mm^3. 30% develop fever or infection when neutropenia lasts for less than 7 days as compared to nearly 100% when it remains low for more than 7 days. Neutropenia less than 500 cells/mm^3 and duration more than 7 days are taken as the critical event while managing patients with febrile neutropenia. Similarly mortality is 47% in those with ANC less than 100 cells/mm^3, as compared to 14% in those with ANC more than 1,000 cells/mm^3.

Besides neutropenia, there are other arms of immunity which could be possibly deranged in these patients such as loss of natural barriers like IV devices or mucositis, low CD4 counts, monocytopenia, hypogammaglobulinemia as seen in patient with chronic lymphocytic leukemia (CLL) or human immunodeficiency virus (HIV), macrophage function defects, malnutrition, etc.

BACTERIAL ETIOLOGY AND ANTIMICROBIAL SUSCEPTIBILITY

Till 1970's, Gram-negative organisms were the leading cause of infection in a neutropenic patient. The first EORTC trial microbiological data on the causative organisms showed that the proportion of Gram-negative to Gram-positive organisms for the period 1973–1976 was 71% vs. 29% which changed to 33% vs. 67% for the period of 1988–1994. With the use of antibiotics to cover the Gram-negative infections, Gram-positive organisms have become the leading cause of infections now currently accounting for more than 60–70% of isolates in the Western World. However, the situation is different in India. In a symposium published in Indian Journal of Cancer in 2014, various centers from different parts of India shared their data on the microbial etiology and antimicrobial susceptibility of infections in cancer patients including children. Summarization of the data suggests that Gram-negative bacteria contribute to 60–90% of infections in various centers. *E. coli, Klebsiella, Pseudomonas,* and *Acinetobacter* are the top four pathogens. Drug resistance in Gram-negative pathogens was very high with 50–80% of the isolates being extended spectrum beta-lactamase (ESBL)-producing; many centers reported carbapenem resistance prevalence to amount up to 30% and some centers even reported colistin resistance. Gram-positive bacteria contributed to 10–40% of infections with methicillin-sensitive *S. aureus* being the predominant pathogen, others being methicillin-resistant *S. aureus* (MRSA) and *Enterococcus*. However for designing the empiric regimen for febrile neutropenia, each center should generate its own data on microbial etiology and antimicrobial susceptibility.

INVASIVE FUNGAL INFECTIONS IN CHILDREN WITH CANCER

The prevalence of invasive fungal infections (IFI) in cancer patients is increasing the risk of IFI in children with cancer depends largely on the type of cancer or hematopoietic stem cell transplantation (HSCT) status (Table 1) and is further modified by the intensity of the chemotherapy regimen, local factors including the health care set up where the children are undergoing chemotherapy, and the use of antifungal prophylaxis. Basically prolonged and profound neutropenia (ANC of ≤500/µL), defects in cell-mediated immunity (lymphopenia due to T cell cytotoxic agents and steroids), and disruption of mucosal barriers (mucositis, presence of central venous catheters) are the main risk factors. The most common fungi causing IFI in this risk group include *Candida* (including azole resistant *C. glabrata, C. krusei,* and

TABLE 1: Approximate risk of IFI in children on cancer chemotherapy or HSCT.

Group	*Risk of IFI*
Allogenic HSCT with GVHD, allogenic HSCT (especially umbilical cord blood transplant, partially matched related donor), AML/MDS treated as AML, relapsed acute lymphatic leukemia, severe aplastic anemia, congenital immunodeficiency	≥10%
Non-Hodgkin's lymphoma, autologous HSCT, new acute lymphatic leukemia	<5%
Hodgkin's lymphoma, solid tumors	Sporadic/rare

(AML: acute myeloid leukemia; GVHD: graft-versus-host disease; HSCT: hematopoietic stem cell transplantation; IFI: invasive fungal infections; MDS: myelodysplastic syndrome)

C. auris), *Aspergillus*, and Mucoraceae. The incidence of other molds including *Fusarium* and *Scedosporium* is also increasing. In a study from Northern India, the prevalence of IFI in children (as defined by EORTC/MSG criteria) with acute leukemia and febrile neutropenia who were not on antifungal prophylaxis was significantly high (23%) with a relatively low mortality rate of 9.5%.

EVALUATION

Clinical and laboratory evaluation should be thoroughly done in every patient with febrile neutropenia.

Clinical

Common sites of infection like oral cavity and periodontal region, GI tract, lungs, skin, IV sites/central line exit sites, perianal and perineal region should be examined. Typical signs of inflammation may be absent in a neutropenic patient in spite of obvious infection and hence patient may have skin infection without typical cellulitis, lung infection without the typical infiltrates on X-ray, meningitis without obvious clinical signs or cerebrospinal fluid (CSF) pleocytosis and urinary tract infection (UTI) without pyuria. Pain may be the only symptom of localization.

Laboratory

Laboratory evaluation includes estimation of complete blood counts, serum creatinine, serum transaminases, and serum electrolytes. These investigations will help define any organ dysfunction and guide therapy while using potentially nephrotoxic antimicrobials like aminoglycosides, amphotericin B, etc. Sending C-reactive protein (CRP) is recommended to estimate the severity of infection and to follow-up response to antimicrobial therapy. Similarly, procalcitonin has been found to be beneficial in differentiating infection from drug fever in oncology patients and follow-up response to therapy.

Most important is to obtain blood cultures. The yield is highest with two blood culture sets taken from two separate venipunctures. Blood from one venipuncture is inoculated in one aerobic and one anaerobic bottle; hence two sets indicate four bottles. The anaerobic culture is important even for picking up facultative anaerobes such as *Enterobacteriaceae* and streptococci apart from the fastidious anaerobes. Cultures in fungal media should be sent if *Candida* is suspected. If there is a central venous catheter then one set should be from the catheter and one from a peripheral vein. The yield of culture depends on the volume of blood inoculated in the culture medium and at least a total of 1% of the circulating blood volume should be collected (40% in adults). Blood cultures should be obtained before the antibiotics are administered or changed. Ideally blood cultures should be done using automated methods as they are quick, better isolation rate, and can tell the differential time taken for positivity when simultaneous cultures are obtained from peripheral site and catheter lumen in a suspected case of catheter-related bloodstream infections. High-grade bacteremia, with more than 500 cfu/mL, is associated with greater morbidity and mortality.

Lastly if possible, quantitative or semi-quantitative culture of catheter tip should be done whenever the catheter is removed for suspected/established line sepsis. Similarly culture from local discharge at IV site infection or local wound should be done whenever present. Routine cultures of urine or stools are not indicated as the yield is poor; however they should be done whenever local urinary or GI infection is suspected. In patients with diarrhea one may need to send tests for *C. difficile* infection and multiplex PCR of stool to detect other pathogens such as norovirus and cryptosporidium which can cause severe diarrhea in immunocompromised as well as modified acid-fast bacilli (AFB) stain to detect other opportunistic pathogens including Microsporidia and Isospora. Routine X-ray of the chest is not indicated unless patient has chest symptoms or the patient is being treated as an outpatient. In patients with respiratory symptoms, there may be a place to send multiplex PCR of nasopharyngeal swab for respiratory viruses if facilities are available.

Patients with persistent fever will need further evaluation including CT of chest to pick up invasive mold infection and biomarkers such as serum or bronchoalveolar lavage (BAL) galactomannan.

INITIAL EMPIRIC ANTIBIOTIC THERAPY

As the course of bloodstream infections in a neutropenic patient can be rapid and fatal, empirical antibiotics are justified in febrile neutropenic patients. The choice of initial antibiotics will depend on the local etiology pattern, previous experience and exposure to antibiotics, and previous colonizing flora if available. A very important consideration is the degree of sickness of the patient; a sick patient with organ dysfunction merits high-end antibiotics at the onset. Other factors include presence of a catheter and toxicities of the drugs used like nephrotoxicity of aminoglycosides used with amphotericin B.

Standard guidelines recommend classifying patients as low-risk or high-risk as shown in Box 1. Guidelines recommend trying oral antibiotics for low-risk adults, however oral antibiotic therapy for low-risk patients is not approved for children. It is also not a viable option in the Indian setting since prevalence of drug resistance to oral antibiotics is extremely high. So

BOX 1: Factors defining patient at low risk to develop severe infection.

- Neutrophil count more than or equal to 100/ mm^3, monocyte count more than or equal to 100/ mm^3
- Duration of neutropenia less than 7 days and recovery expected within 10 days
- Normal results of imaging studies including X-ray of chest
- Normal results of organ function tests
- No catheter-related infection suspected
- Malignancy in remission
- Clinically stable patient without comorbidity

(Excludes pediatric patient for initial oral antibiotic therapy)

parenteral antibiotics are indicated in all settings of childhood febrile neutropenia at least to begin with.

There are two options available for initial antibiotic therapy—(1) de-escalation approach and (2) escalation approach. This approach has been suggested by the European consortium for treatment of infections in cancer patients and suits us better than the IDSA guidelines that are more conservative and have not been revised for the past one decade. The focus is on an appropriate Gram-negative cover since they are the predominant cause of febrile neutropenia in our setting. Since the incidence of infections with Gram-positive infections has declined, vancomycin as a rule should not be used as initial therapy for febrile neutropenia. Infections caused by most of the vancomycin needing organisms are indolent and delaying vancomycin for 2–3 days till culture reports are available does no harm. Penicillin-resistant *S. viridans* may lead to severe infection and need vancomycin, but it is sensitive to most commonly used first-line antibiotics as discussed below. Use of vancomycin as the first-line therapy routinely is likely to do more harm by inducing vancomycin resistance in organisms, especially enterococci. Clinical situations which require vancomycin as first-line therapy are discussed later in the article.

De-escalation Approach

This approach is recommended for sick patients with complicated presentations or organ dysfunction and where there is high likelihood of infection with multi-drug resistant (MDR)/ extremely drug resistance (XDR) pathogens.

Here the antimicrobials recommended are:

- Carbapenems with or without aminoglycoside
- Carbapenem with colistin/polymyxin B
- Any of the above with addition of glycopeptides (vancomycin/teicoplanin) if risk factors are present.

The decision to add aminoglycosides will depend on the rates of aminoglycoside susceptibility at the center/seriousness of infection. In centers where there is high prevalence of carbapenem resistance or where there is history of exposure to carbapenems or known infection/colonization in the index case with carbapenem-resistant bacteria, polymyxins may need to be added to the regimen. Colistin is the preferred polymyxin, but in patients with septic shock where quick attainment of steady state is required or where there is pre-existent renal dysfunction, polymyxin B may be used. In some centers where carbapenem resistance rates are high and patient is extremely sick/carbapenem experienced, one may have to use reserve antimicrobials such as tigecycline/fosfomycin in combination with the polymyxins. This is because here using polymyxin with carbapenems is like using polymyxin monotherapy which is associated with high mortality (Chapter 13).

As discussed earlier, routine use of glycopeptides is not indicated for all sick patients. Addition of glycopeptides for empiric therapy should be considered if there is suspected serious catheter-related infection, unstable patient with hypotension, known colonization with drug-resistant Gram-positive organisms in past, use of quinolones prophylaxis in past, and perhaps fever more than 40°C, and presence of severe mucositis. Vancomycin is the gold standard drug but teicoplanin has also been used widely especially in Europe. Advantages of teicoplanin are reduced infusion related side effects and nephrotoxicity. Linezolid, though effective, is not commonly used due to its myelosuppressive potential.

Escalation Approach

This approach is recommended for stable patients at low-risk for infection with XDR pathogens. In Western literature, monotherapy with ceftazidime and cefepime is indicated in this group of patients. However, these are not viable options in India since the prevalence rates of ESBL pathogens is extremely high even approaching 80%. Hence, the frontline antimicrobial recommended in this setting is a β-lactam-β-lactamase inhibitor (BL-BLI) combination either piperacillin-tazobactam/cefoperazone-sulbactam with or without aminoglycoside. The choice between piperacillin-tazobactam and cefoperazone-sulbactam is center-dependent and is discussed in greater detail in Chapter 8. The addition of an aminoglycoside is again dependent on local susceptibility patterns and recommended for patients with hematologic malignancies; in patients with febrile neutropenia following chemotherapy for solid tumors, monotherapy with BL-BLI combinations can be used.

ANTIBIOTIC THERAPY IN THE FIRST 5–7 DAYS

After starting empirical antibiotics, one has to decide on the follow-up and the duration for which antibiotics need to be continued. The culture reports will be available in the first 48–72 hours. If positive, the drugs should be optimized. If vancomycin is started and the organisms show sensitivity to other drugs, vancomycin should be stopped. If carbapenem-resistant organism has been isolated, therapy should be changed to polymyxin-based combination therapy (with carbapenems/tigecycline/fosfomycin as discussed in chapter 13). If combination therapy was started, one drug may be dropped if susceptibility results so indicate. De-escalation is particularly important to preserve antimicrobial options for future infections.

If the patient shows deterioration, one may have to add or change antibiotics even before 72 hours, otherwise it usually takes 3–5 days for response to the first-line antibiotics. Low-risk patients may show response as early as 2 days. Accordingly the patient may be afebrile in first 3–5 days or the patient may continue to have persistent fever in the first 3–5 days. The approach to both these situations is different as shown in Flowcharts 1 and 2.

- *Patient is afebrile in the first 3–5 days of initial antibiotic therapy (Flowchart 1):* If the causative organism is identified, the antibiotics are adjusted according to the sensitivity pattern. When

Flowchart 1: Management approach in patients afebrile in first 3–5 days after initial empirical antibiotic therapy.

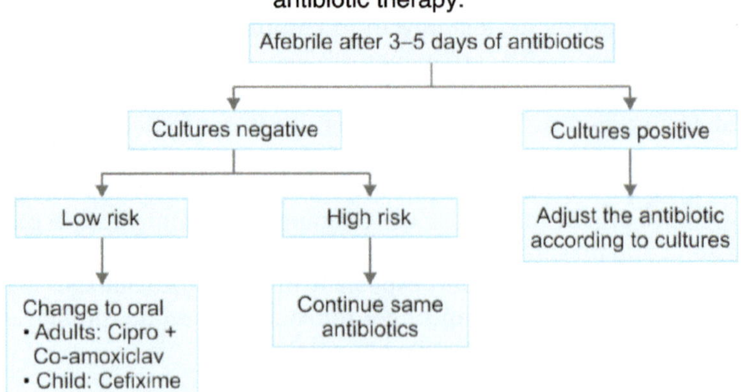

Flowchart 2: Management approach in patients with persistent fever in first 3–5 days after initial empirical antibiotic therapy.

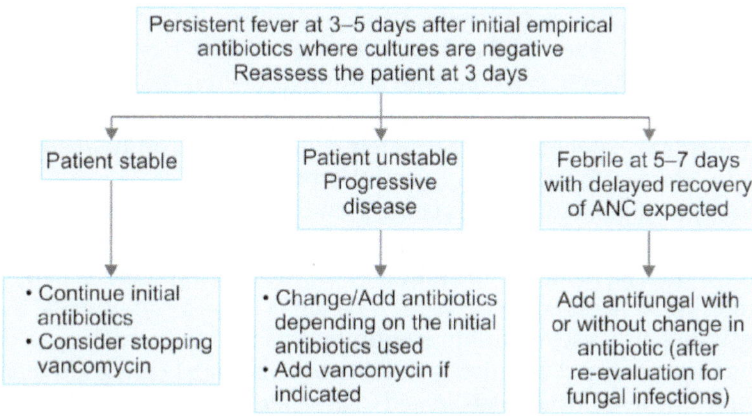

(ANC: absolute neutrophil count)

the cultures are negative and there is no discernible focus of infection and the patient is low-risk to start with and if the neutrophil counts are recovering, one can, after 48–72 hours of IV antibiotics, change to oral antibiotics, i.e. ciprofloxacin plus amoxicillin-clavulanic acid in adults and cefixime in children as studies have shown that the outcome is the same with both approaches. Oral antibiotics are more convenient, cheaper, and acceptable to patients. In patients who were sick at onset or where the neutrophil counts are low, one may continue the same empiric IV antibiotics.

- *Patient has persistent fever in the first 3–5 days of initial antibiotic therapy:* When the cultures are negative and the patient is still febrile on day 3 after the initial antibiotics, possibilities include—(1) the patient has non-bacterial infection; (2) delayed response as some patients may take up to 5 days for the response; (3) infection with drug-resistant organisms; (4) a breakthrough secondary infection; (5) super-added fungal infection; (6) suboptimal antibiotic levels or (7) presence of organ infection like abscess. The patient should be re-evaluated at 72 hours including thorough clinical examination, repeat cultures, serum creatinine, serum transaminases, imaging as deemed appropriate (chest and paranasal sinuses, abdomen), biomarkers such as serum galactomannan/beta-D-glucan, and checking of the catheter site. If the reassessment yields positive result, antibiotics are changed accordingly. If not and the patient is still febrile at 5 days, one has one of the three choices—(1) continue same antibiotics, (2) change/add antibiotics, and (3) add antifungal with or without change in antibiotics (Flowchart 2).
    1. *Continue the same antibiotics:* If the patient is clinically stable, there is no discernible focus and the cultures are negative on reassessment, one can continue the same antibiotics as some patients may respond only on or after 5 days.
    2. *Change/add antibiotics*: If the patient shows progression with new symptoms, diarrhea, abdominal pain, hypotension, new pulmonary infiltrates, and IV line discharge, one has to change or add antibiotics. This will depend on the initial antibiotics used, degree of sickness, and local flora. Usually this entails change to a better Gram-negative cover since most infections in our setting are Gram-negative. If BL-BLI combinations were used, therapy should be changed to carbapenem with or without aminoglycosides/polymyxins.

In settings where resistant Gram-positive infections are common and if glycopeptides were not used initially, they can be added.

3. *Add antifungals*: It has been proved that patients with profound neutropenia of more than 7–10 days who fail to respond to antibiotics for 5–7 days have 30% chances of a fungal infection. Most physicians would start antifungals when the patient is still febrile with neutropenia in spite of adequate antibiotics at the end of 5–7 days. However, if recovery of neutropenia is expected within next few days, one can withhold antifungals.

One has to investigate for fungal infection thoroughly like sinus studies, chest imaging, and biomarkers. Serum galactomannan using a cutoff defined as more than or equal to 0.5 has been found to have good sensitivity (76%) and specificity (86%) for diagnosis of invasive aspergillosis in children as in adults. In children with high-risk of mold infection twice weekly galactomannan estimation is recommended (A II) but is usually not possible due to high cost and availability issues. The use of antifungal prophylaxis also reduces the performance of the serum galactomannan assay. A positive BAL galactomannan ($\geq$1) is a good diagnostic test for invasive pulmonary aspergillosis. In suspected CNS aspergillosis, a CSF galactomannan can be estimated (cutoff of $\geq$0.5). There is limited data about the sensitivity and specificity of the beta-D-glucan test in diagnosis of invasive *Candida* and *Aspergillus* infection in children with some current studies showing high rates of false positivity. CT imaging of chest sinuses is of value in diagnosis of invasive mold infection. However, the characteristic signs of invasive pulmonary aspergillosis including the halo/crescent and reverse halo signs are seen infrequently in children especially those below 5. The usual findings in young children are nonspecific nodules, masses, consolidations, and infiltrates.

In centers where access to biomarkers and imaging is readily available, one may follow the algorithm of pre-emptive antifungals where antifungals are withheld if imaging and biomarkers are negative. In other circumstances, one uses empiric antifungal therapy. In centers where fluconazole is not used for prophylaxis and chances of infection with *Aspergillus fumigatus* or fluconazole-resistant species like *C. krusei* or *C. glabrata* are low, one can use fluconazole as it is cheap, oral, and convenient. However more often than not, where there are chances of resistant *Candida* infection or likelihood of invasive mold infection (respiratory infections or sinusitis), one should use amphotericin B. Liposomal amphotericin is the drug of choice for empiric therapy for febrile neutropenia. However if there are cost issues one may use amphotericin B deoxycholate. Children tolerate amphotericin B deoxycholate (AMB-D) better than adults. Other options for empirical therapy for febrile neutropenia include caspofungin and voriconazole.

DURATION OF ANTIBIOTICS (FLOWCHART 3)

If cultures are positive then antibiotics (whether IV or oral) need to be given for 10–14 days depending on the etiologic organism. In culture negative cases, the most important determinant to decide when to stop antibiotics is neutrophil count as shown in Flowchart 3. When ANC is more than 500 cells/mm^3, the patient is afebrile for more than 2 days, the patient is clinically stable without any complications and no organism is isolated on cultures, one can stop the antibiotics. If the patient is afebrile, but continues to have ANC less than 500 cells/mm^3, one should ideally continue antibiotics for the whole neutropenic period; however this will increase the toxicities, cost, and chances of development of drug resistance. The current consensus, as especially advocated by the European consortium, is to hit hard in the beginning and stop quickly. Hence the antibiotics can be stopped after the patient is healthy and afebrile for at least 48 hours even if the ANC is still low. The patient should be monitored and antibiotics should

Flowchart 3: Duration of antibiotics in febrile neutropenia.

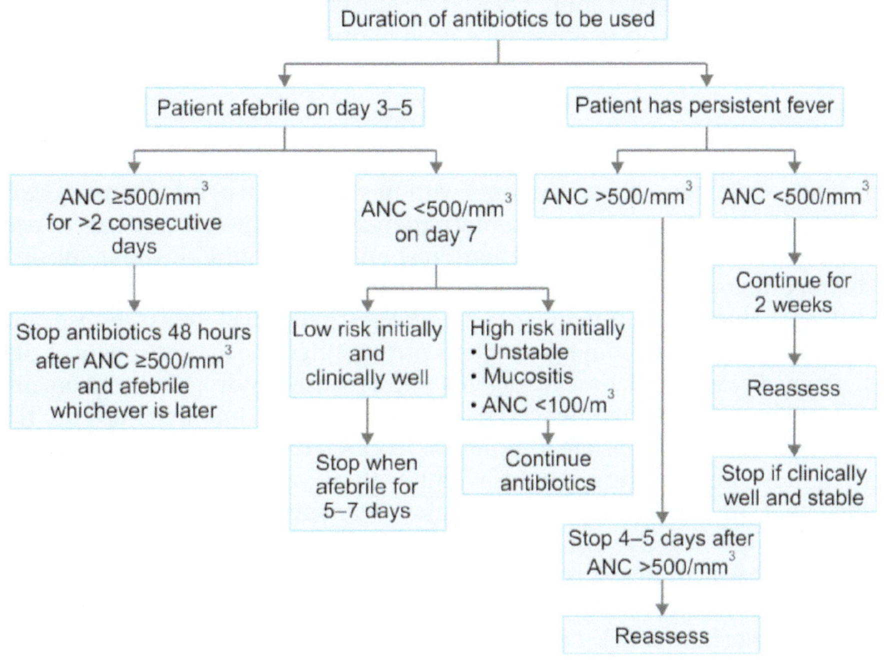

(ANC: absolute neutrophil count)

be restarted after evaluation if the patient develops fever again. In patients with persistent fever, or afebrile patient with unstable condition, mucositis, GI infections, unstable signs, and profound neutropenia one should continue antibiotics for a longer time may be for 2 weeks or more depending on the condition.

The decision as to when to stop antifungal therapy is more difficult to make than when to start it. If the fungus is isolated on cultures, one should continue antifungal accordingly. *Candida* infection should be treated with antifungal for 2 weeks after the blood culture turns negative. For aspergillosis, one has to continue amphotericin B till chest signs are normal, cultures are negative, and imaging shows clearance of infection, which usually will take 4–6 weeks. If the fungus has not been isolated, one can stop antifungals when the patient is clinically well, ANC is more than 500 cells/mm^3, and imaging studies are normal. If the ANC is still low one can continue antifungal for 2 weeks after the patient is clinically well with normal imaging.

For patients who are febrile in spite of ANC more than 500 cells/mm^3, one should rule out other causes of infections like viral infections, fungal infections or mycobacterial infections. One needs to do appropriate cultures, CMV viral load and imaging studies, and clinical evaluation and one can stop antibiotics 5 days after the ANC is more than 500/mm^3.

ANTIVIRAL THERAPY

Antiviral drugs are indicated only for treating definite viral infections like HSV, varicella, cytomegalovirus infection, etc. They are not indicated as empirical therapy or as prophylactic therapy. CMV viremia has emerged as not an uncommon cause of prolonged pyrexia in neutropenia resulting from cancer chemotherapy unlike earlier where it was more commonly seen in stem cell transplant patients. Diagnosis is by doing quantitative viral load. In patients with CMV disease, IV ganciclovir should be started and continued till the viral load is negative. Later patient should be put on maintenance dose of oral valganciclovir till period of intense chemotherapy is over. One should also watch for relapse in future with further chemotherapy.

OUTCOME

Outcome of the febrile neutropenic patients with bacteremia depends on many variables in spite of the best therapy. A study of bacteremic patients with febrile neutropenia done over two decades showed that the percentage of patients responding to antibiotics has gone up recently, reflecting better understanding of the disease and better management options available of late. Patients with sepsis due to *Pseudomonas* or *Enterobacter* species have less response rate (84% vs. 93%) as compared to all other etiological agents put together due to more chances of complex sepsis (with organ disease) with these two agents. Sepsis caused by drug-resistant organisms (e.g. MRSA or penicillin-resistant streptococci) had poor response to initial therapy but responded well with the change to appropriate antibiotics. In cases of sepsis caused by Gram-positive organisms, the response rate was similar whether there was simple sepsis (without major organ involvement) or complex sepsis (with major organ involvement), whereas in cases with sepsis caused by Gram-negative organisms, the response rates were less for complex sepsis as compared to simple sepsis. Response rate was better when the neutrophil count recovered as compared to when it decreased or remained low. Those with shock at presentation fared worse than those who did not have shock. Lastly, the choice of correct antibiotics led to better outcome.

COST CONSIDERATIONS IN FEBRILE NEUTROPENIA

Various studies have shown tremendous scope for cost reduction while treating patients with febrile neutropenia without compromise in the outcome or morbidity. Basic principles of personal hygiene and precautions taken in the hospital by caretakers including health care workers go a long way in preventing episodes of febrile episodes in cancer patients and the ultimate cost of therapy. Besides this, intelligent management of febrile neutropenia episodes can also bring down the cost of therapy.

Correct choice of antibiotics (avoidance of expensive antibiotics like vancomycin and carbapenem when not indicated), correct dose, use of oral antibiotics in low-risk patients (in adults), step down with early discharge after response to initial antibiotics (possible in pediatric patients), avoiding indiscriminate use of antifungals like amphotericin B, reserving use of liposomal amphotericin B only for those who cannot tolerate regular amphotericin B, and avoiding unnecessarily prolonged course of therapy are some of the measures one can use to bring down the cost.

Outdoor therapy and oral antibiotics are two options that bring down the cost of therapy. In pediatric patients outdoor treatment or oral antibiotics as the initial treatment is not recommended as there is very little experience with this mode of therapy in pediatric patients. However in low-risk pediatric patients one can step down to oral drugs and discharge the patient early when the patient becomes afebrile after 48 hours of IV antibiotic therapy. Similarly drugs like vancomycin and carbapenem are often misused as panacea of all "pyrexia of unknown origin (PUO)" in sick children with febrile neutropenia (often without proper cultures), which not only increases the cost but also induces emergence of drug resistance; this is to be condemned. They should be used only when indicated.

PROPHYLAXIS

Antibiotic Prophylaxis

Neutropenia is a good predictor for subsequent episodes of fever and infection. Early afebrile period in a neutropenic patient thus provides an opportunity to start antibiotic prophylaxis to prevent or reduce the chances of subsequent infections. Various drugs have been used for this purpose. Most of the drugs are aimed at selective sterilization of gut, the main source of pathogens in febrile neutropenic patients. Non-absorbable drugs like neomycin, polymyxin, and vancomycin have been found to be inferior to absorbable drugs like trimethoprim-sulfamethoxazole (TMP-SMX) or quinolones. TMP-SMX has been shown to significantly reduce the incidence of fever and infections as compared to placebo. Similarly quinolones have been shown to be better that TMP-SMX and quinolones plus penicillin have been shown to be better than quinolones alone when used prophylactically. Use of antibiotics for prophylaxis however leads to toxicities, marrow suppression, and all of which counter the benefits of reduced infections. The most important problem is emergence of drug-resistant organisms, a situation which is not desirable or acceptable. Moreover these studies of benefits of prophylaxis are from the Western World where there is still good susceptibility to drugs like quinolones. This approach is unlikely to work in India where resistant rates to quinolones and TMP- SMX are high.

Hence routine use of antibiotics for prophylaxis in neutropenic children is not justified. More important than prophylaxis is use of good infection control measures to prevent infections.

Antifungal Prophylaxis

Here again the most important measures includes implementation of the prevention bundle for central venous catheters, avoiding areas of construction, dampness and seepage, and potted plants. Patients undergoing HSCT and even those patients on cancer chemotherapy with severe and prolonged neutropenia should be treated in rooms with positive pressure and high-efficiency particulate air (HEPA) filters.

Not all children with cancer need prophylaxis. There is a general consensus that children undergoing allogenic HSCT, with acute myeloid leukemia (AML), relapsed acute lymphoblastic leukemia (ALL), and severe aplastic anemia should be given antifungal prophylaxis. Patients undergoing autologous HSCT should also receive antiyeast prophylaxis during the neutropenic phase. Newly diagnosed ALL, solid tumors do not merit routine antifungal prophylaxis. Options for antifungal prophylaxis include fluconazole, itraconazole, voriconazole, and posaconazole in those above 13 years, intermittent liposomal amphotericin B, nebulized amphotericin B, and echinocandins. Choice depends on the pattern/prevalence of mold infections, logistics and cost, and is center-dependent; there is no one size fits all approach.

TMP-SMX is indicated for prophylaxis against *Pneumocystis jiroveci* in children with ALL, lymphoma, and those undergoing HSCT.

CONCLUSION

In conclusion, febrile neutropenia is often an emergency while dealing with patients who are immune compromised. This is one situation where empirical antibiotic therapy is perfectly justified and it is often to err on doing more than lose a patient. Unless treated in time with the appropriate antibiotic, the mortality is high and the time available often is in hours and not days.

Proper clinical evaluation may provide some hints as to the type and the site of infection, however the classical signs of inflammation are usually missing in these patients. The main emphasis is on obtaining proper cultures and on starting appropriate antibiotics without waiting for the reports of investigations. One needs to use first-line antibiotics depending on local spectrum and sensitivity and on recent local experience. One needs to modify the drugs depending on the reports of cultures.

RECOMMENDED READING

1. Averbuch D, Orasch C, Cordonnier C, et al. ECIL4, a joint venture of EBMT, EORTC, ICHS, ESGICH/ ESCMID and ELN. European guidelines for empirical antibacterial therapy for febrile neutropenic patients in the era of growing resistance: summary of the 2011 4th European Conference on Infections in Leukemia. Haematologica. 2013;98(12):1826-35.
2. Elting LS, Rubenstein EB, Rolston K, et al. Time to clinical response: an outcome of antibiotic therapy of febrile neutropenia with implications for quality and cost of care. J Clin Oncol. 2000;18:3699-706.
3. Elting LS, Rubenstein EB, Rolston KV, et al. Outcomes of bacteria in patients with cancer and neutropenia: observation from two decades of epidemiological and clinical trials. Clin Infect Dis. 1997;25:247-59.
4. Giamarellou H, Antoniadou A. Infectious complications of febrile leucopenia. Infect Dis Clin North Am. 2001;2:457-82.
5. Groll AH, Castagnola E, Cesaro S, et al. Fourth European Conference on Infections in Leukaemia (ECIL-4): guidelines for diagnosis, prevention, and treatment of invasive fungal diseases in paediatric patients with cancer or allogeneic haemopoietic stem-cell transplantation. Lancet Oncol. 2014;15:e327-40.
6. Hughes WT, Armstrong D, Bodey GP, et al. 2002 guidelines for the use of antimicrobial agents in neutropenic patients with cancer. Clin Infect Dis. 2002;34:730-50.
7. Jones RN. Contemporary antimicrobial susceptibility patterns of bacterial pathogens associated with febrile patients with neutropenia. Clin Infect Dis. 1999;29:495-502.
8. Kanvinde S, Bhargava P, Patwardhan S. Cytomegalovirus infection as a cause of cytopenia after chemotherapy for hematological malignancies. Indian Pediatr. 2013;50(2):197-201.
9. Kern W, Kurrle E. Ofloxacin versus trimethoprim-sulphamethoxazole for prevention of infection in patients with acute leukemia and granulocytopenia. Infection. 1991;19:73-80.
10. Kern WV, Cometta A, Bock RD, et al. Oral versus intravenous empirical antimicrobial therapy for fever in patients with granulocytopenia who are receiving cancer chemotherapy. N Engl J Med. 1999;341:312-8.
11. Klaassen RJ, Goodman TR, Pham B, et al. "Low- risk" prediction rule for pediatric oncology patients with fever and neutropenia. J Clin Oncol. 2000;18:1012-9.
12. Kumar J, Singh A, Seth R, et al. Prevalence and predictors of invasive fungal infections in children with persistent febrile neutropenia treated for acute leukemia: A prospective study. Indian J Pediatr. 2018;85(12):1090-5.
13. Pizzo PA. Fever in immunocompromised patients. N Engl J Med. 1999;341:893-900.
14. Rubin M, Hathorn JW, Marshall D, et al. Gram-positive infections and the use of vancomycin in 550 episodes of fever and neutropenia. Ann Int Med. 1988;108:30-5.
15. Shenep JL, Flynn PM, Baker DK, et al. Oral cefixime is similar to continued intravenous antibiotics in the empirical treatment of febrile neutropenic children with cancer. Clin Infect Dis. 2001;32:36-43.
16. Symposium-Infections in Cancer. Ind J of Cancer 2014; 51(4): 415-496.
17. Zinner SH. Changing epidemiology of infections in patients with neutropenia and cancer: Emphasis on gram-positive and resistant bacteria. Clin Infect Dis. 1999;29:490-4.

Antimicrobial Prophylaxis

32
Chapter

Pramod Kulkarni

INTRODUCTION

Prophylaxis means "Treatment given or action taken to prevent disease" (Latin *pro*—"before" + Greek *phylaxis*—to "guard" or prevent beforehand). Antimicrobial prophylaxis (AP) refers to the prevention of infection using antimicrobial therapy, most commonly "Antibiotics". This preventive intervention may be primary (i.e. at exposure to, before invasion by pathogen) or secondary (i.e. after invasion by pathogen). AP is a valuable arm of antimicrobial therapy in the management of infectious diseases.

Unfortunately, prophylactic use of antibiotics has serious limitations and consequences; especially when used indiscriminately and for prolonged periods as commonly happens in practice such as:

- Overuse and failure of AP
- Potential harm to individual—various adverse drug reactions, drug interactions, and allergic risks
- Waste of resources
- Contribution to increasing antimicrobial resistance (AMR).

A recent review of antibiotic usage reveals sizeable, significantly inappropriate prophylactic use of antibiotic globally. Stark overuse, extended duration, preference for broad spectrum and multiple antibiotics are the highlight of misappropriate pediatric AP. Most inappropriate use of prophylactic antimicrobials occurs in situations of perioperative usage, prevention of infective endocarditis, recurrent urinary tract infections (UTI), and neonatal and critical care infections. Regular periodic critical reassessment of prophylactic antibiotic usage, regional AMR trends, revision of local guidelines/recommendations, and measures to improve adherence to AP regimen are the priority remedial interventions. Emerging evidence, growing awareness, and better understanding of AMR over last decade have significantly changed the approach of global authorities toward AP. Global trends in AP recommendations now reflect less aggressive approach, better definitions of indications, and sparing use of antimicrobial agents. Active immune prophylaxis through appropriate, effective, and up-to-date immunization, and meticulous infection control practices are undoubtedly superior, effective, safe, and desirable preventive measures than AP alone.

Judicious use of chemoprophylaxis is known to reduce serious infections and their consequences in many clinical situations with high risk of infection. In reality, there are only a select few indications having good clinical evidence to support such presumed benefits and are well accepted recommendations for AP.

In office practice and small hospitals, common notable indications of antibiotic prophylaxis with definite potential benefits are: surgical site infections, recurrent UTI, recurrent otitis media, outbreak infections, tuberculosis, perinatal infections, travel infections, contagious serious bacterial infections (SBI) in household, infective endocarditis, rheumatic fever and heart diseases, and opportunistic infections in HIV care.

Additionally, in advanced/specialty care pediatric facilities, healthcare-associated/hospital-acquired infections are emerging as main targets for chemoprophylaxis. Situations with opportunities for AP in these facilities are: healthcare-associated infections (HAI) associated with advanced neonatal care, intensive care, chronic disease care, device and implants, hematopoietic stem cell transplants and organ transplants, hematology, oncology, and immune compromising conditions like primary immune deficiencies. AP in specialty child care at advanced centers is not discussed in detail here and reference to respective specialty and infectious disease resources is recommended.

BASICS

Principles of Antimicrobial Prophylaxis

Successful use of prophylactic antibiotic depends on the following principles:
- The individual patient should be at definite and high risk of infection
- The likely and prevalent infecting organisms and their current susceptibilities should be well-known
- The antimicrobial agent must be rationally selected and has to be effective at the target site
- Prophylaxis should be administered only for shortest possible period of exposure/infection risk
- Other measures of infection control must be followed to reduce size of infective pathogen inoculum
- Existing infection must be treated appropriately and completely with therapeutic regimen prior to AP.

Ideal Antimicrobial Agent for Prophylaxis

The ideal antimicrobial for prophylactic use should have proven efficacy and a therapeutic safety so that its benefits clearly outweigh the risks. It should have good tissue penetration to achieve adequate bactericidal concentrations at the target site under risk of infection. It should have narrowest possible spectrum, no toxicity, few side effects, and should not alter the host flora or induce development of bacterial resistance. It should not be extensively used in therapy. Easy accessibility, affordable cost, acceptability, convenience of administration, and low monitoring needs of the agent are equally desirable characteristics.

Duration and Timing

Duration and timing of AP are dependent on period of high risk. A brief/limited time exposure in a healthy host usually needs short duration AP over few days, e.g. perioperative/surgical site infection (SSI), household/close contacts of outbreak infections or invasive bacterial infections. A high risk of infections due to prolonged but finite time host defense issues like recurrent UTI, otitis media or hematopoietic stem cell transplantation (HSCT) recipients, HIV infected usually need continuous AP for few months. A constant risk of serious infections in a host with significantly impaired specific or general immunity mandates AP over decades or even lifetime, e.g. rheumatic fever, primary immune deficiencies. Prophylaxis aimed at infections with a single exogenous pathogen given over short period of time is likely to be more successful then otherwise.

SURGICAL PROPHYLAXIS

Surgical site infections are one of the most common HAIs. SSIs average 1–5% of common hospital surgeries and are associated with significant morbidity, mortality, and health care expenditure. Patients developing SSIs are 60% more likely to be admitted to an ICU, are more than five times more likely to be readmitted to the hospital and are twice as likely to die as similar patients without SSIs. Prevention of SSI with all relevant measures including judicious perioperative AP is therefore a top priority. At the same time, inappropriate use of perioperative AP can result in *Clostridium difficile* infection and/or adverse drug events at patient level or increase in AMR and health care costs at population level. It should also be remembered that surgical AP is not a replacement of basic infection control measures including hand hygiene to prevent SSI. Even high-end antibiotics will not prevent SSI if the basic infection prevention bundle is not adhered to.

Following categorization of surgical procedures can guide estimation of associated risks of infection.

Clean: Elective, non-traumatic, no acute site inflammation, no break, non gastrointestinal tract (GIT), respiratory tract entry, closed primarily: infection risk less than 2%.

Clean contaminated: Emergency, elective entry to GIT, respiratory tract, minimal noninfected spill, minor break: infection risk less than 10%.

Contaminated: Non-purulent inflammation/infection at site, gross spill, major break, and penetrating trauma less than 4 hours, chronic wound grafting: infection risk~20%.

Dirty: Purulent inflammation/infection of site, preoperative perforation of tract, and penetrating trauma more than 4 hours: infection risk~40%.

Common clean traumatic cuts, lacerations, abrasions, nonextensive superficial burns do not warrant systemic AP. Appropriate asepsis, wound care, topical antibiotic and a keen follow-up are mostly adequate. Systemic AP is indicated for clean/clean contaminated surgical procedures. When antibiotics are used for contaminated and dirty wounds, they are treatment and not prophylaxis.

Choice of Antibiotic

Antibiotics should be chosen on the basis of their effectiveness against the pathogens most likely to be encountered rather than against every possible pathogen. Skin flora (e.g. *Staphylococcus*) is the usual target, so first- or second-generation cephalosporins including cefazolin or cefuroxime are the usual choices. For surgeries in the head and neck, gynecologic tract and colon/rectum addition of metronidazole is recommended. For patients undergoing genitourinary procedures, an antimicrobial effective against the uropathogens in that individual is recommended. Use of vancomycin in addition to the usual drugs is indicated for patients colonized with methicillin-resistant *Staphylococcus aureus* (MRSA). For patients with a history of anaphylaxis or urticaria after penicillin/beta-lactam therapy, vancomycin or clindamycin with or without gentamicin should be used. Use of broad-spectrum antibiotics including beta-lactam (BL) + beta-lactamase

TABLE 1: Doses of antibiotics used for surgical prophylaxis.

Antibiotic	*Pediatric dose*	*Adult/max dose*
Cefazolin	30 mg/kg/dose	2 g
IV cefuroxime	30–50 mg/kg/dose	1.5 g/2 g
Gentamicin	4 mg/kg/dose	4 mg/kg/dose/240 mg
Amikacin	15 mg/kg/dose	15 mg/kg/dose/1 g
Vancomycin	15 mg/kg/ dose	1 g/2 g
Metronidazole	10–15 mg/kg/dose	500 mg
Clindamycin	10–20 mg/kg/dose	600/900 mg

inhibitor (BLI) combinations and carbapenems for routine surgical prophylaxis is not desirable and hence not recommended. If the patient is already on broad-spectrum antibiotics for pre-existing infections (known or suspected), additional surgical AP may not be necessary. Doses should be scheduled for re-dosing just prior to skin incision. Doses of commonly used antibiotics for surgical prophylaxis are listed in Table 1.

Timing and Duration

The most important principle in surgical antibiotic prophylaxis is to ensure high blood levels of effective antibiotic at the time of anticipated wound contamination. The drug should therefore be administered IV within 60 minutes of the skin incision. Studies have shown that administration between 0–30 minutes is better than 30–60 minutes. For antibiotics with longer administration time, e.g. vancomycin infusion must be started 120 minutes prior to the time of skin incision. The antimicrobial should be repeated if the surgery time exceeds two half-lives of the antibiotic, e.g. cefazolin and cefuroxime should be re-dosed for surgery lasting more than 4 hours.

During surgical procedures, the infection risk period is finite and therefore the AP regimen should also be appropriately short/limited duration. A single dose prior to skin incision is usually sufficient. Most studies show no added benefit of extending antimicrobial prophylaxis to more than single dose and in fact contribute to increase in antimicrobial resistance and adverse effects including *C. difficile.*

RECURRENT UTI

Use of continuous antibiotic prophylaxis (CAP) to prevent recurrent UTI in children is an established practice. It is based on concerns about additive renal injury and potential long-term renal dysfunction, and hypertension linked to recurrent UTI. UTI in infants and young children have a high recurrence rate of about 30 to 50%, mostly during subsequent 3–6 months. Children with UTI and vesicoureteral reflux (VUR) show renal parenchymal scarring in 10–15%. About 10% of these children are presumed to develop hypertension and a fewer number, renal insufficiency. AP is therefore warranted.

Children with congenital anomalies of kidney and urinary tract, like VUR detected at antenatal ultrasound screening or at first symptomatic UTI in children are the usual indications for continuous AP for recurrent UTI. It is assumed that continuous antibiotic prophylaxis results in sterile urine which does not cause renal damage with continued reflux and in most cases, reflux is observed to resolve spontaneously.

High risk of AMR development due to long duration of AP and difficult management of resistant breakthrough infections are significant limitations of continuous AP for recurrent UTI.

Current evidence of efficacy and benefits of AP for recurrent UTI is conflicting and controversial. Modest benefits in preventing recurrent febrile/symptomatic UTI episodes are noted without significant benefits in curtailing long-term renal dysfunction and hypertension. Consequently, different regional guidelines vary in considerations and recommendations for CAP. The current IAP guidelines continue to recommend continuous AP for recurrent UTI. Indications include:

- UTI below 1 year of age while awaiting imaging studies
- VUR: For grades I and II, antibiotic prophylaxis until 1 year old. Restart prophylaxis if breakthrough febrile UTI. For grade III–V prophylaxis till age 5 years. If breakthrough, consider surgery. Extend prophylaxis beyond 5 if bladder bowel dysfunction.
- Frequent febrile UTI (3 or more episodes in a year) even if the urinary tract is normal. Here prophylaxis should be continued for 6 months–1 year.
- Antibiotic prophylaxis is not advised in patients with urinary tract obstruction (e.g. posterior urethral valves), urolithiasis, and neurogenic bladder, and in patients on clean intermittent catheterization.

Recommended Agents

The agent should have best urinary concentration and least systemic levels with optimal action against common uropathogens, i.e. Gram-negative enteric bacteria and perineal flora. Any one of following may be given in single daily dose at bedtime:

- Trimethoprim (TMP)–sulfamethoxazole: 2 mg TMP/kg (not for age <2 months)
- Nitrofurantoin: 1–2 mg/kg (not for age <2 months)
- Cephalexin: 10 mg/kg
- Ampicillin: 20 mg/kg
- Amoxicillin: 10 mg/kg.

RECURRENT OTITIS MEDIA

Old studies support modest efficacy of AP with amoxicillin in reducing recurrent episodes of acute otitis media (AOM) in otitis prone children. Alterations in nasopharyngeal flora and colonization with resistant organisms compromise the long-term efficacy of CAP. Increasing coverage with pneumococcal vaccines is reducing the incidence and recurrences of AOM. Tympanostomy tube insertion also modestly reduces recurrent episode of AOM. Other measures include preventing feeding in lying down position and avoiding exposure to indoor air pollution. Therefore, continuous oral AP recommendation is reserved for infrequent situations—3 or more episodes in 6 months or 4 or more episodes in preceding year when other measures have failed. AP for recurrent otitis mostly benefits children less than 2 years age and those at out-of-home child care. AP is targeted at common respiratory pathogens—*Streptococcus pneumoniae, Moraxella catarrhalis,* and non-typable *H. influenzae*. Daily oral administration of amoxicillin 20 mg/kg each evening for 3 to 6 months or winter season is the recommendation.

HOUSEHOLD/OUTBREAK INFECTIONS WITH HIGH RISK/INVASIVE PATHOGENS

Infectious diseases due to invasive pathogen with general risk of severe outcome, high infectivity, rapid/easy spread, and amenable to effective antimicrobial agent are common practice indications for AP (Table 2). Once detected (suspected and/diagnosed) in a household,

TABLE 2: Antimicrobial prophylaxis recommendations for contacts of high risk/invasive infection.

Organism/disease	*AP eligibility/ indications*	*Antimicrobial Agent*	*Route*	*Frequency*	*Daily dose*	*Duration*
Influenza	Only in high-risk contacts within <48 hours of exposure	Oseltamivir	PO	Once a day	3 month–1 year: 3 mg/kg, >1 year and <15 kg: 30 mg, 15 kg–23 kg: 45 mg, 23–35 kg: 60 mg and >35 kg: 75 mg	10 days
Tuberculosis	After exclusion of active TB disease in: 1. All asymptomatic contacts of TB (<6 years age) 2. All neonates of mothers with TB in pregnancy 3. All MT positive children with HIV/immuno-suppressive therapy 4. All HIV-infected children between age 1 year and 5 years	Isoniazid (INH)*	PO	Once a day	10 mg/kg	6 months
Meningococcal disease	Close contacts (>8 hours, <3 feet) of a patient of invasive meningococcal disease or direct exposure to respiratory secretions	Rifampicin *or*	PO	Every 12 hourly	<1 month: 5 mg/kg >1 month: 10 mg/kg	2 days
		Ceftriaxone	IM	Single dose	<15 years: 125 mg >15 years: 250 mg	Only once
Haemophilus influenzae b	Close contact (<10 years age) of a patient of invasive Hib disease-household/ (>4 hours over 5/7 days before hospitalization) Household contacts <18 years age with immune compromise	Rifampicin	PO	Once a day	<1 month: 10 mg/kg >1 month: 20 mg/kg (max 600 mg)	4 days

Contd...

Contd...

Organism/disease	*AP eligibility/ indications*	*Antimicrobial Agent*	*Route*	*Frequency*	*Daily dose*	*Duration*
Cholera	Only if high probability of fecal exposure within 24 hours of index case identification	Azithromycin	PO	Single dose	20 mg/kg max 1 g	Only once
		or Erythromycin	PO	Every 6 hourly	12.5 mg/kg, max 250 mg 4.4 mg/kg max 300 mg	3 days
		or Doxycycline	PO	Single dose		Only once
Pertussis**	Within 21 days of onset of cough in index case Regimen: Same as for treatment	Azithromycin	PO	Once a day	<6 month: 10 mg/kg >6 months: 10 mg/kg max 500 mg 5 mg/kg	5 days D1 followed by D2 through D5
	1. All household contacts, close contacts	Erythromycin	PO	Every 6 hourly	max 250 mg	7–14 days
	2. Non-household contacts at high risk of severe pertussis: Young infants, pregnant women, mod-severe asthma	Clarithromycin	PO	Every 12 hourly	>1 month 15 mg/ kg/day max 1 g	7 days
		TMP + SMX (only if age > 2 months)	PO	Every 12 hourly	8 mg/kg (of TMP) max 320 mg	14 days
Diphtheria**		Erythromycin *or*	PO	6 hourly	40–50 mg/kg Max: 2 g	7 days
		Benzathine penicillin	IM	Once	600,000 unit if <27 kg 1.2 million unit if ≥27 kg	

(SMX: sulfamethoxazole; TMP: trimethoprim)

*alternate regimes considered now include daily INH and rifampicin for 3 months, daily rifampicin for 4 months, daily INH and weekly rifapentine for 12 weeks.

**For pertussis and diphtheria immunization in the nonimmunized/partially immunized contacts is also recommended.

community or locale; prompt and correct preventive interventions along with AP can potentially curtail the spread of infection.

Apart from appropriate index case diagnosis of high-risk infection and its management, identification and evaluation of primary contacts and high-risk population for early pathogen-specific chemoprophylaxis are responsibilities of the pediatrician. Prompt notification to and involvement of local public health systems to investigate, control, and manage the outbreak at community level is a universal regulatory mandate.

MALARIA

Malaria is a common and life-threatening disease transmitted in many tropical and subtropical areas. Travelers from other non-malarious regions having none or partial specific immunity are at risk of severe malaria during visit to any of these 91 countries and territories with high transmission of malaria. Residents of malaria endemic regions including India are immune to severe malaria due to repeated clinical and subclinical malaria episodes, hence do not require prophylaxis. However people of Indian origin who have been residing in non-malaria endemic countries for a long time need prophylaxis before visiting India.

Simultaneous adherence to personal protective measures against mosquito bites is equally important. No antimalarial prophylactic regimen gives complete protection, but good chemoprophylaxis (adherence to the recommended drug regimen) significantly reduces the risk of fatal malaria disease. For travelers to India, options include daily doxycycline, weekly mefloquine or daily atovaquone and proguanil.

Up-to-date knowledge of travel destination malaria transmission status, prevalent *Plasmodia* species with drug susceptibility/resistance and best personal protective measures are essentials of AP advice (Table 3). Such updated information is freely accessible at local/national health agency and WHO and Centers for Disease Control and Prevention (CDC) websites. Attention to adverse effects, drug interactions and intolerance risk of antimalarials is indispensable [WHO, National Vector Borne Disease Control Program (NVBDCP), CDC].

INFECTIVE ENDOCARDITIS

Infective endocarditis (IE) is a life-threatening complication with potential to significantly impair the long-term prognosis in children with cardiac disease. Prevention of IE in susceptible children with congenital cardiac malformations and acquired heart diseases is the oldest, most common, evaluated, established, and standard indication of AP over many decades.

The guidelines are under regular expert revisions and the current American Heart Association (AHA) guidelines (2007) have major changes in recommendations. The new conservative approach for AP is based on widely accepted evidence to focus on optimal oral hygiene more than episodic chemoprophylaxis before potential bacteremic orodental and other non-dental invasive procedures, solely to prevent IE.

Recommendations for AP for IE have now been restricted to considerably narrower group of children having certain cardiac abnormalities with *high risk of adverse outcome* and for certain *dental procedures*. Prophylaxis is no longer recommended for procedures involving the gastrointestinal, genitourinary tracts or upper/lower respiratory tract; solely to prevent infective endocarditis. No significant change was reported in infective endocarditis hospitalization rates after implementation of these revised IE prophylaxis guidelines, over 11 years in USA.

TABLE 3: Recommendations for travel prophylaxis of malaria.

Indications	*Antimalarial agent*	*Route*	*Frequency*	*Dose*	*Timing and duration*
All travelers to malaria endemic areas coming from non-malaria area	Doxycycline OR	PO	Once a day	2.2 mg/kg, max. 100 mg	2 days before, through 4 weeks after travel
Consider prevalent *Plasmodium* species, local drug sensitivity/resistance status Always with personal protective measures	Atovaquone + Proguanil (combination) Pediatric tablet: 62.5 mg ato. + 25 mg proguanil Adult tablet: 250 mg ato. + 100 mg proguanil	PO	Once a day	5–8 kg: ½ pediatric tablet >8–10 kg: ¾ pediatric tablet >10–20 kg: 1 pediatric tablet >20–30 kg: 2 pediatric tablet >30–40 kg: 3 pediatric tablet >40 kg: 1 adult tab	2 days before, through 7 days after travel
Only in mefloquine sensitive areas	Mefloquine	PO	Once a week	5 mg/kg (base), max 300 mg	2 weeks before, through 4 weeks after travel
Only in chloroquine sensitive area	Chloroquine	PO	Once a week	5 mg/kg of base weekly	2 weeks before, through 4 weeks after travel
Only for short travel to vivax area	Primaquine	PO		≤9 kg: 5 mg/kg >9–19 kg: ¼ tablet >19–30 kg: ½ tablet >30–45 kg: ¾ tablet >45 kg: 1 tablet Each tablet: 250 mg salt 5 mg/kg (base), max 300 mg 0.5 mg/kg (base) max. 30 mg	2 days before, through 7 days after travel

TABLE 4: Regimens for antimicrobial prophylaxis for a dental procedure.

Situation	*Agent*	*Route*	*Regimen: Single dose 30 to 60 min Before Procedure*
Oral	Amoxicillin	PO	50 mg/kg max 2 g
Unable to take orally	Ampicillin	IM/IV	50 mg/kg max 2 g
Allergic to penicillin	Cephalexin/Cefuroxime *or* Clindamycin *Or* Azithromycin/ Clarithromycin	PO PO PO	50 mg/kg max 2 g 20 mg/kg max 600 mg 15 mg/kg max 500 mg
Allergic to penicillin/ ampicillin *and* unable to take oral medication	Cefazolin *or* Ceftriaxone *or* Clindamycin	IM/IV IM/IV IM/IV	50 mg/kg max 1 g 50 mg/kg max 1 g 20 mg/kg max 600 mg

Cardiac conditions associated with the highest risk of IE:

- Acquired valvular heart disease with stenosis or regurgitation
- Prosthetic valve replacement or repair
- Previous infective endocarditis
- Completely repaired structural congenital heart defect with prosthetic material or device during the first 6 months after the procedure (period of complete endothelialization)
- Congenital heart disease (CHD)
  - Unrepaired cyanotic CHD, including palliative shunts and conduits
  - Unrepaired acyanotic CHD except isolated ostium secundum atrial septal defect (ASD)
  - Repaired CHD with residual defect(s) at the site or adjacent to a prosthetic patch/device.
- Hypertrophic cardiomyopathy
- Cardiac transplantation with subsequent cardiac valvulopathy.

Dental procedures for which endocarditis prophylaxis is reasonable for above patients

- All dental procedures that involve manipulation of gingival tissue or the periapical region of teeth or perforation of the oral mucosa, biopsies, suture removal, and placement of orthodontic bands.

Procedures and events not requiring prophylaxis: Routine anesthetic injections through non-infected tissue, dental radiographs, placement/adjustments of removable appliances, placement of orthodontic brackets, shedding of deciduous teeth, and bleeding from trauma to the lips or oral mucosa.

Regimes for prevention of IE are listed in Table 4.

RHEUMATIC FEVER

Group A streptococcal (GAS) infections, mainly tonsillopharyngitis, have potential risk of late immune-mediated complications. Rheumatic fever (RF) is the most significant of these which may result in permanent damage to cardiac structures and function. It can complicate

TABLE 5: Chemoprophylaxis for recurrences of acute rheumatic fever.

Drug	*Route*	*Dose*	*Frequency*
Penicillin G benzathine	IM	1.2 million U: Wt. >27 kg 600,000 U: Wt.<27 kg	Every 3/4 week
or			
Penicillin V	Oral	250 mg	Twice a day
or			
Sulfadiazine or sulfisoxazole	Oral	0.5 g: Wt. <27 kg 1.0 g: Wt. >27 kg (60 lb)	Once a day
Erythromycin	Oral	250 mg	Twice a day
Azithromycin	Oral	250 mg (6 mg/kg)	Once a day
Clarithromycin	Oral	15 mg/kg	Twice a day

TABLE 6: Duration of prophylaxis for people who have had acute rheumatic fever (ARF): Recommendations of the American Heart Association.

Category	*Duration*
Rheumatic fever without carditis	5 years since last episode of ARF or until 21 years of age, whichever is longer
Rheumatic fever with carditis but without residual heart disease (no valvular disease)	10 years since last episode of ARF or until 21 years of age, whichever is longer
Rheumatic fever with carditis and residual heart disease (persistent valvular disease)	10 years since last episode of ARF or until 40 years of age, whichever is longer; consider lifelong prophylaxis for people with severe valvular disease or likelihood of ongoing exposure to group A streptococcal infection

symptomatic as well as subclinical GAS infections and predispose to added cardiac risk at each recurrence.

Primary prevention of first attack of RF is reliably achieved by optimum antibiotic therapy and eradication of GAS from site. A complete 10 days oral penicillin regimen or single IM benzathine penicillin appropriate for weight is mostly effective.

Secondary prevention of RF is crucial on account of very high risk of subsequent recurrences of GAS infections over next years to decades. A continuous AP is recommended for at risk individuals with well-documented history of RF and/or confirmed rheumatic heart disease.

A long-acting benzathine G penicillin administered deep IM every 3 weekly, in weight adjusted dose is the preferred regimen. Oral penicillin V, sulfadiazine, sulfisoxazole, and macrolides are options to be considered only in compelling situations of injectable penicillin intolerance (Tables 5 and 6).

PROPHYLAXIS FOR OPPORTUNISTIC INFECTIONS IN HIV

Opportunistic infections (OIs) are defined as infections that are more frequent or more severe because of immunosuppression. HIV-induced progressive cellular immunodeficiency is a major risk factor for most common infections and specific opportunistic infections. Opportunistic infections have significant association with and negative impact on course and outcome of untreated HIV infection.

Effective prevention of OIs in children living with HIV involves four interventions:

1. Early and effective antiretroviral therapy prevents or restores HIV-induced immuno-deficiency. Anti-retroviral therapy (ART) is the best and priority preventive intervention.
2. Active immune-prophylaxis through vaccination for vaccine preventable diseases.
3. Specific chemoprophylaxis for select pathogen on long-term basis.
4. Prevention of environmental exposure to transmissible pathogen by specific measures.

After launch of highly active antiretroviral therapy (HAART) in 1990's, the opportunistic infection incidence rates in HIV have reduced dramatically, yet the higher risk, burden and pattern remain unaltered. The American guidelines by National Institutes of Health (NIH), CDC, and HIV Medicine Association (HIVMA) of Infectious Diseases Society of America (IDSA) and Pediatric Infectious Diseases Society (PIDS) were released in 2013 and are updated regularly with new recommendations.

Antimicrobial prophylaxis for OI in HIV is started in conjunction with ART and with decline of cell-mediated immunity as defined by age-dependant CD4 values in cell counts/percentages.

Primary AP for *Pneumocystis jirovecii* (PJP), tuberculosis, Mycobacterium avium complex, and toxoplasmosis is generally recommended in the presence of immunosuppression. Primary AP is generally *not* recommended for vaccine preventable infections due to *Streptococcus pneumoniae*, *H. influenzae* B, *Salmonella*, *Neisseria*, Hepatitis B, Influenza, and *Varicella*. Primary AP is generally *not* recommended for candidiasis, bartonellosis, cytomegalovirus, HSV, cryptosporidiosis, cryptococcosis, coccidioidomycosis, and histoplasmosis where monitoring for serological conversion, clinical disease, and pre-emptive/definitive treatment as needed is advocated.

Details of primary antimicrobial prophylaxis for common opportunistic infections in children with HIV are given below in Table 7. Secondary antimicrobial prophylaxis (after occurrence of particular OI) for OI in HIV children is generally recommended in select situations of persistent risk of immunosuppression due to inadequate ART, recurrent, severe, disseminated, and persistent infections, and specific pathogen. The details of secondary chemoprophylaxis in HIV are freely accessible on HIV resource websites.

PROPHYLAXIS FOR OCCUPATIONAL EXPOSURE TO BLOOD-BORNE PATHOGENS

Though this is strictly not in the purview of antimicrobial prophylaxis, it is discussed here since it can impact physicians/pediatricians involved with the care of children/patients with infection with HIV and blood-borne pathogens. Though exposure to HBV and HCV does not entail use of antimicrobials it is still discussed for sake of completion.

Postexposure Prophylaxis for Exposure to HBV

The risk of transmission varies from 22% to 30% for hepatitis B e-antigen (HBeAg) positive source and 1–6% for HBeAg negative source. The efficacy of postexposure prophylaxis (PEP) (from perinatal data) with the HBV vaccine alone is 70–75% and that with HBV vaccine + hepatitis B immune globulin (HBIg) is 85–95% (Table 8).

TABLE 7: Primary antimicrobial prophylaxis for common opportunistic infections in children with HIV.

Infection	*Recommendation*	*First choice*	*Alternative*	*Review for change*
Pneumocystis jiroveci Pneumonia	• All HIV-infected/ indeterminate infants 4–6 weeks to 12 months (regardless of CD4 cell count/%) • HIV-infected children: 1 to <6 years with CD4 count <500 cells/mm^3 or % <15% • HIV-infected children: 6 years and above with CD4 count <200 cells/mm^3 or %<15%	TMP–SMX (Co-trimoxazole): PO TMP 2.5–5 mg/kg/dose with SMX 12.5–25 mg/kg/ dose twice per day Dosing based on TMP Max total daily dose: 320 mg TMP and 1,600 mg SMX Other dosing schemes— • Given 3 days per week on consecutive/alternate days • Given 2 days per week on consecutive/ alternate days • Total daily single dose each day	• Dapsone PO Children ≥1 month: 2 mg/kg (max 100 mg) once daily or 4 mg/kg (max 200 mg) once weekly • Atovaquone PO (with food) Children 1–3 months and 2–12 years: 30–40 mg/kg once daily 4–24 months: 45 mg/kg once daily ≥13 years: 1,500 mg once daily • Pentamidine: aerosolized Children ≥5 years: 300 mg every month via respigard II nebulizer	Discontinuing primary prophylaxis: (not in HIV infected children <1 year) After ≥6 months of cART • Aged 1 to <6 years: CD 4% ≥15%/count ≥500 cells/ mm^3 for >3 consecutive months, or • Aged ≥6 years: • CD4 % ≥15%/count ≥200 cells/mm^3 for >3 consecutive months • Restarting primary prophylaxis: • Aged 1 to <6 years: CD4% <15%/ count <500 cells/ mm^3 • Aged ≥6 years: CD4% <15%/count <200 cells/ mm^3
Mycobacterium avium complex (MAC)	Children: <1 year with CD4 count <750 cells/mm^3 • 1 to <2 years with CD4 count <500/mm^3 • 2 to <6 years with CD4 count <75/mm^3 • ≥6 years with CD4 count <50 cells/mm^3	• Clarithromycin PO 7.5 mg/ kg (max 500 mg) twice daily *or* • Azithromycin PO 20 mg/kg (max 1,200 mg) once weekly	• Azithromycin PO 5 mg/kg (max 250 mg) once daily • Rifabutin PO (Children aged >5 years) 300 mg once daily with food	Discontinuing prophylaxis: (Do not discontinue in children <2 years) After ≥6 months of cART and • 2 to <6 years with CD4 count >200/mm^3 for >3 consecutive months • ≥6 years with CD4 count >100/mm^3 for >3 consecutive months • Restarting primary prophylaxis: • 2 to <6 years with CD4 count <200/mm^3 • ≥6 years with CD4 count <100/mm^3

Contd...

Contd...

Infection	*Recommendation*	*First choice*	*Alternative*	*Review for change*
Toxoplasmosis	Positive IgG antibody to *Toxoplasma* and severe immunosuppression: HIV-infected children <6 years with CD4% <15% HIV-infected children ≥6 years with CD4 count <100 cells/mm^3	TMP–SMX PO: 150/750 mg/m^2 BSA once daily Acceptable alternative schedules: • TMP–SMX 150/750 mg/m^2 BSA/dose 3 times weekly, on three consecutive day/week • TMP–SMX 75/375 mg/m^2 BSA/dose twice daily every day • TMP–SMX 75/375 mg/m^2 BSA/ dose twice daily 3 times weekly on alternate days	Children aged ≥1 month: • Dapsone PO: 2 mg/kg or 15 mg/m^2 BSA *plus* • Pyrimethamine PO: 1 mg/kg (max 25 mg) once daily plus • Leucovorin PO 5 mg every 3 days Children 1–3 months, and >24 months: • Atovaquone 30 mg/kg once daily Children aged 4–24 months: • Atovaquone 45 mg/kg once daily, with or without • Pyrimethamine 1 mg/kg or 15 mg/m^2 BSA plus (max 25 mg) once daily	Discontinuing primary prophylaxis: (not in children <1 year) • After ≥6 months of cART, and • 1 to <6 years; CD4% ≥15% for >3 consecutive months • ≥6 years; CD4 count >200/ mm^3 for >3 consecutive months Restarting primary prophylaxis: • 1 to <6 years with CD4% <15% • ≥6 years with CD4 count <100 to 200/mm^3
			• Leucovorin 5 mg every 3 days	
Bacterial Infections *S. pneumoniae* and other invasive bacteria	Vaccines routinely recommended for primary prophylaxis. Additional primary prophylaxis indication • Hypogammaglobulinemia (IgG <400 mg/dL)	Pneumococcal, meningococcal, and Hib vaccines • Intravenous immune globulin (400 mg/kg every 2 to 4 weeks)	TMP–SMX PO 75/375 mg/m^2 BSA/per dose twice daily	Discontinuing primary prophylaxis: • Resolution of hypogamma-globulinemia • Restarting primary prophylaxis: • Relapse of hypogamma-globulinemia

Contd...

Contd...

Infection	*Recommendation*	*First choice*	*Alternative*	*Review for change*
Influenza A and B	Pre-exposure chemoprophylaxis after careful consideration of risks vs. benefits • HIV with severe immuno-suppression during influenza virus circulation Postexposure chemoprophylaxis: • HIV with severe immuno-suppression regardless of influenza vaccination status • HIV with moderate immunosuppression if Influenza vaccination is contraindicated or unavailable; or documented Low influenza vaccine effectiveness in the current influenza season; and • Exposure within 48 hours to a suspected/confirmed case of influenza	Oseltamivir PO <3 months: not recommended 3 months to <1 year: 3 mg/kg/dose, once daily ≥1 year to 12 years; Weight-band dosing: ≤15 kg: 30 mg once daily >15 kg to 24 kg: 45 mg once daily ≥25 kg to 34 kg: 60 mg once daily ≥35 kg: 75 mg once daily ≥13 years: 75 mg once daily Zanamivir inhaled ≥5 years, 10 mg (2 inhalations) once daily	None	Duration: Pre-exposure AP—continue for the duration of influenza virus circulation in the community Duration of AP depends on the degree of immunosuppression—type of exposure, influenza vaccine—timing and effectiveness • Influenza vaccination given after contact, AP duration: 2 weeks after vaccination • Exposure to a household contact, AP: 7 days. • Institutional outbreak—14 days or 7 days after onset of symptoms in the last person infected, whichever is longer Oseltamivir Dosing adjustments—premature infants and renal dysfunction
Cytomegalo-virus (CMV)	Primary prophylaxis can be considered but not usually recommended for: • CMV antibody positivity and • Severe immuno-suppression: ≥6 years: CD4 cell count <50/mm^3 <6 years: CD4 percentage <5%	Valganciclovir PO • Older children —adult dose (BSA based), tablets 900 mg once daily with food • 4 months–16 years, oral solution 50 mg/mL dose in milligrams = 7 x BSA x CrCl (up to max CrCl—150 mL/min/1.73 m^2) (max 900 mg/day) once daily with food	N/A	Discontinuing primary prophylaxis: • Children ≥6 years; CD4 cell count >100/mm^3 • Children <6 years CD4 percentage >10% Restarting primary prophylaxis: • ≥6 years: CD4 cell count <50 cells/mm^3 • <6 years CD4 percentage <5%

Contd...

Contd...

Infection	*Recommendation*	*First choice*	*Alternative*	*Review for change*
Varicella-zoster virus (VZV) Primary (Postexposure) prophylaxis	HIV children with substantial exposure to varicella or zoster, Susceptible to varicella with any of: No verified history of varicella or zoster Seronegative for VZV Lack of evidence of vaccination Limit to severely immuno-compromised, (CDC Category—Immunologic 3, clinical Ca and high HIV RNA plasma viral load (BIII). Start acyclovir at first appearance of rash	Varicella ZIG IM 125 IU/10 kg (maximum 625 IU), Ideally within 96 hours: Up to 10 days after exposure	IVIG If varicella ZIG cannot be administered within 96 hours (up to 10 days), 400 mg/kg once ideally be administered within 96 hours Acyclovir PO When passive immunization is not possible, beginning 7–10 days after exposure 20 mg/kg /dose (maximum dose 800 mg), QID for 7 days	N/A

(ARV: antiretroviral; BSA: body surface area; cART: combination antiretroviral therapy; CrCl: (estimated) creatinine clearance; DOT: directly observed therapy; HBV: hepatitis B virus; IGRA: interferon-gamma release assay; QID: four times daily; TB: tuberculosis; TMP–SMX: trimethoprim–sulfamethoxazole)

TABLE 8: Postexposure prophylaxis for exposure of HBV.

Sl. No.	*Vaccination and antibody status of exposed person*	*Treatment when source is HBsAg positive*	*Treatment when source is unknown or not available for testing*
1.	Unvaccinated	Check anti-HBs. If negative HBIG x 1* and initiate hepatitis B vaccine series	Initiate vaccination
2.	Previously vaccinated		
	A. Known responder**	No treatment	No treatment
	B. Known non-responder	HBIG x 1 and initiate re-vaccination or HBIG x 2	No treatment
	C. Antibody response unknown	Vaccine booster dose and anti-HBs levels 1 month later	Vaccine booster dose and anti-HBs levels 1 month later
	D. Partially vaccinated	Give booster dose and test exposed person for anti-HBs 1 month later	Complete series

*Dose Hepatitis B immunoglobulin (HBIG) of 0.06 mL/kg (max 5 mL) or 500 IU IM at a site distant from the vaccine as soon as and preferably within 24 hours of exposure but not more than 7 days after exposure

**Responder is one who has an anti-HBs level of more than 10 IU/ mL at any time previously.

The exposed should refrain from donating blood for next 6 months and should be tested for HBsAg after 3 months of exposure. Anti-HBs status 1–2 months after last vaccine dose should be determined if indicated.

Postexposure Prophylaxis for Exposure to HCV

The risk of transmission is 1.8% following needle stick injury and is negligible following mucous membrane exposure. There is no effective PEP as of date but the focus should be on early detection of infection since many effective drugs are available. The exposed should be tested for serum glutamic oxaloacetic transaminase (SGOT) and serum glutamic pyruvic transaminase (SGPT) as well as HCV RNA at 4 weeks, and HCV antibodies at 12 weeks. If the SGPT is elevated then HCV RNA testing should be done.

Postexposure Prophylaxis for Exposure to HIV

Blood or visibly bloody fluids or other potentially infectious material (e.g. semen; vaginal secretions; breast milk; and cerebrospinal, synovial, pleural, peritoneal, pericardial, and amniotic fluids) are the only source fluids that carry meaningful risk. Exposure to saliva, tears, sweat, or non-bloody urine or feces does not require PEP. The risk of transmission of HIV following percutaneous exposure is around 0.3% and following mucosal exposure is 0.09%.

While the National AIDS Control Organization of India recommends two- or three-drug regime based on the severity of exposure and HIV status of the host, international guidelines recommend three-drug regime for all irrespective of mucosal/percutaneous exposure, severity of the exposure, and the status of disease in the host. The common international regimes include two nucleoside reverse transcriptase inhibitors (NRTIs) (tenofovir and emtricitabine) with either a boosted protease inhibitor (PI) (atazanavir/lopinavir) or integrase strand inhibitors (raltegravir/dolutegravir) starting as soon as possible after exposure but not later than 24 hours after exposure and continued for a period of 28 days. See chapter 34 for doses. The health care worker should be counseled about importance of adherence to the regime and side effects. Complete blood counts, liver and renal function tests should be done 2 weeks after initiation of therapy. HIV antibody test should be done 3 months after exposure. Health care workers who are pregnant/intolerant to the drugs or exposed to drug resistant HIV should be referred to a specialist. The same regime can be given to adolescents or adults with history of sexual exposure to a person with suspected or confirmed HIV infection if started within 36 hours of exposure.

RECOMMENDED READING

1. Bates KE, Hall M, Shah SS, et al. Hill Trends in infective endocarditis hospitalisations at United States children's hospitals from 2003 to 2014: impact of the 2007 American Heart Association antibiotic prophylaxis guidelines. Cardiology in the Young. 2017;27(4):686-90.
2. Bratzler DW, Dellinger EP, Olsen KM, et al. American Society of Health-System Pharmacists (ASHP); Infectious Diseases Society of America (IDSA); Surgical Infection Society (SIS); Society for Healthcare Epidemiology of America (SHEA). Clinical practice guidelines for antimicrobial prophylaxis in surgery. Surg Infect (Larchmt). 2013;14:73-156.
3. Craig JC, Simpson JM, Williams GJ, et.al. Prevention of Recurrent Urinary Tract Infection in Children with Vesico-ureteric Reflux and Normal Renal Tracts (PRIVENT) Investigators. Antibiotic prophylaxis and recurrent urinary tract infection in children. N Engl J Med. 2009;361:1748-59.
4. Ehrenkranz NJ. Antimicrobial prophylaxis in surgery: mechanisms, misconceptions, and Mischief. Infect Control Hosp Epidemiol. 1993;14:99-106.
5. Gerber MA, Baltimore RS, Eaton CB, et al. Prevention of rheumatic fever and diagnosis and treatment of acute Streptococcal pharyngitis: a scientific statement from the American Heart Association Rheumatic Fever, Endocarditis, and Kawasaki Disease Committee of the Council on Cardiovascular Disease in the Young, the Interdisciplinary Council on Functional Genomics and Translational Biology, and the Interdisciplinary Council on Quality of Care and Outcomes Research: endorsed by the American Academy of Pediatrics. Circulation. 2009;119(11):1541-51.
6. Huf*n*agel M, Versporten A, Bielicki J, et al. High rates of prescribing antimicrobials for prophylaxis in children and neonates: results from the antibiotic resistance and prescribing in European children point prevalence survey. J Pediatric Infect Dis Soc. 2018.
7. Indian Society of Pediatric Nephrology. Revised statement on management of urinary tract infections. Indian Ped. 2011;48:709-17.
8. Kesler RW, Guhlow LJ, Saulsbury FT. Prophylactic antibiotics in pediatric surgery. Pediatrics. 1982;69:1-3.
9. Kimberlin DW, Brady MT, Jackson MA (Eds). Red Book (2018). Report of the Committee on Infectious Diseases, 31st edition. US: American Academy of Pediatrics; 2018.
10. Sandora TJ, Fung M, Melvin P, et al. National variability and appropriateness of surgical antibiotic prophylaxis in US children's hospitals. JAMA Pediatrics.2016;170:570-6.
11. Siberry GK, Abzug MJ, Nachman S, et al. Panel on Opportunistic Infections in HIV-Exposed and HIV-Infected Children, National Institutes of Health, Centers for Disease Control and Prevention, HIV Medicine Association of the Infectious Diseases Society of America, Pediatric Infectious Diseases Society, American Academy of Pediatrics. Guidelines for the prevention and treatment of opportunistic infections in HIV-exposed and HIV-infected children. Pediatr Infect Dis J. 2013;32 Suppl 2:i-KK4.
12. Weber DJ, Rutala WA. Occupational Health Update: Focus on Preventing the Acquisition of Infections with Pre-exposure Prophylaxis and Postexposure Prophylaxis. Infect Dis Clin North Am. 2016;30: 729-57.
13. Williams G, Craig JC. Long-term antibiotics for preventing recurrent urinary tract infection in children. Cochrane Database Syst Rev. 2011;(3):CD001534.
14. Wilson W, Taubert KA, Gewitz M, et al. American Heart Association. Prevention of infective endocarditis: guidelines from the American Heart Association. J Am Dent Assoc. 2008;139:3S-24S.

Antimalarial Therapy

33

Chapter

Ritabrata Kundu, Krishnendu Mondal, Ashok Kapse, Tanu Singhal

INTRODUCTION

Malaria is an important public health problem with a reported 300–500 million cases per year and 1 million deaths. Around 90% of the deaths occur in children of Sub Saharan Africa. Around 1.5 million cases of malaria are reported in India every year with 50% being *Plasmodium falciparum*. The increasing resistance in malaria vectors to insecticides, rising cases of malaria due to *P. falciparum* and increasing resistance in *P. falciparum* to antimalarial in India is a matter of serious concern.

ANTIMALARIAL DRUGS

Chloroquine

Chloroquine belongs to group of 4-aminoquinolines; the other antimalarial in this group is amodiaquine.

Mechanism of Action

The malaria parasite utilizes hemoglobin for its amino acid requirements. Hemoglobin digestion releases large quantities of heme; free heme is toxic to malarial parasites. To protect them parasite convert toxic heme into an innocuous crystal called as hemozoin. Chloroquine binds to heme and thereby prevents it from being incorporated into the hemozoin crystal.

Antimalarial Activity

Chloroquine is active against all stages of schizonts of *Plasmodium malariae, Plasmodium ovale* and against chloroquine-sensitive strains of *P. falciparum* and *Plasmodium vivax*. It also has gametocytocidal activity against *P. vivax, P. malariae, P. ovale* as well as immature gametocytes (stages 1–3) of *P. falciparum*. The drug is inactive against hypnozoites and hence needs to be combined with primaquine to achieve radical cure of *P. vivax* and *P. ovale*.

Resistance Status

P. falciparum: Barring certain parts of globe (Central America, and the Caribbean) falciparum has acquired a significant resistance to chloroquine.

P. vivax: Although there are isolated reports of emerging resistance in *P. vivax* from certain quarters (Papua New Guinea) the species in general is sensitive to chloroquine.

Pharmacokinetics

Chloroquine has excellent oral bioavailability; a single dose of 10 mg/kg achieves therapeutic level for *P. vivax* and chloroquine-sensitive *P. falciparum* parasites within 30 min. Parenterally, the drug achieves dangerously high levels; therefore, it should always be used with great caution. Parenteral chloroquine is no longer used today. The drug is preferentially concentrated in erythrocytes and this concentration is enhanced in parasitized erythrocytes. The drug has a high capacity for binding to the melanin-containing tissues of the skin and eye. Chloroquine is eliminated slowly and has an elimination half-life of around 10 days; however, it may be detected in blood for up to 56 days.

Therapeutic Uses

Chloroquine is the first line treatment for *P. vivax* infection; though there are few reports suggesting emergence of resistance in this species, yet in most cases resistance is sporadic and inconsistent and hence does not warrant change in treatment policies.

Due to widespread resistance, chloroquine is no more recommended as first line treatment for *P. falciparum* malaria. However, in areas where resistance level is low; it may still be an effective drug for *P. falciparum* malaria; provided it is used in combination with other antimalarials. Even in areas of low resistance it might be safer to use a more effective drug for severe or complicated malaria and in vulnerable populations like small children and pregnant women.

Owing to prolonged duration of action chloroquine used to be a favorite drug for malarial chemoprophylaxis; however, with advent of extensive resistance, the drug has lost this utility.

No abortifacient or teratogenic effects have been reported with chloroquine; therefore, it is the safest antimalarial for treatment of malaria during pregnancy.

Dosage

Oral: Orally chloroquine should be prescribed in doses of 25 mg per kg as base, to be given over a period of three days. The ceiling dose is 1,500 mg of the base. Drug could be used in one of the following two regimens:

- First regimen consists of 10 mg of base per kg as first dose, followed by 5 mg/kg 6–8 hours later and 5 mg/kg on each of the following 2 days.
- A more practical regimen is 10 mg/kg of base on the first and second days and 5 mg/kg on the third. Though this regimen is pharmacokinetically bit inferior, clinical results are similar and is recommended by the national program.

Parenteral: This route is no longer used due to possibility of serious adverse effects including cardiac arrest and also because safer parenteral options including the artemisinins are available.

Side Effects

Serious adverse reactions to chloroquine are rare at the usual antimalarial dosages; transient headaches, nausea, and vomiting, gastrointestinal symptoms and "blurred vision" may occur following chloroquine administration, this could be avoided by administering the dose after a meal. Dark skinned people could suffer from intolerable pruritis, and as it may compromise compliance; it is advisable to use an alternative effective drug in the event of reinfection. Antihistamines are futile for chloroquine induced pruritis; however, calamine lotion may alleviate it. Chloroquine may precipitate attacks of acute porphyria and psoriasis in susceptible individuals.

Irreversible visual impairment resulting from accumulation of chloroquine in the retina was a rare but recognizable complication of long-term chloroquine prophylaxis. Cumulative total doses of 1 g of base per kg body weight or 50–100 g of base have been associated with retinal damage.

Over Dosage

Chloroquine has a low safety margin, as little as twice the therapeutic dose ingestion (3–4 g in adults) may culminate into acute toxicity. Accidental over dosage may happen due to inadvertent use of the double strength preparation of tablets containing 300 mg of base instead of the single strength tablets having 150 mg of base. Poisoning may result in cardiovascular failure with hypotension and cardiac arrhythmias rapidly progressing to cardiovascular collapse, convulsions, cardiorespiratory arrest, and death. Diazepam, adrenaline and mechanical ventilation constitute modern management of chloroquine toxicity. Diazepam competes with chloroquine for benzodiazepine receptors in cardiac myocytes while adrenaline counteracts the chloroquine effects on myocardium and vasculature.

Contraindications

Chloroquine is contraindicated in persons with known hypersensitivity, with a history of epilepsy, and those suffering from psoriasis. The drug can be used in G6PD deficiency.

Availability

This is a very cheap drug and readily available in all suitable forms like tablets, syrup, drops and injections. Tablets containing 150 mg or 300 mg of chloroquine base as phosphate or sulfate, syrup containing 10 mg base per mL and drops containing 50 mg base per mL are available.

Quinine

Extracts of cinchona bark; quinine and its congener quinidine are effective antimalarial drugs.

Mechanism of Action

Like chloroquine, quinine also interferes with parasitic metabolism of heme; quinine opposes polymerization of hemin into hemozoin.

Antimalarial Activity

Quinine has blood schizonticidal activity against all malarial species including chloroquine and antifolate resistant strains. However, it is relatively less effective against *P. vivax*. It is active against gametocytes of all species excluding *P. falciparum*. The drug is devoid of hypnozoitocidal activity.

Though significant resistance to quinine has not yet occurred some decrease in sensitivity to quinine has been detected in areas of South-East Asia where it has been extensively used for malaria therapy. Poor compliance and incomplete treatment are responsible for this decreased sensitivity. There is some cross resistance between quinine and mefloquine, suggesting that the wide use of quinine in Thailand might have influenced the development of resistance to mefloquine in that country.

Pharmacokinetics

Quinine has excellent oral bioavailability and peak plasma concentrations are reached within 1–3 h. It readily crosses the placental barrier and is found in cerebrospinal fluid. Quinine is extensively metabolized in the liver, has an elimination half-life of 10–12 h in healthy individuals and is subsequently excreted in the urine.

Some of the pharmacokinetic characteristics are affected by age of the patient, and also by malaria. The volume of distribution is less in young children than in adults. In patients with acute malaria, the volume of distribution is reduced and systemic clearance is slower than in healthy subjects, these changes are proportional to the severity of the disease.

Indications

The use of quinine for severe falciparum malaria has now been supplanted by the artemisinin derivatives since randomized controlled trials have shown superior efficacy of artemisinin derivatives as compared to quinine. For uncomplicated falciparum malaria in chloroquine resistant areas quinine is often used but there are problems with compliance due to troublesome side effects. Quinine should always be used in combination with other antimalarial drugs such as tetracycline, clindamycin and pyrimethamine-sulfadoxine (SP). Quinine is inferior to chloroquine, mefloquine and artemisinin derivatives in the treatment of vivax malaria and is best avoided for *P. vivax* infections.

Use in Pregnancy

Quinine is safe in pregnancy. Combination of quinine and clindamycin is the drug of choice for uncomplicated falciparum malaria in the first trimester when the artemisinin derivatives cannot be used. Studies have shown that therapeutic doses of quinine do not induce labor and that the stimulation of contractions and evidence of fetal distress associated with the use of quinine are in fact due to fever and other effects of malarial disease. The risk of quinine-induced hypoglycemia is, however, greater than in nonpregnant women, particularly in severe disease.

Dosage

Quinine can be given by the oral, intravenous or intramuscular routes. Quinine should not be given alone for the treatment of malaria as short courses, e.g. 3 days, owing to the possibility of recrudescence and resistance.

Parenteral: If parenteral therapy is indicated as in severe malaria quinine should be given intravenously as 10 mg/kg of salt by slow infusion in isotonic fluid or 5% dextrose saline slowly over 4 h every 8 hourly. A loading dose of 20 mg/kg is recommended for severe and complicated malaria. The loading dose should be avoided if there is reliable evidence that the patient has received quinine or halofantrine or mefloquine in the past 24 hours (both halofantrine and mefloqune produce additive cardiac toxicity). If facilities for intravenous infusion are not available quinine can be given intramuscularly (IM) in the same dosage with the same therapeutic results. In this case the drug should be diluted to a concentration of 60 mg/mL and divided into two halves, one half being delivered into each anterior thigh. Whenever parenteral quinine is used, oral treatment should be resumed as soon as the patient is able to take it, and continued for the completion of the course. In situations where infusion need is beyond 48 hours or in renal failure the dose should be reduced to half. Total duration of therapy is 7 days. A second drug such as doxycycline, clindamycin, SP should be added once the patient starts taking orally.

Oral: Quinine, 10 mg of salt per kg three times daily for 7 days. As discussed earlier quinine should be combined with single dose pyrimethamine-sulfadoxine (1 mg/kg of pyrimethamine) or tetracycline (5 mg/kg 6 hourly for 7 days) or doxycycline (2 mg/kg twice a day for 7 days) or clindamycin (20–40 mg/kg divided in 3 daily doses for 5 days). Tetracyclines cannot be used in children aged less than 8 years. A single gametocidal dose of primaquine (0.75 mg/kg) should be given in falciparum malaria at end of therapy to interrupt transmission as quinine is not effective against gametocytes of *P. falciparum.*

Side Effects

Cinchonism, a symptom complex characterized by tinnitus, hearing impairment, and sometimes vertigo or dizziness, occurs in a high proportion of treated patients. Symptoms appear even at the lower limit of the therapeutic range of the drug. These symptoms are usually reversible and rarely constitute a reason for withdrawing the drug but do reduce compliance with 7 days therapy.

Serious side effects with parenteral quinine are rare if it is administered properly. Severe hypotension may develop if the drug is injected too rapidly. Quinine produces prolongation of the QTc interval in the electrocardiograph (ECG) but significant conduction or repolarization abnormalities are rare and iatrogenic dysrhythmias are extremely uncommon in normal hearts. Routine ECG monitoring during quinine infusion is not required if there is no evidence of preexisting heart disease. Quinine is known to produce hypoglycemia through stimulatory action on the pancreatic β cells. Hypoglycemia is particularly common in children and pregnant women. Frequent blood glucose monitoring is a must. Care should be taken to monitor and treat for hypoglycemia in children administered IM quinine as they may not have an IV access for IV fluids.

Quinine produces hemolysis in G6PD deficiency; it also produces hemolysis in non-G6PD deficient patients by a still not well-elucidated immune mechanism. Hemolysis and hemoglobinuria at presentation is not a contraindication to quinine if the patient is not known to G6PD deficient. If hemolysis develops during quinine therapy, it may be advisable to shift to artemisinin derivatives.

Toxicity

A single dose of quinine of more than 3 g is capable of causing serious and potentially fatal intoxication. Intoxication has three main elements:

1. Central nervous system depression and seizures
2. Dysrhythmias, hypotension and cardiac arrest
3. Blindness.

Contraindications

Quinine is contraindicated in persons: with known hypersensitivity, with underlying cardiac disorders, on cardiosupressant drugs and with G6PD deficiency. Thrombocytopenia, jaundice, renal failure, hypotension are not contraindications for quinine administration. Administration of mefloquine prior to quinine administration is not a contraindication to use of quinine but ECG monitoring is desirable and the loading dose should be avoided.

Formulations

Tablets of quinine hydrochloride, quinine dihydrochloride or quinine sulfate containing 100 mg and 300 mg quinine salt is available. Injectable solutions of quinine hydrochloride, quinine dihydrochloride or quinine sulfate containing 82%, 82% and 82.6% quinine base, respectively.

Pyrimethamine—Sulfadoxine or Sulfalene

Synergistic combinations that act against the parasite-specific enzymes, dihydropteroate synthase (DHPS) and dihydrofolate reductase (DHFR) constitute effective antimalarial drugs. Because trimethoprim has a much lower affinity than pyrimethamine for the parasite dihydrofolate reductase enzyme, cotrimoxazole the combination of sulfamethoxazole and trimethoprim has weak antimalarial properties and therefore should not be used for the treatment of malaria.

Mechanism of Action

Folate metabolism is the target of several antimalarials as well as drugs used against other pathogens. Due to its high rate of replication the malaria parasite has a high demand for nucleotides as precursors for DNA synthesis and thus is particularly sensitive to antifolates. The malaria parasite synthesizes folates de novo and is unable to utilize exogenous folates. In contrast human beings must obtain preformed folates and cannot synthesize folate. The inability of the parasite to utilize exogenous folates makes folate biosynthesis a good drug target. Folate is synthesized from 3 basic building blocks, guanosine triphosphate (GTP), para-aminobenzoic acid (PABA), and glutamate, in a pathway involving 5 enzymes. One of these enzymes, DHPS, is inhibited by sulfa-based drugs. DHFR is a ubiquitous enzyme that participates in the recycling of folates by reducing dihydrofolate to tetrahydofolate. The tetrahydrofolate is then oxidized back to dihydrofolate as it participates in biosynthetic reactions (e.g. thymidylate synthase). Inhibiting DHFR will prevent the formation of thymidylate and lead to an arrest in DNA synthesis and subsequent parasite death. Pyrimethamine and proguanil are the two most common DHFR inhibitors used as antimalarials. These drugs inhibit DHFR from the parasite to a greater degree than the host enzyme and thus show a selective toxicity towards the parasite.

Antimalarial Activity

Pyrimethamine-sulfadoxine is schizontocidal for *P. falciparum;* it is devoid of hypnozoitocidal activity and gametocytocidal activity. They however have been shown to be sporontocidal in animal models. Antifolates have inherently weak blood schizonticidal effects against *P. vivax.*

Resistance Status

P. falciparum: The long half-life of sulfa drug-pyrimethamine combinations provides a potent selective pressure for parasite resistance in areas of high transmission, therefore, where ever drug has been in extensive use significant resistance evolved within short time. There is no cross resistance with the 4-aminoquinolines, mefloquine, quinine, halofantrine or the artemisinin derivatives.

P. vivax: Combination is inherently less effective against *P. vivax.*

Pharmacokinetics

Sulfadoxine, sulfalene and pyrimethamine are highly bound to protein with relatively long mean elimination half-lives of around 180 h, 65 h and 95 h, respectively. All three drugs cross the placental barrier and are also detected in breast milk.

Indications

Chemotherapy: Sulfa drug-pyrimethamine combinations are effective against *P. falciparum* and have been successfully used in uncomplicated falciparum malaria in areas with resistance to chloroquine. However, with use resistance to these agents rapidly appears and they soon lose their utility. These drugs should be used in combination therapy with artemisinin derivatives only in areas where there is no significant resistance to these drugs. Sulfadoxine-pyrimethamine is the most widely used formulation; sulfalene-pyrimethamine has been largely used in the Indian subcontinent. Although comparative data is lacking; it is generally assumed that these two formulations are equipotent. Folic acid, even in physiological doses, can antagonize the action of sulfadoxine hence it has been suggested that folic acid supplements should be delayed for 1 week after sulfa drug–pyrimethamine treatment to avoid an inhibitory effect on antimalarial efficacy. Pyrimethamine-sulfadoxine should not be used for management of vivax malaria or for mixed infection.

Chemoprophylaxis: Sulfa drug–pyrimethamine combinations are no longer recommended for chemoprophylaxis because of the risk of severe adverse reactions.

Use in Pregnancy

Studies in Kenya and Malawi have shown that administration of a full adult treatment dose of sulfadoxine-pyrimethamine at the first attendance at an antenatal clinic during the second trimester of pregnancy and repeated once at the beginning of the third trimester is effective in clearing or preventing placental infection and peripheral parasitemia with *P. falciparum* and reducing the risk of low birth weight. Following these reports, several national malaria control programs have adopted this intermittent regimen for the prevention of malaria during pregnancy. No teratogenic effects were ever noted with use of sulfa drug-pyrimethamine combinations for malaria treatment in pregnant women; while there is a theoretical risk of jaundice among premature babies born to mothers given sulfa drugs late in the third trimester; increased incidence of kernicterus has not been observed.

Use in Lactating Women

Both pyrimethamine and sulfadoxine are excreted in small amounts in breast milk.

Diarrhea and rash have been reported in nursing infants exposed to sulfonamides through breast milk; however, these reports are rare, and more serious adverse reactions have not been documented. Thus, sulfonamide excretion in breast milk does not appear to pose a significant risk for most infants. Pyrimethamine is considered safe during breast feeding.

Dosage

Sulfadoxine-pyrimethamine and sulfalene-pyrimethamine are recommended as single dose therapy calculated as 1.25 mg/kg of pyrimethamine.

Side Effects

Sulfa drug-pyrimethamine combinations are generally well tolerated when used at the recommended doses for malaria therapy; however, in a person allergic to sulfa drugs, serious hypersensitivity reactions involving skin could occur. Serious events usually occur following multiple doses, it is rare when drug is used in a single dose. Life-threatening events, like erythema multiforme (Stevens-Johnson syndrome) and toxic epidermal necrolysis, have been reported in 1 in 5,000 to 1 in 8,000 people taking the drug for weekly chemoprophylaxis. The combination is therefore no longer recommended for prophylactic use.

Contraindications

The use of sulfadoxine- or sulfalene-pyrimethamine combinations is contraindicated in persons with known hypersensitivity to sulfa drugs or pyrimethamine, in persons with severe hepatic dysfunction, in G6PD deficiency and in infants less than 2 months of life.

Formulations

Formulations available are as follows:

- Tablets containing 500 mg of sulfadoxine and 25 mg of pyrimethamine.
- Syrup containing 250 mg of sulfadoxine and 12.5 mg of pyrimethamine.
- Ampoules containing 500 mg of sulfadoxine and 25 mg of pyrimethamine in 2.5 mL of injectable solution (Not available in India).

Mefloquine

Mefloquine is a 4-quinoline methanol chemically related to quinine.

Mechanism of Action

Mechanism of action is same as that of chloroquine. Mefloquine binds hemin and there by foils parasite attempt to form hemozoin crystal.

Antimalarial Activity

Mefloquine is a potent long-acting blood schizonticide active against *P. falciparum* resistant to 4-aminoquinolines and sulfa drug-pyrimethamine combinations. It is also highly active against *P. vivax* and, *P. malariae* and most probably *P. ovale*. It does not have gametocytocidal activity and is ineffective against the hepatic stages of malaria parasites.

Resistance Status

P. falciparum: Owing to its long elimination half-life and consequent prolonged sub-therapeutic concentrations in the blood, the development of resistance is a likely occurrence especially in areas of high transmission. Since the late 1980s, resistance of *P. falciparum* to mefloquine has developed in South-East Asia. More than 50% of patients have recrudescence of parasitemia within 28 days after a dose of 15 mg/kg. The sensitivity of *P. falciparum* populations recrudescing after treatment with mefloquine is substantially reduced compared with the original population. *P. falciparum* resistance to mefloquine is also accompanied by cross resistance to halofantrine and reduced sensitivity to quinine. Resistance to mefloquine is also being reported in India from various places including around Mumbai.

Pharmacokinetics

Mefloquine has a long elimination half-life, varying between 10 days and 40 days in adults. Elimination half-life tends to be shorter in children and pregnant women. The pharmacokinetic parameters of mefloquine are changed in acute falciparum malaria; the drug reaches a higher serum level, probably due to a contraction of the apparent volume of distribution.

Indications

Chemotherapy: Drug should be reserved for known or suspected uncomplicated chloroquine-resistant falciparum malaria, sensitive to mefloquine and only as a companion drug with the artemisinin derivatives. In Thailand, introduction of combination therapy of mefloquine and artesunate significantly decreased mefloquine resistance that had been observed when mefloquine was used alone.

Chemoprophylaxis: Mefloquine is drug of choice as chemoprophylactic agent for travelers to areas with significant risk of chloroquine-resistant falciparum malaria.

Dosage

Treatment: 15–25 mg of mefloquine base per kg. For many years, the standard dose of mefloquine for treatment of uncomplicated malaria has been 15 mg/kg, however, development of resistance forced to increase the dose to 25 mg/kg. The bioavailability of mefloquine considerably improves if it is taken after food; drinking of water before drug administration also improves oral bioavailability. The higher dosage of mefloquine (25 mg/kg) is associated with greater drug intolerance, especially vomiting in young children. If vomiting occurs within 1 hour of drug intake, a full dose needs to be repeated. Vomiting after 1 hour does not require repeat therapy. Tolerability could substantially be improved by administrating drug as divided doses of 15 mg/kg and 10 mg/kg 8 hours apart.

Chemoprophylaxis: 5 mg of mefloquine base per kg weekly, maximum 250 mg of base per week. To achieve an optimal efficacy chemoprophylaxis should at least be started 2–3 weeks before departure and continued for 4 weeks after return.

Use in pregnancy: While mefloquine may be given with confidence for both chemoprophylaxis and treatment during the second and third trimesters of pregnancy, it should be avoided during the first trimester.

Lactating women: Mefloquine is excreted in breast milk in small amounts, however, circumstantial evidence suggests that no adverse effects occur in breastfed infants whose mothers are taking mefloquine.

Side Effects

Mefloquine has high potential for adverse effects. Side effects comprise of: gastrointestinal, neuropsychiatric, and cardiac problems.

Gastrointestinal problems: Vomiting, diarrhea and abdominal pain may occur in some of the patients. Vomiting is three times more common with higher doses (25 mg/kg body weight), splitting the dose significantly reduces vomiting.

Neuropsychiatric problems: These include affective disorders, anxiety disorders, hallucinations, sleep disturbances including nightmares and, in a few people, overt psychosis, toxic encephalopathy, convulsions and acute brain syndrome. Neuropsychiatric problems are higher in Caucasians and Africans compared to Asians. The frequency of neuropsychiatric adverse reactions is reported to be more common following mefloquine treatment than prophylactic use, and is proportional to the dose taken with a usual incidence of 1 in 15,000.

Cardiovascular effects: Bradycardia and sinus arrhythmia have been reported in certain patients treated with mefloquine.

Drug Interactions

Concomitant administration of mefloquine with other related compounds such as quinine, quinidine and chloroquine may produce ECG abnormalities and increase the risk of convulsions. In general, mefloquine should not be administered within 12 hours of the last dose of quinine. The use of halofantrine after mefloquine causes significant lengthening of the QTc interval and has been linked with cardiac arrests in patients treated with both drugs. Halofantrine should, therefore, not be used in persons who have recently received mefloquine.

Concerns were raised that coadministration of mefloquine, with drugs which are used to treat cardiovascular disease such as anti-arrhythmic drugs, β-adrenergic blocking agents and calcium channel blockers as well as antihistamines, tricyclic antidepressants and phenothiazines might contribute to the prolongation of the QTc interval. However, no evidence of such drug interaction has been reported to date and comedication with such drugs is no longer contraindicated.

Contraindications

The use of mefloquine is contraindicated in persons with a history of allergy to mefloquine, with a history of severe neuropsychiatric disease, and those receiving halofantrine treatments.

Formulations, Cost Considerations and Comparisons

Tablets containing 274 mg of mefloquine hydrochloride, equivalent to 250 mg of mefloquine base are available. Because of its high cost, increasing prevalence of resistance and potentially serious side effects mefloquine is not a favored antimalarial drug as a single agent, its main use these days is as an add on drug with artemisinin compounds. The unavailability of standalone preparations of oral artemisinin derivatives in India has prevented use of this drug in treatment.

It is however the preferred drug for chemoprophylaxis for travelers visiting chloroquine resistant *P. falciparum* endemic areas.

Artemisinin Compounds

Artemisinin (qinghaosu) is the antimalarial principle isolated from Chinese herb *Artemisia annua L.* It is a sesquiterpene lactone with a peroxide bridge linkage. Artemisinin is poorly soluble in oil or water but the parent compound has yielded many derivatives like dihydroartemisinin, artemether, arteether, and artesunate, which have circumvented the solubility problem.

Mechanism of Action

Chemical structure of artemisinin compound contains a labile peroxide bridge. Hemozoin catalyzes the decomposition of this labile bridge. The process of decomposition generates free oxygen radicals, which are toxic to parasite membrane.

Antimalarial Activity

Artemisinin derivatives are very potent and most rapidly acting blood schizonticidal drugs. They act on all stages of the parasites of all species including trophozoites, schizonts and mature schizonts. Compounds are devoid of hypnozoitocidal action, but have considerable gametocytocidal activity against all *Plasmodium* species.

Resistance Status

The fertile ground for antimalarial drug resistance in South-East Asia has seen the emergence of artemisinin resistance. This has manifested in the form of increase in parasite clearance times and has been associated with *K13* mutations. A recent paper has described the emergence of artemisinin resistance in Eastern India.

Disposition

All derivatives are metabolized to a common bioactive metabolite, dihydroartemisinin.

Indications

The antimalarial activity of artemisinin and its derivatives is extremely rapid and most patients show clinical improvement within 1–3 days of treatment, therefore, these drugs are recommended for both uncomplicated as well severe falciparum malaria. Though these compounds have excellent antimalarial activity they are beset with problem of high recrudescence rate. Recrudescence rate is related to length of treatment and is unacceptably high when duration of therapy is lesser than 5 days particularly if drugs are used as monotherapy. Monotherapy with these drugs is therefore not recommended. Artemisinin compounds have been successfully used in combination with mefloquine, sulfadoxine-pyrimethamine, lumefantrine, piperaquine, clindamycin and doxycycline.

Artemisinin compounds can also be used equally successfully for treatment of malaria due to *P. vivax, P. malariae* or *P. ovale* and are especially indicated for mixed infection with *P. falciparum* and *P. vivax.*

Chemoprophylaxis: There is no rationale at present for using artemisinin compounds for chemoprophylaxis.

Use in pregnancy: Preclinical studies have consistently shown that artemisinin and its derivatives do not exhibit mutagenic or teratogenic activity, therefore, these compounds are drugs of choice for severe malaria and can be used for treatment of uncomplicated malaria during the second trimester and third trimester of pregnancy in areas of multiple drug resistance. However, owing to lack of data, their use in the first trimester is yet not recommended for uncomplicated malaria, but may be used for complicated malaria since here the benefits outweigh the risks.

Side Effects

Experience indicates that artemisinin and its derivatives are the least toxic of the antimalarial drugs, few significant adverse effects being associated with their use.

Animal studies have demonstrated severe neurotoxicity following parenteral administration of very high doses of artemether or arteether. Such effects have not been observed with oral administration of any artemisinin derivative or with intravenous artesunate in extensive clinical trials in China, Myanmar, Thailand and Vietnam. In prospective studies involving more than 10,000 patients or in the more than two million people who have received these drugs, there is no clinical evidence of serious neurotoxicity.

Minor adverse effects may include headache, nausea, vomiting, abdominal pain, itching, drug fever and dark urine.

Contraindications

There are no absolute contraindications to these drugs, however, due to lack of enough safety data, drugs should preferably be avoided during first trimester of pregnancy.

Formulations and Dosage

Three artemisinin compounds: artesunate, artemether, and arteether are available in the Indian market.

Artesunate:

- *Formulations*: Artesunate is available for use as oral tablet, IV or (IM) intramuscular injection and rectal suppository. Tablets contain 50 mg of sodium artesunate, while ampoules for IM or IV injection have 60 mg of sodium artesunate in 1 mL of injectable solution. Rectal capsules containing 100 mg or 400 mg of sodium artesunate are available in China but not in India.
- *Dosage (Uncomplicated malaria)*: 4 mg/kg once a day for 3 days, plus mefloquine (15 mg or 25 mg of base per kg) as a single dose or split dose on the second and/or third day.
  Recent studies in Africa have demonstrated that combinations of artesunate (oral administration of 4 mg/kg daily for 3 days) plus a single dose of sulfadoxine-pyrimethamine on the first day are highly efficacious, although efficacy appears to be reduced in areas with preexisting moderate levels of sulfadoxine-pyrimethamine resistance.
- *Dosage (severe malaria)*: 2.4 mg/kg by the IM or IV route followed by 2.4 mg/kg at 12 h and 24 h, then 2.4 mg/kg daily. The dose is 3 mg/kg in children weighing less than 20 kg. Once the patient can swallow, the daily dose can be given orally as 4 mg/kg/day. If the second drug is clindamycin or doxycycline treatment duration is 7 days. If the combination drug is SP or mefloquine three days treatment is adequate. Treatment from parenteral artesunate can also be shifted to oral artemether and lumefantrine combination.

Artemether:

- *Formulations*: Artemether is an oil-soluble methyl ether derivative of dihydroartemisinin and available as ampules of injectable solution for IM injection containing 80 mg in 1 mL. It is also available as an oral combination with lumefantrine.
- *Dosage (uncomplicated malaria)*: Given as artemether-lumefantrine (in the ratio of 1: 6, 20 mg of artemether and 120 mg of lumefantrine) with artemether as 1.7 mg/kg/dose twice daily for 3 days.
- *Dosage (Severe malaria)*: 3.2 mg/kg by the IM route as a loading dose on the first day, followed by 3.2 mg/kg daily. It may then be shifted to oral combinations of 3 days of artemether, lumefantrine as discussed earlier. It is less efficacious the artesunate for severe malaria.

Arteether:

- *Formulation*: Arteether is the oil-soluble ethyl derivative of dihydroartemisinin and is available as ampoules containing 150 mg of arteether in 2 mL of injectable solution in India.
- *Dosage*: 3 mg/kg/day by the IM route for 3 days.

Arterolane:

- *Formulation*: Arterolane maleate is available as tablet coformulated with piperaquine (150 mg of arterolane and 750 mg of piperaquine)
- *Dosage*: It can be used in treatment of uncomplicated malaria as one tablet daily for 3 days.

Primaquine

Mechanism of Action

Primaquine is supposed to damage parasite mitochondria. Drug is believed to compete with dihydroorotate dehydrogenase enzyme, which is involved in pyrimidine synthesis.

Antimalarial Activity

Primaquine is an 8-aminoquinoline compound. Drug is highly active against hypnozoites of the relapsing malarial parasites, *P. vivax* and *P. ovale* and gametocytes of all malaria species. It is also effective against the asexual forms of *P. vivax* and hence combination of chloroquine and primaquine is like combination therapy for vivax malaria.

Resistance Status

P. vivax: There are geographical variations in the sensitivity of hypnozoites of *P. vivax* to primaquine. The parasites from the southern regions of South-East Asia and Oceania are the least susceptible while *P. vivax* from India seems to be the most sensitive. Chesson strain of *P. vivax* is relatively resistant to primaquine and requires longer treatment courses. The anti-relapse effect of primaquine is related to the total dose rather than the duration of treatment.

Pharmacokinetics

Primaquine is readily absorbed when taken, peak plasma concentrations occur within 1–3 hours. Primaquine is rapidly metabolized in the liver and only a small amount is excreted unchanged in the urine, suggesting extensive intrahepatic recycling.

Indications

- *Antirelapse treatment in P. vivax and P. ovale infections*: Primaquine may be given concurrently with an active blood schizonticide, such as chloroquine, from the first day of treatment for the prevention of relapse. 0.3 mg/kg body weight for 14 days is mandatory for this purpose; previously recommended 5 days treatment with primaquine was derived largely on the basis of empirical views, and exerts little or no anti-relapse activity. In areas with primaquine resistance higher daily doses of 0.5 or 0.75 mg/kg/day for 2 weeks may be used. G6PD deficiency should be excluded before standard therapeutic doses of primaquine are given as anti-relapse therapy. In patients with mild G6PD deficiency primaquine may be given as once weekly dose of 0.75 mg/kg for 8 weeks. Patients should be instructed to stop treatment and seek medical advice if they have abdominal pain, become weak or pale, or notice darkening of the urine.
- *Gametocytocide*: Gametocytocidal treatment is given with an objective to eliminate residual gametocytes after effective blood schizonticidal treatment; it is given in falciparum malaria when quinine or artemisinin derivatives are used for therapy. A single dose of 0.25 mg/kg is

sufficient for this purpose as recently recommended by World Health Organization (WHO) (the National Control Program however still recommends 0.75 mg/kg for this purpose). Primaquine may be given concurrently with the schizonticidal drug but should not be administered until the condition of the patient stabilizes. Testing for G6PD deficiency is not required.
- *Chemoprophylaxis*: Primaquine also has a causal chemoprophylactic activity but, until recently this property had not been evaluated due to the prevailing view that primaquine was too toxic for routine chemoprophylaxis. Recent studies in Irian Jaya and Kenya have now shown that daily doses of 0.5 mg/kg can be effective in protecting both adults and children against falciparum and vivax infections.
- *Use in pregnancy:* Fetus is relatively deficient in G6PD hence primaquine is contraindicated during pregnancy.

Side Effects

- *GI disturbances*: May cause anorexia, nausea, vomiting, abdominal pain and cramps. These symptoms are dose related and are relatively rare at therapeutic doses. Gastric intolerance can be minimized by administering the drug with food.
- *Hematological disturbances*: Primaquine is known to cause methemoglobinemia, leukopenia and suppression of myeloid series. In higher doses primaquine causes severe suppression of bone marrow. Primaquine does not normally cause granulocytopenia at the doses recommended for malaria therapy. Primaquine can induce severe hemolysis in G6PD deficient person. It is usually self-limiting but blood transfusions may be necessary in severe cases.
- *Over dosage*: Gastrointestinal symptoms, weakness, methemoglobinemia, cyanosis, hemolytic anemia, jaundice and bone marrow depression may occur with over dosage. There is no specific antidote and treatment is symptomatic.

Contraindications

Primaquine is contraindicated in pregnancy, lactating mothers and in infants below 1 year and in individuals with G6PD deficiency. The drug is also contraindicated in conditions predisposing to granulocytopenia, including active rheumatoid arthritis and lupus erythematosus.

Drug Interactions

Primaquine should not be administered with any other drug that may induce hematological disorders, like sulfadoxine + pyrimethamine, chloramphenicol.

Formulations

Drug is available only in tablet formulation containing 2.5 mg, 7.5 mg and 15 mg of drug.

Tafenoquine

Tafenoquine is a 5-phenoxy derivative of primaquine. It has a very long elimination half-life (14 days as compared to 6 hours of primaquine). The drug is a vast improvement over parent compound: it is 7 times more active as hypnozoitocide, 14 times more effective as causal prophylactic, and 100 times more potent as blood schizontocide. Drug is better tolerated than primaquine but like parent compound does cause hemolysis in a G6PD deficient person. Tafenoquine has a great potential as antimalarial drug.

Doxycycline

Doxycycline is derived from oxytetracycline, and has an identical spectrum of activity. Doxycycline, like tetracyclines, is used as an add-on drug with quinine or artemisinin derivatives. In contrast to tetracycline, doxycycline can also be used for chemoprophylaxis.

Doxycycline is readily and almost completely absorbed from the gastrointestinal tract and absorption is not significantly affected by the presence of food in the stomach or duodenum. Milk and milk products decrease drug absorption. Adverse effects include gastrointestinal irritation, phototoxic reactions (increased vulnerability to sunburn), transient depression of bone growth and discoloration of teeth and permanent enamel hypoplasia. As with tetracycline, esophageal ulceration can be prevented if the oral dose is washed down with copious amounts of water. Other gastrointestinal symptoms can be reduced if doxycycline is taken with a meal. Milk products must be avoided since they reduce absorption. Doxycycline is contraindicated in pregnancy and in nursing mothers.

The dose for treatment is doxycycline 3.5 mg/kg body weight in two divided doses for 7 days. The dose for prophylaxis is 100 mg per day for adults and 1.5 mg/kg/day for children to be started 1 week before departure and continued for 4 weeks after return.

Clindamycin

Antimalarial Activity

Clindamycin is a semisynthetic antibiotic derived from lincomycin. Like tetracycline, it is an efficient but slow acting blood schizonticide. Clindamycin has excellent oral bioavailability.

Indications

As with doxycycline, clindamycin provides another option as an add-on drug with quinine or artemisinin with an advantage that it could be used in children and pregnant women unlike doxycycline. It should not be used alone for the treatment of malaria because of its slow action.

Dosage

Clindamycin 20 mg/kg/day (1,200 mg/day) twice daily for 7 days. Clindamycin should be administered with food and copious amounts of water.

Side Effects

Nausea, vomiting, abdominal pain or cramps and diarrhea may occur with clindamycin uses. *Pseudomembranous colitis*, a potentially fatal condition caused by *Clostridium difficile* toxin, may develop in some cases.

Contraindications

Clindamycin is contraindicated in patients with hypersensitivity to clindamycin or lincomycin, in those with a history of gastrointestinal disease, particularly colitis and those with severe hepatic or renal impairment.

Formulations

Clindamycin is available as capsules containing 75 mg, 150 mg or 300 mg of clindamycin base as hydrochloride.

Malarone (Atovaquone + Proguanil)

Mechanism of Action

Atovaquone inhibits mitochondrial respiration.

Antimalarial Activity

Atovaquone has a weak antimalarial activity against blood stages of *P. falciparum* parasite (trophozoite, gametocytes). Used alone, the drug has very high recrudescence rate. However, it has a synergistic effect with proguanil and this combination is highly efficacious against *P. falciparum* including strains that are resistant to chloroquine and mefloquine.

Pharmacokinetics

Atovaquone is absorbed slowly from the gastrointestinal tract and is subject to wide individual variability. Absorption is greatly increased if the drug is taken with a fatty meal.

Indications

Atovaquone is used for the treatment of uncomplicated multidrug resistant falciparum malaria only in combination with proguanil (Malarone). Dose for adults is 1 g of atovaquone plus 400 mg of proguanil (4 tablets) daily for 3 days. Atovaquone reduced fetal body weight in rabbits; hence it should not be given in pregnancy. The pediatric dose is weight dependent; 5–8 kg dose: 125 mg/50 mg PO qid × 3 days; (9–10 kg): 187.5 mg/75 mg PO qid × 3 days (11–20 kg): 250 mg/100 mg PO qid × 3 days (21–30 kg): 500 mg/200 mg PO qid × 3 days (31–40 kg): 750 mg/300 mg PO qid × 3 days (>41 kg): 1,000 mg/400 mg PO qid × 3 days.

Atovaquone and proguanil is also used for chemoprophylaxis of malaria in areas with multidrug resistant *P. falciparum* such as the Thai-Myanmar border. It can also be used as an alternative for mefloquine and doxycycline in case these drugs are not tolerated. Prophylaxis should be started 1 day prior to departure and continued for 7 days after return. For adults the dose is 250 mg of atovaquone plus 100 mg of proguanil (one tablet) daily. Pediatric dose is (5–8 kg): 31.25 mg/12.5 mg PO qid; (9–10 kg): 46.9 mg/18.7 mg PO qid; (11–20 kg): 62.5 mg/25 mg PO qid; (21–30 kg): 125 mg/50 mg PO qid; (31–40 kg): 187.5 mg/75 mg PO qid; (>41 kg): 250 mg/100 mg PO qid.

Side Effects

Adverse effects include abdominal pain, nausea, vomiting, diarrhea, headache, anorexia, coughing and maculopapular rash.

Drug Interactions

With rifampicin, atovaquone increases rifampicin levels while its own concentration decreases. It also increases concentration of zidovudine and didanosine.

Formulations and Availability

Film-coated tablets containing 250 mg of atovaquone and 100 mg of proguanil hydrochloride (adult strength). Pediatric tablets contain 62.5 mg of atovaquone and 25 mg of proguanil hydrochloride. Drug is unavailable in India.

CHOICE OF ANTIMALARIAL THERAPY (TABLE 1)

Uncomplicated Malaria

Treatment objective: The objective of treatment in uncomplicated malaria is to cure infection and hence prevent morbidity and progression to severe disease. The public health goal is to reduce transmission of infection to others and reduce the infectious reservoir. An equally important secondary goal is to prevent emergence of resistance to antimalarials. Speed of response, adverse effect profile and tolerability of medications are also important issues.

Empirical therapy for uncomplicated malaria: Earlier the National Malaria Eradication Program had recommended presumptive diagnosis of malaria in any case of fever, collection of blood smears and administration of initial dose of chloroquine (4 tablets in adults and 10 mg/kg in children) to all patients pending reports of blood smears. Therapy was completed if smears are positive. In high-risk areas full dose, i.e. 25 mg/kg of chloroquine or 10 tablets were offered as presumptive therapy. There were considerable drawbacks in this approach. It is interesting to note that in the first half of 2006, out of 27.35 million blood smear examinations throughout the country the slide positivity rate (SPR) was found to be only 1.3%. Extrapolating from these data it is evident that the use of presumptive treatment of malaria had the potential for facilitating resistance by greatly increasing the number of patients who are treated unnecessarily. Further complete and successful antimalarial therapy is possible only when the parasite species are known. Hence the National Vector Borne Disease Control program issued revised guidelines in 2011. All efforts should be made to establish a diagnosis of malaria by microscopic or rapid antigen detection methods prior to starting therapy. The algorithm for diagnosis is depicted in Flowchart 1.

TABLE 1: Therapy of malaria.

Situation	*Treatment*
Uncomplicated *P. vivax* malaria	Chloroquine (10 mg/kg of base loading, and then 10 mg/kg and 5 mg/kg after 24 hours and 48 hours (25 mg/kg, maximum total dose is 1,500 mg of base) with primaquine (0.3 mg/kg/day for 14 days, no ceiling dose). In chloroquine resistant areas antimalarial activity (ACT) can be used.
Uncomplicated *P. falciparum* malaria	ACT (3 days treatment) with single gametocidal dose of primaquine (0.75 mg/kg)
Mixed infection (*P. vivax* + *P. falciparum*) cases	Full course of ACT (like falciparum malaria) and primaquine 0.25 mg per kg body weight daily for 14 days (like vivax malaria)
Severe malaria (Falciparum/ Vivax)	Intravenous (IV) artesunate 2.4 mg/kg loading dose and then 2.4 mg/kg 12 hours later and then once daily. The dose in children with weight less than 20 kg is 3 mg/kg. Once the patient is taking orally therapy should be switched to ACT (artesunate–SP/artemether lumefantrine) or chloroquine (for vivax). Primaquine should be given if vivax malaria.

Flowchart 1: National Vector Borne Disease Control Program (NVBDCP) algorithm for diagnosis and treatment of malaria.

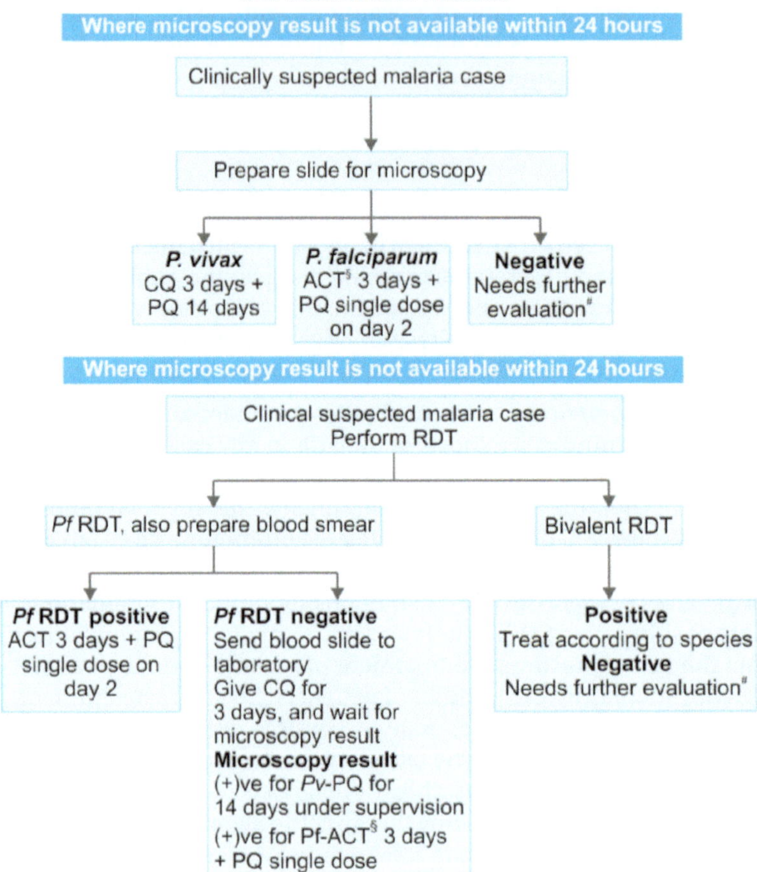

§ACT recommended in NE states is AL while in rest of India it is AS+SP

#Look for other causes of fever; repeat blood slide examination after an appropriate interval

(CQ: chloroquine; PQ: primaquine; NVBDCP: National Vector Borne Disease Control Program; RDTs: rapid diagnostic tests)

Therapy of uncomplicated vivax malaria: Since *P. vivax* in India is susceptible to chloroquine, chloroquine is the drug of choice. Chloroquine should not be given empty stomach and fever should be brought down before administration of chloroquine. If vomiting occurs within 45 minutes of chloroquine administration the dose should be repeated after giving domperidone or other antiemetics. This should be followed by primaquine 0.3 mg/kg/day for 14 days for radical cure. In areas with resistance to primaquine or where relapses have occurred despite standard doses, higher doses of 0.5–0.75 mg/kg should be given. Screening for G6PD deficiency is recommended prior to starting primaquine and close supervision is needed to detect any complications. In case of mild G6PD deficiency primaquine can be given as a weekly dose of 0.6–0.8 mg/kg for 8 weeks with close medical supervision for potential primaquine induced hemolysis. Primaquine should not be given to pregnant women, lactating women with infants below 6 months and infants below 6 months. In these patients, weekly suppressive therapy with chloroquine 10 mg/kg of base may be given for a few months to prevent relapse followed by primaquine when it is no longer contraindicated.

Therapy of uncomplicated falciparum malaria: Therapy has been complicated by widespread resistance in *P. falciparum*. Chloroquine resistance in India is widespread. Resistance to SP is slowly emerging and is widespread in the North Eastern States. There are pockets of mefloquine resistance as well.

The World Health Organization (WHO) now advocates combination therapy for treatment of uncomplicated falciparum malaria. Antimalarial combination therapy (ACT) is the simultaneous use of two or more blood schizontocidal drugs with independent modes of action and thus unrelated biochemical targets in the parasite. Drug combinations such as sulfadoxine-pyrimethamine, sulfalene-pyrimethamine, proguanil-dapsone, chlorproguanil-dapsone and atovaquone-proguanil have linked drug targets and not considered as ACT. The rationale for combining antimalarials with different modes of action is twofold:

- The combination is often more effective
- In the event that a mutant parasite that is resistant to one of the drugs arise de novo during the course of the infection, the parasite will be killed by the other drug.

This mutual protection is thought to prevent or delay the emergence of resistance. To realize the two advantages, the partner drugs in a combination must be independently effective. The possible disadvantages of combination treatments are the potential for increased risk of adverse effects and the increased cost. WHO advocates one of the following is recommended for ACT:

- Artemether + lumefantrine
- Artesunate + amodiaquine
- Artesunate + mefloquine
- Dihydroartemisinin + piperaquine
- Artesunate + sulfadoxine + pyrimethamine

Artemisinin and its derivatives are preferred as combination therapy agents as they produce rapid clearance of parasitemia and rapid resolution of symptoms. They reduce parasite numbers by a factor of approximately 10,000 in each asexual cycle, which is more than other current antimalarials (which reduce parasite numbers 100–1,000-fold per cycle). Artemisinin and its derivatives are eliminated rapidly and hence there is risk of recrudescence. When given in combination with rapidly eliminated compounds (doxycycline, clindamycin), a 7-day course of treatment with an artemisinin compound is required; but when given in combination with slowly eliminated antimalarials, shorter courses of treatment (3 days) are effective. In 3-day ACT regimens, the artemisinin component is present in the body during only two asexual parasite life-cycles (each lasting 2 days, except for *P. malariae* infections). This exposure to 3 days of artemisinin treatment reduces the number of parasites in the body by a factor of approximately one hundred million ($10^4 \times 10^4 = 10^8$). However, complete clearance of parasites is dependent on the partner medicine being effective and persisting at parasiticidal concentrations until all the infecting parasites have been killed. Thus the partner compounds need to be relatively slowly eliminated. As a result of this the artemisinin component is "protected" from resistance by the partner medicine provided it is efficacious and the partner medicine is partly protected by the artemisinin derivative. It has been shown in numerous RCTs that artemisinin based combination therapy significantly reduces treatment failure, recrudescence and gametoctye carriage as compared to monotherapy with amodiaquine, mefloquine and SP. Courses of ACTs of 1–2 days are not recommended; they are less efficacious, and provide less protection of the slowly eliminated partner antimalarial. Non-artemisinin based combination therapies (chloroquine and SP, amodiaquine and SP) are inferior to artemisinin based combination therapies and not recommended.

Various options for artemisinin based combination therapy include artemether-lumefantrine, artesunate-mefloquine, artesunate-amodiaquine and artesunate-SP. The choice depends on the prevalence of resistance to the partner drug. Therapy is likely to succeed only if the 28-day cure rate to monotherapy with the partner drug exceeds 80%.

As per the national program the first option for treatment of uncomplicated falciparum malaria is artesunate (4 mg/kg for 3 days) with SP (1.25 mg/kg of pyrimethamine on day 1). In the North Eastern States, artemether lumefantrine is the recommended therapy. A single gametocidal dose of primaquine 0.75 mg/kg (WHO recommends 0.25 mg/kg) should be given to interrupt transmission.

It must be remembered that efficacy of the partner drug of artemisinin is vital for ACT to succeed. If partner drugs of artemisinin compounds continue to be available and used as monotherapy as they are today, there will compromise the effectiveness of ACT due to increase in resistance to partner drug.

Therapy of uncomplicated mixed malaria: Therapy should be as for uncomplicated falciparum malaria with artemisinin-based combination therapy. Artemisinin based therapy with primaquine is noninferior to chloroquine with primaquine for treating vivax malaria. However, here partner drugs with longer half-life such as piperaquine and mefloquine are better in reducing the risk of recrudescence of the vivax component as compared to the rapidly eliminated lumefantrine. However, dihydroartemisinin-piperaquine and artesunate-mefloquine are not available commercially. Arterolane-piperaquine is another newly introduced combination which may be used in adults (pediatric dosage guidelines not available). Artemisinin combination with SP should be avoided as *P. vivax* has developed resistance to most antifolates. Quinine containing regimes should be avoided as it is inherently less active against *P. vivax*. Radical therapy with primaquine for 14 days must be given.

Complicated or Severe Malaria

The description of complicated or severe malaria has been described in Box 1.

BOX 1: Criteria for severe malaria.

Impaired consciousness: A Glasgow coma score <11 in adults or a Blantyre coma score <3 in children.
Prostration: Generalized weakness so that the person is unable to sit, stand or walk without assistance.
Multiple convulsions: More than two episodes within 24 h.
Acidosis: A base deficit of >8 mEq/L or, if not available, a plasma bicarbonate level of <15 mmol/L or venous plasma lactate ≥5 mmol/L. Severe acidosis manifests clinically as respiratory distress (rapid, deep, labored breathing).
Hypoglycemia: Blood or plasma glucose <2.2 mmol/L (<40 mg/dL).
Severe malarial anemia: Hemoglobin concentration ≤5 g/dL or a hematocrit of ≤5% in children <12 years of age (<7 g/dL and <20%, respectively, in adults) with a parasite count >10,000/µL.
Renal impairment: Plasma or serum creatinine >265 µmol/L (3 mg/dL) or blood urea >20 mmol/L.
Jaundice: Plasma or serum bilirubin >50 µmol/L (3 mg/dL) with a parasite count >100,000/ µL.
Pulmonary edema: Radiologically confirmed or oxygen saturation <92% on room air with a respiratory rate >30/min, often with chest in drawing and crepitations on auscultation
Significant bleeding: Including recurrent or prolonged bleeding from the nose, gums or venipuncture sites; hematemesis or melena.
Shock: Compensated shock is defined as capillary refill ≥3s or temperature gradient on leg (mid to proximal limb), but no hypotension. Decompensated shock is defined as systolic blood pressure <70 mmHg in children or <80 mm Hg in adults, with evidence of impaired perfusion (cool peripheries or prolonged capillary refill).
Hyperparasitemia: P. falciparum parasitemia >10%.

Treatment Objectives

The main objective is to prevent the patient from dying. Secondary objectives are prevention of recrudescence, transmission or emergence of resistance and prevention of disabilities.

Empirical therapy: The outcome of severe malaria depends on rapidity with which treatment is instituted. Hence if clinically suspected, the first dose of antimalarial should be given pending laboratory reports. However, all efforts should be made to confirm the diagnosis by repeated blood smear examinations and or rapid antigen detection tests. Antimalarials should be stopped if repeated smears are negative and an alternative diagnosis has been established.

Specific antimalarial therapy: Initial treatment of complicated or severe malaria is the same whether the culprit species is *P. falciparum or P. vivax.* Two options are available: parenteral quinine or artemisinin derivatives. Artemisinin derivatives are easier to administer as compared to quinine, equivalent in cost and more efficacious.

In a systematic review of artesunate for severe malaria, eight randomized controlled trials with a total of 1,664 adults and 5,765 children directly compared parenteral artesunate with parenteral quinine. The trials were conducted in various African and Asian countries between 1989 and 2010. In comparison with quinine, parenteral artesunate reduced mortality from severe malaria by about 40% in adults (RR: 0.61; 95% CI: 0.50–0.75, five trials, 1,664 participants), and reduced mortality from severe malaria by about 25% in children (RR: 0.76; 95% CI: 0.65–0.90, four trials, 5765 participants). The use of artesunate in children was associated with a small increase in neurological sequelae in children at the time of hospital discharge (RR: 1.36; 95% CI: 1.01–1.83, three trials, 5,163 participants), most of which however, slowly resolved, with little or no difference between artesunate and quinine 28 days later. The WHO guideline development group considered that the small increase in neurological sequelae at discharge after treatment with artesunate was due to the delayed recovery of the severely ill patients, who would have died had they received quinine. This should not be interpreted as a sign of neurotoxicity.

Intravenous artesunate is thus the preferred drug for management of severe or complicated malaria and should be given as a bolus of a freshly prepared solution and never as infusion. Artesunate is dispensed as a powder of artesunic acid, which is dissolved in sodium bicarbonate (5%) to form sodium artesunate. The solution is then diluted in approximately 5 mL of 5% dextrose and given by IV injection or by IM injection into the anterior thigh (if IV access is not available). Care should be taken to use established brands as some preparations of artesunate may be of substandard quality. If artesunate is not available, IM artemether is the next best option. Randomized controlled trials have shown artemether to be inferior to artesunate in severe malaria but more efficacious than quinine. Quinine should only be used if either of these artemisinin derivatives is not available.

Combination therapy of artesunate with quinine or clindamycin or doxycycline in the acute phase is of no added benefit and should be avoided and may actually cause cardiac complications.

Once the patient is better therapy should be switched to oral. For falciparum malaria artemisinin based combination therapy can be given with a single gametocidal dose of primaquine (0.75 mg/kg). For complicated vivax, therapy can be either switched to oral chloroquine or artemisinin-based combination therapy and primaquine for 14 days.

Supportive therapy: Supportive therapy and management of complications are important components of management of severe malaria. It will not be discussed further.

Recurrence of Malaria

Recurrence of vivax malaria: Recurrence within 28 days may be due to inadequate treatment or drug resistance or use of artemisinin derivatives (which are rapidly eliminated from the body). If chloroquine was used then history of vomiting after the drug should be determined. The patient should be retreated with a drug from a different class (if chloroquine was used in adequate doses artemisinin derivatives should be given) and vice versa. Recurrence after 28 days can be due to relapse (if inadequate doses of primaquine were used) or reinfection or less commonly recrudescence. Differentiation between relapse and reinfection can only be by molecular tests which are not commercially available. These recurrences should be treated with chloroquine in appropriate doses especially if artemisinin derivatives were used the first time. Higher doses of primaquine may be used. Some patients with repeated episodes of vivax despite appropriate therapy may be placed on weekly suppressive therapy with 10 mg/kg of the base for 3–6 months.

Recurrence of falciparum malaria: Recurrence within 28 days indicates a recrudescence and should be treated with an alternative ACT effective in that region. Unfortunately, the only ACT commercially available for children is artemether-lumefantrine. Therefore, here a combination of quinine with clindamycin or doxycycline may have to be used or artemether-lumefantrine may be reused. In adults arterolane-piperaquine is a possible alternative. Recurrence after 28 days is usually a reinfection and can be treated with the same regime as given the first time.

Chemoprophylaxis of Malaria

Chemoprophylaxis for malaria is indicated for people from non-endemic countries travelling to India. The options include daily doxycycline (if given for less than 6 weeks) or weekly mefloquine (if given for more than 6 weeks). Atovaquone-proguanil is another option but not available in India. For doses please refer to the individual sections.

CONCLUSION

Management of malaria is a dynamic topic with changing resistance patterns, changing policies and availability of new drugs. All efforts should be made towards establishing a definitive diagnosis, refraining from unnecessary empiric therapy and judiciously using drugs as per recommendations to prevent development of drug resistance.

RECOMMENDED READING

1. World Health Organization. Guidelines for treatment of malaria. 3rd edition. [online] Available from https://www.who.int/malaria/publications/atoz/9789241549127/en/. [Accessed December, 2018].
2. Government of India. Guidelines for diagnosis and treatment of malaria 2014. [online] Available from http://www.mrcindia.org/Diagnosis%20of%20Malaria%20pdf/Guidelines%202014.pdf. [Accessed December, 2018].
3. Graves PM, Choi L, Gelband H, et al. Primaquine or other 8-minoquinolines for reducing Plasmodium falciparum transmission. Cochrane Database Syst Rev. 2018;2:CD008152.
4. Esu E, Effa EE, Opie ON, et al. Artemether for severe malaria. Cochrane Database Syst Rev. 2014;(9):CD010678.
5. Gogtay N, Kannan S, Thatte UM, et al. Artemisinin-based combination therapy for treating uncomplicated Plasmodium vivax malaria. Cochrane Database Syst Rev. 2013;(10):CD008492.

6. Sinclair D, Donegan S, Isba R, et al. Artesunate versus quinine for treating severe malaria. Cochrane Database Syst Rev. 2012;(6):CD005967.
7. Tickell-Painter M, Maayan N, Saunders R, et al. Mefloquine for preventing malaria during travel to endemic areas. Cochrane Database Syst Rev. 2017;10:CD006491.
8. Uthman OA, Graves PM, Saunders R, et al. Safety of primaquine given to people with G6PD deficiency: systematic review of prospective studies. Malar J. 2017; 16(1):346.
9. Song T, Chen J, Huang L, et al. Should we abandon quinine plus antibiotic for treating uncomplicated falciparum malaria? A systematic review and meta-analysis of randomized controlled trials. Parasitol Res. 2016;115(3):903-12.
10. Warrell DA, Giles HM. Treatment and prevention of malaria. Essential Malariology, 4th edition. London: Edward Arnold; 2000. pp. 268-312.
11. Bruce-Chwatt LJ, et al. Chemotherapy of malaria, revised 2nd edition. Geneva: World Health Organization; 1987.
12. Fontanet AL, Johnston DB, Walker AM, et al. High prevalence of mefloquine-resistant falciparum malaria in eastern Thailand. Bull World Health Organ 1993;71(3-4):377-83.
13. Weinke T, Trautmann M, Held T, et al. Neuropsychiatric side effects after the use of mefloquine. Am J Trop Med Hyg. 1991;45(1):86-91.
14. De Vries PJ, Dien TK. Clinical pharmacology and therapeutic potential of artemisinin and its derivatives in the treatment of malaria. Drugs. 1996;52(6):818-36.
15. Ha V, Nguyen NH, Tran TB, et al. Severe and complicated malaria treated with artemisinin, artesunate or artemether in Viet Nam. Trans R Soc Trop Med Hyg. 1997;91(4):465-7.
16. Severe falciparum malaria. World Health Organization, Communicable Diseases Cluster. Trans R Soc Trop Med Hyg. 2000;94(Suppl 1):S1-90.
17. Gogtay NJ, Desai S, Kamtekar KD, et al. Efficacies of 5-and 14-day primaquine regimens in the prevention of relapses in *Plasmodium vivax* infections. Ann Trop Med Parasitol. 1999;93(8):809-12.
18. Baird K. Randomized, double-blind, placebo controlled evaluation of Malarone for prophylaxis of *P. vivax* and *P. falciparum* in non-immune transmigrants to Irian Jaya. ASTM Standardization News, Houston, TX; 2000.
19. Radloff PD, Philipps J, Nkeyi M, et al. Atovaquone and proguanil for *Plasmodium falciparum* malaria. Lancet. 1996;347(9014):1511-4.
20. Das S, Saha B, Hati AK, et al. Evidence of Artemisinin-Resistant *Plasmodium falciparum* Malaria in Eastern India. N Engl J Med. 2018;379(20):1962-4.

Antiretroviral Therapy

34

Chapter

Ira Shah, Vishrutha Karkera

INTRODUCTION

India has the burden of having third largest human immunodeficiency virus (HIV) epidemic in the world. In 2015, HIV prevalence in India was 0.2% which remained almost constant as of 2017 Joint United Nations Programme on HIV/acquired immunodeficiency syndrome (AIDS) (UNAIDS) data. As per the 2015 estimate, the total number of people living with HIV (PLHIV) in India is 2,110,000 and of these 6.47% are children less than 15 years of age. Among these 1,070,000 including 57,230 children are receiving antiretroviral therapy (ART) as on December 2016. The National AIDS Control Organization (NACO) launched in 1992 is carrying out a comprehensive program for prevention and control of HIV/AIDS in India. The current objective of NACO IV is to reduce new infections by 50% and to provide comprehensive care, support, and treatment to all persons living with HIV/AIDS.

This chapter discusses ART of HIV in children and prevention of parent to child transmission of HIV. Opportunistic infection (OI) prophylaxis and postexposure prophylaxis is discussed in Chapter 32 and treatment of OIs is dealt with in individual chapters.

ANTIRETROVIRAL DRUGS

Antiretrovirals (ARVs) are a group of drugs that are used in the treatment of children living with HIV to decrease the viral burden. They are potent inhibitors of viral replication. These drugs fall into three major classes: (1) nucleoside and nucleotide analogue reverse transcriptase inhibitors (NRTIs and NtRTIs), (2) non-nucleoside analogue reverse transcriptase inhibitors (NNRTIs), and (3) protease inhibitors (PIs) along with pharmacokinetic enhancers. There are two new classes of drugs now approved for treatment of HIV in children. They are the entry and fusion inhibitors and integrase strand transfer inhibitors (INSTIs).

Nucleoside Reverse Transcriptase Inhibitors

The NRTIs were the first class of ARV drugs that became available for treatment of HIV. They inhibit the reverse transcriptase enzyme. They have activity against both HIV-1 and HIV-2. Dual NRTI is the backbone of current combination of various ARV therapies.

Drugs in this class include:

- Zidovudine (AZT/ZDV)
- Lamivudine (3TC)

- Stavudine (d4T)
- Didanosine (ddI)
- Abacavir (ABC)
- Emtricitabine (FTC)
- Tenofovir disoproxil fumarate (TDF): It is a NtRTI. It also acts against hepatitis B.
- Tenofovir alafenamide (TAF): TAF has less bone and renal toxicity than TDF, but equal antiviral efficacy.

The drugs stavudine and didanosine are no longer recommended for use in children due to their toxicity profile.

Non-nucleoside Reverse Transcriptase Inhibitors

The NNRTIs were the second class of anti-HIV agents to be developed. The parent compounds are the active moieties, and are therefore immediately active on entering the cell. The NNRTI class of drugs rapidly reduce viral load (VL); however, drug resistance develops quickly after initiation of monotherapy and cross-resistance between drugs in this class is common. There are currently three NNRTIs used for treatment of HIV infection. They are only active against HIV-1.

- Nevirapine (NVP)
- Efavirenz (EFV)
- Etravirine: Used in children more than 6 years of age and is considered a "second-generation" NNRTI, in part because it retains activity against HIV-1 isolates which are resistant to other NNRTIs.
- Rilpivirine (only approved for use in adults).

Protease Inhibitors

The PIs inhibit the protease enzyme. Virions are produced, but they are incomplete and noninfectious. PIs were the third class of ARVs to be developed. They are highly potent. They are active against both HIV-1 and HIV-2. PIs have a high genetic barrier to resistance, and PI resistance at regimen failure is uncommon.

The various PIs used for treatment of HIV infection are:

- Ritonavir (RTV)
- Lopinavir (LPV)
- Amprenavir
- Atazanavir (ATZ)
- Darunavir
- Tipranavir
- Fosamprenavir

Boosted Protease Inhibitors

Low-dose RTV, a potent PI, acts as a potent inhibitor of the cytochrome P450 3A4 (CYP3A4) isoenzyme, thereby inhibiting the metabolism of other PIs. It has been used in low doses combined with another PI as a "pharmacokinetic booster", increasing drug exposure by prolonging the second drug's half-life. Boosted PI-based regimens are commonly used in treatment of adults, but adequate pediatric data are only available for coformulated lopinavir/ritonavir in children older than 2 weeks of age and for atazanavir, fosamprenavir, darunavir, and tipranavir with low-dose ritonavir in children age more than 6 years.

New Classes of Antiretroviral Drugs

Entry Inhibitors

These agents inhibit viral binding or fusion to host target cells. T-20 (enfuvirtide) is the drug currently used and has to be given subcutaneously twice daily and is to be used only in children more than 6 years of age. It prevents virus-cell fusion. It is used as part of salvage regime in patients who have multi-ART regime failures.

CCR5 Coreceptor Antagonist

Maraviroc blocks the chemokine CCR5 coreceptor on the CD4 cell surface thereby preventing HIV from entering the cell. This was the first ARV drug to be developed that does not actually target the virus itself. This drug is approved for use in children more than 2 years of age. Maraviroc is effective as part of combination therapy in patients with multidrug-resistant HIV-1. Before starting treatment with this drug, however, it is necessary to check for CCR5 or CXCR4 virus tropism. CCR5 antagonists will be inactive against CXCR4-tropic virus and mixed/dual tropic HIV virus. There are considerable interactions with both PI and NNRTI classes, requiring alteration in maraviroc dosing depending on other drugs in the regimen.

Integrase Strand Transfer Inhibitors

They block the integrase enzyme thereby preventing incorporation of viral deoxyribonucleic acid (DNA) into human genome. Raltegravir, dolutegravir, elvitegravir, and bictegravir are INSTIs. These drugs have been found to be useful in the treatment of patients with multidrug-resistant HIV-1. Raltegravir is Food and Drug Administration (FDA)-approved for treatment of HIV-infected full-term neonates, infants, and children. Raltegravir has a favorable safety profile and lacks significant drug interactions. Dolutegravir has recently been approved by the FDA for use in children weighing more than 30 kg. The drug has a very favorable safety profile and can be dosed once daily in treatment of INSTI-naive patients.

Pharmacokinetic Enhancers

Cobicistat

It is used in adolescents and adults as a pharmacokinetic enhancer (boosting agent) of selected PIs and the integrase inhibitor elvitegravir. Cobicistat is not interchangeable with RTV. It is approved in children less than 18 years of age.

DOSAGE RECOMMENDATIONS OF VARIOUS ANTIRETROVIRALS

Dosing of various ARVs are as per weight or surface area in children. The doses are depicted in Table 1.

ANTIRETROVIRAL THERAPY

Currently, highly active combination antiretroviral therapy (HAART) regimens including at least three drugs are recommended; such regimens have been associated with enhanced survival,

TABLE 1: Dosing of various ARVs.

NRTI	
Zidovudine (ZDV/ AZT)	Neonates <30 weeks: Birth 4 weeks: 2 mg/kg/dose 12 hourly for 4 weeks Age 4 weeks to 8–10 weeks: 3 mg/kg/dose 12 hourly Age >8–10 weeks: 12 mg/kg/dose 12 hourly Neonate >30 weeks to <35 weeks: 2 mg/kg/dose 12 hourly for 2 weeks; 3 mg/kg/dose 12 hourly till 6–8 weeks and 12 mg/kg/dose 12 hourly for age >6–8 weeks ≥35 weeks: 4 mg/kg/dose 12 hourly for 4 weeks Continuation: 12 mg/kg/dose 12 hourly Pediatric dose: 4 kg to ≤9 kg: 12 mg/kg/dose 12 hourly 9 kg to <30 kg: 9 mg/kg/dose 12 hourly ≥30 kg: 300 mg 12 hourly (oral dose as per BSA:180–240 mg/m^2) Adult: 300 mg 12 hourly
Lamivudine (3TC)	Neonatal dose (<4 weeks): 2 mg/kg 12 hourly Pediatric dose: ≥4 weeks to <3 months: 4 mg/kg 12 hourly ≥3 months to <3 years: 5 mg/kg 12 hourly, up to 150 mg ≥3 years: 5 mg/kg 12 hourly up to 150 mg or 10 mg/kg once daily up to 300 mg
Emtricitabine (FTC)	Neonatal dose (0 to <3 months): 3 mg/kg once daily <3 months to 17 years: 6 mg/kg once daily (maximum dose of oral solution is 240 mg) Adults: 200 mg once daily capsule
Abacavir (ABC)	8 mg/kg every 12 hours (max 600 mg) or 16 mg/kg. Not approved for infants <3 months.
Tenofovir (TAF) alafenamide	Children, adolescent weighing >25 kg This drug is used as fixed dose combination tablet Emtricitabine (200 mg) + TAF (25 mg) 1 tab once daily Emtricitabine (200 mg) + rilpivirine (25 mg) + TAF (25 mg) 1 tab once daily
Tenofovir disoproxil fumarate (TDF)	Pediatric dose (>2 years to <12 years): 8 mg/kg once daily (maximum 300 mg per day) >12 years: 300 mg once daily
NNRTI	
Nevirapine (NVP)	Age <1 month: 6 mg/kg/dose twice daily Age >1 month: 300–400 mg/m^2 in 2 divided doses to max 400 mg (give a lead in dose for first 15 days at half the recommended dose to watch for Steven-Johnson syndrome
Efavirenz (EFV)	Age ≥3 years and weight ≥10 kg: 10 to <15 kg: 200 mg at bedtime 15 to <20 kg: 250 mg at bedtime 20 to <25 kg: 300 mg at bedtime 25 to <32.5 kg: 350 mg at bedtime 32.5 to <40 kg: 400 mg at bedtime ≥40 kg: 600 mg at bedtime Capsule may be administered by sprinkling the content into an age appropriate food. Weight bands approximate a dose of EFV 367 mg/m^2 (max 600 mg)

Contd...

Contd...

Etravirine (ETR/ ETV)	Age 6–18 years: 16 kg to <20 kg: 100 mg twice daily 20 kg to <25 kg: 125 mg twice daily 25 kg to <30 kg: 150 mg twice daily ≥30 kg: 200 mg twice daily
Rilpivirine (RPV)	Not approved for use in children Adolescent (weight ≥35 kg) and adults: 25 mg once daily
PI	
Nelfinavir (NFV)	2 years and above: 45–55 mg/kg twice daily Adults: 1,250 mg twice daily
ATZ (Atazanavir)	Age ≥3 months: Powder formulation 5 to <15 kg: Atazanavir 200 mg plus ritonavir 80 mg both once daily with food 15 to <25 kg: Atazanavir 250 mg plus ritonavir 80 mg both once daily with food Age ≥6 years: Capsule formulation 15 to <35 kg: Atazanavir 200 mg plus ritonavir 100 mg, both once daily with food >35 kg: Atazanavir 300 mg plus ritonavir 100 mg, both once daily with food
Darunavir (DRV)	Age 3 to <12 years: 10 to <11 kg: Darunavir 200 mg plus ritonavir 32 mg 11 to <12 kg: Darunavir 220 mg plus ritonavir 32 mg 12 to <13 kg: Darunavir 240 mg plus ritonavir 40 mg 13 to <14 kg: Darunavir 260 mg plus ritonavir 40 mg 14 to <15 kg: Darunavir 280 mg plus ritonavir 48 mg 15 to <30 kg: Darunavir 375 mg plus ritonavir 48 mg 30 to <40kg: Darunavir 450 mg plus ritonavir 100 mg ≥40 kg: Darunavir 600 mg plus ritonavir 100 mg Give twice daily with food
Lopinavir/ritonavir (LPVr)	14 days and above: 300 mg/75 mg lopinavir/ritonavir per m^2 of body surface area twice daily
Fosamprenavir (FPV)	≥6 months to 18 years: Give twice daily <11 kg: Fosamprenavir 45 mg/kg plus ritonavir 7 mg/kg 11 kg to <15 kg: Fosamprenavir 30 mg/kg plus ritonavir 3 mg/kg 15 kg to <20 kg: Fosamprenavir 23 mg/kg plus ritonavir 3 mg/kg ≥20 kg: Fosamprenavir 18 mg/kg plus ritonavir 3 mg/kg (max: fosamprenavir 700 mg plus ritonavir 100 mg twice daily)
Tipranavir (TPV)	2 years to 18 years: Tipranavir 375 mg/m^2 plus ritonavir 150 mg/m^2 twice daily
INSTIs	
Raltegravir (RAL)	Birth to 4 weeks: 1.5 mg/kg/dose once daily for 1 week and 3 mg/kg/dose twice daily for next 4 weeks >4 weeks: 6 mg/kg/dose twice daily (max: tablet is 300 mg twice daily)
Fusion inhibitors	
Enfuvirtide (T-20)	6 years and above: 2 mg/kg (maximum dose 90 mg) twice daily subcutaneously
CCR5 receptor antagonist	
Maraviroc (MVC)	For use in treatment experienced children ≥2 years and weight ≥10 kg Dose when used along with potent CYP 3A inhibitors/inducers (EVG/r, PIs): 10 to <20 kg: 50 mg BD 20 to <30 kg: 75 mg BD 30 to <40kg: 100 mg BD >40 kg: 150 mg BD

Contd...

Contd...

	Dose when used along with drugs that are not potent CYP 3A inhibitors/inducers (NRTIs, T-20, TPV/r, NVP, RAL): 10 to <20 kg: Not recommended 20 to <30kg: Not recommended 30 to <40 kg: 300 mg BD >40 kg: 300 mg BD

(BSA: body surface area; INSTIs: integrase strand transfer inhibitors; NNRTI: non-nucleoside analogue reverse transcriptase inhibitor; NRTI: nucleoside reverse transcriptase inhibitor; PI: protease inhibitor)

reduction in OIs, improved growth and neurocognitive function, and improved quality of life in children. ART does not cure HIV infection and requires very close adherence in order to be effective and prevent emergence of resistance and thus the patient has to be prepared for lifelong treatment in order to optimally control the virus replication.

Goals of Pediatric Antiretroviral Therapy

The aims of treatment with ARV drugs in HIV-infected children are to achieve and sustain full HIV ribonucleic acid (RNA) VL suppression and minimize short- and long-term ARV drug toxicity. At the time of ART initiation, CD4 cell count and plasma VL should be measured to establish a baseline to monitor ART benefit. For monitoring ART toxicity complete blood count, serum electrolytes, creatinine, glucose, hepatic transaminases, urinalysis, and serum lipids (cholesterol and triglycerides) should be measured.

Duration of Antiretroviral Therapy

Human immunodeficiency virus infection cannot be eradicated by the ARV drugs that are currently available. Proviral DNA persists in sanctuary sites such as the central nervous system (CNS) and testis, while continued production of drug-sensitive virus has been demonstrated in children on HAART with plasma levels of HIV RNA below the limit of detection of current clinical assays (<50 copies/mL). Consequently, VL increases to pretreatment levels within 1–2 weeks of stopping therapy, making lifelong treatment necessary. Also error-prone reverse transcriptase enzyme leads to mutations in the virus that prevent its eradication.

When to Start Antiretroviral Therapy?

Although implementing ART is complex, a number of guidelines are available to help practitioners to select effective regimens for particular patients. The current guidelines for starting ART have been simplified. As per World Health Organization (WHO) July 2017 update on HIV treatment and care, ART should be initiated in everyone living with HIV at any CD4 cell count and regardless of WHO clinical stage.

Which Antiretroviral Therapy Regimens?

Triple combination therapy is recommended for treating all HIV infected children. All possible OIs should be treated first ideally prior to starting ART. HLA-B*5701 genotype prior to abacavir therapy should be done. For treatment naïve children ARV regimen to be considered is dual NRTI backbone of any regimen in combination with one active drug from following classes: NNRTI,

TABLE 2: Preferred and alternative first-line regimens for children according to the WHO November 2015 consolidated guidelines.

Age group	*Preferred first-line regimens*	*Alternative first-line regimens in children*
Children <3 years	ABC (or AZT) + 3TC + LPV/r	ABC (or AZT) + 3TC+ NVP
Children 3 years to <10 years	ABC + 3TC + EFV	ABC + 3TC + NVP AZT +3TC +EFV (or NVP) TDF+ 3TC (or FTC)+ EFV (or NVP)
Adolescents	TDF + 3TC (or FTC) + EFV	AZT +3TC +EFV (or NVP) TDF or ABC+3TC or FTC+DTG* or EFV_{400}* or NVP

[ABC: abacavir; AZT: zidovudine; DTG: dolutegravir; EFV: efavirenz; EFV_{400}: efavirenz at lower dose (400 mg/kg/day); FTC: emtricitabine; LPV/r: lopinavir-ritonavir; NVP: nevirapine; 3TC: lamivudine; TDF: tenofovir disoproxil fumarate]

*Safety profile and efficacy data on use of DTG and EFV_{400} in people with human immunodeficiency virus/tuberculosis coinfection and children less than 12 years are not yet available.

a boosted PI or INSTIs (Table 2). There are currently eight NRTIs which are FDA approved for use in children aged less than 13 years. Dual NRTIs backbone regimen includes zidovudine with lamivudine or emtricitabine combination due to favorable safety profile and extensive experience and abacavir plus lamivudine or emtricitabine for children aged more than or equal to 3 months. Tenofovir alafenamide and emtricitabine as fixed dose combination tablet along with INSTI or NNRTI (single tablet) is indicated in children more than or equal to 25 kg weight or more than or equal to 6 years with estimated creatinine clearance more than or equal to 30 mL/min. Tenofovir disoproxil fumarate with lamivudine or emtricitabine combination is FDA approved for use in children more than or equal to 2 years. However, risk of decreased bone mineral density versus benefits should be considered.

Response to Antiretroviral Therapy in Children

Within 1 month of starting effective ART in children, plasma HIV RNA VL decreases substantially and the CD4 count starts to rise. Infants, who frequently start from a VL of between 10^5 copies/mL and 10^7 copies/mL, can take many months to become undetectable. As per new WHO recommendations, routine VL testing is encouraged at 6 months and 12 months after initiating ART and if the patient is stable on ART (i.e. on ART for at least 1 year, no current illness or pregnancy, good understanding of lifelong adherence, and evidence of treatment success which is two consecutive VL measures below 1,000 copies/mL), then every year thereafter. WHO recommend CD4 cell count every 6 months until stable on ART, following which CD4 cell count monitoring can be withheld in patients who are virally suppressed and stable on ART.

Drug-drug Interactions

CYP3A is the most important enzyme for metabolism of drugs in general, and for anti-HIV drugs in particular. It metabolizes all currently available PIs and NNRTIs. PIs are substrates of CYP3A and are often also inhibitors of these enzymes. The NNRTIs are not only substrates of CYP3A but they are also able to induce this enzyme. As a result plasma levels of the drug itself will decrease before reaching steady-state (7–14 days). Both nevirapine and efavirenz are inducers of CYP3A; when combined with PIs, the plasma levels of most PIs (i.e. indinavir, saquinavir, amprenavir, atazanavir, and lopinavir) will decrease.

Some anticonvulsants are strong enzyme inducers: phenytoin, phenobarbital, and carbamazepine. Plasma levels of PIs or NNRTIs will decrease when combined with these anticonvulsants. On the other hand, PIs increase plasma levels of carbamazepine which enhances the risk for toxicity.

Concomitant use of antihistaminic agents such as astemizole or terfenadine along with boosted PIs and NNRTIs has been associated with severe and life-threatening reactions such as cardiac arrhythmias.

Nevirapine based ARV regimen along with itraconazole or ketoconazole may decrease the concentration of these antifungals to subtherapeutic levels. Thus, alternative antifungal agents such as flucytosine or fluconazole should be used for adequate treatment of fungal infections among people with HIV.

Combination of EFV with the antimalarial amodiaquine has been associated with significant increase in liver transaminases. PIs should not be used with halofantrine and lumefantrine.

Boosted PIs and statin combination may increase the risk of myopathy and rhabdomyolysis. Thus, alternative cholesterol lowering agents should be used.

Potential drug interactions to be considered when using ARV drugs and direct acting antiviral agents (DAAs) for hepatitis C infection. Treatment with ribavirin and pegylated interferon alpha-2a along with zidovudine is associated with increased risk of anemia and hepatic decompensation.

Dolutegravir should not be simultaneously administered with cation-containing antacids, laxatives, and multivitamins due to risk of chelation. Dolutegravir should be administered 2 hours before or 6 hours after taking medications containing polyvalent cations.

Antitubercular Treatment and Antiretroviral Therapy

When treating TB patients living with HIV, TB treatment should be initiated first, followed by ART as soon as possible, i.e. within 2–8 weeks. The most important drug interaction is between rifampicin and ARV drugs. Rifampicin being a potent CYP3A enzyme inducer and by P-glycoprotein mediated efflux mechanism lowers the ARV drug levels, especially significant reduction in PIs level (except RTV, which partially reverses this effect) and moderate reductions in NVP, NRTIs, and EFV drug levels. Rifampicin also causes significant reduction in plasma concentration of dolutegravir. The choice of ART regimen in TB coinfection should be carefully considered. However, 2NRTIs backbone is maintained, along with third drug being super-boosted PI or EFV or NVP at maximum dose. If VL is less than 100,000 copies/mL, then triple NRTI therapy is an option in children.

If patient is receiving a boosted PI, rifampicin may need to be substituted with rifabutin and if rifabutin is not available, PI based regimen is used doubling the standard dose of LPV/r or increasing the boosting dose of RTV for the duration of TB treatment. In case multi- or extensively drug-resistant TB treatment, there is limited information on drug interactions of ARV drugs with new drugs like bedaquiline and delamanid. As bedaquiline is primarily metabolized by CYP3A4, concomitant use with EFV, and PIs should be undertaken with extreme caution and close monitoring.

Adverse Effects of Antiretroviral Therapy

Antiretrovirals are potentially toxic drugs and have several adverse effects (AEs). However, overall benefits of viral suppression and improved immune function far outweigh the risk associated with ARV. AEs to the tune of 30% may be seen in patients on ART and may be a major factor for poor adherence. Fortunately, current ARV regimens are associated with fewer serious and intolerable AEs than regimens used in the past. The common AEs of ARVs are depicted in Table 3.

Antiretroviral drug-associated AE can vary from mild to life-threatening illness (hypersensitivity reaction and symptomatic hepatotoxicity). Drug-related toxicity can be acute (occurring soon after drug administration), subacute (occurring within 1–2 days of administration) or late (after prolonged drug administration, like dyslipidemia).

Changing Antiretroviral Therapy

Antiretroviral therapy regimen may be changed in the following circumstances:
- Failure of current regimen
- Toxicity or intolerance to current regimen.

TABLE 3: Adverse effects of antiretroviral drugs.

NRTI	ABC: Hypersensitivity reaction ZDV: Severe anemia, leukopenia, lactic acidosis, severe hepatomegaly with steatosis, lipoatrophy, lipodystrophy, myopathy TDF: Hypophosphatemia, elevated creatinine and osteoporosis, fatty liver, lactic acidosis, proteinuria
NNRTI	EFV: Persistent CNS toxicity (dizziness, insomnia, abnormal dreams), anxiety, depression, confusion, seizure, hypersensitivity reactions, hepatotoxicity, gynecomastia NVP: Hepatotoxicity, hypersensitivity reaction, including Stevens–Johnson syndrome (SJS) ETV: Hypersensitivity reaction RPV: Not to be used in patients with high viral load
PI	LPV/r: ECG abnormalities (PR and ORS interval prolongation, torsades de pointes), hepatotoxicity, pancreatitis, dyslipidemia, diarrhea ATV/r: ECG abnormalities, nephrolithiasis, indirect hyperbilirubinemia DRV/r: Hypersensitivity reactions, hepatotoxicity
INSTI	DTG: Hypersensitivity reactions, hepatotoxicity, insomnia, neuropsychiatric symptoms, elevated creatinine RAL: Rhabdomyolysis, myopathy, myalgia, hepatitis, hepatic failure, severe skin rash and hypersensitivity reaction
Pharmacokinetic enhancers	COBI: Elevated creatinine RTV: GI intolerance (nausea, vomiting, diarrhea), hyperlipidemia, hepatitis, hyperglycemia, fat maldistribution, SJS
Entry and fusion inhibitor	T-20: Local injection site reaction, hypersensitivity reaction, increased risk of bacterial pneumonia MVC: Hepatotoxicity, postural hypotension, fever, rash

(CNS: central nervous system; ECG: electrocardiography; INSTI: integrase strand transfer inhibitors; GI: gastrointestinal; NNRTI: non-nucleoside analogue reverse transcriptase inhibitor; NRTI: nucleoside reverse transcriptase inhibitor; PI: protease inhibitor)

TABLE 4: WHO definition of clinical, immunological, and virological failure for the decision to switch ART regimens.

Failure	*Definition*	*Comment*
Clinical failure	New or recurrent clinical event indicating severe immunodeficiency, WHO clinical stage 4 condition in adults and adolescents whereas WHO clinical stage 3 and 4 clinical conditions with the exception of TB in children after 6 months of effective treatment	The condition must be differentiated from immune reconstitution inflammatory syndrome (IRIS) occurring after initiating ART For adults, certain WHO clinical stage 3 conditions (pulmonary TB and severe bacterial infections) may also indicate treatment failure
Immunological failure	Adults and adolescents: CD4 count $\leq$250 cells/mm^3 following clinical failure* or Persistent CD4 levels <100 cells/mm^3 Children: <5 years: Persistent CD4 levels below 200 cells/mm^3 >5 years: Persistent CD4 levels below100 cells/mm^3	Without concomitant or recent infection to cause a transient decline in the CD4 cell count Current WHO clinical and immunological criteria have low sensitivity and positive predictive value for identifying individuals with virological failure
Virological failure	Viral load above 1,000 copies/mL based on two consecutive viral load measurements in 3 months, with adherence support following the first viral load test	An individual must be taking ART for at least 6 months before it can be determined that a regimen has failed

*Previous guidelines defined immunological failure based on a fall from baseline, which is no longer applicable in the context of CD4-independent treatment initiation. The option of CD4 cell count at or below 250 cells/mm^3 following clinical failure is based on an analysis of data from Uganda and Zimbabwe.

Treatment Failure

Poor adherence, inadequate drug levels, prior existing drug resistance, drug-drug interaction or inadequate potency of the drugs chosen can all contribute to ARV treatment failure. Treatment failure is considered as either clinical failure, immunological failure or virological failure (Table 4).

When to Switch Antiretroviral Drugs for Treatment Failure?

Available drug regimens, viral resistance profiles, previous treatment, adherence issues, and readiness of the family and child to switch; all need to be considered. Adding or substituting single drugs in a failing ART regimen without resistance testing risks giving the new drug as effective monotherapy which may result in rapid development of further resistance. It is therefore recommended that all changes in therapy with detectable viremia be preceded by resistance testing unless it is unequivocal that there is no cross-resistance with previous drugs received. Ideally resistance testing should be performed while the patient is still on the old regimen, or within a few weeks of stopping. Expert opinion should be sought in interpreting resistance genotypes. The general rule is to change all the drugs in the regimen after first-line ART failure with resistance. The new regimen should include at least two, preferably three, fully active ARV drugs based on past treatment history and resistance pattern for durable and potent virologic suppression. The new WHO recommendations include use of DRV/r or RAL with LPV/r as alternative ART regimens for adults and adolescents. For children after failure of first-line LPV/r-based regimen, RAL-based second-line regimen is recommended. Failure of an NNRTI-based regimen is often as a result of viral drug resistance, and switching to a boosted PI or an INSTI-based regimen is appropriate. Failure of a boosted PI-based regimen is more likely to be because of poor adherence than resistance. If resistance is detected, a switch to an NNRTI-based regimen or another PI without overlapping resistance may be appropriate. If resistance is not detected, continuing the PI with enhanced adherence support should be considered. Any change in regimen should be preceded by a thorough reassessment of adherence, and a plan for adherence monitoring of the new regimen.

CONCLUSION

Antiretroviral treatment reduces illness and mortality among children living with HIV. With a gamut of ARV drugs and multiple treatment regimens to select from, treatment of HIV-infected children is complex and difficult. Due to the availability of newer classes of drugs and newer drugs in existing classes, it has become possible for the better management of children even with extensive drug resistance disease. In addition, adherence issues, lifelong therapy and evolution of resistance indicate that therapy should be given under consultation from expert who deals with management of these children.

PREVENTION OF PARENT-TO-CHILD TRANSMISSION—GUIDELINES FROM NACO

Human immunodeficiency virus can be transmitted from an HIV-positive woman to her child during pregnancy, childbirth, and breastfeeding. Mother-to-child transmission (MTCT) which is also known as "vertical transmission" accounts for most infections in children (0–14 years). Without treatment, the likelihood of the virus passing from mother-to-child is 15% to 45%. However, with ART for the mother and a short course of ARV drugs for the baby this risk is reduced to below 5%. Around 1.4 million HIV infections among children were prevented between 2010 and 2018 due to the implementation of prevention of mother-to-child transmission (PMTCT) services. In India, the PPTCT program was launched in the the year 2002 with an aim to prevent the perinatal transmission of HIV from an HIV infected pregnant mother to her newborn baby. Prevention of parent-to-child transmission (PPTCT) as advocated by NACO is discussed here; for other strategies readers are referred to specialized texts and guidelines.

Management of the Mother

The program entails counseling and testing of pregnant women in the integrated counseling and testing centers (ICTCs). In 2014, all pregnant women who are HIV positive are initiated on lifelong ART, irrespective of CD4 count and WHO clinical staging. The recommended first-line regimen for HIV-infected pregnant women is tenofovir (TDF) (300 mg) + lamivudine (3TC) (300 mg) + efavirenz (EFV) (600 mg) (if there is no prior exposure to NNRTIs (NVP/EFV) at any gestational age. HIV-infected pregnant women who have had previous exposure to single dose NVP (or EFV) for PPTCT prophylaxis in prior pregnancies, an NNRTI-based ART regimen may not be fully effective due to persistence of archived mutation to NNRTIs. Thus, these women will require a protease-inhibitor based ART regimen viz: TDF + 3TC + LPV/r. The dose is TDF + 3TC

(1 tablet daily) + LPV (200 mg)/r (50 mg) (2 tablets twice daily). However, the great majority of HIV infections in India are due to HIV-1, there are small foci of HIV-2 infection as well, primarily in western India. HIV-2 will also progress to AIDS, although progression is generally much slower. HIV-2 has the same modes of transmission as HIV-1, but has been shown to be much less transmissible from mother-to-child (transmission risk 0–4%). NNRTI drugs, such as NVP and EFV, are not effective against HIV-2 infection. Therefore, for women who are infected with HIV-2 alone should follow standard adult guidelines for HIV-2 treatment which consists of 2NRTIs + LPV/r. Prophylaxis with AZT (instead of syrup NVP) to be given to babies in mothers with HIV-2.

At the time of delivery, MTCT risk is increased by prolonged rupture of membranes, repeated per vaginal examinations, assisted instrumental delivery (vacuum or forceps), invasive fetal monitoring procedures (scalp/fetal blood monitoring), and episiotomy. Safe delivery techniques should be followed to reduce the transmission during delivery. Cesarean sections in HIV-positive pregnant women should be performed for obstetric indications only. This is unlike the resource replete setting where women with VL of more than 1,000 copies at term are delivered by elective cesarean section.

Human Immunodeficiency Virus-Exposed Infant

As per PPTCT guidelines, HIV-exposed infant should be started on postpartum ARV prophylaxis for minimum of 6 weeks (Table 5). Exclusive breastfeeds up to 6 months and continued breastfeeds in addition to complementary feeds after 6 months up to 1 year for early infant diagnosis (EID) negative babies and up to 2 years for EID positive babies who receive pediatric ART. Only in situations where breastfeeding cannot be done (maternal death and severe maternal illness) or individual mother's choice (at her own risk), then exclusive replacement feeding may be considered. Exclusive replacement feeding should be done only when AFASS criteria is fulfilled (A-Affordable F-Feasible A-Acceptable S-Sustainable S-Safe). Mixed feeding should not be done at any cost within the first 6 months (feeding breastfeeds and replacement feeds simultaneously in the first 6 months, which leads to mucosal abrasions in the gut of the baby facilitating HIV virus entry through these abrasions).

Early infant diagnosis at 6 weeks of age; repeat testing at 6 months, 12 months, and 6 weeks after cessation of breastfeeds. As per 2016 WHO recommendations, HIV virologic testing should be used to diagnose HIV infection among infants and children younger than 18 months and that ART should be started without delay while a second specimen is collected to confirm the

TABLE 5: Dose and duration of infant daily nevirapine (NVP) prophylaxis.

Birth weight (kg)	*Daily NVP dose in mg*	*NVP dose in mL (10 mg/mL)*	
Less than 2 kg	2 mg/kg once a day	0.2 mL/kg once a day	Start within 6–12 hours of delivery Up to 6 weeks, irrespective of whether the baby is exclusively breastfed or exclusively replacement fed. The duration may be extended to 12 weeks if the mother had not received ART for at least 24 weeks, including women initiated on ART during labor and if she is breastfeeding the child
2–2.5 kg	10 mg once a day	1 mL once a day	
More than 2.5 kg	15 mg once a day	1.5 mL once a day	

(ART: antiretroviral therapy)

initial positive virological test result. Co-trimoxazole prophylaxis from 6 weeks of age till age of 1 year or till the diagnosis of HIV is excluded. The diagnosis of HIV can be considered excluded if the HIV virologic test is negative at age 4 months in non-breastfed infants or 6 weeks after stopping breastfeeds in breastfed infants. Confirmation of HIV status of all babies at 18 months using all three antibody (rapid) tests.

RECOMMENDED READING

1. Aidsinfo. (2018). Guidelines for the use of antiretroviral agents in pediatric HIV Infection. [online] Available from https://aidsinfo.nih.gov/guidelines [Accessed January, 2019].
2. Avert. (2018). Prevention of Mother-to-child Transmission (PMTCT) of HIV. [online] Available from https://www.avert.org/professionals/hiv-programming/prevention/prevention-mother-child [Accessed January, 2019].
3. Caldwell CB, Oxtoby MJ, Simonds RJ, et al. 1994 revised classification system for human immunodeficiency virus infection in children less than 13 years of age. MMWR CDC Surveill Summ. 1994;43:1-10.
4. Hirsch MS, Burn-Vezinet F, Clotet B, et al. Antiretroviral drug resistance testing in adults infected with human immunodeficiency virus type-1: 2003 Recommendations of an International AIDS Society—USA Panel. Clin Infect Dis. 2003;37:113-28.
5. NACO. (2003). Prevention of Parent-to-Child Transmission (PPTCT). [online] Available from http://naco.gov.in/prevention-parent-child-transmissionpptct [Accessed January, 2019].
6. NACO. (2017). Office Memorandum: Revised guidelines on initiation of antiretroviral therapy (ART). [online] Available from http://naco.gov.in/sites/default/files/Scan_OM%20CST.pdf [Accessed January, 2019].
7. NACO. (2018). National Guidelines for HIV-1 Viral Load Laboratory Testing. [online] Available from http://naco.gov.in/sites/default/files/NationalGuidelinesForHIV-1ViralLoadLaboratoryTestingApril2018%20%282%29.pdf [Accessed January, 2019].
8. PENTA Steering Committee, Welch S, Sharland M, et al. PENTA 2009 guidelines for the use of antiretroviral therapy in pediatric HIV-1 infection. HIV Med. 2009;10:591-613.
9. Shah I, Dhabe H, Lala M, et al. Assessment of adherence to antiretroviral therapy in HIV infected children—A preliminary Indian study. Mumbai: Pedicon; 2007.
10. Shah I. Adverse effects of antiretroviral therapy in HIV-1 infected children. J Trop Pediatr. 2006;52(4):244-8.
11. Shah I. Antiretroviral therapy (ART). In: Shah I, Shah NK, Manglani M (Eds). IAP Speciality Series on Pediatric HIV. Mumbai: Indian Academy of Pediatric; 2007.
12. Shah I. Lactic acidosis in HIV infected children due to antiretroviral therapy. Indian Pediatr. 2005;42:1051-2.
13. Shah I. Pediatric HIV in India—Current Issues. JK Science. 2006;8:183-4.
14. Swaminathan S, Ramachandran G, Hemanth Kumar AK, et al. Factors influencing plasma nevirapine levels: a study in HIV-infected children on generic antiretroviral treatment in India. J Antimicrob Chemother. 2011;66(6):1354-9.
15. UNAIDS. (2018). Miles to go: Global AIDS update 2018. [online] Available from http://www.unaids.org/en/site-search#?cludoquery=Miles%20to%20go%3A%20global%20AIDS%20update%202018&cludopage=1&cludorefpt=Miles%20to%20go%20-%20Global%20AIDS%20update%202018%20%7C%20UNAIDS&cludorefurl=http%3A%2F%2Fwww.unaids.org%2Fen%2F20180718_GR2018 [Accessed January, 2019].
16. WHO. (2016). Consolidated guidelines on the use of antiretroviral drugs for treating and preventing HIV infection: Recommendations for a public health approach—Second edition. [online] Available from https://www.who.int/hiv/pub/arv/arv-2016/en/ [Accessed January, 2019]

17. WHO. (2017). transition to new antiretrovirals in HIV programmes. [online] Available from https://www.who.int/hiv/pub/toolkits/transition-to-new-arv/en/ [Accessed January, 2019].
18. WHO. (2017). What's new in treatment monitoring: viral load and cd4 testing. [online] Available from https://www.who.int/hiv/pub/arv/treatment-monitoring-info-2017/en/ [Accessed January, 2018].
19. WHO. (2018). Updated recommendations on first-line and second-line antiretroviral regimens and post-exposure prophylaxis and recommendations on early infant diagnosis of HIV [online] Available from https://www.who.int/hiv/pub/guidelines/ARV2018update/en/ [Accessed January, 2019].
20. WHO. Mother-to-child transmission of HIV. [online] Available from https://www.who.int/hiv/topics/mtct/en/ [Accessed January, 2019].

Anthelminthic Therapy

35

Chapter

S Balasubramaniam, Sumanth Amperayani

INTRODUCTION

Parasitic infections of the gastrointestinal (GI) tract occur in all geographic regions of the world and produce a substantial morbidity in children. Prevalence is highest in the economically deprived regions of the world, notably in the tropics. There has been controversy regarding the clinical relevance of many of these common intestinal parasitic infections, which often appear to coexist with their hosts without causing significant clinical problems. However, recent studies confirm the importance of many of these infections, particularly in immunocompromised children with severe undernutrition or human immunodeficiency virus (HIV) infection. In this chapter, we shall discuss the pharmacology of the commonly used antihelminthic drugs followed by brief discussion on the treatment of commonly occurring helminthic infections in India.

CLASSIFICATION OF ANTIHELMINTHIC DRUGS

Anthelmintics are classified based upon their chemical structures.

- Piperazines: For example, diethylcarbamazine (DEC) citrate, piperazine citrate
- Benzimidazoles: For example, albendazole, mebendazole, thiabendazole
- Heterocyclics: For example, oxamniquine, praziquantel
- Natural products: For example, ivermectin, avermectin
- Vinyl pyrimidines: For example, pyrantel, oxantel
- Amides: For example, niclosamide
- Nitro derivative: For example, niridazole
- Imidazo thiazole: For example, levamisole.

Benzimidazoles

The benzimidazoles, albendazole, and mebendazole, have broad-spectrum activity against roundworm, whipworm, hookworm, and pinworm species. They act on the parasite by binding to tubulin (a protein that is the main constituent of the microtubules of living cells), inhibit microtubule assembly, decrease glucose absorption, and inhibit fumarate reductase.

Albendazole

Pharmacokinetics: It is poorly soluble in water, but well absorbed with a fatty meal. It is rapidly metabolized in the liver to the active form, albendazole sulfoxide, which has a serum half-life of 8–9 hours, and is excreted by the kidneys. It is usually very well-tolerated as a single dose or daily for 3 days.

Indications: It is the drug of choice for ascariasis, hookworm, pinworm, trichuriasis, trichinosis, filariasis (along with DEC), cysticercosis, and hydatid disease. It can also be used as an alternative drug for cutaneous and visceral larva migrans. Prolonged high-dose regimens of albendazole constitute the most effective medical treatment of larval cestode disease caused by *Echinococcus granulosus*, *E. multilocularis*, and *E. vogelii.*

Dose: 200 mg/day (2–5 years)/400 mg/day above 5 years and for tissue infection 15 mg/kg/day (maximum 800 mg/day).

Mebendazole

Indications: It is the drug of choice for trichuriasis/whipworm infestations. It can be used as an alternative drug to albendazole for roundworm and pinworm infections. It is less effective than albendazole for hookworm infections.

Dose: 100 mg Q12 hourly for 3 days. For enterobiasis, 100 mg once, may be repeated after 2–4 weeks. Single dose of 500 mg can be used for trichuriasis.

Adverse effects: Diarrhea, nausea, and pain in abdomen. Allergic reactions, hair loss, and granulocytopenia occur with high doses. It should be used with caution in patients with liver disease.

Pyrantel Pamoate

Pyrantel is a depolarizing neuromuscular blocking agent which paralyzes worms until they are expelled in feces. Pyrantel pamoate is active against *Ascaris* and *Enterobius*, only partially effective against hookworm and ineffective against *Trichuris* and *Strongyloides.*

Indications

It can be used as an alternative drug to albendazole/mebendazole for roundworm or pinworm infections.

Dose

Dose is 11 mg/kg (maximum dose is 1 g), and can be repeated after 2 weeks for pinworm infections.

Levamisole

Levamisole is an immune stimulant which is effective against *Ascaris* and hookworm, and may be more effective for intestinal obstruction from roundworms, since it acts by paralyzing the myoneural junction of the worm.

Indications

Hookworm, roundworm infestation.

Dose

For roundworm in children from 1 month to 18 years, 2.5–3 mg/kg (maximum 150 mg) as a single dose. For hookworm in children from 1 month to 18 years, 2.5 mg/kg (maximum 150 mg) as a single dose repeated after 7 days if severe.

Ivermectin

Spectrum of Activity and Pharmacokinetics

Ivermectin has broad-spectrum activity against helminths and filariasis, but is the drug of choice against strongyloidiasis. It is also effective against *Sarcoptes scabiei* and pediculosis. Ivermectin is well absorbed orally, accumulating in adipose tissue, metabolized in the liver, highly protein bound with a serum half-life of 12 hours and excreted in stool. It is generally well tolerated, with occasional abdominal distension, chest tightness, or wheezing.

Dose

0.15–0.4 mg/kg/dose oral single dose. For severe crusted scabies in immunodeficient patients, 2 doses of 0.2 mg/kg separated by 2 weeks.

Indications

It is the drug of choice for *Strongyloides stercoralis* and onchocerciasis, cutaneous larva migrans, and along with albendazole for bancroftian and brugian filaria. It can also be used as alternative therapy for roundworm, *Trichuris*, scabies and pediculosis.

Adverse Effects

Adverse effects are mild pruritus, giddiness, abdominal pain, transient electrocardiographic (ECG) changes, reactions due to degeneration products of microfilariae, arthralgia, skin rash, and Steven-Johnson syndrome. Adverse effects are caused by reactions to the release of endosymbiotic bacteria from dying parasites. This Mazzotti-type reaction can occur in onchocerciasis and filariasis and consists of fever, pruritus, urticaria, headache, myalgia, joint and bone pain, and tender lymphadenopathy. It should be used with caution in liver disorder and loiasis. It is not recommended for children weighing less than 15 kg or less than 5 years. Increases the effect warfarin [increased international normalized ratio (INR)].

Nitazoxanide

Nitazoxanide is a new broad-spectrum antimicrobial agent with activity against nematodes, trematodes, anaerobic bacteria, and protozoal parasites such as cryptosporidium. It is metabolized in blood to tizoxanide, which inhibits the key enzyme pyruvate ferredoxin oxidoreductase of target organisms, and is excreted in urine and feces. In view of this wide spectrum of action, single-dose therapy in combination with other drugs is under investigation for community treatment programs.

Indications

It is the drug of choice for cryptosporidiosis. It is also an alternative choice in giardiasis, and *Fasciola hepatica* infections. It is in clinical trials for hepatitis C in combination with peginterferon alfa-2a.

Dose

- 12–47 months, 100 mg
- 4–11 years, 200 mg
- More than 11 years, 500 mg Q 12 h for 3 days oral.

Praziquantel

This antihelminthic drug has predominant activity against the cestodes and trematodes.

Indications

It is the drug of choice for schistosomiasis, intestinal forms of *Taenia saginata, T. solium.* It is an alternative drug for neurocysticercosis (NCC) and echinococcosis.

Dose

20 mg/kg once oral (tapeworm), Q4h × 3 doses (schistosomiasis), Q8h × 6 doses (other flukes), Q8h × 14 days (cysticercosis).

Adverse Effects and Precautions

Adverse effects are bitter taste, nausea, pain in abdomen, headache, dizziness, sedations, and rashes. Fever and body aches can occur as a reaction to dead parasites. Patients with NCC are often concomitantly receiving antiepileptics and are at risk of therapeutic failure with praziquantel. Phenytoin, carbamazepine, and dexamethasone induce metabolism and reduce its bioavailability.

Niclosamide

This drug is mainly effective against the cestodes.

Indications

It is indicated for *Hymenolepis nana, T. saginata,* and *T. solium.*

Dose

50 mg/kg once oral (tapeworm) above 18 years.

Precautions

Not effective against larval worms. Fears of developing cysticercosis in *T. solium* infections have proved unfounded. All the same, an antiemetic can be given before treatment and a laxative can be given 2 hours after niclosamide.

Diethylcarbamazine

Diethylcarbamazine is a piperazine derivative used primarily in the treatment of selected human filarial infections. For lymphatic filariasis and loiasis, relatively low-dose microfilaricidal regimens are often used in the developing world as part of mass treatment campaigns. In the treatment of an individual patient, however, the aim is macrofilaricidal activity with the use of multiple aggressive courses of therapy. Because of frequent unacceptable side effects in treating

Onchocerca volvulus, DEC should not be used for microfilaricidal treatment of this parasite and ivermectin has become the drug of choice. DEC is ineffective against *Mansonella* species and should not be used to treat visceral larva migrans. DEC, which should be taken after a meal, is absorbed readily, is distributed into all body compartments, and undergoes renal excretion with a serum half-life of 8 hours. The mechanism of action is not documented clearly.

Dose

Dose is 3–6 mg/kg/day.

Adverse Effects

Side effects most commonly seen include nausea, dizziness, headache, visual disturbances, and fever. Transient microscopic hematuria is common. The GI tract side effects are dose-related, and some patients cannot tolerate the dose of 9 mg/kg/day. In patients with lymphatic filariasis, the death of adult worms often results in lymphadenopathy or lymphangitis, frequently in the genital region. Encephalopathy can occur after treatment for loiasis in people with high microfilarial counts.

DRUG TREATMENT FOR INDIVIDUAL HELMINTHIC INFECTIONS

Treatment of helminthic infections in India is depicted in Table 1.

TABLE 1: Treatment of helminthic infections in India.

Helminth	*Primary drug*	*Alternative(s)*	*Comment*
Roundworm (*Ascaris*)	Single-dose albendazole	Mebendazole, pyrantel pamoate, ivermectin, nitazoxanide	
Hookworm (*Ancylostoma, Necator*)	Albendazole	Mebendazole, pyrantel pamoate	Daily for 3 days Ivermectin ineffective
Pinworm (*Enterobius*)	Single-dose albendazole	Single-dose pyrantel or mebendazole	Repeat in 2 weeks Treat all family members Reinfection common
Whipworm (*Trichuris*)	Mebendazole 100 mg twice daily	Albendazole 200–400 mg daily/ivermectin 0.2 mg/kg daily	Treat for 3 days
Trichinellosis (*Trichinella*)	Albendazole 400 mg twice daily for 8–14 days	Mebendazole 500 mg thrice daily for 10 days	Concomitant prednisolone 40–60 mg daily
Strongyloides	Ivermectin for 2 days	Albendazole twice daily for 7 days (not very effective)	For hyperinfection repeat after 15 days
Cutaneous *Larva migrans*	Ivermectin for 1–2 days	Albendazole twice daily for 3 days	
Visceral *L. migrans*	Antihistaminics and steroids Albendazole/mebendazole twice daily for 5 days		Antihelminthics controversial
Hymenolepiasis nana	Praziquantel	Niclosamide	
Taenia saginata and *T. solium*	Praziquantel	Niclosamide	

MASS COMMUNITY ANTIHELMINTHIC TREATMENT

Empiric deworming refers to use of anthelminthic drugs to reduce the prevalence of infection due to soil-transmitted helminths in endemic areas. Infestation due to soil-transmitted helminths has been associated with morbidity including delays in growth and cognitive development, particularly among children 2–12 years of age. Such reductions in prevalence by mass therapy are generally temporary; mass drug administration interrupts parasite life cycles but does not halt them completely as the risk for reinfection is high. Thus, the degree of benefit depends on patient characteristics, regional parasite species, and burden of infection. Mass treatment protocols may reduce the risk of drug resistance by only repeating treatment at intervals greater than the nematode generation time. Albendazole and praziquantel have broad-spectrum anthelminthic activity against ascariasis, trichuriasis, enterobiasis, hookworm, giardiasis, strongyloidiasis, and schistosomiasis at relatively low cost and with low rates of resistance.

The United Nations Children's Fund (UNICEF), the World Bank, and World Health Organization (WHO) promote routine mass anthelminthic treatment programs as a cost-effective intervention. School-based programs are also popular. Old school of thought that deworming should not be done in children under 2 years of age (as well as in pregnancy and lactation) stays invalid now as a WHO Informal Consultation states that children over 12 months of age should be included in deworming campaigns using praziquantel and albendazole/mebendazole on the basis of improved safety data and risk-benefit analysis.

The data on efficacy for population deworming are mixed. The greatest benefit of deworming appears to be among young children who undergo screening prior to treatment. The WHO has stated that, overall, mass treatment is not beneficial at a population level, but the WHO continues to recommend this approach since studies suggest that the children who are infected do benefit.

Studies performed in India during the 1990s suggested that deworming of malnourished children 1–5 years of age was associated with average weight gain of nearly 1 kg. Subsequently, a meta-analysis including 42 trials noted no association between deworming and child cognition, school attendance, or school performance. Evidence for improvement in weight, hemoglobin level, and cognition was greatest among children screened for helminth infection prior to treatment. Thereafter, the largest single trial addressing population deworming was published in 2013; it included 1 million preschool children in north India treated every 6 months for 5 years. This trial noted no effect on weight gain or mortality; decline in the levels of worm infestation was observed, and compliance with treatment was high.

Finally, whatever said and done, control of intestinal parasites is more than a question of mass chemotherapy, and is influenced by social and cultural factors that affect human behavior, such as treatment seeking and promiscuous defecation. Areas with high prevalence of helminth infection require a number of public health measures beyond preventive treatment, including safe drinking water, basic sanitation, and health education. There is certainly no logic in periodic antihelminthic administration to children belonging to good socioeconomic status.

NEUROCYSTICERCOSIS

Introduction

Cysticercosis is caused by the larval stage of the pork tapeworm *T. solium*. Clinical syndromes related to this parasite include NCC and extraneural cysticercosis. NCC, in turn, is divided into parenchymal and extraparenchymal forms. Extraparenchymal forms include intraventricular, subarachnoid, spinal, and ocular disease.

It is important to understand the staging of the disease for charting out treatment. Stages of cysticercosis include an initial (viable) phase, a degenerating phase, and a nonviable phase.

- Viable cysticerci are round, hypodense lesions (usually 5-20 mm in diameter) on computed tomography (CT) that do not enhance after contrast administration. Viable cysticerci do not cause much inflammation in surrounding tissues.
- Cysticerci that enhance after contrast administration reflect degeneration. The cyst wall increases in density and is often accompanied by edema; such findings reflect the host inflammatory response against the parasite and are frequently associated with seizures. In many cases, enhancing cysticerci retain features of viable cysticerci.
- Nonviable cysticerci are solid, calcified nodular lesions (usually 2-4 mm in diameter; range 1-10 mm); they are usually nonenhancing but may be associated with perilesional edema in some cases. They are also associated with seizures.

Neurocysticercosis is often associated with increase in intracranial tension. Causes of elevated intracranial pressure may be numerous cysticerci (cysticercal encephalitis) or associated with extraparenchymal disease include obstructive hydrocephalus (associated with intraventricular disease) and communicating hydrocephalus (associated with subarachnoid disease).

Treatment

Principles: Treatment is indicated for viable/degenerating cysts and not viable cysts. The recent Infectious Diseases Society of America (IDSA) guidelines published in 2018 detail the current consensus about treatment of NCC. Recent randomized controlled trials have established the striking superiority of combination therapy with albendazole and praziquantel over albendazole alone in producing radiologic resolution of parenchymal cysts. Steroids are indicated in the management of NCC to reduce the edema associated with the cysticidal action of the antihelminthic drugs. Generally, prednisolone at the rate of1 mg/kg/day or dexamethasone at the rate of 0.1 mg/kg/day is started 1 day prior to initiating therapy, continued for duration of the therapy and then tapered over a few days. Steroids tend to decrease praziquantel levels. Prior to initiation of therapy for cysticercosis, all patients should have an ophthalmologic examination to exclude ocular cysticercosis as inflammation around degenerating cysticerci in the eye during antiparasitic therapy can threaten vision. Antiparasitic therapy is generally contraindicated in NCC patients with signs or symptoms of elevated intracranial pressure, regardless of the cause. Such patients should be assessed regarding the need for antiparasitic therapy only after appropriate intervention to reduce the pressure. The initial approach in such patients consists of managing acute symptoms such as increased intracranial pressure (via surgical intervention to remove an obstructing cysticercus or placement of an external ventricular drain/shunt and/or corticosteroids usually dexamethasone 0.2-0.4 mg/kg/day) and seizures (via antiseizure drug therapy), if present. Thereafter, a determination should be made regarding the approach to management of antiparasitic and anti-inflammatory therapy; clinical decisions should be tailored to individual patient circumstances. Anticonvulsants are commonly used in treatment. The choice of anticonvulsant drug should be guided by local availability, cost, drug interactions, and potential side effects. Most reports on management of seizures in the setting of NCC describe use of phenytoin or carbamazepine. Newer therapies (such as levetiracetam) are likely to be similarly effective and perhaps better tolerated, often with fewer drug-drug interactions. Seizures may recur for long periods of time. Anticonvulsant therapy is recommended till there is evidence of neuroradiologic resolution and seizures have not occurred for 6 months if it is a single lesion or 1-2 years for multiple lesions. Calcified cysts may require prolonged use of anticonvulsants.

Parenchymal neurocysticercosis: The preferred drug regime is albendazole 15 mg/kg/day in 2 daily doses (max 800 mg) + praziquantel 50 mg/kg/day in 3 daily doses for 10 days with dexamethasone 0.1 mg/kg starting 1 day prior to therapy and continuing for 10 days and then slow taper.

- If there are multiple cysts then the duration of therapy may be extended to more than 30 days.
- If there are only 1–2 cysts in magnetic resonance imaging (MRI) then only albendazole 15 mg/kg (maximum 1,200 mg) with steroids may be used for 10 days.
- Retreatment after 6 months if viable cysts remain
- Antiseizure medication for up to 2 years if needed
- If only calcified cysts then no antiparasitic medication and only antiepileptics if needed for minimum 1 year.

Subarachnoid NCC: Placement of a *ventriculoperitoneal* (VP) shunt and if needed control of raised *intracranial pressure* (ICP) with steroids is mandatory before starting therapy.

- Recommended treatment is albendazole 15 mg/kg/day (maximum 1,200 mg) for 30 days and dexamethasone 0.1 mg/kg/day for 30 days and then very slow taper. This regime may need to be repeated or given continuously for months according to clinical and MRI evaluation. If albendazole is used for prolonged periods, complete blood count (CBC) and liver function test (LFT) should be monitored every 2 weeks.
- Long courses of albendazole and praziquantel may be tried for refractory disease. The dose of albendazole may be increased to 1,200 mg/day.

Intraventricular NCC: Neuroendoscopic removal of the cyst:

- If no access to removal then use albendazole and dexamethasone for prolonged periods as for subarachnoid NCC and place VP shunt prior to starting therapy.

Extra central nervous system NCC:

- No treatment generally needed, if asymptomatic
- If symptomatic, surgical excision is treatment of choice (medical treatment may be tried)

The complex management of NCC needs consultation with a neurologist, neurosurgeon, and an expert in infectious diseases.

HYDATID CYST

Echinococcosis is caused by infection with the tapeworm *Echinococcus*, which belongs to the family Taeniidae. Four species of *Echinococcus* cause infection in humans. *E. granulosus* and *E. multilocularis* are the most common, causing cystic echinococcosis (CE) and alveolar echinococcosis (AE), respectively.

The available options of treatment are: (1) percutaneous intervention, (2) surgery, (3) drug therapy, and (4) observation alone (for dead calcified cysts). The appropriate approach depends on the size, location, and clinical picture.

Liver Cysts

Percutaneous intervention and albendazole: Percutaneous aspiration-injection-reaspiration (PAIR) is recommended for uncomplicated larval cysts in the liver. It consists of puncture (P) and needle aspirate (A) of cyst content followed by instillation (I) of hypertonic saline (15–30%) or absolute alcohol, waiting 20–30 minutes, then re-aspirating (R) with final irrigation. Adjunctive drug therapy with albendazole for 28 days should be administered to minimize risk of secondary echinococcosis from spillage.

Surgery and albendazole: It is the treatment of choice for management of complicated cysts (e.g. ruptured cyst, cysts with biliary fistulae, cysts compressing vital structures, cysts with secondary infection or hemorrhage) and for management of cysts with many daughter vesicles that are not suitable for percutaneous treatment. Adjunctive drug therapy should be administered to minimize risk of secondary echinococcosis from seeding of protoscolices in the abdominal cavity in the event of fluid spillage. This adjunctive drug therapy reduces the risk of recurrent disease by inactivating protoscolices. It also softens the cyst, facilitating removal. The optimal duration of treatment is uncertain; in general, treatment should be initiated at least 4 days prior to surgery (the WHO suggests 4–30 days preoperatively) and should be continued for at least 1 month (albendazole) or 3 months (mebendazole) following surgery. Some use praziquantel in addition to albendazole, though synergism is not documented. Every effort should be made to avoid fluid spillage, which can lead to secondary seeding of infection and/or anaphylaxis. For circumstances in which intact removal of the cyst is not feasible, a protoscolicidal agent such as 20% hypertonic saline should be injected into the cyst prior to removing the contents. The solution should be in contact with the germinal layer for at least 15 minutes. Albendazole, ivermectin, and praziquantel solutions have been used as protoscolicidal agents in research basis. Formalin has been associated with sclerosing cholangitis and should not be used.

Drug therapy alone: Drug therapy alone may be indicated for cysts smaller than 5–10 cm. The dose is 15 mg/kg/day, divided into two doses, to maximum 400 mg orally twice daily with food given for 30 days at a stretch and for a total of three times with a 2-week gap between each course. Mebendazole may be used as an alternative therapy but it is less well absorbed than albendazole.

Watchful waiting: This is for asymptomatic and calcifying cysts.

Pulmonary Cyst

Surgical resection is the treatment of choice. Preoperative albendazole should be avoided. It may however be given postoperatively 400 mg twice daily for 28 days. Ruptured and complicated cysts may require longer therapy.

Disseminated Disease

- Albendazole 400 mg twice daily till clinical response
- Periodic debulking surgery if possible.

FILARIASIS

Filariasis is caused by nematodes (roundworms) that inhabit the lymphatics and subcutaneous tissues. Three species cause lymphatic filariasis: *Wuchereria bancrofti*, *Brugia malayi*, and *Brugia timori*.

The treatment of choice for lymphatic filariasis is DEC dosed at 6 mg/kg/day given either as single dose or in 2–3 divided doses for a period of 12 days. Recent studies indicate that addition of doxycycline 3 mg/kg/day for a maximum dose of 200 mg for 6 weeks improves the lymphedema. Patients with tropical pulmonary eosinophilia (TPE) due to *W. bancrofti* infection should be treated with 14–21 days of DEC (6 mg/kg/day).

For eradication of lymphatic filariasis, yearly mass drug administration is recommended. A recent trial demonstrated superior efficacy of three drug combination with albendazole 400 mg with DEC 6 mg/kg/dose and ivermectin 150 μg/kg/dose in eradication of microfilaria as compared to single or dual therapy. Mass drug treatment programs with DEC are not recommended in areas that are endemic for onchocerciasis or loiasis since DEC can cause blindness/encephalopathy due to rapid destruction of these pathogens.

RECOMMENDED READING

1. AAP Redbook. Elk Grove Village, IL: American Academy of Pediatrics; 2018.
2. Allen HE, Crompton DW, de Silva N, et al. New policies for using antihelminthics in high risk groups. Trends Parasitol. 2002;18:381-2.
3. Brunetti E, White AC Jr. Cestode infestations: hydatid disease and cysticercosis. Infect Dis Clin North Am. 2012;26:421-35.
4. Gilbert DN, Chambers HF, Eliopoulos GM, Saag MS, Pavia AT (Eds). Sanford Guide for Antimicrobial Therapy. Sperryville, VA, USA: Sanford; 2018.
5. King CL, Suamani J, Sanuku N, et al. A Trial of a triple-drug treatment for lymphatic filariasis. N Engl J Med. 2018;379(19):1801-10.
6. Welch VA, Ghogomu E, Hossain A, et al. Mass deworming to improve developmental health and wellbeing of children in low-income and middle-income countries: a systematic review and network meta-analysis. Lancet Glob Health. 2017;5(1):e40-e50.
7. White AC, Coyle CM, Rajshekhar V, et al. Diagnosis and treatment of neurocysticercosis: 2017 Clinical Practice Guidelines by the Infectious Diseases Society of America (IDSA) and the American Society of Tropical Medicine and Hygiene (ASTMH). Am J Trop Med Hyg. 2018;98(4):945-66.
8. World Health Organization. Guidelines for the Evaluation of Soil-transmitted Helminthiasis and Schistosomiasis at Community Level: a Guide for Managers of Control Programmes. Geneva: WHO; 1998.

Antiviral Therapy

Chapter 36

Vijay Yewale

INTRODUCTION

The close relationship between the viral replicative cycle and host-cell metabolism is primarily the reason why development of safe and effective antiviral agents has lagged behind development of other antimicrobial agents such as antibiotics. Since the first antiviral drug, idoxuridine, was approved in 1963, 90 antiviral drugs categorized into 13 functional groups have been formally approved for the treatment of nine human infectious diseases. Antiviral drugs have been approved to treat human infections caused by human immunodeficiency virus (HIV), hepatitis B virus (HBV), hepatitis C virus (HCV), cytomegalovirus (CMV), herpes simplex virus (HSV), respiratory syncytial virus (RSV), varicella-zoster virus (VZV), and parainfluenza virus. Agents approved in children and used in treatment of viral infections with the exception of HIV are discussed here. Antivirals against HIV are discussed in Chapter 34.

AGENTS USED IN THE TREATMENT OF HSV AND VZV INFECTIONS

Acyclovir

Mechanism of Action

Acyclovir is phosphorylated to monophosphate form by viral thymidine kinase (TK) and to triphosphate form by cellular enzymes. This triphosphate form inhibits DNA polymerase and viral replication. It also is incorporated into the viral DNA and acts as a chain terminator to inhibit replication.

Spectrum of Activity

Antiviral spectrum is limited to herpes viruses. It is active against HSV type 1, type 2, VZV, and EBV in descending order of susceptibility. It also has some effect on CMV.

Resistance

It is by one of the three mechanisms:

1. Absence or partial production of TK: HSV
2. Altered thymidine kinase substrate specificity: VZV
3. Altered viral DNA polymerase: VZV.

Prevalence of acyclovir-resistant HSV is 1% but as high as 10–20% in immunocompromised hosts. Acyclovir resistant VZV is unusual.

Pharmacokinetics

Oral bioavailability is 10–30% and decreases with increasing dose. Peak plasma concentration is 0.4–0.8 µg/mL after 200 mg dose and 0.8–1.6 µg/mL after 800 mg dose. Bioavailability is less with liquid preparation. Peak plasma levels after 5 mg/kg IV over 1 hour are 9.8 µg/mL and 20 µg/mL after 10 mg/kg dose. Acyclovir is distributed widely in body fluids including vesicular fluid, aqueous humor, CSF, and salivary and vaginal secretions. Also concentrated in breast milk, amniotic fluid, and placenta. The mean plasma half-life (t½) of elimination is 2.5 hours. It is 4 hours in neonates and increases to 20 hours in anuric patients. It is excreted almost unchanged in urine. Dose modification is required in renal failure.

Dosage

- *Topical acyclovir*: 5% ointment every 3 to 4 hours for 7 days.
- *Oral acyclovir*: 200 mg capsule or 800 mg tablet or 400 mg/5 mL suspension.

Adverse Effects

- *Topical acyclovir*: Pain, local irritation or local rash due to polyethylene glycol base.
- *Systemic acyclovir*: Nausea, diarrhea, rash or headache. Neutropenia in neonates put on oral after IV acyclovir treatment. Extravasations can cause inflammation, ulceration, and necrosis of surrounding tissue. Neurotoxicity associated with lethargy, tremors, seizures, and coma. Renal toxicity in patients with poor hydration, rapid IV infusion, in those with prior renal disease, and in those on other nephrotoxic drugs. Renal toxicity including renal tubular damage, crystalline nephropathy or interstitial nephritis may occur in 5% patients.

Valacyclovir

It is a prodrug form of acyclovir or the hydrochloride salt of the ester of acyclovir. After oral administration, valacyclovir is absorbed rapidly and is metabolized by first pass through intestinal tract and by liver into acyclovir and L-valine. The relative bioavailability of acyclovir increases 3 to 5 times to 70% following valacyclovir administration. Valacyclovir is converted rapidly and virtually completely to acyclovir and therefore has the same mechanism of action and resistance as acyclovir.

It is used as an alternative to oral acyclovir as better bioavailability and less frequent primary VZV and zoster (1,000 mg tid for 5 days). Liquid formulation not available and pediatric dosing not standardized.

Penciclovir

Spectrum of Activity

- Selective activity against herpes viruses similar to that of acyclovir. Inhibits HSV-1, HSV-2, and VZV at increasing concentration in plasma. Negligible activity against CMV.
- Inhibits HBV also.

Mechanism of Action and Resistance

Like acyclovir, phosphorylated to triphosphate and inhibits viral DNA polymerase. It is 100 times less potent than acyclovir triphosphate in inhibiting DNA polymerase but an antiviral effect is achieved because of its presence in high concentrations for a prolonged period in virus-infected cells. Resistance is minimal and is by production of deficient or altered TK activity.

Pharmacokinetics

Poorly absorbed after oral administration. Information on intravenous use in pediatric patients is not available. Penciclovir 1% cream is not absorbed systemically.

Clinical Indications

Cream for the treatment of herpes labialis lesions on lips and face. At the onset of lesions, every 2 hours while awake for 3 to 5 days.

Famciclovir

It is the prodrug of penciclovir. Famciclovir undergoes rapid transformation to penciclovir and then acts like penciclovir.

Pharmacokinetics

Absorbed rapidly after oral administration. Excellent bioavailability of 77%. Administration with food reduces peak plasma levels but does not alter bioavailability. Metabolized in liver by deacetylation and oxidation to form penciclovir. Elimination t½ is 2 to 3 hours. Excreted by filtration and active tubular secretion by kidneys. Nonrenal clearance by fecal excretion of one-third drug.

TREATMENT OF INFECTIONS CAUSED BY HSV

Factors considered in the treatment of HSV infections include site of infection, the immune status of the host and whether the infection is primary or secondary.

Gingivostomatitis and Orolabial HSV Infections

Oral therapy started within 3 days of symptoms of primary HSV gingivostomatitis shortens duration of fever, lesions, and viral shedding. Oral treatment for 7–10 days with acyclovir, valacyclovir, or famciclovir. Topical acyclovir decreases slightly healing time and viral shedding in mucocutaneous lesions in primary infection with HSV. No clinical benefit except mild soothing effect in patients with recurrent herpes simplex lesions.

Acyclovir: Adults 200 mg 5 times a day for 10 days and in children 15 mg/kg/dose (max 200 per dose) 5 times a day for 10 days. Recurrent HSV 800 mg tds for 2 days *or* 400 mg tds for 5 days. Suppressive therapy is 400 mg bd. Valacyclovir dose needed for treatment of primary disease (1,000 mg twice daily for 7–10 days) and recurrent HSV infections (500 mg twice daily), herpes labialis (2 g twice daily for 1 day). Famciclovir adult dose for primary dose is 500 mg twice daily for 7 days or 1,500 mg single dose or 750 mg twice daily for 1 day.

Genital HSV Infections

Oral acyclovir is generally used. Famciclovir and valacyclovir offer the advantage of less frequent dosing. Topical acyclovir is not recommended. In patients with frequent recurrences, especially in HIV-infected patients, suppressive therapy may be used.

HSV Infections of the Central Nervous System

These have to be treated with IV acyclovir. The dose in infants is 20 mg/kg 8 hourly, children below 12 years is 15–20 mg/kg/dose 8 hourly and in children more than 12 years is 12.5 mg/kg/dose 8 hourly. The dose calculation in obese patients is uncertain. Treatment duration is for 14–21 days.

Neonatal HSV Infections

Intravenous acyclovir in high dose (20 mg/kg/dose thrice daily) for 14 days in skin and mucous membrane disease and 21 days in disseminated and CNS disease. In fact in CNS disease, PCR in CSF should be done near day 21 and, if positive, treatment should be continued for another 7 days. Continuous suppressive therapy with oral acyclovir at the rate of 900 mg/m^2/day in three divided doses for 6 months reduces cutaneous recurrences after neonatal infection when given after intravenous therapy has been completed.

Prophylaxis for HSV

Prophylaxis with acyclovir is routinely given to patients with acute lymphoblastic leukemia on chemotherapy and recipients of HSCT who are seropositive for HSV to reduce the incidence of severe HSV disease. In acute leukemia, this for duration of intense chemotherapy and in HSCT from the time of start of conditioning till engraftment occurs. The oral dose in children is 60–80 mg/kg/day in 2-3 divided doses and IV dose is 250 mg/m^2 8 hourly. In adults and children above 40 kg the dose is 400–800 mg twice daily or 250 mg/m^2 12 hourly. Valacyclovir may also be used in adult doses of 500 mg once or twice daily and in children less than 40 kg as 250 mg twice daily.

TREATMENT OF CHICKENPOX

Immunocompetent Children and Adolescents

Acyclovir and its congeners reduce duration of fever, mean number of lesions, and the time to crusting by 2 days in children, adolescents, and adults with primary VZV infection if started within the first 24 hours after appearance of the lesions. For healthy children below 12 years, varicella is typically self-limited and antiviral treatment is generally not recommended but may be offered.

Antiviral therapy is recommended in:

- Unvaccinated adolescents more than 13 years of age since the disease are likely to be more severe in these individuals
- Children with chronic skin disorders or chronic pulmonary disorders
- Children on intermittent oral or inhaled steroids
- Children on salicylates.

Oral acyclovir in children—20 mg/kg/dose (max dose 800 mg) 4 times a day for 5 days. In adults, 800 mg five times daily for 5 days. Oral valacyclovir 20 mg/kg/dose (max 1,000 mg) three times a day. Valacyclovir not recommended in children below 2 years as safety and efficacy have not been established. In adults, famciclovir 500 mg thrice daily may be used but evidence is lacking.

Immunocompromised Children

Children on high dose corticosteroids for more than 14 days, HIV-infected children, and children with malignancy with chickenpox of any severity should preferably be treated with intravenous acyclovir at the rate of 1,500 mg/m^2 or 30 mg/kg/day in three divided doses. IV therapy continued until no new lesions appear followed by oral treatment until crusting of all the lesions. However, this may not always be logistically possible since it would entail admission to a negative pressure room and substantial expense. In such a situation, oral acyclovir should be started irrespective of duration of disease with a close watch for complications.

Individuals with Complications

Any patient with severe varicella including pneumonia or encephalitis should be treated with IV acyclovir at the rate of 1,500 mg/m^2 or 30 mg/kg/day in 3 divided doses for 7 to 10 days. Dose adjustment is required for children with reduced renal function.

VZV Infections in Newborn

Newborns with VZV disease in mother within 5 days before and 2 days after delivery are at the greatest risk of severe disease. Babies exposed to maternal varicella in this period should be given varicella zoster immunoglobulin (VZIG) at the rate of 1 mL/kg as soon as possible. Other indications for VZIG are exposure to varicella in preterm babies more than 28 weeks whose mothers do not have varicella zoster immunity and preterm babies less than 28 weeks and less than 1,000 g regardless of maternal history of varicella or vaccination. In case, these neonates develop disease they should be treated with IV acyclovir at 10–12 mg/kg thrice daily for 7–10 days.

Prophylaxis for Chickenpox

Acyclovir can be used as postexposure prophylaxis in neonates/pregnant women and immunocompromised if VZIG is not available or affordable. Here the treatment doses should be started 7–9 days after exposure and continued for 7 days. Acyclovir/valacyclovir is also indicated for prevention of recurrences in patients with prior history of varicella and who undergo HSCT. Here doses of acyclovir in children (<40 kg) are 60–80 mg/kg/day in 2–3 divided doses and in adults 800 mg twice daily for 1 year after transplant. Valacyclovir may also be used in doses of 500 mg twice daily in adults and 250 mg twice daily in children.

TREATMENT OF HERPES ZOSTER

Antiviral therapy is indicated for patients aged more than 50 years, moderate-to-severe rash or pain, involvement of face/eye, acute complication of infection or immunocompromised host. Acyclovir treatment decreases length of time for new vesicle formation, number of days to crusting, days of acute discomfort, and reduction of complication in immunocompromised. Treatment should be started with oral acyclovir/valacyclovir in same doses as used in chickenpox started within 72 hours of onset of lesions for 7–10 days. IV acyclovir is recommended in the treatment of immunocompromised children with herpes zoster (HIV infected children, children with recent organ transplantation, children on cancer chemotherapy) and ophthalmic involvement.

DRUGS FOR TREATMENT OF CMV INFECTIONS

Ganciclovir

Mechanism of Action

Phosphorylated by TK in HSV-infected cells and by protein kinases encoded by *UL97* gene in CMV-infected cells. The active form, i.e. ganciclovir triphosphate, is incorporated into viral DNA, where it slows and stops viral DNA chain elongation and produces short and noninfectious viral DNA fragments. It also inhibits DNA polymerase.

Spectrum of Activity

Ganciclovir has selective activity against herpes viruses, with uniquely potent antiviral activity against CMV at a very low concentration. HSV-1, HSV-2, VZV, EBV, HHV-6, HHV-7, and HHV-8 are also inhibited. In vitro activity against HBV and adenoviruses.

Resistance

Resistance is seen in 8–38% especially in children who have undergone HSCT and have been treated in the past. Resistant strains emerge either quickly after a few weeks of therapy or slowly after therapy. There are two mechanisms:

1. Point mutation or deletion in UL97 gene reducing phosphorylation of ganciclovir—common and the strains remain susceptible to foscarnet and cidofovir.
2. Point mutation in viral polymerase *UL54* gene. They are resistant to foscarnet and cidofovir as well.

Pharmacokinetics

After IV administration widely distributed. CSF (levels up to 70% of plasma) and brain (38%). Aqueous, vitreous, and subretinal fluid levels are like serum levels. Excreted by kidneys and needs dose modification. Oral bioavailability is poor; 5% and is better if administered with food.

Dosage

Solution for IV use 10 mg/mL over 1 hr; Also available as 250 mg, 500 mg capsule.

Therapy of disease: Involves induction and maintenance. Induction—5 mg/kg/dose bid for 2 to 3 weeks and then maintenance dose of 5 mg/kg/day. In neonatal CMV disease, 6 mg/kg/dose bid for 6 weeks.

Preemptive treatment: 5 mg/kg/dose bid for 7 to 14 days followed by maintenance for 2–5 weeks till PCR negative.

Prophylaxis: 5 mg/kg/day for 3–6 months (Valganciclovir may be more convenient).

Adverse Effects

Local phlebitis, irritation, blistering or ulceration. Dose-dependent reversible neutropenia seen in one-third to one-half patients who receive treatment for over 2 weeks. Thrombocytopenia especially in AIDS patients on antiretroviral therapy. Monitor CBC 2–3/week and discontinue if absolute neutrophil count (ANC) less than 500–750 or platelets less than 25,000. Granulocyte-colony stimulating factor (G-CSF) can be used to treat neutropenia. Headache, behavioral changes, psychosis, seizures, and coma.

Valganciclovir

Prodrug of ganciclovir, metabolized rapidly to ganciclovir in the body. Well absorbed after oral administration and hydrolyzed in intestine and liver to ganciclovir. Bioavailability is high 60% as compared to 6–9% of ganciclovir. Absorption is enhanced with ingestion of food. Excreted by kidneys.

It is FDA approved and a more convenient alternative to IV ganciclovir for therapy in CMV retinitis in AIDS patients and for prophylaxis and preemptive therapy in transplant patients. Also useful for maintenance therapy once induction therapy with IV ganciclovir is complete. A randomized controlled trial in neonatal CMV disease showed that follow-up therapy with oral valganciclovir for 6 months following 6 weeks IV therapy showed superior hearing outcomes as compared to placebo.

Adult doses for treatment are 900 bid and maintenance dose is 900 mg qd. Available as 450 mg tablets. The tablets have to be swallowed whole and ideally cannot be crushed or broken. A liquid pediatric formulation is not available in India, though it is available abroad. The pediatric dose for prophylaxis is calculated on the basis of body surface area and creatinine clearance and is 7 X BSA in m^2 X creatinine clearance or 15 mg/kg 12 hourly.

Side effects are similar to IV ganciclovir and there is complete cross-resistance with ganciclovir.

Foscarnet

Mechanism of Action

Does not require phosphorylation and directly inhibits viral DNA polymerase.

Spectrum of Activity

Selectively inhibits herpes viruses as well as most but not all acyclovir resistant HSV and VZV and most but not all ganciclovir-resistant CMV. When combined with ganciclovir, has a synergistic effect against CMV and, with zidovudine, synergistic against HIV. Also active against HIV and HBV.

Pharmacokinetics

Cerebrospinal fluid levels are 60% of plasma levels. Vitreous concentration same or slightly higher than plasma. 80% excreted unchanged by kidney. 20% deposited in bones and teeth and remains for months. Oral foscarnet has poor bioavailability.

Clinical Indications

Used as a second-line agent for therapy of ganciclovir-resistant CMV infections and acyclovir-resistant HSV infections. Not used as primary therapy due to unfavorable side effect profile.

Dosage

For HSV: 60 mg/kg/dose tid for 3 weeks for induction

For CMV: 90 mg/kg IV 12 hourly for 14 days and then 90 to 120 mg/kg/day for maintenance Infusions should be given slowly over 1–2 hours (no faster than 1 mg/kg/min).

Adverse Effects

Renal toxicity in one-third of patients. Occurs after 1st week of therapy and is reversible. Serum creatinine should be monitored 1–3 times/week and treatment stopped if more than 2.9 mg/dL. Concomitant nephrotoxic drugs increase risk of nephrotoxicity. Hypocalcemia, hypercalcemia, hypophosphatemia, hyperphosphatemia, hypokalemia, and hypomagnesemia (Monitor electrolytes 1–2/ week). Other side effects include perioral tingling, numbness, paresthesia of the limbs and tetany or seizures, and cardiac dysrhythmias.

Cidofovir

Mechanism of Action and Resistance

Selectively inhibits viral DNA polymerase. Phosphorylated by cellular enzymes and does not need TK. Resistance by mutation in viral DNA polymerase.

Spectrum of Activity

Broad-spectrum against all DNA viruses. Most specific and potent against CMV especially ganciclovir-resistant strains. Very active against VZV and HSV-1 and acyclovir-resistant, TK-deficient strains of HSV-1.

Pharmacokinetics

Not well absorbed orally (bioavailability is 5%). Alkoxyalkyl esters of cidofovir, with better absorption will be available soon. Aerosolized form is being developed. Poor CSF concentration. Mainly excreted by kidney unchanged. t½ is short but intracellular t½ is long (17 to 65 hours).

Clinical Indications

As a second-line agent for ganciclovir and foscarnet resistant CMV, HSV, and VZV infections.

Dosage

5 mg/kg once weekly for 2 weeks for induction and 5 mg/kg once in 2 weeks for maintenance. Probenecid given 3 hours before and then 2 hours and 8 hours after completion of IV cidofovir to reduce the risk of nephrotoxicity. Hydration with normal saline mandatory before cidofovir.

Adverse Effects

Nephrotoxicity is frequent 30–50% (proteinuria, azotemia, proximal tubular dysfunction). It is dose-dependent, increased with other nephrotoxins, and reduced with hydration and probenecid. Use of cidofovir is contraindicated with other nephrotoxic drugs such as aminoglycosides, amphotericin B, foscarnet, and nonsteroidal anti-inflammatory drugs (NSAIDs). One week wash out period is recommended before cidofovir is given. Other side effects are neutropenia and metabolic acidosis.

TREATMENT OF CMV INFECTIONS

Congenital CMV Infection

Treatment of symptomatic infants with antiviral improves long-term audiologic and neurodevelopmental outcome. Symptomatic infants (sepsis-like syndrome, pneumonia, severe hepatitis, myocarditis, neurologic dysfunction, enterocolitis, refractory thrombocytopenia, sight threatening retinitis) and asymptomatic infants with isolated hearing loss/CNS involvement should be treated with antiviral drugs. Initial therapy is with ganciclovir for 6 weeks and then oral valganciclovir for 6 months. Intravitreal ganciclovir is indicated in babies with retinitis.

Immunocompetent Children with Postnatal CMV Infection

No antiviral treatment is recommended. Treatment is recommended only in preterm or very low birth weight infants who have symptomatic CMV disease such as anemia, hepatosplenomegaly, and thrombocytopenia/pneumonia. IV ganciclovir if unable to take orally 6 mg/kg per dose 12 hourly. Oral valganciclovir 15–16 mg/kg per dose 12 hourly (but oral formulation not available in India). Duration of therapy—3 weeks or longer in some infants. Monitoring during treatment—clinical response and weekly quantitative CMV viral load. CBC, platelet count and aspartate aminotransferase (AST), and alanine aminotransferase (ALT) for bone marrow and hepatic toxicity.

Immunocompromised Children with End-organ CMV Disease

Antiviral treatment is recommended in immunocompromised children (hematopoietic stem cell transplant recipient, HIV infected, cancer chemotherapy) with CMV end-organ disease. IV ganciclovir 5 mg/kg/day 12 hourly should be started for 2 to 3 weeks and when CMV—PCR negative, therapy should be switched to 5 mg/kg daily as maintenance for a few weeks. Oral valganciclovir can be used for initiation of therapy in stable children (e.g. HIV with CMV retinitis) and for maintenance therapy in children who can tolerate oral medication. In patients who do not show reduction in viral load after 2 weeks of therapy or in whom clinical symptoms progress despite starting ganciclovir, resistance should be suspected, genetic studies for resistance sent and therapy with foscarnet/cidofovir initiated. Unfortunately, these drugs are not easily available in India.

Preemptive Therapy

Early or preemptive therapy means initiating treatment in immunocompromised patients with virologic markers (PCR or antigen) of CMV but no active disease. Preemptive therapy now favored over prophylaxis in patients with allogenic HSCT and high-risk lung, liver, heart, and kidney transplant patients. This involves sending CMV viral loads on a weekly basis at least for the first 100 days post-transplant and starting therapy if the plasma viral loads are more than 1,000 copies/mL. Ganciclovir is initial therapy of choice but valganciclovir can also be used in stable patients who can tolerate oral medication.

Prophylaxis

Prophylaxis is indicated in transplant recipients (HSCT and solid organ) who are at high risk for CMV disease (seropositive donors and seronegative recipients) and those who have received highly immunosuppressive therapy including anti-thymocyte globulin (ATG). Here ganciclovir or valganciclovir may be used as once daily dose for 3–6 months. Letermovir is a new drug that has been recently approved for prevention of CMV infection and disease in HSCT recipients. The advantage is that it is less myelotoxic than ganciclovir/valganciclovir.

DRUGS FOR TREATMENT OF INFLUENZA

Amantadine and Rimantadine

These drugs act on the M2 protein in the cell membrane of the influenza A virus, inhibiting replication, uncoating, and assembly of the virus. Resistance is frequent and rapid and occurs by change in the M2 viral protein by mutation. These drugs have almost become redundant in the treatment of influenza as the currently circulating influenza viruses including novel H1N1 and H3N2 are almost always resistant to these drugs. Highly pathogenic avian influenza virus (H5N1) is also resistant. These drugs are no longer recommended by the WHO in management of current day influenza infections.

Oseltamivir and Zanamivir (Neuraminidase Inhibitors)

These drugs are the cornerstone in management of current day influenza virus infections.

Mechanism of Action and Resistance and Spectrum of Activity

Potent and specific inhibitors of the neuraminidase of influenza A (including H5N1) and B viruses. They act by inhibition of influenza virus neuraminidase. Influenza virus neuraminidase is responsible for virus assembly and release and oseltamivir inhibits this process. Resistance is by mutation in the hemagglutinin and/or neuraminidase. Resistance has not been recognized in influenza B virus to date but is being reported in influenza A virus.

Pharmacokinetics

Zanamivir: Inhaled dry powder. 4 to 17% of drug is absorbed systemically. Oral bioavailability is very low. IV preparation is under trial.

Oseltamivir: Good oral bioavailability—70 to 80% absorbed. Prodrug form is metabolized by the liver esterases to active parent compound, carboxylate. No interaction with P450 system. Food does not decrease bioavailability but reduces the risk of gastrointestinal intolerance. Eliminated unchanged in urine.

Dosage

Zanamivir: 5 mg/dose two such inhalations bid for 5 days. Not FDA approved but effective for prophylaxis in the dose of 10 mg once daily.

Oseltamivir: (75 mg capsule or 12 mg/mL liquid). For treatment dose for more than 13 years/>35 kg is 75 mg BD. For less than 15 kg—30 mg BD, 15–24 kg—45 mg BD, 25–34 kg—60 mg BD. Therapy needs to be continued for 5 days. For severe illness, immunocompromised patients double the usual recommended dose may also be used and treatment continued for 10 days. However a recent randomized controlled trial failed to show additional benefit with double dose. For prophylaxis, oseltamivir is approved as a once daily dose (i.e. half the therapeutic dose) of 75 mg once daily for at least 10 days. The drug should be started within 2 days of exposure. The duration of protection lasts for as long as dosing is continued and therefore in community outbreaks it may and can be safely given for up to 6 weeks.

Adverse Effects

Oseltamivir is known to cause neurologic and GI side effects. Occasional bronchospasm has been reported following inhalation of zanamivir.

Indications for Use

Therapeutic: The exact role of neuraminidase inhibitors in management of influenza is uncertain. Manufacturer sponsored trials in 1999 demonstrated that neuraminidase inhibitors reduce morbidity and duration of influenza related illness by 24–48 hours. They reduce infectivity and slow down virus transmission. They are most beneficial when given within the first 48 hours of illness.

A 2006 meta-analysis showed that they also reduce the likelihood of development of complications like pneumonia and mortality. A 2014 Cochrane meta-analysis showed no reduction in pneumonia and mortality and increased side effects if given for prophylaxis. Then came another meta-analysis in 2015 published in the Lancet that oseltamivir reduces symptoms, pneumonia, and hospitalization in adults but increase nausea and vomiting. So the jury is still out as far as the efficacy of neuraminidase inhibitors in reducing complications of influenza.

Given the controversy about the benefits of the drug and the risk of promoting resistance with unrestricted use, when should these drugs be used for suspected/confirmed influenza? For any patient presenting with influenza-like illness, the treatment strategy depends on two factors: the severity of illness and the likelihood of complications.

In patients with mild disease who are not at risk for complications, only symptomatic treatment is indicated. Antibiotics and antivirals should not be prescribed. Patients should be counseled about the red flag signs and asked to seek medical care in the event these occur. These patients should be asked to stay at home till they are afebrile to prevent disease transmission to others.

Patients with influenza-like illness (ILI) who are at high risk for complications (aged more than 65, immunocompromised, pregnant women, morbid obese and those with severe comorbidities) should be started on antiviral therapy irrespective of the severity of disease. The use of antivirals in all children below the age of 5 (a risk group for severe disease) or with flu-like illness is however debatable. These children may present with multiple episodes of flu-like illness in the season and how many episodes would one use antivirals? Hence some discretion in use of antivirals in children below the age of 5 with mild illness is advised and watchful waiting is definitely an option.

For patients who present with symptoms of severe illness or who have complications, antiviral treatment with oseltamivir should be started without delay. Definitive diagnosis of influenza by molecular tests is not a pre-requisite to start antiviral treatment in this setting. This is because by the time results are available the disease may have progressed and also because negative molecular tests do not rule out influenza. However now tests on GeneXpert platform are available that have a turnaround time of just 1–2 hours.

Intravenous peramivir is a new drug that has received approval for treatment of influenza infections and has been demonstrated to be noninferior to oral oseltamivir.

Prophylactic: Prophylactic antivirals are indicated in patients who are exposed to influenza and have high risk of developing complications. These include the immunocompromised, pregnant women, those with chronic comorbid conditions, and the morbidly obese. Risk of developing resistance is a danger of this approach and this approach is now no longer recommended by the WHO.

DRUGS EFFECTIVE AGAINST RNA VIRUSES

Ribavirin

Mechanism of Action and Resistance

Interferes with viral mRNA synthesis. Resistance is rare.

Spectrum of Activity

Broad-spectrum antiviral active against orthomyxoviruses (Influenza A and B), paramyxoviruses (Parainfluenza, RSV, measles), arenaviruses (Lassa fever virus), bunyavirus (encephalitis), hantavirus, togaviruses (HCV), and enteroviruses (polio, coxsackie B).

Pharmacokinetics

Administered by aerosol, orally or intravenously. Absorbed when used as aerosol. Bioavailability 33 to 45% after oral dose. CSF levels 70% of plasma levels. Metabolized by liver and 40% excreted by kidney. Concentrated in erythrocytes and t½ in RBCs is 40 days.

Clinical Indications

- Aerosol for treatment of RSV bronchiolitis/pneumonia in specific children including age less than 6 weeks, congenital heart disease, chronic lung disease, preterm infants, immunocompromised children, cystic fibrosis, and children with neurologic or neuromuscular disorders. No benefit in mild disease or when started late.
- Oral therapy for infections with RSV, parainfluenza, measles in immunocompromised patients especially those who have undergone HSCT or on intensive cancer chemotherapy.
- As oral treatment of HCV when combined with interferon-α produces a sustained decrease in HCV RNA levels, improves systemic symptoms, and improves liver histology.

- As intravenous therapy for hemorrhagic fevers including Lassa fever, hemorrhagic fever renal syndrome (hanta virus), Crimean-Congo hemorrhagic fever, Ebola virus disease, and adenovirus disease. Oral ribavirin may be of benefit prophylactically in individuals exposed to hemorrhagic fevers.
- Tried in SSPE in combination with interferon-α; benefits but does not cure.

Dosage

Bronchiolitis: 6 g dissolved in 300 mL sterile water and administered by a small particle aerosol generator (SPAG-2) over 18 hrs for 3 to 7 days. Can be delivered by mask, oxygen hood or through ventilator.

For RSV, parainfluenza pneumonia: Dose is 10–30 mg/kg/day in 2–3 divided doses for 5–10 days.

HCV: 600 mg bid for 24 to 48 weeks.

Lassa fever: 2 g loading (25 to 33 mg/kg) followed by half the dose qid for 4 days and then half of this dose tid for 3 days.

Adverse Effects

Aerosolized ribavirin can cause anorexia, nausea, and bronchospasm. Environmental exposure to aerosolized ribavirin by health workers can cause headache, conjunctivitis, and bronchospasm. Ribavirin may get precipitated in ventilator tubings. Oral and intravenous ribavirin can cause dose related hemolytic anemia. *Very highly teratogenic* (category X) and pregnant health care workers should take care while caring for a patient on inhalation ribavirin therapy.

Lamivudine

Mechanism of Action and Resistance

It is a nucleoside analog that inhibits HIV reverse transcriptase and HBV DNA polymerase. Resistance occurs by mutation in the HBV DNA polymerase.

Spectrum of Activity

Active against HIV and HBV.

Pharmacokinetics

Following oral administration, it is rapidly absorbed with a bioavailability of 80%. It is widely distributed in a volume comparable to total body water. Plasma half-life is 9 hours. 70% is excreted unchanged in urine. 3 mg/kg per day provides plasma levels comparable to adults.

Clinical Indications

Chronic hepatitis B (CHB): It suppresses HBV DNA levels and is associated with biochemical normalization and histological improvements in inflammation and progression of fibrosis. A minority of patients develop HBeAg seroconversion, i.e. loss of HBeAg, and development of anti-HBe antibodies. In most patients, viremia returns to pretreatment levels after discontinuation of lamivudine, sometimes in association with hepatitis flare. A major limitation with use of lamivudine is rapid emergence of mutations (YMDD mutants). Lamivudine therapy can benefit patients with decompensated cirrhosis and extend the transplantation free time. Combined use of interferon-α with lamivudine generally shows no greater efficacy than monotherapy with interferon-α, although combination therapy may be associated with higher HBe seroconversion.

HIV: See section on antiretroviral therapy (Chapter 34).

Adefovir Dipivoxil

Adefovir dipivoxil has recently been approved for the treatment of CHB. Adefovir dipivoxil is the oral prodrug of adefovir, a nucleotide analog of adenosine monophosphate. In vivo, adefovir dipivoxil is converted to the parent compound, adefovir, and through two phosphorylation reactions, to adefovir diphosphate, the active intracellular metabolite that interacts with the HBV polymerase. Adefovir diphosphate acts as a competitive inhibitor and chain terminator of HBV replication.

Two large randomized controlled trials have demonstrated that adefovir dipivoxil in a dose of 10 mg per day is effective in patients with HBeAg-positive or HBeAg-negative CHB. Also, adefovir dipivoxil effectively suppresses lamivudine-resistant HBV in patients with CHB after liver transplantation, compensated or decompensated liver disease, and co-infection with HIV. Adefovir is well-tolerated, reduces HBV DNA levels, and normalizes ALT levels. But sustained response with HBeAg to anti-HBe seroconversion is rarely obtained and HBsAg loss is exceptional. The response is maintained during therapy, which needs to be continued indefinitely in the majority of patients since withdrawal of treatment is generally followed by a rapid reactivation of hepatitis B.

CONCLUSION

Several new antiviral agents are under development. Identification of agents with improved pharmacokinetics, greater potency, and/or improved toxicity profile will make antiviral therapy more satisfactory. Prodrugs can be used to improve bioavailability. Newer drug delivery techniques are being identified. Combination therapy is being studied to increase antiviral activity, reducing drug dosage and toxicity.

RECOMMENDED READING

1. Bowman LJ, Melaragno JI, Brennan DC. Letermovir for the management of cytomegalovirus infection. Expert Opin Investig Drugs. 2017;26:235-41.
2. Bryson YJ. Antiviral Agents. In: Feigen RD, Cherry JD (Eds). Textbook of Pediatric Infectious Diseases, 4th edition. Philadelphia: WB Saunders Company; 1998. pp. 2660-90.
3. Chemaly RF, Shah DP, Boeckh MJ. Management of respiratory viral infections in hematopoietic cell transplant recipients and patients with hematologic malignancies. Clin Infect Dis. 2014;59 Suppl 5:S344-51.
4. Dobson J, Whitley RJ, Pocock S, et al. Oseltamivir treatment for influenza in adults: a meta-analysis of randomised controlled trials. Lancet. 2015;385(9979):1729-37.
5. Gani R, Hughes H, Fleming D, et al. Potential impact of antiviral drug use during influenza pandemic. Emerg Infect Dis. 2005;11:1355-6.
6. James SH, Kimberlin DW. Neonatal herpes simplex virus infection: epidemiology and treatment. Clin Perinatol. 2015;42(1):47-59.

7. Jefferson T, Jones MA, Doshi P, et al. Neuraminidase inhibitors for preventing and treating influenza in healthy adults and children. Cochrane Database Syst Rev. 2014;(4):CD008965.
8. Karnsakul W, Schwarz KB. Hepatitis B and C. Pediatr Clin North Am. 2017;64(3):641-58.
9. Kimberlin DW, Brady MT, Jackson MA (Eds). Red Book (2018). Report of the Committee on Infectious Diseases, 31st edition. US: American Academy of Pediatrics; 2018.
10. Kotton CN. CMV: Prevention, diagnosis and therapy. Am J Transplant. 2013;13:24-40.
11. Lee J, Park JH, Jwa H, et al. Comparison of efficacy of intravenous peramivir and oral oseltamivir for the treatment of influenza: Systematic review and meta-analysis. Yonsei Med J. 2017;58(4):778-85.
12. Lim Y, Lyall H. Congenital cytomegalovirus—who, when, what-with and why to treat? J Infect. 2017;74:S89-S94.
13. Sauerbrei A. Diagnosis, antiviral therapy, and prophylaxis of varicella-zoster virus infections. Eur J Clin Microbiol Infect Dis. 2016;35(5):723-34.
14. Writing Committee of the WHO Consultation on Clinical Aspects of Pandemic (H1N1) 2009 Influenza. Clinical Aspects of Pandemic 2009 Influenza A (H1N1) Virus Infection. NEJM. 2010;362:1708-19.

Antifungal Therapy

37 Chapter

Tanu Singhal

INTRODUCTION

With the advent of newer and ever more potent chemotherapeutic, immunosuppressive, and antimicrobial regimens, complications due to fungal pathogens are on the rise. Concurrently, great advances have been made in the field of antifungal drugs. Newer antifungal drugs have been discovered and older drugs are re-formulated. This review discusses the pharmacology and clinical use of various systemic antifungal drugs.

CLASSES OF ANTIFUNGAL DRUGS

- Polyenes (Amphotericin B)
- Azoles
- Echinocandins
- Nucleoside analogs.

Polyenes (Amphotericin B)

The oldest antifungal class is the polyene macrolides including amphotericin B and nystatin. Amphotericin B deoxycholate (AMB-D) has been the "gold standard" for the treatment of invasive fungal infections (IFIs) and the yardstick to measure efficacy of new agents. Lipid formulations available are amphotericin B colloidal dispersion (ABCD), lipid complex formulation (ABLC), and small unilamellar liposomal formulation (L-AMB). However, cost/adverse effects of the liposomal preparations and availability of the new azoles and echinocandins have reduced the use of amphotericin B and its derivatives.

Mechanism of Action

The main mechanism of action is binding to ergosterol, the principal sterol in the fungal cell membrane. This binding leads to cell death by depolarization of the membrane with subsequent increase in membrane permeability. A contributory mechanism of action may be the generation of oxidative metabolites which is implicated to cause in vitro functional stimulation of phagocytes. In addition to fungal ergosterol, amphotericin B also binds to cholesterol in human cell membranes, possibly accounting for its toxicity.

Lipid formulations of amphotericin B are taken up by activated monocytes and macrophages and transported to the site of infection where phospholipases release the free drug. They are better tolerated than the conventional deoxycholate preparation because the lipid stabilizes the drug in a self-associated state so that it cannot interact with human cell membrane cholesterol.

Spectrum of Activity

Most *Candida* species, *Aspergillus, Cryptococcus neoformans,* Zygomycetes, *Blastomyces dermatitidis, Coccidioides immitis, Histoplasma capsulatum, Paracoccidioides brasiliensis, Sporothrix schenckii,* and *Penicillium marneffei.*

Does not cover Candida lusitaniae, some *C. auris, Fusarium, Trichosporon, Pseudallescheria boydii, and Scedosporium prolificans.*

Resistance to amphotericin B has been produced in vitro, and resistant strains have been isolated from patients who have received long-term therapy with AMB-D. Fluconazole-resistant strains of *C. albicans* that were cross-resistant to amphotericin B have been isolated from a few immunocompromised patients. *C. neoformans* isolates resistant to fluconazole and amphotericin B have also been documented. Fungi resistant to AMB-D are also resistant to lipid formulations.

Pharmacokinetics

Absorption of amphotericin B from the gastrointestinal (GI) tract is negligible. After intravenous infusion of the conventional deoxycholate formulation, the drug is released from its carrier, distributes predominantly (≥90%) with lipoproteins, and is taken up preferentially by organs of the mononuclear phagocytic system (MPS). The drug follows biphasic elimination from plasma with an initial half-life of 24–48 hours, followed by a terminal half-life of up to 15 days. Tissue accumulation and redistribution into the plasma pool apparently account for most amphotericin B disposition, since the drug is only very slowly excreted into urine and bile and since no metabolites have been identified. Cerebrospinal fluid (CSF) concentrations are only 2–4% of serum concentrations, so this drug is a poor choice for monotherapy in meningitis.

Lipid formulations of amphotericin B are important therapeutic advances because they reduce nephrotoxicity while preserving antifungal activity of the parent compound. The plasma pharmacokinetics of ABCD is not markedly different from those of conventional amphotericin B. The ABLC is taken up more rapidly by the MPS; the L-AMB is characterized by comparatively higher peak plasma levels and prolonged circulation in plasma. The lipid formulations spare the kidney thus reducing nephrotoxicity but at the same time are ineffective in treating renal fungal infections.

Clinical Uses

- Amphotericin B is the treatment of choice for invasive and life-threatening fungal infections, including blastomycosis, coccidioidomycosis, paracoccidioidomycosis, cryptococcosis, histoplasmosis, mucormycosis, and sporotrichosis.
- For aspergillosis, voriconazole is now preferred to amphotericin B.
- For candidemia in non-neutropenic adults, the echinocandins are preferred to amphotericin B due to similar efficacy but lower toxicity. However, in non-neutropenic children where data on echinocandins is limited amphotericin B/fluconazole are the preferred drugs. Liposomal amphotericin B is the drug of choice for treatment of central nervous system (CNS). *Candida* infections and *Candida* endocarditis along with flucytosine in both children and adults.

AMB-D is the drug of choice for neonatal candidiasis and in treatment of fluconazole resistant urinary tract infections.

- Amphotericin B is the preferred agent for treatment of pregnant women with IFIs due to concerns regarding the use of azole antifungal agents during pregnancy.
- Intravenous amphotericin B (especially lipid formulations) is the preferred agent for empiric therapy in febrile neutropenic patients in both adults and children.
- Amphotericin B is also used for the treatment of certain protozoal infections, including leishmaniasis (single dose of liposomal amphotericin B 10 mg/kg is drug of choice) and amebic meningoencephalitis.
- Liposomal amphotericin B has also been used to prevent fungal infections in high-risk patients including recipients of stem cell transplants either given as intermittent therapy or as nebulization.

Dosage

Dosage of conventional amphotericin B: For AMB-D the initial test dose is 0.1 mg/kg body weight (minimum 1 mg). Some authorities do not recommend a separate test dose, but do use a cautious infusion of the first dose (quasi test dose). Prediction of allergic responses to subsequent doses cannot be done on the basis of allergic response to the test dose as the two do not always correlate. The daily dose is 0.6–1 mg/kg. For seriously ill patients, the daily dose may be gradually increased up to an absolute maximum of 1.5 mg/kg. The higher dosage level may be given on alternate days. The drug should be diluted in 5% dextrose (recommended concentration 10 mg/100 mL). Studies have shown that rapid infusion (over 1–2 hours) is as safe and well tolerated as prolonged (over 3–6 hours) infusion of conventional amphotericin B and greatly facilitates outpatient and home administration of the drug. Rapid infusion should *not* be used in patients with azotemia (creatinine clearance < 25 mL/min), hyperkalemia, or dose more than 1 mg/kg, or in patients who receive drug therapy via a central catheter that extends into the right heart. Administration of normal saline at the rate of 10 mL/kg prior to amphotericin B reduces nephrotoxicity. Rigors respond to pethidine. There is no benefit in premedicating with hydrocortisone/paracetamol and hydroxyzine prior to administration.

Dosage of lipid formulations: Lipid preparations are conventionally used in dosages of 3–5 mg/kg/day which has equivalent efficacy as 1 mg/kg/day of AMB-D. However, a large multicenter maximum tolerated dose study of L-amphotericin B (ambisome) using doses of 7.5–15 mg/kg/day found a nonlinear plasma pharmacokinetic profile and no demonstrable dose-limiting nephrotoxicity or infusion-related toxicity.

- *Amphotericin B colloidal dispersion*: Initial test dose 2 mg over 10 minutes then 3–4 mg/kg daily as a single dose; maximum 6 mg/kg daily
- *Lipid complex formulation*: The initial test dose is 1 mg over 15 minutes then 5 mg/kg daily.
- Liposomal formulation (L-AMB; Ambisome): Test dose 1 mg over 10 minutes then 3–5 mg/kg daily. Higher doses up to 10 mg/kg/day may be needed in mucormycosis. A new indigenous liposomal formulation is now available which needs sonication prior to administration. This preparation can be dosed as 1–3 mg/kg/day (higher doses recommended for mucormycosis).

Duration of Therapy

The optimal duration of amphotericin B therapy is unknown. It depends on the clinical indication, the extent of infection, degree of immunosuppression, and graft function (in post-transplant patients). No specific total dose is recommended.

Adverse Effects

Infusion-related adverse events are fairly common with conventional amphotericin B (50–90%). These are characterized by nausea and vomiting, diarrhea, epigastric pain, febrile reactions, headache, myalgia, dyspnea, and tachypnea. In one large comparative trial, during initial infusion without premedication, L-AMB recipients experienced significantly less fever and chills than AMB-D recipients (fever, 16.9% versus 43.6%, respectively; chill 18.4% versus 54.4%, respectively). Infusion-related events connected with ABCD and ABLC appear to be considerably more common than those associated with L-AMB and similar in frequency to infusion-related events associated with AMB-D. Fever and chills associated with the lipid-based drugs tend to occur mainly after the first two infusions and are less frequent with subsequent infusions. Infusion-related hypoxia has been documented in as many as 25% of ABCD and ABLC recipients but is usually reversible and without long-term sequelae. Prophylactic antipyretics, antihistaminics, steroids, and meperidine partially ameliorate these reactions with conventional and lipid-based products.

Rapid infusion of AMB-D has been associated with a more severe reaction consisting of hypotension, bronchospasm, hypokalemia, arrhythmias, and shock. It may be difficult to determine whether these severe reactions indicate intolerance or hypersensitivity to amphotericin B. Anaphylaxis and anaphylactoid reactions have been reported in people taking all formulations of amphotericin B.

Nephrotoxicity is the other major dose-limiting toxicity of amphotericin B occurring in 30–50% cases. The manifestations of nephrotoxicity are azotemia, decreased glomerular filtration, loss of urinary concentrating ability, renal loss of sodium, potassium, and magnesium, and renal tubular acidosis. The renal injury reduces erythropoietin production and leads to a normochromic normocytic anemia. Nephrotoxicity associated with AMB-D appears to involve several mechanisms including direct vasoconstrictive effects on renal arterioles and lytic action on renal tubular cell membranes. Renal function usually improves within a few months of discontinuing therapy, but some impairment may remain. Sodium and water repletion (10–15 mL/kg) prior to the infusion helps in reducing nephrotoxicity. The serum creatinine and electrolytes (K, Mg) should be monitored regularly at least twice a week and potassium and magnesium supplemented. A rise in serum creatinine beyond 2.5 mg/dL may be an indication to switch to the lipid-based agents. Nephrotoxicity is less common with all three lipid formulations of amphotericin B than with AMB-D. In comparative studies, the respective rates of nephrotoxicity (defined as twice baseline serum creatinine) are: ABLC ~25%, ABCD ~15%, L-AMB ~20%, and AMB-D ~30–50%. Importantly, in open-label studies, administrations of lipid-based amphotericin B drugs are reported to stabilize or even improve renal function in patients with pre-existing renal insufficiency. In addition, individuals receiving concurrent nephrotoxic agents (e.g. cyclosporine, aminoglycosides) are less likely to have renal dysfunction when receiving lipid formulations compared to AMB-D.

Amphotericin B intravenous infusion has also been associated with anemia, headache, thrombophlebitis, and GI effects (indigestion, loss of appetite, nausea, vomiting, diarrhea, stomach pain). Less frequently, blurred or double vision, cardiac arrhythmias, leukopenia, polyneuropathy, seizures, and thrombocytopenia have been reported. Other adverse events associated with lipid-based products have included elevations in liver transaminases, alkaline phosphatase, and serum bilirubin levels. Liver function test abnormalities have been noted in 25–50% of patients treated with L-AMB but these findings are reversible without drug discontinuation in the majority of patients.

Drug Interactions

Close monitoring is required with concomitant administration of nephrotoxic drugs or cytotoxic agents. Drugs that increase the risk of nephrotoxicity of AMB include aminoglycosides, cyclosporin, tacrolimus, vancomycin, pentamidine isethionate, and polymyxins. Drugs that increase the risk of hypokalemia due to AMB include systemic corticosteroids and adrenocorticotropic hormone (ACTH), thiazide, and loop diuretics. AMB may increase the toxicity of cardiac glycosides and skeletal muscle relaxants (by virtue of hypokalemia) and that of flucytosine by reducing renal excretion and increased cellular uptake of flucytosine. Concomitant administration of zidovudine and amphotericin B may be associated myelotoxicity and nephrotoxicity. Amphotericin B coadministered with blood dyscrasia causing medications, bone marrow depressants, or radiation therapy may increase chance of anemia or other hematologic effects. Dosage reduction may be required.

Contraindications

Amphotericin B deoxycholate and alternative formulations of amphotericin B are contraindicated in patients allergic to amphotericin B or any of formulation components. Extreme caution should be exercised when using AMB-D in patients with renal impairment.

Which Formulation to Use?

With the exception of neonates, renal infections, cryptococcosis, lipid formulations are the drugs of choice owing to reduced toxicity and superior efficacy. However, there are cost constraints with their use; also children may tolerate AMB-D better than adults. So, in resource-limited setting, treatment with the conventional preparation can be initiated but therapy should be switched to lipid formulations if nephrotoxicity develops.

The most suitable of all lipid formulations is liposomal form (lowest toxicity and best efficacy); in fact, in the current era, the other lipid formulations of ABCD and ABLC are not easily available and do not offer much cost advantage as compared to L-AMB.

Azoles

Unlike amphotericin B, the antifungal azoles are synthetic compounds. The azoles are classified as imidazoles (miconazole and ketoconazole) or triazoles according to whether they contain two or three nitrogen atoms, respectively, in the five-membered azole ring. The triazoles can be further classified as first-generation triazoles (itraconazole, fluconazole) and second-generation (voriconazole, ravuconazole, posaconazole). The new azole isavuconazole has been recently introduced.

The chemical structures and pharmacologic profiles of ketoconazole and itraconazole are similar. Ketoconazole is now infrequently used and will not be discussed further. Fluconazole is unique because of its comparatively small molecular size and lower lipophilicity. Voriconazole is a second-generation triazole and a synthetic derivative of fluconazole. Voriconazole combines the broad-spectrum of antifungal activity of itraconazole with the increased bioavailability of fluconazole.

Mechanism of Action

The azoles inhibit ergosterol synthesis through an interaction with C-14 alpha demethylase, a cytochrome P-450 dependent enzyme that is necessary for the conversion of lanosterol to ergosterol. The depletion of ergosterol alters membrane fluidity, thereby reducing the activity of membrane-associated enzymes and leading to increased permeability and inhibition of cell growth and replication. The potential for similar interactions in mammalian cells with enzymes dependent on cytochrome P-450 also mediates some of the major toxic effects and drug interactions of the azoles. One important distinction between the triazoles and imidazoles is the greater affinity of the former for fungal as compared with mammalian cytochrome P-450 enzymes.

Other antifungal effects of azoles include the inhibition of endogenous respiration, a toxic interaction with membrane phospholipids, and the inhibition of the morphogenetic transformation of yeasts to the mycelial form.

Itraconazole and Fluconazole

Spectrum of Activity

Principally active against dermatophytes, *Candida* species, *C. neoformans, T. beigelii,* and dimorphic fungi (*B. dermatitidis, H. capsulatum, C. immitis, P. brasiliensis, S. schenckii*). Only itraconazole is active against *Aspergillus* and dematiaceous molds and both itraconazole and fluconazole have no activity against *Fusarium* and Zygomycetes.

Resistance

Resistance in *Candida* spp. to azoles is increasing. In a recent study on ICU-associated candidemia from India, fluconazole resistance was 12%. Some species including *C. glabrata, C. krusei,* and *C. auris* are almost universally resistant; now resistance is being reported even in *C. albicans* and *C. tropicalis*. Aspergillus resistance to itraconazole is on the rise. Resistance in *Cryptococcus* has also been reported.

Pharmacokinetics

Itraconazole is a weak base and requires an acid environment for optimal solubilization and absorption. Itraconazole is available abroad as a capsule, as an oral cyclodextrin formulation which has superior bioavailability, and as an intravenous formulation. Only the capsule form is available in India. The bioavailability of capsular itraconazole is two to three times higher when taken with fatty food than when taken on an empty stomach. The peak plasma concentrations of itraconazole are three to five times higher after 7–14 days of treatment (steady state) than after a single dose. A loading dose of 200 mg of itraconazole three times daily for 3 days is recommended in patients with serious infections to reduce the time until steady-state concentrations are attained. Itraconazole are extensively bound (>99%) to plasma proteins, but unbound drug distributes well throughout most tissues including the brain but not in nonproteinaceous body fluids. Itraconazole is extensively metabolized in the liver and excreted almost exclusively in the feces and urine. The terminal elimination half-lives for itraconazole at steady-state conditions are 7–10 hours and 24–42 hours, respectively. The half-life increases with increases in the dose from 100 mg to 400 mg daily, suggesting that the metabolic pathways in the liver are saturable within the therapeutic dose range. Because little itraconazole is excreted in the urine, the doses need not be changed in patients with renal impairment. In addition, drug is not removed by hemodialysis.

Fluconazole is available as both an oral and an intravenous formulation. In contrast to itraconazole, the absorption of oral fluconazole is not altered by the presence of food or gastric acidity. Peak plasma concentrations of fluconazole are proportional to the dose occur within 2–4 hours after oral administration, and are approximately 2–2.5 times higher at steady state (which occurs about 6–10 days after treatment is begun) than after single doses. As with itraconazole, the administration of a loading dose of fluconazole is recommended. Fluconazole resembles flucytosine in that both are highly water soluble, minimally bound to plasma proteins, and distributed in a volume that approximates that of total body water. The concentrations of fluconazole in most body tissues and fluids usually exceed 50% of the corresponding plasma concentrations and are especially high in CSF and urine. The peak CSF concentrations in patients with fungal meningitis range from approximately 70 to 90% of peak plasma concentrations. Similarly, urinary concentrations of fluconazole may exceed 100 μg/mL which is much higher than those of other oral azoles. In contrast to the imidazoles and itraconazole, fluconazole is minimally metabolized; approximately 80% of an administered dose is excreted unchanged in the urine. The terminal elimination half-life increases from approximately 30 hours in patients with normal renal function to 98 hours in patients with severe renal impairment (glomerular filtration rate <20 mL/minute). Consequently, the dose should be reduced in patients with glomerular filtration rates below 50 mL/minute. Fluconazole is effectively removed during hemodialysis and to a lesser extent during peritoneal dialysis.

Clinical Uses

Fluconazole:

- Fluconazole may be used in treatment of proven or suspected candidemia in non-neutropenic adults and children. However as per current guidelines, the echinocandins are the drugs of choice in adults due to superior efficacy as compared to fluconazole. The guidelines for children are, however, recommend use of fluconazole as empirical therapy in patients who are not critically sick and when infection is acquired in units with low rates of fluconazole resistance.
- It is the preferred drug in initial management of oropharyngeal and esophageal candidiasis and also in all invasive/deep seated *Candida* infections after initial therapy with amphotericin B/echinocandins if the isolate is susceptible to fluconazole. It can also be used instead of topical therapy in management of vulvovaginal candidiasis (single dose) or as pulse therapy in *Tinea corporis, Pityriasis versicolor,* and onychomycosis.
- It is the drug of choice for meningeal and nonmeningeal coccidial infections and *Trichosporon* infections.
- It is also indicated for consolidation/maintenance therapy of cryptococcal meningitis and also for induction therapy in resource-limited settings.
- In the prophylactic setting, it is effective for preventing *Candida* infections in acute leukemia, bone marrow transplant, liver transplant patients, neonates and those with recurrent vulvovaginal candidiasis, in primary prevention of cryptococcosis and histoplasmosis in *acquired* immune deficiency syndrome (AIDS) patients, and in secondary prevention of cryptococcosis and *coccidioidomycosis* in human immunodeficiency virus (HIV) infected patients.

Itraconazole:

- It is indicated for dermatophytic infections, *Pityriasis versicolor,* and all forms of cutaneous and mucosal *Candida* infections but not for invasive *Candida* infections.
- It is an approved agent for *Aspergillus* infections especially allergic bronchopulmonary aspergillosis, chronic cavitary pulmonary aspergillosis, and chronic noninvasive/

granulomatous *Aspergillus* sinusitis. With availability of voriconazole, it is no longer the drug of choice for managing invasive pulmonary aspergillosis.
- It is the therapy of choice for nonmeningeal and non-life-threatening paracoccidioidomycosis, blastomycosis, sporotrichosis, and histoplasmosis.
- Intravenous itraconazole is an approved agent for febrile neutropenia but not commonly used due to nonavailability of the intravenous formulation.
- It is also approved for antifungal prophylaxis in hematopoietic stem cell transplant (HSCT) recipients.

Dosage

Fluconazole: 6–12 mg/kg/day
- *Oropharyngeal candidiasis*: Oral or IV 3–6 mg/kg on 1st day then 3 mg/kg daily for 7–14 days
- *Esophageal candidiasis*: 3–6 mg/kg/day for 14–21 days
- *Invasive candidiasis and cryptococcal infections*: Oral or IV loading 12 mg/kg daily (maximum 800 mg) and then 6 mg/kg/day (maximum 400 mg). In neonates, 25 mg/kg loading and then 12 mg/kg/day
- *Cryptococcosis*: Dose varying from 3 mg/kg/day to 12 mg/kg/day (200–1,200 mg) depending on the stage of therapy.
- *Antifungal prophylaxis in immunocompromised patients*: Oral or IV 6 mg/kg/day; maximum 400 mg daily; neonates, 3–6 mg/kg given IV three times a week till IV access is present.

Itraconazole: The recommended dose of the capsule formulation is 5–8 mg/kg/day (100–400 mg/day) with a loading dose of 4 mg/kg three times daily for the first 3 days in serious infections.
- *Oropharyngeal candidiasis*: 100 mg daily (200 mg daily in immunocompromised) for 15 days
- *Vulvovaginal candidiasis*: 200 mg twice daily for 1 day
- *Pityriasis versicolor*: 200 mg daily for 7 days
- For doses in dermatophytosis see Chapter 24
- *Histoplasmosis*: 200 mg one to two times daily
- *Systemic aspergillosis, candidiasis, and cryptococcosis including cryptococcal meningitis where other antifungal drugs inappropriate or ineffective*: 200 mg once daily (candidiasis 100–200 mg once daily) increased in invasive or disseminated disease and in cryptococcal meningitis to 200 mg twice daily
- *Maintenance in AIDS patients to prevent relapse of underlying fungal infection and prophylaxis in neutropenia when standard therapy inappropriate*: 200 mg once daily, increased to 200 mg twice daily if low plasma-itraconazole concentration
- *Systemic aspergillosis, candidiasis, and cryptococcosis including cryptococcal meningitis where other antifungal drugs inappropriate or ineffective*: IV 200 mg every 12 hours for 2 days, then 200 mg once daily for maximum 12 days.

Adverse Reactions

Fluconazole: It is a well-tolerated drug even in doses as high as 1,200 mg/day in adults and 12 mg/kg/day in children. In adults receiving 100–400 mg/day, the incidence of serious adverse effects or laboratory abnormalities leading to discontinuation of the drug is 2.8%. Nausea, vomiting, diarrhea, and other GI symptoms are seen in less than 5%, skin rash and headache in less than 2%, and reversible asymptomatic elevations of hepatic transaminases in less than 7%. Severe side effects including liver failure and exfoliative dermatitis have been reported anecdotally.

Itraconazole: It is well-tolerated like fluconazole (discontinuation needed in only 4% of those receiving up to 400 mg/day). Nausea, vomiting (10%), hypertriglyceridemia (9%), hypokalemia (6%), elevated liver enzymes (5%), rash or pruritus (2%) are reported. There are rare reports of heart failure and hence prescribe with caution to patients at high-risk of heart failure with poor ventricular function, and those being treated with negative inotropic drugs.

Drug Interactions

These are a major problem with the use of azoles in Table 1 for details.

TABLE 1: Drug interactions of triazoles.

Mechanism and drug involved	*Triazole involved*	*Comment*
Decreased absorption of triazole Antacids, H_2 antagonists, omeprazole, sucralfate, didanosine, grapefruit juice	Itra	Take them at least 2 hours apart
Increased metabolism of triazole INH, rifampicin, rifabutin, phenytoin, phenobarbital, carbamazepine	Itra, flu, vori	Potential for therapy failure, increased potential for hepatotoxicity
Increased concentration of coadministered drug through inhibition of its metabolism by triazole		
Terfenadine, astemizole, cisapride, pimozide, quinidine	Itra, flu, vori	Concomitant use prohibited
Lovastatin, simvastatin, atorvastatin	Itra, flu, vori	Concomitant use prohibited
Phenytoin	Itra, flu, vori	Monitor levels
Benzodiazepines	Itra, flu, vori	Monitor closely
Carbamazepine	Flu	Monitor closely
Haloperidol	Itra	Monitor closely
Rifampicin, rifabutin	Itra, flu	Monitor closely
Clarithromycin	Itra	Monitor closely
Indinavir	Itra	Monitor closely
Ritonavir, NNRTI	Vori	Monitor closely
Vinca alkaloids	Itra, vori	Avoid concomitant use
Busulfan	Itra	Avoid concomitant use
All- trans-retinoic acid	Flu	Monitor closely
Nifedipine, felodipine	Itra, flu	Monitor closely
Cyclosporin A, tacrolimus	Itra, flu, vori	Monitor serum levels
Sulfonyl urea drugs, warfarin, prednisolone	Itra, flu, vori	Monitor closely
Digoxin, quinidine	Itra	Monitor levels
Zidovudine, theophylline	Flu	Monitor closely

(INH: isoniazid; NNRTI: non-nucleoside reverse-transcriptase inhibitors)

Voriconazole

Spectrum of Activity

Effective against a wide variety of fungi comprising many *Candida* species including some *C. krusei* but not *C. glabrata* (mainly fungistatic), *T. beigelii, C. neoformans, Aspergillus* species (fungicidal), *Fusarium* species, and most dimorphic fungi. It is not effective against Zygomycetes.

Pharmacokinetics

Voriconazole is almost completely absorbed after oral administration but should be given empty stomach. It is distributed well with tissue and CSF levels several times the plasma levels. It is extensively metabolized by the liver and is both an inhibitor and a substrate of enzymes CYP2C19, CYP2C4, and CYP2C4. As a result of point mutation in the genes encoding these enzymes, patients are either poor or extensive metabolizers of voriconazole. The levels can be up to four times higher in patients who are deficient in this gene as compared to homozygous subjects. 20% non-Indian Asians and 5% of whites are deficient. Owing to problems in voriconazole metabolism, therapeutic drug monitoring (TDM) of voriconazole levels is recommended. The recommended drug level is 1-6 mcg/mL. Voriconazole metabolism is nonlinear in adults with an approximately threefold increase in its area under the concentration-time curve after a 33% increase in dosage. Children eliminate voriconazole more rapidly than adults and hence per kg dosage in children is much higher than adults.

Clinical Use

Voriconazole has been approved in children older than 2 years.

- It is the drug of choice for invasive aspergillosis (superior to conventional amphotericin B).
- Though it is approved for management of *Candida* infections, it does not offer any significant advantage over the cheaper fluconazole. As per guidelines, voriconazole should not be used for fluconazole resistant *Candida*. Its niche use is in oral step down therapy for *C. krusei* if it demonstrates susceptibility to voriconazole.
- Other indications include fusariosis, scedosporiosis, and as salvage therapy for invasive and refractory fungal infections.
- In patients with fever and neutropenia, it did not meet the noninferiority criteria as compared to liposomal amphotericin B for the composite end point but showed lesser breakthrough infections and lesser toxicity.
- It is also indicated and used for prophylaxis of fungal infections in high-risk patients especially HSCT recipients. It is an attractive option in children where posaconazole cannot be used but has substantial interactions with immunosuppressive agents, such as cyclosporine and tacrolimus.

Dosage

The dosage in adults is 6 mg/kg/dose BD (twice a day) for 1 day followed by maintenance of 4 mg/kg/dose BD (400 mg twice a day on day 1 and then 200 mg twice daily). In children, drug elimination is quicker and higher doses are recommended (Table 2).

In patients with renal insufficiency, no dosing changes are required for the oral preparation; however, due to the renal clearance of the IV carrier, individuals with creatinine clearances of less than 30 mL/min should receive the oral preparation. Those with mild-to-moderate hepatic

TABLE 2: Dosage of voriconazole in children.	
2–12 years 12–14 years (weight <50 kg)	IV 9 mg/kg/dose twice daily day 1 and then 8 mg/kg/dose twice daily Oral 9 mg/kg twice daily
12–14 years >50 kg ≥ 15 years	6 mg/kg twice daily on day 1 And then 4 mg/kg twice daily or 200 mg twice daily

(IV: intravenous)

dysfunction should receive half the maintenance dose. As mentioned earlier, TDM is indicated 7 days after starting therapy. The recommended therapeutic levels are 1-6 μg/mL.

Adverse Effects

Important side effects include transient dose-related visual disturbances, such as altered enhanced perception of light, blurred vision (25-45%), hallucinations or confusion (10%), skin reactions (10%), and transient liver enzyme abnormalities (10-20%). The drug should be used cautiously in patients with liver dysfunction. Periostitis can occur with long-term use.

Drug Interactions

Very significant (*See* Table 1).

Posaconazole

Posaconazole is a new expanded spectrum triazole agent with a spectrum as wide as amphotericin B.

Spectrum of Activity

Posaconazole is active against *Candida* species, *Aspergillus*, Zygomycetes, and cryptococci. Additionally, it is effective against less common fungal pathogens with intrinsic resistance to other antifungal agents including *Fusarium*, chromoblastomycosis, coccidioidomycosis, and other fungi.

Pharmacokinetics

The drug is available in India as an oral suspension. It is absorbed better if given along with food/ fatty meal or nutritional supplements. Dividing the daily oral dose increases total exposure to the drug. However, absorption is erratic and unpredictable and hence TDM is recommended. The tablet form of the drug is available in Western countries and has more predictable absorption. Now an intravenous formulation has become available. The drug is extensively distributed in all body tissues and has a long half-life of 35 hours. Age, race, gender, renal, and hepatic function do not affect its elimination and no dosage adjustments are required.

Indications

Posaconazole is approved in children older than 13 years for the following indications:

- Prevention of fungal infections in high-risk patients including acute myeloid leukemia (AML), myelodysplastic syndrome, and recipients of HSCT. IV posaconazole has currently been approved only for the prophylactic indication

- As combination/salvage/switch over therapy for mucormycosis
- As salvage therapy of IFIs including aspergillosis, fusariosis, chromoblastomycosis, infections with pigmented fungi (*Cladophialophora bantiana*), and coccidioidomycosis. The mortality in patients with refractory aspergillosis treated with posaconazole was 42% compared with 26% in an external control group
- Posaconazole has also demonstrated efficacy in management of oropharyngeal candidiasis.

Dosage

Posaconazole is approved in patients older than 13 years of age where the prophylactic dose is 200 mg thrice daily and the therapeutic dose is 400 mg twice daily (in patients who have poor oral intake, it should be given as 200 mg four times daily). No dose adjustments are needed for patients with renal or hepatic dysfunction; the drug is not removed by hemodialysis. As mentioned earlier, TDM is recommended, for prophylaxis the level should be more than 0.7 μg/mL and for therapy more than 1 μg/mL.

Adverse Effects

Nausea, vomiting, diarrhea, and mild elevation of liver enzymes are common side effects. Rarely, the drug can cause severe hepatic dysfunction and liver failure.

Drug Interactions

Posaconazole only inhibits the cytochrome P450 3A4 enzyme and none of the other cytochrome P450 enzymes and thus has limited potential for drug interactions as compared to other azoles. Its use is contraindicated with certain cytochrome P450 3A4 substrates, such as ergot alkaloids, quinidine, astemizole, terfenadine, cisapride, halofantrine, and pimozide due to effect on prolongation of the QT interval. Use of anticonvulsants and rifampicin reduce posaconazole exposure and hence their concomitant use should be avoided.

Isavuconazole

It is a new generation azole with good activity against both *Aspergillus* and *Mucor*, with better and more predictable bioavailability as compared to voriconazole/posaconazole and has been approved in adults for treatment of invasive aspergillosis and mucormycosis.

Echinocandins

The echinocandins are a new class of antifungal lipopeptides. Three echinocandin compounds are now licensed for use including caspofungin, micafungin, and anidulafungin. These agents have similar pharmacologic properties; they possess potent, broad-spectrum, fungicidal in vitro activity against *Candida* spp. and potent inhibitory activity against *Aspergillus* spp. and have demonstrated antifungal efficacy against these organisms in various animal models and in patients.

Mechanism of Action

They inhibit the synthesis of 1,3-β-D-glucan, a polysaccharide in the cell wall of many pathogenic fungi. Along with chitin, rope-like glucan fibrils are responsible for the cell wall's strength and shape are essential in maintaining osmotic integrity of the fungal cell, and play an important role in cell division and cell growth. As 1,3-β-D-glucan is a selective target present only in fungal cell walls and not in mammalian cells, echinocandins have few adverse effects.

Spectrum of Activity

- *Candida* (fungicidal), *Aspergillus* (fungistatic), *pneumocystis*
- Not *C. neoformans*, *Fusarium*, zygomycetes.

Pharmacokinetics

Echinocandins are available only in parenteral form, have favorable pharmacokinetic properties, and are targeted for once daily dosing. They are distributed well into all tissues including the brain but not in CSF and urine. The pharmacokinetics of the echinocandins is compared in Table 3.

TABLE 3: Pharmacokinetics and dosage of the echinocandins.

	Caspofungin	*Micafungin*	*Anidulafungin*
T½ in hours	9–11	11–17	24–26
Protein binding	96–97	99.8	84
Metabolism	Metabolized, spontaneous degradation	Via COMP	Slow degradation
Dose change in liver disease: Mild Moderate Severe	 None Decrease dose No data	 None None No data	 None None None
Loading dose	Required	Not required	Required
Infusion times	60 minutes	60 minutes	91–182 minutes
Storage after reconstitution	48 hours	Can be used up to 48 (96) hours	Used within 24 hours
Protection from light	Not required	Required	Not required
Volume of diluent	250 mL	100 mL	115 (100 + 15) for 50 mg 280 (250 + 30) mL for 100 mg 560 (500 + 60) mL for 200 mg
Adult dose	70 mg loading and then 50 mg OD	100 mg OD	200 mg loading and then 100 mg OD
Pediatric dose	70 mg/m^2 loading and then 50 mg/m^2	2–4 mg/kg OD	Not approved, but 1.5 mg/kg
Neonatal dose	25 mg/m^2 (some have used up to 5 mg/kg)	10–12 mg/kg	Not approved

(COMP: Catechol O methyltransferase; OD: once a day)

Clinical Use

- They are the drug of choice in management of candidemia in adults. In studies comparing caspofungin with liposomal amphotericin B for candidemia, caspofungin was as efficacious with lower toxicity. In a comparative trial with fluconazole in invasive candidiasis in mainly non-neutropenic patients, anidulafungin was superior to fluconazole. Micafungin in comparative trials with liposomal amphotericin B and caspofungin was noninferior. Hence, in candidemia in adults in both neutropenic/non-neutropenic patients, echinocandins have supplanted amphotericin B as drug of choice due to similar efficacy and lower toxicity. The importance of echinocandins has increased further in the era of *C. auris* as this fungal species is sometimes only susceptible to the echinocandins. Echinocandins may also be used in other deep-seated *Candida* infections for initial therapy in place of amphotericin B with the exception of CNS, eye, and kidneys. All the echinocandins are similar in efficacy in management of candidemia. However, in the presence of liver dysfunction, anidulafungin is the preferred choice. Anidulafungin also has the lowest minimum inhibitory concentrations (MICs), especially in biofilms; however, the clinical benefit of this phenomenon has still to be demonstrated. The drug interactions are also least with anidulafungin.
- The role of echinocandins in neonatal and pediatric invasive candidiasis is debatable. This is because there is limited data in children. Moreover, in neonates where renal and CNS involvement are common, the echinocandins are at a disadvantage. However, echinocandins are indicated in salvage therapy for *Candida* infections in neonates and children that are resistant to other agents, chiefly *C. auris*. The author has successfully treated resistant neonatal invasive candidiasis with caspofungin.
- Echinocandins have been demonstrated as noninferior to fluconazole in management of oropharyngeal candidiasis. However, anidulafungin has been seen to be associated with higher relapse rates as compared to fluconazole.
- Caspofungin and anidulafungin are approved for salvage treatment of *Aspergillus* infections either alone or in combination with other agents like amphotericin B and voriconazole.
- Though *Mucor* is inherently resistant to the echinocandins, caspofungin has been used in combination with amphotericin B for treatment of mucormycosis.
- Caspofungin has been approved for empirical therapy of febrile neutropenia.
- Micafungin has also been approved as prophylaxis for fungal infections in patients who have undergone stem cell transplant.
- Caspofungin has been used as salvage therapy for pneumocystis pneumonia not responding to cotrimoxazole.

Dosage and Administration

See Table 3.

Adverse Reactions

It is a well-tolerated drug with side effects serious enough to cause discontinuation seen only in 5%. The most frequently reported side effects include elevated transaminases, GI upset, headaches, and occasionally histamine-mediated symptoms. Injection site reactions may be seen and are more common with caspofungin. Micafungin can cause benign liver tumors in rats.

Drug Interactions

Caspofungin levels are decreased by carbamazepine, dexamethasone, efavirenz, nevirapine, phenytoin, and rifampicin (initially increased and then reduced). Hence, consider increasing the dose of caspofungin. The plasma concentration of caspofungin is increased by cyclosporin.

Micafungin and anidulafungin have fewer drug interactions as compared to caspofungin. Cyclosporin increases anidulafungin levels but the significance of this is not known. Micafungin can increase nifedipine and cyclosporine levels.

Flucytosine

Flucytosine [5-fluorocytosine, (5-FC)] is a low-molecular-weight, synthetic, fluorinated pyrimidine-analog. Its advantage lies in the fact that it has the least drug interactions as compared to all the other classes of antifungal drugs.

Mechanism of Action

5-fluorocytosine is rapidly converted into 5-fluorouracil (5-FU) in susceptible fungal cells. 5-FU inhibits fungal protein synthesis after getting incorporated within fungal deoxyribonucleic acid (DNA) in place of uridylic acid as well as inhibits fungal DNA synthesis by inhibiting thymidylate synthetase. The toxicity of flucytosine seems to be due to its conversion to 5-FU.

Spectrum of Activity

Candida, C. neoformans. 5-FC has little or no antiaspergillus activity. Organisms develop resistance very quickly if used as monotherapy.

Pharmacokinetics

Flucytosine is readily absorbed from the GI tract, has negligible protein binding, and distributes evenly into tissues and body fluids. It undergoes negligible hepatic metabolism and is eliminated predominantly in active form in urine. Based on an elimination half-life of 3–6 hours in patients with normal renal function, flucytosine usually is administered in 3–4 equally divided doses. It is available in oral and parenteral forms

Clinical Use

When flucytosine is used in combination with amphotericin B, the chances of resistance developing to flucytosine are less. Also, the antifungal activity of amphotericin B is enhanced especially in sites where penetration of amphotericin B is poor (CSF, heart valves, and vitreal body). It is indicated as a companion to AMB in induction therapy of cryptococcal meningitis and in invasive deep-seated *Candida* infections (endocarditis and meningitis)

Dosage

100 mg/kg/day in 3–4 divided doses. Monitoring of plasma concentration is essential to avoid toxicity and blood sample should be taken 2 hours post dosage. Levels of 40–60 μg/mL are desirable.

Adverse Reactions

It is very toxic. Nausea, vomiting, diarrhea, rashes, hallucinations, convulsions, headache, sedation, vertigo, alterations in liver function tests (hepatitis and hepatic necrosis reported), and blood disorders including thrombocytopenia, leucopenia, and aplastic anemia reported. It can cause colitis and also peripheral neuropathy.

Drug Interactions

Renal excretion of flucytosine is decreased and cellular uptake is increased by amphotericin (toxicity possibly increased). Close monitoring is required with concomitant administration of nephrotoxic drugs or cytotoxics. Plasma concentration of flucytosine possibly reduced by cytarabine.

ANTIFUNGAL AGENTS AT A GLANCE

See Table 4.

TREATMENT OF FUNGAL INFECTIONS

See Table 5.

ANTIFUNGAL PROPHYLAXIS

Antifungal prophylaxis in neonates is discussed in Chapter 28. The role of antifungal prophylaxis in critically sick children in the pediatric intensive care unit (ICU) is controversial and not routinely recommended.

The main role of antifungal prophylaxis is in children undergoing cancer chemotherapy and HSCT. Systematic review suggests that antifungal prophylaxis in allogeneic HSCT patients reduces incidence of IFI as well as fungal and all-cause mortality whereas in acute leukemia it reduced IFI and fungal-related mortality. There is a general consensus that children undergoing allogeneic HSCT, with AML/relapsed (*acute lymphoblastic leukemia*) ALL and severe aplastic anemia should be given antifungal prophylaxis. Patients with hematologic malignancies including leukemia, lymphoma, and myeloma undergoing autologous HSCT should also receive

TABLE 4: Antifungal agents at a glance.

	Fluconazole	*AMB-D*	*L-AMB*	*Voriconazole*	*Posaconazole*	*Echinocandins*
Candida	+	++	++	++	++	+++
Aspergillus	No	Yes	Yes	Yes	Yes	Yes
Mucor	No	Yes	Yes	No	Yes	No
Cryptococcus	Yes	Yes	Yes	Yes	Yes	No
Route available	IV, PO	IV	IV	IV, PO	PO, IV	IV
Adverse effects	++	++++	++	++	++	+
Drug interactions	++	+	+	+++	++	+

(AMB-D: amphotericin B deoxycholate; IV: intravenous; L-AMB: small unilamellar liposomal formulation; PO: per os)

TABLE 5: Treatment of fungal infections.

Type of fungal infection	*Drug of choice*	*Alternative drug*	*Comments*	*Duration of therapy*
Candida				
Suspected/confirmed invasive candidiasis in adults	Echinocandin	Amphotericin B/ fluconazole	Change in the recent guidelines that recommend echinocandins for all patients irrespective of level of sickness, azole exposure	Treat for 2 weeks after last negative culture Remove all intravascular catheters Do retinoscopic examination
Suspected/confirmed invasive candidiasis in children/neonates	Fluconazole *or* Amphotericin B	Echinocandin	Amphotericin B preferred as limited data on echinocandins in children AMB-D preferred to L-AMB in neonates	In neonates, treat for 3 weeks after last negative culture Look closely for CNS and eye involvement in neonates
Pyelonephritis	Fluconazole	Amphotericin B deoxycholate	Echinocandins and lipid amphotericin B not recommended	2 weeks Important to differentiate colonization from true infection
CNS candidiasis	L-AMB and flucytosine Followed by fluconazole	Fluconazole	Echinocandins not recommended as they do not cross the blood-brain barrier	Treat till complete clinical, CSF, and radiologic resolution
Endocarditis	L-AMB with 5-FC and then step down to fluconazole	Double dose echinocandins and then step down to fluconazole	Surgery is strongly recommended	6 weeks intensive therapy and then lifelong azoles
Osteomyelitis	L-AMB followed by fluconazole or fluconazole alone	AMB-D or echinocandin followed by fluconazole		Prolonged treatment of up to 6–12 months and surgical debridement is often needed

Contd...

Contd...

Type of fungal infection	*Drug of choice*	*Alternative drug*	*Comments*	*Duration of therapy*
Septic arthritis	L-AMB followed by fluconazole or fluconazole alone	AMB-D or echinocandin followed by fluconazole	Drainage of affected joint is necessary. For hip joint, open drainage is needed. For prosthetic joint infection, removal of joint is required	6 weeks therapy
Chronic disseminated candidiasis	Fluconazole alone for stable patients For sick patients, L-AMB or AMB-D followed by fluconazole	Echinocandin followed by fluconazole	Transition to fluconazole once patient is stable	Several months till all lesions have resolved radiologically. Treatment should continue till period of immunosuppression is over
Oropharyngeal candidiasis	Fluconazole orally or clotrimazole suspension	Voriconazole/posaconazole/itraconazole/echinocandin/AMB-D	Mild disease use topical therapy and moderate-to-severe disease use fluconazole Use other drugs in fluconazole refractory disease	7–14 days
Esophageal candidiasis	Fluconazole	Itraconazole/posaconazole/voriconazole Echinocandin	Oral fluconazole treatment of choice	14–21 days
Candida from respiratory secretions	Treatment generally not recommended			
Febrile neutropenia				
Empirical therapy	L-AMB or caspofungin	AMB-D Voriconazole		

Contd...

Contd...

Type of fungal infection	*Drug of choice*	*Alternative drug*	*Comments*	*Duration of therapy*
Aspergillosis				
Invasive aspergillosis	Voriconazole	L-AMB or caspofungin or micafungin or posaconazole or itraconazole	Consider surgical intervention Role of combination therapy with voriconazole and anidulafungin in some patients. If breakthrough on prophylaxis, switch to agent of another class	At least 6–12 weeks, in immunosuppressed patients continue till immunosuppression is over. For successfully treated patients, resume antifungal therapy once immunosuppression recommences
Aspergilloma	Role of medical therapy uncertain	Itraconazole or voriconazole	Surgical resection therapy of choice	
Allergic bronchopulmonary aspergillosis	Itraconazole	Voriconazole or posaconazole	Corticosteroids are mainstay of therapy	
Mucormycosis	L-AMB in maximally tolerated doses	AMB-D Posaconazole	Surgical resection important and treatment of underlying predisposing factor such as control of diabetes	Treat till clinical resolution and stabilization of radiologic lesions and underlying risk factor is corrected, at least 4 weeks
Cryptococcosis				
Cryptococcal meningitis	AMB-D and flucytosine followed by fluconazole	L-AMB followed by fluconazole Fluconazole and flucytosine	Manage intracranial pressure	Initial induction therapy for 2 weeks in HIV and 4–6 weeks in non-HIV and then consolidation with fluconazole for 10 weeks and then maintenance for 1 year or longer
Pneumocystis jiroveci pneumonia	TMP-SMX dosed at 15–20 mg/kg of TMP per day in 3–4 divided doses	Primaquine and clindamycin Caspofungin	Adjunct use of steroids in patients with severe PCP especially in the HIV infected	14 days in HIV infected and 21 days in the non-HIV infected

(AMB-D: amphotericin B deoxycholate; CFS: cerebrospinal fluid; CNS: central nervous system; 5-FC: 5-fluorocytosine; HIV: human immunodeficiency virus; L-AMB: small unilamellar liposomal formulation; TMP-SMX: trimethoprim-sulfamethoxazole)

TABLE 6: Antifungal prophylaxis in cancer chemotherapy and HSCT.

Drug choices	*Dose*	*Comments*
Fluconazole	6–8 mg/kg/day (maximum 400 mg) once daily	Most commonly recommended drug for children No protection against molds Interactions with vincristine/anticancer drugs
Itraconazole	5 mg/kg/day Q 12 hourly	Superior to fluconazole but more side effects Food interactions, need for TDM Drug interactions Nonavailability of syrup formulation Not commonly used
Voriconazole	In children below 12 years/<50 kg 8–9 mg/kg twice daily In children >12 years/>50 kg 400 mg twice daily on day 1 and then 200 mg twice daily	No protection against *Mucor* Need for TDM Drug interactions with many drugs chiefly cyclosporine and tacrolimus But the only oral mold active agent for children Adverse effects with prolonged therapy
Posaconazole (above 13 years)	Oral: 200 mg thrice daily IV: 300 mg twice daily on day 1 and then 300 mg once daily	Superior to fluconazole and itraconazole in adults with AML/MDS but more serious adverse effects Cannot be given in children below 13 years Food interactions and unpredictable pharmacokinetics for syrup Tablet form not available in India IV posaconazole is better Adverse effects and drug interactions
Amphotericin B deoxycholate	0.2 mg/kg/day	Noninferior to fluconazole But significantly more toxic May be an option in resource-limited setting
Liposomal amphotericin B	1 mg/kg alternate day 2.5 mg/kg twice weekly	Noninferior to fluconazole More toxic Administration problems
Aerosolized amphotericin B	12.5 mg on 2 consecutive days of week	Only effective for pulmonary molds Need for special nebulizer Cough may interrupt therapy Need to be combined with IV fluconazole for *Candida* protection
Micafungin	1 mg/kg/day (maximum dose 50 mg)	Noninferior to fluconazole Minimal adverse effects, no drug interactions IV route
Caspofungin	70 mg/m^2 day 1 and then 50 mg/m^2/day	Noninferior to itraconazole Minimal adverse effects, no drug interactions IV route

(AML: acute myeloid leukemia; IV: intravenous; MDS: myelodysplastic syndrome; TDM: therapeutic drug monitoring) antiyeast prophylaxis during the neutropenic phase. Newly diagnosed ALL, solid tumors do not merit routine prophylaxis.

Studies on fluconazole prophylaxis in allogeneic HSCT recipients have demonstrated reduced risk of both early and late candidiasis, gut-related *graft-versus-host disease* (GVHD), and mortality. However, the main limitation of fluconazole is no effect on molds. Subsequently, several agents including AMB-D, aerosolized amphotericin B, L-AMB, itraconazole, voriconazole, posaconazole, micafungin, and caspofungin have been evaluated against fluconazole. All these agents have limitations of cost, adverse effects, need for TDM, drug interactions, and nonavailability of pediatric data. There is no one size fits all drug. Hence, choice of antifungal prophylaxis varies between centers. Indian studies report a high incidence of mold infections in this predisposed population and hence need for a mold active agent is important. Table 6 discusses the choices for antifungal prophylaxis in children. In HSCT, the duration of prophylaxis is variable with either stopping prophylaxis with engraftment or continuing till immunosuppression is stopped in patients with GVHD or high-risk for GVHD (mismatched, unrelated, haploidentical or umbilical cord transplants).

CONCLUSION

The prognosis of several serious fungal infections has improved substantially as newer, less toxic antifungal drugs have become available, but still the invasive mycoses have remained difficult to treat. As new antifungal drugs are released and more data about combination regimens become available, we can look forward to more effective and better-tolerated treatments for candidiasis, aspergillosis, and other invasive mycoses.

RECOMMENDED READING

1. Como JA, Dismukes WE. Oral azole drugs as systemic antifungal therapy. New Eng J Med. 1994;330:263-72.
2. Dvorak CC, Fisher BT, Sung L, et al. Antifungal prophylaxis in pediatric hematology/oncology: new choices & new data. Pediatr Blood Cancer. 2012;59:21-6.
3. Groll AH, Castagnola E, Cesaro S, et al. Fourth European Conference on Infections in Leukaemia (ECIL-4): guidelines for diagnosis, prevention, and treatment of invasive fungal diseases in paediatric patients with cancer or allogeneic haemopoietic stem-cell transplantation. Lancet Oncol. 2014;15:e327-40.
4. Groll AH, Gea-Banacloche JC, Glasmacher A, et al. Clinical pharmacology of antifungal compounds. Infect Dis Clin North Am. 2003;17:159-91.
5. Hoesley CJ, Dismukes WE. New antifungal agents: emphasis on lipid formulations of amphotericin B. Clinical updates National Foundation for Infectious Diseases. 1999;II(2).
6. Pappas PG, Kauffman CA, Andes DR, et al. Clinical practice guideline for the management of candidiasis: 2016 Update by the Infectious Diseases Society of America. Clin Infect Dis. 2016;62(4): 409-17.
7. Patterson TF, Thompson GR 3rd, Denning DW, et al. Practice guidelines for the diagnosis and management of aspergillosis: 2016 Update by the Infectious Diseases Society of America. Clin Infect Dis. 2016;63(4):433-42.
8. Saag MS, Graybill RJ, Larsen RA, et al. Practice guidelines for the management of cryptococcal disease. Infectious Diseases Society of America. Clin Infect Dis. 2000;30:710-8.
9. Steinbach W. Antifungal agents in children. Paed Clin North Am. 2005;52:895-915.
10. Tomblyn M, Chiller T, Einsele H, et al. Guidelines for preventing infectious complications among hematopoietic cell transplantation recipients: a global perspective. Biol Blood Marrow Transplant. 2009;15:1143-238.

Antimicrobial Therapy of Assorted Infections

38
Chapter

Nigam Prakash Narain, Atul Kulkarni, Mahesh S Kore

ANTIMICROBIAL THERAPY OF VISCERAL LEISHMANIASIS (KALA-AZAR)

INTRODUCTION

Kala-azar [visceral leishmaniasis (VL)] is a disease of the reticuloendothelial system seen in tropical countries caused by members of the *Leishmania donovani* complex (a protozoan parasite) and transmitted by the bite of an insect vector, sandfly. The disease is characterized by irregular bouts of fever, substantial weight loss, hepatosplenomegaly, and progressive anemia. If left untreated, the fatality rate can be as high as 100% within 2 years. In India most of the cases of kala-azar are reported from Bihar, Jharkhand, Uttar Pradesh, and West Bengal. Widespread resistance to standard therapy with antimony compounds has made the treatment of kala-azar extremely complex. However, many new advances holding great promise have been made in the treatment of kala-azar in the recent years.

ANTILEISHMANIAL DRUGS

Antimony Compounds

For more than 60 years, pentavalent antimony compounds meglumine antimoniate and sodium stibogluconate (SSG) were the cornerstone of treatment for kala-azar worldwide. SSG (antimony 100 mg/mL) had been used widely in children with kala-azar in a dose of 20 mg/kg intramuscular (IM) daily for 30 days with initial response rates more than 90–95%. Most children improved and became afebrile within less than a week, whereas hematological restoration and significant subsidence of splenomegaly usually occurred within 2 weeks.

However, there were certain disadvantages to this drug, namely parenteral administration, long duration of therapy and frequent adverse effects. Systemic toxicity normally relates to the total dose administered and is usually reversible. The main adverse effects are ECG changes, increased transaminases, chemical pancreatitis, and pneumonitis. In order to decrease the adverse effects observed with this drug, efforts are on to develop lipid formulations of antimonials. A novel liposome-based meglumine antimonial formulation appears to be a promising product for the treatment of kala-azar.

However, in India and particularly in Bihar, parasite resistance to antimony compounds has emerged as a major problem. The reported prevalence of drug resistance to antimony compounds in Bihar is over 65%. Hence these drugs are no longer used in the treatment of kala-azar in India.

Pentamidine

A diamidine derivative, pentamidine isoethionate, has been used in the treatment of antimonial resistant kala-azar. It is given in a dose of 4 mg/kg, thrice weekly intravenous (IV)/IM for 6 weeks. However, the drug has many significant and some irreversible adverse effects including nephrotoxicity, bone marrow suppression, hypoglycemia, diabetes mellitus, pancreatitis, and arrhythmia-related sudden death.

The drug achieves poor response rates approximately 75% when used as a second-line drug in antimonial resistant cases; this has been a major factor in its limited use in the treatment of kala-azar.

Amphotericin B

It is the treatment of choice for kala-azar now. With this drug, 98% long-term cure rates have been obtained in both antimonial-unresponsive and previously untreated patients. It intercalates with the parasite ergosterol, and leads to damage to the cell membrane of the parasites. The drug is administered as 1 mg/kg on an alternate day schedule over a 30 day period. Daily therapy with 1 mg/kg/day for 2 weeks is also effective and well-tolerated. Standard protocols for hydration, premedication, and monitoring should be followed. The disadvantages of the drug include expense; infusion-related side effects, nephrotoxicity and need for prolonged hospitalization for IV administration and renal function monitoring.

In an effort to limit the toxicity associated with this drug and to shorten the duration of treatment, lipid associated formulations (amphotericin B colloidal dispersion, amphotericin B lipid complex, and liposomal amphotericin B) have been used and have proved to be highly effective and better tolerated than conventional amphotericin B. In India, long-term cure rates above 90–95% have been achieved with these formulations. However, respiratory distress has been observed in children under 6 years. These lipid formulations allow administration of considerably higher daily doses and simultaneously appear to target infected tissue macrophages via enhanced phagocyte uptake. Two regimens are commonly employed: A 5-day regimen of daily infusion at 3 mg/kg or a 10-day regimen with infusions on day 1–5 and on day 10. In 1997, US Food and Drug Administration (FDA) approved liposomal amphotericin B in the dose of 3 mg/kg on days 1–5, 14, and 21 for the treatment of visceral leishmaniasis (VL) in immunocompetent children.

However, in developing countries where the need is greatest, the use of these lipid formulations is prohibitively expensive. To reduce the cost, the simple mixing of amphotericin B with a commercially available fat emulsion has been proposed (at 2 mg/kg on alternate days for a total duration of 10 days). It has proved to be more affordable and equally effective.

Owing to the effectiveness, ease of use and assured compliance, a single-dose regimen of liposomal amphotericin B in a dose of 10 mg/kg administered as an infusion IV over 2 hours has been assessed in patients in Indian children with cure rates approaching 100%. This single dose therapy has been recommended by the World Health Organization (WHO) and has been included in the therapy of choice in the program for kala-azar elimination by National Vector Borne Disease Control Program (NVBDCP).

Miltefosine

It is the first orally effective drug against kala-azar. It is a phosphorylcholine ester of hexadecanol, a membrane active phospholipid. The drug has a long half-life in the range of 150–200 hours. The antileishmanial activity of miltefosine is related to a direct cytotoxic effect on the parasite and to the activation of cellular immunity against the parasitic infection. Leishmania have high levels of etherlipids on the surface and miltefosine acts on key enzymes involved in the later steps of metabolism of ether lipids. In vitro studies demonstrate that miltefosine stimulates T cells and macrophages to secrete activating cytokines including interferon (IFN) gamma and enhances macrophage production of microcidal reactive nitrogen and oxygen intermediates.

The recommended dose in children aged 2–12 years is 2.5 mg/kg/day for a period of 28 days. In patients aged more than 12 years with weight less than 25 kg the daily dose is 50 mg while in those above 12 years and weighing more than 25 kg the daily dose is 50 mg twice daily. The most important adverse effect of miltefosine is vomiting and diarrhea which may be seen in 20–40% of patients. There may be a rise in serum levels of aspartate aminotransferase (AST), alanine aminotransferase (ALT), creatinine and blood urea nitrogen (BUN). Grade III hepatotoxicity and renal damage has also been reported. These adverse effects usually occur in the first 2 weeks of therapy and are reversible in the face of continued treatment or after discontinuation of treatment. Overall, miltefosine is well tolerated in adults with considerably fewer adverse effects as compared to antimonials and amphotericin B.

Treatment with miltefosine with this regimen has been almost 100% effective and well tolerated in phase I/II studies conducted in India among antimonial resistant and untreated kala-azar patients. It is now approved for use in all cases of kala-azar in patients more than 2 years of age. It is contraindicated in pregnant, lactating women, and women of childbearing age who refuse contraception because of its teratogenic effects in animal studies. Miltefosine is available in India by the trade name of impavido (zentaris) as 10, 50, and 100 mg capsules.

Aminosidine (Paromomycin)

This is an amino glycoside antibiotic administered once daily, usually by the IM route. Combined with antimonials, paromomycin (12–18 mg/kg for 21 days) allows a reduction in the duration of the therapy and may be more efficient than antimonials alone in areas with high levels of antimonial resistance. Aminosidine also appears to be active when used alone in some Indian studies. However, it's potential for causing ototoxicity and nephrotoxicity is of concern. In the current era combination therapy of miltefosine and paromomycin for 10 days has also been used in India.

AGENTS UNDER EVALUATION

Sitamaquine

Sitamaquine (WR6026), an 8-aminoquinoline, first reported in 1994, may be a promising oral drug. Sitamaquine (1 mg/kg/day for 4 weeks) when administrated to 8 patients provided a 50% cure rate. More recently, a phase 2 dose-escalating trial was performed in Brazil. Cure rates for patients treated for 28 days were 0% and 67% at 1 mg/kg/day and 2 mg/kg/day, respectively. Further studies are needed to determine the efficacy and toxicity profile of this agent.

Interferon Gamma

Interferon gamma is a potent macrophage activator with synergistic activity with antimonials in mice. IFN gamma alone has limited efficacy in human VL.

In recent trials, daily IFN-gamma injections combined with pentavalent antimonial agents were shown to accelerate the clinical response and achieve a long-term cure in approximately two-third of cases unresponsive to treatment with antimonial compounds alone. However, in a randomized controlled study conducted in India where resistance to pentavalent antimonial agents is high, the same combination given for 28 days failed to show such adjunctive activity in terms of long-term cure. The high cost of IFN gamma precludes its widespread use in the developing world.

Allopurinol

At the beginning of the 1980s, nonrandomized trials showed that a combination of antimonials and allopurinol (15 mg/kg/day) was efficacious in treating VL. Recently, a randomized trial in patients with antimonial-unresponsive VL suggested that combined therapy with allopurinol plus pentamidine provided higher cure rate than with pentamidine alone. Allopurinol is not recommended as monotherapy.

RECOMMENDATIONS FOR THERAPY

The NVBDCP in its 2015 guidelines has made the following recommendations for the treatment of kala-azar in India:

- The first line is single dose liposomal amphotericin B @ 10 mg/kg
- If L-AMB cannot be given then options include:
  - Oral miltefosine for 28 days (contraindicated below 2, in pregnant and lactating women and women of childbearing age who refuse contraception and HIV-infected patients), (dosage mentioned earlier)
  - Oral miltefosine and IM paromomycin @ 11 mg/kg/day for 10 days
  - Amphotericin B deoxycholate @ 1 mg/kg alternate day for 30 days or 15 doses
- Amphotericin B lipid emulsion (Amphomul) in a dose of 15 mg/kg single dose has been introduced on a pilot basis in 2 districts (one each in Bihar and Jharkhand) under supervision of the Indian Council of Medical Research (ICMR).

MONITORING TREATMENT IN KALA-AZAR

The term *apparent cure* at the end of treatment on day 30 requires the absence of fever, general clinical improvement, a decrease in spleen size, and a parasite-free splenic or bone marrow aspirate smear. *Definitive cure* measured 6 months after treatment requires that the patient be healthy with no symptoms or signs of relapse. *Relapse* is defined as reappearance of signs and symptoms with positive parasite in bone marrow or splenic aspirates after initial cure with WHO recommended dosage of SSG usually within 6 months. *Primary unresponsiveness* is no clinical or parasitological improvement during or after the first course of treatment with SSG. *Secondary unresponsiveness* occurs during relapse after one or more courses of apparently successful treatment.

Evaluation of effectiveness of therapy of kala-azar is very important. Response to therapy can be assessed clinically and by repeat bone marrow or splenic examination. Although rK39 test is an excellent test for making a diagnosis of kala-azar, it cannot be used in predicting response to therapy or relapses, as immunoglobulin G antibodies persist in blood for long time after successful treatment. A latex agglutination test (KATEX), based on the detection of antigen in urine of the patients with VL, has been described to have a specificity of ~100% and a sensitivity of 47.7–100%. The test becomes negative after successful therapy. Polymerase chain reaction (PCR) can be used to make a definitive diagnosis of kala-azar, and in 85% patients it turns negative at the end of treatment and in 97% at 3 months.

ANTIMICROBIAL THERAPY OF RICKETTSIAL INFECTIONS

INTRODUCTION

Rickettsial diseases are group of specific communicable diseases caused by obligate intracellular gram-negative bacilli and transmitted to man by arthropod vectors. Among the various types of rickettsial infections, scrub typhus, Indian tick typhus, murine flea born typhus, and Q fever are reported from India.

THERAPY

Rickettsial infections respond dramatically well to treatment. Treatment should be initiated immediately in persons with signs and symptoms suggestive of rickettsial disease without waiting for diagnostic confirmation. Delay in diagnosis and treating rickettsial disease may result in increased severity and times may prove fatal. Treatment should not be discontinued solely on the basis of negative test result. Due to the nonspecific signs and symptoms of rickettsial diseases, early empiric treatment for rickettsial diseases often needs to be administered concomitantly with empiric treatment for other conditions in the differential diagnosis. For example, for a patient in whom meningococcal disease and tick-borne rickettsial disease are being considered, administering antibacterial therapy to treat potential *Neisseria meningitidis* infection in addition to administering doxycycline to treat rickettsial agents is appropriate while awaiting additional diagnostic information.

The drugs for rickettsial infections are easily available and are not expensive. Tetracycline, doxycycline, chloramphenicol, and azithromycin are the drugs advocated for the treatment of rickettsial infections. Though these drugs are routinely used, limited evidence and data are available with randomized controlled trials.

Doxycycline is the drug of choice for treatment of all rickettsial diseases in patients of all ages including children aged below 8 years, and dose of doxycycline (oral or IV) is 2.2 mg/kg/dose twice daily (maximum dose 200 mg/day, i.e. 100 mg twice daily). Intravenous therapy is indicated for more severely ill patients who require hospitalization, and in patients who are vomiting or obtunded. Intravenous doxycycline is given as infusion over 1–2 hours. Rapid administration should be avoided.

Fever typically subsides within 24–48 hours after treatment when the patient receives doxycycline in the first 4-5 days of illness. Lack of a clinical response within 48 hours of early treatment with doxycycline could be an indication that the condition is not a rickettsial disease, and alternative diagnoses or coinfection should be considered. Severely ill patients might require more than 48 hours of treatment before clinical improvement is noted, especially if they have multiple organ dysfunction.

The recommended duration of therapy is at least 3 days after subsidence of fever and until evidence of clinical improvement is noted, typically the minimum total course of treatment is 5–7 days. Severe or complicated disease could require longer treatment courses.

Doxycycline in Children

The American Academy of Pediatrics and Centre for Disease Control and Prevention (CDC) recommend doxycycline as the treatment of choice for children of all ages with suspected tick-borne rickettsial disease. Previous concerns about tooth staining in children aged below 8 years stem from experience with older tetracycline class drugs that bind more readily to calcium than newer members of the drug class, such as doxycycline. Doxycycline used at the dose and duration recommended for treatment of Rocky Mountain spotted fever (RMSF) in children aged below 8 years, even after multiple courses, did not result in tooth staining or enamel hypoplasia in a retrospective cohort study of 58 children who received doxycycline before the age of 8 years, compared with 213 children who had not received doxycycline. These results support the findings of a study published in 2007 reporting no evidence of tooth staining among 31 childrens with asthma exacerbation who were treated with doxycycline. The use of doxycycline to treat children with suspected rickettsial disease should no longer be a subject of controversy.

Alternative Antibacterial Agents to Doxycycline

Tetracyclines, including doxycycline, are the only antibacterial agents recommended for treatment of all tick-borne rickettsial diseases. Alternative effective drugs are macrolides (oral clarithromycin or oral/IV azithromycin), chloramphenicol, and rifampicin.

Azithromycin 10 mg/kg daily for 3–5 days and clarithromycin 15 mg/kg/day in two divided doses are effective treatment for rickettsial disease. A recent meta-analysis has shown no difference in outcomes between doxycycline, tetracycline, and azithromycin in scrub typhus. Data about chloramphenicol was scanty. Chloramphenicol has been used to treat RMSF; however, epidemiologic studies using CDC case report data suggest that patients with RMSF treated with chloramphenicol are at higher risk for death than persons who received a tetracycline. A recent randomized controlled trial in mild scrub typhus demonstrated rifampicin to be noninferior to doxycycline. However routine use of rifampicin is not recommended in India and it should be reserved for its antitubercular activity.

Rickettsial strains with reduced susceptibility to doxycycline are reported and alternative drugs can be used in such a situation. Doxycycline resistance should be suspected in patients with confirmed rickettsial disease who do not respond doxycycline.

Many classes of broad-spectrum antibacterial agents that are used empirically to treat febrile patients, such as beta-lactams, aminoglycosides, and sulfonamides, are not effective against tick-borne rickettsial diseases. Although some fluoroquinolones have in vitro activity against rickettsiae, their use for treatment of certain rickettsial infections has been associated with delayed subsidence of fever, increased disease severity, and longer hospital stay.

Sulfonamide antimicrobials are associated with increased severity of rickettsial diseases. Experimental and accumulated anecdotal clinical data suggest that treatment of patients with RMSF with a sulfonamide drug can result in increased disease severity and death. In some patients treated with sulfonamide or beta-lactam drugs, diagnosis and appropriate treatment of rickettsia illness was delayed because the development of a rash was mistaken for a drug eruption rather than recognized as a manifestation of rickettsial illness.

MANAGEMENT OF COMPLICATIONS AND ADJUVANT THERAPY

Rickettsial disease can be associated with encephalitis, pulmonary involvement, renal failure, and myocarditis. These should be managed symptomatically. Patients with rickettsial encephalitis may be treated with methylprednisolone 30 mg/kg for 3–5 days.

PREGNANCY AND LACTATION

Use of tetracycline class drugs has generally been contraindicated during pregnancy because of concerns about potential risk to the musculoskeletal development of the fetus, cosmetic staining of primary dentition in fetuses exposed during the second or third trimester, and development of acute fatty liver of pregnancy in the mother. Controlled studies to assess the safety of doxycycline use in pregnant women have not been conducted, and available data are primarily observational. An expert review on doxycycline use during pregnancy however concluded that therapeutic doses were unlikely to pose a substantial teratogenic risk; however, the data were insufficient to conclude that no risk exists. The risk for cosmetic staining of the primary teeth by doxycycline could not be determined because of limited data. No reports of maternal hepatic toxicity associated with doxycycline use have been published.

Doxycycline has been used successfully to treat tick-borne rickettsial diseases in several pregnant women without adverse effects to the mother; however, follow-up to address adverse effects to the fetus was limited. Chloramphenicol is a potential alternative treatment for RMSF during pregnancy; however, care must be taken when administering the drug late during the third trimester of pregnancy because of the theoretical risk for gray baby syndrome.

Doxycycline is excreted into breast milk at low levels; however, the extent of absorption by nursing infants is unknown. Short-term use of doxycycline as recommended for the treatment of tick-borne rickettsial disease is considered probably safe during lactation on the basis of available literature and expert opinion. Although doxycycline is not specifically addressed, tetracycline is listed by the American Academy of Pediatrics Committee on Drugs as "usually compatible with breastfeeding". Azithromycin can be used during pregnancy and lactation.

PREVENTIVE THERAPY AFTER TICK BITE

Studies of preventive antibacterial therapy for rickettsial infection in humans are limited. Available data do not support prophylactic treatment for rickettsial diseases in persons who have had recent tick bites and are not ill.

TREATMENT OF ASYMPTOMATIC PERSONS SEROPOSITIVE FOR RICKETTSIAL DISEASE

Treatment of asymptomatic persons seropositive for rickettsial diseases is not recommended regardless of past treatment status. Anti-rickettsial antibodies can persist in the absence of clinical disease for months to years after primary infection; therefore, serologic tests cannot be used to monitor response to treatment for tick-borne rickettsial diseases.

CONCLUSION

Doxycycline is the drug of choice and is safe in the recommended doses even in young children, pregnant and lactating mothers. Other alternative drugs like macrolides, chloramphenicol, and fluoroquinolones are inferior choices. It is imperative to have a high index of suspicion for rickettsial disease and make clinical diagnosis on basis of history and physical findings. Therapeutic trial with specific agent is justified because a delay in initiating treatment proves costly. Rapid and favorable response is suggestive of correct diagnosis.

ANTIMICROBIAL THERAPY OF LEPTOSPIROSIS

INTRODUCTION

Leptospirosis is a zoonosis, caused by pathogenic spirochetes of genus *Leptospira* mainly seen in tropical regions. Animals like rodents, swine, horse, goat, cattle, dogs, and sheep are natural hosts. Rodents are main reservoirs; they shed the organisms in urine throughout life and the organism remains alive in soil for months. It is transmitted by animal urine coming in contact with breaks in skin, or mucous membranes of the eye, mouth or nose. Transplacental transmission can occur. Farmers, sewer workers, and waders or swimmers in fresh water are at high-risk of contracting the disease. The disease can present as an undifferentiated febrile illness or a severe illness with multiorgan dysfunction (Weil's disease). *Leptospira* is an organism which is very susceptible to most antibiotics including those that are routinely used in an acute febrile illness. In that respect, it differs from rickettsia.

TREATMENT

Mild Cases

Doxycycline is an effective drug and can be safely administered even to children below 8 years and the usual dose is 3–4 mg/kg/day (maximum of 200 mg daily). Other alternatives include amoxycillin in a dose of 50 mg/kg in three divided daily doses or ampicillin in a dose of 100 mg/kg/day in divided doses. Treatment is for 7 days. In patients who are allergic to penicillin, one can treat with azithromycin (dose 10 mg/kg on day 1 followed by 5 mg/kg for 4 days).

Severe Cases

The drug of choice is penicillin G (dose 20,000 to 40,000 units/kg/day in six equally divided doses, maximum 6–12 million units daily) for 7 days. However penicillin G is not readily available. Another alternative is ceftriaxone 80–100 mg/kg/day once or twice daily (maximum 4 g) or cefotaxime 100–150 mg/kg/day in three divided doses for 7 days. For children with beta-lactam hypersensitivity, azithromycin 10 mg/kg/IV on day 1 then 5 mg/kg/IV on subsequent day or doxycycline 4 mg/kg IV/day in divided doses (maximum 200 mg/day) can be used. *Jarisch-Herxheimer reaction* is an acute response to clearance of spirochetes from circulation presenting with fever, rigors, and hypotension and may occur after initiation of antimicrobial therapy.

Acute respiratory distress syndrome is common in severe leptospirosis. There were uncontrolled studies suggesting benefit of high dose methylprednisolone at 30 mg/kg in patients with leptospirosis and pulmonary involvement when started early in the course of the disease. A recent randomized controlled trial however failed to show benefit of steroids in severe leptospirosis and in fact increased the risk of nosocomial infections. Hence the decision to use steroids should be on a case-by-case basis.

PREVENTION

Prophylactic strategies against leptospirosis following exposure to flood water have been often studied. A Cochrane review published in 2009 failed to show any benefit with doxycycline prophylaxis. However, recent quasi randomized study from Thailand with single dose of doxycycline 200 mg in people exposed to flood water showed 75% efficacy against leptospira infection, 85% efficacy against clinical leptospirosis, and 92% efficacy against clinical leptospirosis in patients who had a laceration.

Hence it is now recommended that patients having significant exposure to flood water should be given prophylaxis. Options include doxycycline 200 mg single dose in adults and 3 mg/k g in children. Although doxycycline can be given in younger children as well, the other option is to use azithromycin 10 mg/kg single dose. However, questions remain. What degree of exposure needs prophylaxis? What about repeated exposure? In people with repeated exposure weekly prophylaxis with doxycycline 200 mg has been suggested.

ANTIMICROBIAL THERAPY FOR BRUCELLOSIS

INTRODUCTION

Brucellosis is a zoonotic infection transmitted to humans by contact with fluids from infected animals (sheep, cattle, goats, pigs, or other animals) or derived food products, such as unpasteurized milk and cheese. *Brucella abortus* preferentially infects cattle, *B. melitensis* sheep and goats, *B. suis* infect pigs, *and B. canis* infect dogs. All these species can infect humans with *B. melitensis* being the most common. Human brucellosis is known for protean manifestations. The symptoms and signs most commonly reported are fever, fatigue, malaise, chills, sweats, headaches, myalgia, arthralgia, splenomegaly, hepatomegaly, and weight loss. Brucellosis is invariably underdiagnosed and treated as enteric fever, tuberculosis, malaria, and juvenile idiopathic arthritis (JIA).

TREATMENT

The goal of brucellosis therapy is to control the illness and prevent complications, relapses, and sequelae. Important principles of brucellosis treatment include use of antibiotics with activity in the acidic intracellular environment (doxycycline and rifampicin), use of combination regimens, and prolonged duration of treatment. Monotherapy and regimens shorter than 6 weeks are not accepted treatment strategies for brucellosis.

Treatment strategies depend on age of the child and severity of disease and are discussed in Tables 1 and 2. Broadly speaking in nonlocalizing disease, treatment is with trimethoprim-sulfamethoxazole (TMP-SMX) with rifampicin in children below 8 years and doxycycline with rifampicin above 8 years. Addition of aminoglycosides (gentamicin or streptomycin) to this backbone is indicated in children with complications or localizing disease. If streptomycin is used than 2 weeks therapy is recommended and if gentamicin is used than 7 days is usually

TABLE 1: Treatment of brucellosis.

	Children <8 years	*Children >8 years*
Non-localizing disease	TMP-SMX and rifampicin for 6 weeks	Doxycycline for 6 weeks and either aminoglycosides (streptomycin for 2 weeks/ gentamicin for 5–7 days) OR doxycycline and rifampicin for 6 weeks*
Spondylitis/sacroileitis/arthritis	TMP-SMX and rifampicin for 3 months and gentamicin for 7 days	Doxycycline and rifampin for 3 months and gentamicin for 7 days**
Neurobrucellosis	TMP-SMX and rifampicin and ceftriaxone for at least 6 weeks or till CSF normal	Doxycycline and rifampin and ceftriaxone for at least 6 weeks or CSF normal
Endocarditis Surgery almost always needed	TMP-SMX and rifampicin for 6 weeks to 6 months and gentamicin for 2–4 weeks	Rifampicin and doxycycline and TMP-SMX for 6 weeks to 6 months and gentamicin for 2–4 weeks

(TMP-SMX: trimethoprim-sulfamethoxazole)
*Meta-analysis shows that doxycycline with aminoglycoside is a superior regime than doxycycline and rifampicin.
** Can use a combination of quinolones with rifampicin for 3 months.

TABLE 2: Doses of antibrucella drugs.

Drug	*Dose in mg/kg/day*	*Maximum dose/day*
TMP-SMX	TMP 10 mg/kg/day in two doses	TMP—480 mg
Doxycycline	2–4 mg/kg/day in two doses	200 mg
Gentamicin	5 mg/kg once daily	240 mg
Streptomycin	15–20 mg/kg/day	1,000 mg
Rifampicin	15–20 mg/kg/day once daily	900 mg
Ciprofloxacin	20–30 mg/kg/day in two doses	1,500 mg
Ceftriaxone	100 mg/kg/day in two divided doses	4,000 mg

(TMP-SMX: trimethoprim-sulfamethoxazole)

sufficient. Quinolones can also be used in case of allergy or toxicity. In general triple drug therapies have superior sterilizing activity than dual regimes. Duration of therapy varies from 6 weeks to 6 months depending on site of disease.

Relapse

Patients should be monitored for relapse. Relapse rates rate from 5 to 10%. Relapse of symptoms should prompt assessment for a focal lesion. While antimicrobial susceptibility should be performed on any culture isolate, development of resistance is rare. Most relapses can be treated successfully with a repeat course of the recommended regimen for sufficient time.

RECOMMENDED READING

1. Brett-Major DM, Coldren R. Antibiotics for leptospirosis. Cochrane Database Syst Rev. 2012;(2):CD008264.
2. Brett-Major DM, Lipnick RJ. Antibiotic prophylaxis for leptospirosis. Cochrane Database Syst Rev. 2009;(3):CD007342.
3. Bukhari EE. Pediatric brucellosis. An update review for the new millennium. Saudi Med J. 2018;39(4):336-41.
4. Centre for Disease Control and Prevention (CDC). Rickettsial Diseases. [online] Available from http://www.cdc.gov/ncidod/diseases/sunmenus/sub_rickettsial.htm. [Accessed January 2018].
5. Chusri S, McNeil EB, Hortiwakul T, et al. Single dosage of doxycycline for prophylaxis against leptospiral infection and leptospirosis during urban flooding in southern Thailand: a non-randomized controlled trial. J Infect Chemother. 2014;20:709-15.
6. Davidson RN, Croft SL, Scott A, et al. Liposomal Amphotericin B in drug-resistant visceral Leishmaniasis. Lancet. 1991;337:1061-2
7. Dietze R, Carvalho SF, Valli LC, et al. Phase 2 trial of WR6026, an orally administered 8-aminoquinoline, in the treatment of visceral Leishmaniasis caused by Leishmania chagasi. Am J Trop Med Hyg. 2001;65:685-9.
8. El Sayed I, Liu Q, Wee I, et al. Antibiotics for treating scrub typhus. Cochrane Database Syst Rev. 2018;9:CD002150.
9. Herwaldt BL. Leishmaniasis. Lancet. 1999;354:1191-9.
10. Jha TK. Evaluation of Allopurinol in the treatment of kala-azar occurring in North Bihar, India. Trans R Soc Trop Med Hyg. 1983;77:204-7.
11. Meng F, Pan X, Tong W. Rifampicin versus streptomycin for brucellosis treatment in humans: A meta-analysis of randomized controlled trials. PLoS One. 2018;13(2):e0191993.
12. Murray HW. Treatment of visceral Leishmaniasis (kala-azar): a decade of progress and future approaches. Int J Infect Dis. 2000;4:158-77.
13. NVBDCP. Operational guidelines on kala azar elimination in India 2015. [online] Available from www.nvbdcp.gov.in [Accessed December 2018].
14. Pandey K, Pal B, Siddiqui NA, et al: Efficacy and safety of Liposomal Amphotericin B for Visceral Leishmaniasis in Children and Adolescents at a Tertiary Care Center in Bihar, India. Am J Trop Med Hyg. 2017;97(5):1498-502.
15. Pappas G, Akritidis N, Bosilkovski M, et al. N Engl J Med. 2005;352(22):2325-36.
16. Rathi N, Kulkarni A, Yewale V, et al. IAP Guidelines on Rickettsial diseases. Indian Pediatrics. 2017;54:223-9.
17. Rathi NB, Rathi AN, Goodman MH. Rickettsial diseases in Central India: proposed clinical scoring system for early detection of spotted fever. Indian Pediatr. 2011;48:867-72.
18. Rodrigo C, Lakshitha de Silva N, Goonaratne R, et al. High dose corticosteroids in severe leptospirosis: a systematic review. Trans R Soc Trop Med Hyg. 2014;108(12):743-50.
19. Sundar S, Agrawal G, Rai M, et al. Treatment of Indian visceral Leishmaniasis with single or daily infusions of low dose Liposomal Amphotericin-B: randomized trial. BMJ. 2001;323:419-22.
20. Sundar S, Agrawal S, Pai K, et al. Detection of leishmanial antigen in the urine of patients with visceral leishmaniasis by a latex agglutination test. Am J Trop Med Hyg. 2005;73(2):269-71.
21. Sundar S, Gupta LB, Rastogi V, et al. Short course, cost-effective treatment with Amphotericin B-fat emulsion cures visceral Leishmaniasis. Trans R Soc Trop Med Hyg. 2000;94:200-4.
22. Sundar S, Jha TK, Thakur CP, et al. Oral Miltefosine for Indian Leishmaniasis. N Engl J Med. 2002;347:1739-46.
23. Sundar S, More D, Singh M, et al. Failure of Pentavalent Antimony in Visceral Leishmaniasis in India: Report from the Center of the Indian Epidemic. Clin Infect Dis. 2000;31:1104-7.
24. Sundar S, Murray HW. Cure of antimony-unresponsive Indian visceral Leishmaniasis with Amphotericin B lipid complex (ABLC). J Infect Dis. 1996;173:762-6.

25. Sundar S, Murray HW. Effect of treatment with interferon-gamma alone in visceral Leishmaniasis. J Infect Dis. 1995;172:1627-9.
26. Thakur CP, Kanyok TP, Pandey AK, et al. Treatment of visceral Leishmaniasis with injectable Paromomycin (Aminosidine). An open-label randomized phase-II clinical study. Trans R Soc Trop Med Hyg. 2000;94:432-3.
27. Thakur CP, Singh RK, Hassan SM, et al. Amphotericin B deoxycholate treatment of visceral Leishmaniasis with newer modes of administration and precautions: a study of 938 cases. Trans R Soc Trop Med Hyg. 1999;93:319-23.
28. Watt G, Kantipong P, Jongsakul K, et al. Doxycycline and rifampicin for mild scrub-typhus infections in northern Thailand: a randomised trial. Lancet. 2000;356(9235):1057-61.
29. Yousefi-Nooraie R, Mortaz-Hejri S, Mehrani M, et al. Antibiotics for treating human brucellosis. Cochrane Database Syst Rev. 2012;10:CD007179.

Rational Antimicrobial Therapy—Illustrative Cases

39 Chapter

Tanu Singhal

INTRODUCTION

We have till this point deliberated a great deal on individual antimicrobials and antimicrobial therapy of common childhood illnesses. However, it is not often easy to make a choice in the practical setting. The objective of this chapter is to critically assess the choice of antimicrobials in various common case scenarios and suggest what might be the right choice in that setting. These cases progress from simple to increasingly complex settings.

CASE 1

A 1-year-old child, with normal weight for age, presents with loose stools of 1-day duration. Stools are watery and 15–20 times per day. There is mucous but no blood. The child has fever up to 101°F, is vomiting and not accepting orally. She is brought to hospital and found to have some dehydration. She is admitted and treatment with intravenous (IV) fluids, IV amikacin, and IV metronidazole is started. Stool routine examination showed 5–6 white blood cell (WBC) and 2–3 red blood cell (RBC) per high power field and cysts characteristic of *Entamoeba histolytica.*

Is antimicrobial therapy needed and is the choice appropriate?

The possible etiologies of acute watery diarrhea of the above description in an infant are predominantly viruses and *E. coli*. Antibiotics are not of any value in therapy of diarrhea caused by these organisms. Few fecal WBC and RBC can be present in any infective diarrhea and do not indicate invasive diarrhea meriting antibiotic therapy. The presence of cysts of *E. histolytica* is not indicative of amoebic dysentery as these might represent nonpathogenic *E. histolytica dispar*. For diagnosis of amoebic dysentery, it is essential to demonstrate the trophozoite form in a fresh stool sample. *E. histolytica* is responsible for less than 3% of diarrhea in children below age 5 even in developing countries.

Antibiotics are definitely indicated in the management of bloody diarrhea usually caused by *Shigella*. But even for *Shigella*, aminoglycosides are inappropriate agents and do not work in vivo despite in vitro susceptibility. Recommended therapeutic agents for bloody diarrhea are azithromycin, cefixime, or quinolones. Oral colistin is often used for diarrhea but is not of any therapeutic benefit.

To conclude this case and most cases of diarrhea do not merit any antibiotic therapy. Use of antibiotics only increases cost of therapy, adverse effects, and contributes to antibiotic resistance.

CASE 2

A 4-year-old child presents with fever, coryza, cough, and difficulty in swallowing. His younger sib had a similar illness few days back. On examination, he has enlarged congested tonsils and small cervical nodes. A throat swab culture is sent and he is started on oral amoxicillin. Two days later he is slightly better and throat swab culture shows beta-hemolytic *Streptococcus* resistant to penicillin. Antibiotics are changed to coamoxiclav, which is then continued for the next 5 days.

This clinical presentation is typical of a viral upper respiratory tract infection because of associated cough and coryza, presence of a similarly sick contact in the family and absence of features typical of a bacterial sore throat such as pus points on the tonsils or flushing of the tonsillar anterior pillar.

Is sending a throat swab culture and starting antibiotics justified?

About 15% of the normal population carries beta-hemolytic streptococcus in its throat as a normal commensal. A throat swab should be restricted to patients who present with a presumptive diagnosis of bacterial sore throat else it may pick up those cases where beta-hemolytic *Streptococcus* is only a commensal and hence lead to unjustified antibiotic therapy. This is what has happened in the index case.

Comment on the antibiotic sensitivity report of the isolate

Group A beta-hemolytic streptococcus is universally sensitive to penicillin with no resistance reported till date. Hence, the laboratory should be asked to recheck the sensitivity report. Antibiotic therapy was not justified in this case right from the beginning and changing to coamoxiclav is even worse!

CASE 3

A 6-year-old child presents with progressively increasing fever and cough of 5 days duration. There is no associated coryza. He has been taking antipyretics and cough suppressants with no improvement. On examination he has mild tachypnea and few scattered crepitations. The complete blood count shows hemoglobin (Hb) of 10 g/dL, a TLC of 14,000 with 60% polymorphs. Chest X-ray (CXR) shows a few scattered infiltrates. He is put on tablet cefixime in a dose of 10 mg/kg/day. 2 days later he is not better.

What is the diagnosis and what are the likely organisms?

This is a case of community-acquired pneumonia (CAP). The most common causes of CAP in children, above the age of 5 years are *Streptococcus pneumoniae, Mycoplasma pneumoniae,* and respiratory viruses. The white cell count is not a reliable indicator of etiology in this setting.

Comment on choice of antibiotics and what would be a rational choice?

In the absence of definitive etiologic diagnosis, antibiotics in CAP are prescribed on the basis of epidemiologic information and the clinical presentation. This usually means cover for *Pneumococcus* and/or *M. pneumoniae.* In the index case, the initial antibiotic should at least cover *Pneumococcus.* Cefixime a third-generation cephalosporin has poor activity against *S. pneumoniae.* An acceptable drug would be amoxicillin. In the event of nonresponse in 48–72 h or deterioration, antibiotic therapy may be switched to an antibiotic effective against *M. pneumoniae* such as azithromycin or clarithromycin. If the index case would be sick and requires inpatient care then one may use a dual cover for both pathogens right at onset. In this scenario, IV ceftriaxone or high-dose amoxicillin with azithromycin or clarithromycin is justified.

CASE 4

A 10-year-old child from Mumbai presents with high-grade fever of 6 days duration. He has poor appetite and has a toxic look. Physical examination is unremarkable. CBC shows an Hb of 10 g%, TLC of 5,400 with 60% polymorphs, no eosinophils, and normal platelets. Malarial parasites are not seen on peripheral smear. A presumptive diagnosis of enteric fever is made, blood culture is sent and treatment with IV ceftriaxone and amikacin is initiated.

Comment on the choice for empirical antibiotic therapy

Since there is increasing resistance to quinolones in *Salmonella enteritica*, quinolones have become redundant in the use of enteric fever in today's scenario. There is return of susceptibility to first-line drugs including amoxicillin, chloramphenicol, and cotrimoxazole. Based on current susceptibility patterns, cefixime or ceftriaxone or azithromycin is the drugs of choice for management of enteric fever. Despite in vitro susceptibility, amikacin does not have any in vivo activity against *Salmonella* and hence is not indicated in this patient.

Blood culture grows *Salmonella* susceptible to ceftriaxone, azithromycin, and first-line drugs. It is nalidixic acid resistant. It is day 4 of ceftriaxone therapy. Fever continues to be high but toxicity is less and oral intake has improved. Parents are very anxious and so oral azithromycin has been added to the regime.

Defervescence in typhoid fever takes time. Most studies indicate that the mean time is around 5–7 days. With beta-lactam therapy, delayed defervescence may also be related to poor intracellular penetration of the drug. If the patient is improving clinically then it may be worthwhile to wait rather than escalate therapy. In a recent randomized controlled trial in adults in Nepal, use of ceftriaxone or cefixime with azithromycin resulted in faster fever clearance as against use of ceftriaxone or cefixime alone by only 8 h (88 h vs 95 h) though bacterial eradication had been superior with the combination.

The patient is afebrile by day 7 with combination therapy. How should therapy be continued?

Here we can continue oral therapy with a single drug. Since the relapse rate is lesser and duration of therapy is shorter with azithromycin, oral azithromycin in a dose of 20 mg/kg (maximum dose 1 g) can be continued for a total period of 7–10 days.

CASE 5

A 5-year-old child presents to the outpatient department with fever of 3 days duration. He has pallor and spleen tip is palpable. Peripheral smear shows *Plasmodium vivax*. He is stable has no complicating features. He is given oral artemether lumefantrine in appropriate doses for 3 days. 3 weeks later he presents with repeat episode of vivax malaria.

Is this recrudescence or relapse or reinfection and why did this happen?

Since this episode happened within 28 days of the first episode, it is most likely recrudescence from the asexual blood phase protozoa. The drug of choice for uncomplicated malaria in our country is chloroquine. Though artemisinin-based therapy is also effective in vivax malaria, recrudescence rates are high with artemether lumefantrine as artemether is rapidly eliminated from the body. Hence, ACT including dihydroartemisinin piperaquine (currently not available in our country) would be better. It is also possible that the bioavailability of artemether lumefantrine may have been compromised, if it was not given with a fatty meal. It should also be noted that primaquine was not given. Apart from activity against the liver hypnozoites, primaquine also acts against the merozoites and thus acts as combination therapy for vivax malaria. Hence giving primaquine would have reduced the risk of both recrudescence and relapse.

How should this patient be treated now?

This patient should be now treated with oral chloroquine at 10 mg/kg loading and then 10 mg/kg at 24 h and 5 mg/kg at 48 h. Primaquine should be given at 0.3 mg/kg/day for 14 days after testing for glucose-6-phosphate dehydrogenase (G6PD).

The same patient presents 2 months later with another episode of vivax malaria. What is this and how should it be treated?

This episode can be a relapse (relapses can occur despite primaquine). This can also be a reinfection, if the patient is staying in a malaria endemic area. True differentiation is possible only by genetic studies, which are not commercially available. We can retreat with chloroquine and then give a higher dose of primaquine (0.5–0.75 mg/kg for 14 days) in this setting. Another option is to put the patient on weekly chloroquine suppressive prophylaxis at 5 mg/kg of base weekly for 3–6 months.

CASE 6

A 10-year-old child develops severe chickenpox followed by necrotizing fasciitis. He is started on meropenem and vancomycin.

Comment on the initial treatment

First, surgical debridement is crucial for good outcomes. The likely pathogens causing necrotizing fasciitis in setting of chickenpox are *Streptococcus pyogenes* and possibly *Staphylococcus aureus*. Ideal therapy here is a combination of ceftriaxone and clindamycin. Clindamycin is particularly important to reduce toxin production. Meropenem and vancomycin in this setting is not only irrational use of antibiotics but is also therapeutically inferior since it does not contain a toxin inhibitor.

The necrotic tissue is debrided and the culture grows methicillin sensitive *S. aureus* (MSSA). The blood culture also grows MSSA. How should therapy be modified?

Though the empiric regime covers MSSA to a fair extent, it is important to optimize therapy now that cultures are available. This is particularly important since there is bacteremia. Ceftriaxone, while fair for treating soft tissue, bone, and joint infections due to MSSA, is not enough for bacteremia. The optimum drug for treating MSSA are first-generation cephalosporins like cefazolin or cloxacillin. While cloxacillin has conventionally been regarded as the gold standard drug, need for frequent administration, cost and erratic availability are disadvantages. Recent retrospective studies have shown cefazolin as equally effective for treatment of MSSA infections with the exception of those of the central nervous system (CNS). A randomized controlled trial comparing cloxacillin and cefazolin is in the offing. IV cefazolin should be given for 2 weeks since there is MSSA bacteremia. Blood cultures should be repeated 72 h after starting optimum therapy to document clearance and careful search should be done for other sites of infection such as endocarditis, osteomyelitis, and arthritis.

CASE 7

A 7-year-old presents with pyrexia of unknown origin for the past 1 month. Extensive evaluation is done and finally a contrast computed tomography (CT) shows necrotic mediastinal nodes with no pulmonary lesions. Tuberculosis (TB) is suspected and the patient is started on the first-line regime with isoniazid, rifampicin, pyrazinamide, and ethambutol.

Comment on the initial management

While the diagnosis does appear to be TB, we should have tried to establish microbiologic diagnosis. A search can be made for peripheral nodes example supraclavicular nodes, which are simpler to biopsy. In the absence of such nodes, an attempt should be made for CT-guided biopsy of the lymph nodes or bronchoscopic biopsy. The limitations to these methods are availability, cost, and invasiveness. Since there are no parenchymal lesions, gastric or bronchoscopic lavage is likely to have a poor yield. So in the real world setting, many children with a similar presentation may have empiric antitubercular therapy started.

However, 4 weeks later there is no response to therapy and ofloxacin and streptomycin is added to the regime.

This approach is not justifiable. Possible reasons for nonresponse could be inadequate doses, poor compliance, and alternative diagnosis such as lymphoma or drug resistant TB. In case, it is something like a lymphoma, this therapy change is likely to delay the diagnosis further apart from being of no therapeutic value. In case of drug resistant TB adding two drugs to a failing regime is incorrect. In fact, neither ofloxacin nor streptomycin are currently recommended as second-line drugs for TB. So here, all efforts should be made for establishing the diagnosis even if it needs invasive methods and referral to a higher center. The lymph node should be sampled and sent for histopathology, TB culture, and Xpert *Mycobacterium tuberculosis* (MTB)/ Rif.

The lymph node histopathology shows caseating granulomas and the Xpert is positive for MTB complex, and there is no rifampicin resistance. Fever continues. Should more anti-TB drugs or steroids added to the regime?

It is sometimes possible to get a clinical response after even 8 weeks. Since we have confirmed diagnosis of TB and the sensitivity of Xpert for diagnosing rifampicin resistance is more than 98%, we can continue first-line treatment with antipyretics and counsel parents. There is no role for adding steroids or other anti-TB drugs at this time.

CASE 8

A primigravida undergoes an emergency lower segment cesarean section (LSCS) at 38 weeks of gestation for fetal distress. The duration of membrane rupture is 1 h. The baby is 2.2 kg with no birth asphyxia. He is kept in the neonatal intensive care unit (NICU) of a tertiary hospital for routine monitoring of blood sugars and also given IV cefotaxime for 3 days and discharged on day 5.

Comment on choice of antibiotic for prophylaxis of neonatal sepsis

Prophylactic antibiotics are often administered to neonates in the presence of maternal fever or signs of chorioamnionitis or prolonged rupture of membranes till neonatal sepsis has been excluded by relevant tests. In the index case, as none of these factors are present, there is no indication for antibiotic therapy and so the issue of choice of antibiotic becomes irrelevant. In fact, such practice can prove dangerous at times (see further). This baby also did not merit stay in the neonatal unit and should have been roomed in with the mother. Keeping the baby in the nursery is associated with exposure to drug-resistant pathogens.

This child is readmitted on day 7 with fever, irritability and excessive crying. The fontanelle is bulging and the skin is mottled. Septic screen is positive and cerebrospinal fluid (CSF) is suggestive of pyogenic meningitis. CSF and blood cultures have been sent and child started on IV ceftazidime and amikacin. Is the choice of antibiotic appropriate?

This baby has sepsis, meningitis, and early septic shock. The likely etiologic agents are *E. coli* and *Klebsiella* of possible nosocomial origin. Additionally, the organism could be an extended spectrum beta-lactamase producer since the child may have acquired infection in the NICU of a tertiary care hospital and there is history of exposure to third-generation cephalosporins. Hence, we need an antibiotic that will provide a good cover for an extended-spectrum beta-lactamase (ESBL) producing *E. coli* and *Klebsiella* and cross the CNS. Also the infection is very serious with a high risk of immediate mortality and long-term morbidity. Therefore, it is important to get the antibiotic right the first time, as there is no room for upgradation in case of nonresponse or after receiving culture reports. Ceftazidime is inappropriate in this respect that it does not cover for ESBL.

What should be the appropriate antibiotic in this scenario?

Available options for treating ESBL infections include cefepime, beta-lactam–beta-lactamase inhibitor combinations and carbapenems. Cefepime a fourth-generation cephalosporin has some stability against ESBL but is susceptible to an inoculum effect. If the organism burden is high, the minimum inhibitory concentration (MIC) rises; it is therefore not recommended for serious ESBL infections with high organism burden as in this scenario. The beta-lactam–beta-lactamase inhibitor combinations also exhibit the inoculum effect; and the beta-lactamase inhibitor does not cross the CNS. Hence, they too are inappropriate in this scenario. The carbapenems are the drugs of choice for serious ESBL infections and cross the CNS. Imipenem cilastatin should not be used for treating meningitis due to risk of seizures. Therefore, the choice is meropenem in maximum permissible doses (40 mg/kg 8 hourly) for a period of 3 weeks. Once culture reports are available, antibiotics can be suitably de-escalated.

Should meropenem be given as monotherapy or as combination therapy?

Meropenem is a very broad-spectrum drug and can be safely given as monotherapy. There is no need to add an aminoglycoside to the regimen. Meropenem does not cover methicillin-resistant *S. aureus* (MRSA) and hence, if MRSA is of concern vancomycin or linezolid may be added to broaden the empirical spectrum. However, the scenario described above is in all likelihood the consequence of a gram-negative infection so empirical MRSA cover is probably not justified unless the unit in which the baby was kept has a high incidence of MRSA infection.

CASE 9

A 7-year-old child presented to the hospital with severe abdominal pain of 3 days duration associated with fever and vomiting. On examination, he has tachycardia, tachypnea, fever, and hypotension. The abdomen shows board like rigidity with absent bowel sounds. A diagnosis of acute appendicitis with perforation, secondary bacterial peritonitis with septic shock and acute respiratory distress syndrome is made and the child resuscitated with fluids, antibiotics (cefotaxime and metronidazole), ventilated and taken for urgent surgical exploration. Postoperatively, he is on the ventilator, has a jugular central venous line and urinary catheter. He steadily improves and by day 7 inotropes have been stopped and there is no fever. However, weaning from the ventilator is still not possible. Tracheal cultures are sent, there is no leukocytosis or new infiltrates on the CXR. Tracheal cultures show *Pseudomonas aeruginosa*, colony count 10^5/mL sensitive to carbapenems. Antibiotics are changed to meropenem.

Is this change of antibiotics appropriate?

There is no evidence of ventilator-associated pneumonia as there is no fever or leukocytosis or purulent secretions or new CXR infiltrates. There is an alternative cause for inability to wean the patient from the ventilator. Sending tracheal secretions for culture was not indicated and the *Pseudomonas* is a colonizer. Hence, change of antibiotics is not justified.

About 5 days later this child is still on the ventilator and starts running fever. Tracheal secretions increase in quantity and are purulent. CBC shows a count of 16,000 with 80% polymorphs and CXR shows right lower zone consolidation. Tracheal secretions again grow *P. aeruginosa* 10^5/mL but now resistant to meropenem and only sensitive to colistin. How should this infection be treated?

This child now definitely has a ventilator-associated pneumonia. Unfortunately due to inappropriate antibiotic therapy, earlier a valuable treatment option is lost. Carbapenem resistance in *Pseudomonas* occurs readily following drug pressure due to induction of carbapenemases or activation of the drug efflux pump that pumps the meropenem out of the bacterial cell. Treatment options now are confined to colistin. The microbiology laboratory should also be asked to check for sensitivity to imipenem, if not already done as sometimes there may be discordance in sensitivity to different carbapenems due to different mechanisms of resistance. This case shows us clearly why not to mess with antibiotics in a desperate situation and land up into a situation where nothing will work!

CASE 10

A 7-year-old child is admitted to the ICU with severe dengue fever with shock. He is resuscitated with fluids and inotropes and intensively monitored. He has an indwelling central line, an arterial line and an indwelling urinary catheter but is not on the ventilator. Is also on cefotaxime and amikacin, which had been started empirically on admission and have still been continued Patient improves gradually but by day 7 starts running low grade fever again after a 3-day intervening afebrile period. Clinically, he is nontoxic. Nosocomial infection is thought of and complete blood count, paired cultures (central line and peripheral blood), urine routine and urine cultures, CXR, and CBC sent. CBC, CXR, and urine routine are normal, central line culture shows coagulase negative *Staphylococcus* (CONS) and urine culture shows *Candida albicans* 1,000 colonies/mL. Peripheral blood culture is sterile. He is put on IV vancomycin and IV fluconazole but fever persists even 48 h later.

Comment on line of management and choice of antimicrobials

This child should not have received cefotaxime and amikacin in the first instance. If they were started before establishing a diagnosis of severe dengue, they should have been stopped once a diagnosis was made. Administration of these antibiotics will lead to selection of resistant organisms in the child and consequent risk of infection with more resistant organisms. Later, a positive central line culture alone is poorly predictive of a catheter related bloodstream infection especially if the pathogen is CONS and more likely to represent colonization of the catheter. Similarly colonization of the urinary tract with *Candida* is fairly common in a catheterized patient on broad-spectrum antibiotics. In the absence of local symptoms and normal urine routine as in the index case the *Candida* is also a colonizer.

What should be the line of management in this scenario?

The index case is nontoxic, stable and has no leukocytosis. He probably does not need the central line and indwelling catheter at this juncture. It will therefore be appropriate to remove both the catheters, stop the broad-spectrum antibiotics and observe. This is sufficient to get rid of both the colonizers (CONS and *Candida*). If fever persists, a fresh search for etiology can be made. However, if the same index case had accompanying toxicity and organ dysfunction with fever, nosocomial infection is high on the cards. The child then should be started empirically on broad-spectrum antibiotics based on the local experience with the ICU flora and sensitivity and may include a beta-lactam–beta-lactamase inhibitor combination or carbapenem. In this setting, even antifungal therapy may have to be considered since isolation of *Candida* from a nonsterile site could represent invasive candidiasis in this setting.

RECOMMENDED READING

1. Crump JA, Barrett TJ, Nelson JT, et al. Reevaluating fluoroquinolone breakpoints for *Salmonella enterica* serotype typhi and for non-typhi salmonellae. Clin Infect Dis. 2003;37:75-81.
2. Davis JS, Turnidge J, Tong S. A large retrospective cohort study of cefazolin compared with flucloxacillin for methicillin-susceptible *Staphylococcus aureus* bacteraemia. Int J Antimicrob Agents. 2018;52(2): 297-300.
3. Fagon JY. Hospital-acquired pneumonia: diagnostic strategies: lessons from clinical trials. Infect Dis Clin North Am. 2003;17:717-26.
4. Falagas ME, Kasiakou SK. Colistin: the revival of polymyxins for the management of multidrug-resistant gram-negative bacterial infections. Clin Infect Dis. 2005;40:1333-41.
5. Gerdes JS. Diagnosis and management of bacterial infections in the neonate. Pediatr Clin North Am. 2004;51:939-59.
6. Gogtay N, Kannan S, Thatte UM, et al. Artemisinin-based combination therapy for treating uncomplicated *Plasmodium vivax* malaria. Cochrane Database Syst Rev. 2013;(10):CD008492.
7. Kapil A, Renuka, Das B. Nalidixic acid susceptibility test to screen ciprofloxacin resistance in *Salmonella typhi*. Indian J Med Res. 2002;115:49-54.
8. Lundstrom T, Sobel J. Nosocomial candiduria: a review. Clin Infect Dis. 2001;32:1602-7.
9. Martin SI, Kaye KM. Beta-lactam antibiotics: newer formulations and newer agents. Infect Dis Clin North Am. 2004;18:603-19.
10. Martin SI, Kaye KM. Beta-lactam antibiotics: newer formulations and newer agents. Infect Dis Clin North Am. 2004;18:603-19.
11. McIntosh K. Community-acquired pneumonia in children. N Engl J Med. 2002;346:429-37.
12. Mermel LA, Farr BM, Sheretz RJ, et al. Guidelines for the Management of Intravascular Catheter-Related Infections. Clin Infect Dis. 2001;32:1249-72.
13. Parry CM, Hien TT, Dougan G, et al. Typhoid fever. N Eng J Med. 2002;347:1770-82.
14. Paterson DL, Bonomo RA. Extended-spectrum beta-lactamases: a clinical update. Clin Microbiol Rev. 2005;18:657-86.
15. Rodrigues C, Shenai S, Mehta A. Enteric fever in Mumbai, India: the good news and the bad news. Clin Infect Dis. 2003;36:535.
16. Shulman ST, Bisno AL, Clegg HW, et al. Clinical practice guideline for the diagnosis and management of group A streptococcal pharyngitis: 2012 Update by the Infectious Diseases Society of America. Clin Infect Dis. 2012;55(10):1279-82.
17. WHO. 2005. The treatment of diarrhea. A manual for physicians and other senior health workers. 2005 WHO/CDD/SER/80.2. [online] Available from: http://apps.who.int/iris/handle/10665/43209 [Accessed January, 2019].
18. Working Group on Tuberculosis, Indian Academy of Pediatrics (IAP). Consensus statement on childhood tuberculosis. Indian Pediatr. 2010;47(1):41-55.
19. World Health Organization. Guidelines for treatment of malaria, 3rd edition. [online] Available from: https://www.who.int/malaria/publications/atoz/9789241549127/en/ [Accessed January, 2019].
20. Zmora N, Shrestha S, Neuberger A, et al. Open label comparative trial of mono versus dual antibiotic therapy for typhoid fever in adults. PLoS Negl Trop Dis. 2018;12(4):e0006380.

Antimicrobial Formulary

Chapter 40

Suhas Prabhu, Jeeson Unni

TABLE 1: Antibacterial agents.

Name	*Formulations*	*Dosage and interval*	*Adverse effects*	*Drug interactions*
Penicillins A. Penicillinase susceptible Amoxicillin	Inj: 250, 500 mg. Cap/Tab/DT: 125, 250, 500 mg. Syp: 125, 250 mg/5 mL Drp: 100 mg/mL	Oral: N; 10–20 mg/kg bd >1 week 10–15 mg/kg tds If penicillin resistance suspected 20–30 mg/kg tds Inj: 30–50/kg tds M: 500 mg bd or tds In uncomplicated gonorrhea: 3 g with 1 g probenecid	Anaphylactic, allergic reactions, drug fever, rash, (especialy with infection mononucleosis), urticaria, perioral edema, nausea, epigastric distress, diarrhea less common	Probenecid increases amoxicillin levels
Ampicillin	Inj: Vial 250, 500, 1,000 mg. Cap/Tab/DT: 125, 250, 500 mg. Syr: 125, 250 mg/5 mL. Drp: 100 mg/mL	IV N: 50 mg/kg bd 1–4 weeks 37.5–50 mg/kg qds. Up to 100 mg/kg qds in Group B *Streptococcus* infection or meningitis. >4 weeks 50–100 mg/kg qds. Oral: 12.5–25 mg/kg qds (up to 100 mg/kg qds in serious infections) M = 12,000	Nausea, epigastric distress, diarrhea, anaphylactic and allergic reactions, drug fever, rash (especialy with infection mononucleosis), urticaria	Chloroquine reduces ampicillin absorption. Probenecid increases ampicillin levels. Prolongation of prothrombin time with warfarin. With allopurinol increased frequency of skin rashes

Contd...

Contd...

Name	*Formulations*	*Dosage and interval*	*Adverse effects*	*Drug interactions*
Penicillin G	Inj: 500,000 units/ vial (300 mg) Tab: 200,000, 400,000, 800,000 units *600 mg = 1,000,000 units (1 megaU) or 1 unit = 1,666 mg*	Inj IV: N: 25 mg/ kg bd. 1–4 weeks 25 mg/ kg tds. >4 weeks 25 mg/ kg qds. Serious infections: N: 50 mg/kg bd 1–4 weeks 50 mg/ kg tds >4 weeks 45–75 mg/kg qds. Double dose in meningitis q 4 hourly, max single dose 2.4 g (approx 40 L units) and a max daily dose of 14.4 g (approx 2–3 million units)	Anaphylactic and allergic reactions, drug fever, rash, urticaria, joint pains, serum sickness, Jarisch-Herxheimer reaction, neutropenia, encephalopathy, convulsions after high doses	Guar gum reduces absorption, probenecid (20 mg/kg bd M = 1,000 mg) delays excretion
Phenoxymethyl penicillin	Tab: 125 mg 250 mg	Oral: <1 year old 62.5 mg qds 1–5 yrs 125 mg qds, 6–12 years 250 mg qds, 12–18 years old 500 mg qds. 750 mg qds for severe infections. Rheumatic fever/postsplenectomy prophylaxis —500 mg/day in 2 divided doses	As above	Guar gum, neomycin, reduce absorption. Probenecid (20 mg/kg bd M = 1,000 mg) delays excretion
Procaine penicillin (usually in combination with penicillin G)	Inj: Procaine penicillin 300,000 units + penicillin G 100,000 units. Procaine penicillin 600,000 units + penicillin G 400,000 units. Procaine penicillin 800,000 units + penicillin G 200,000 units	60 mg/kg/50,000 units/kg od IM M = 2,400 mg	As above. Additionally procaine sensitivity possible	Probenecid (20 mg/kg bd M = 1000 mg) delays excretion
Benzathine penicillin	Inj: 600,000 units, 12,000,000 units and 24,000,000 units	<2 years 60,000 units/kg, 2–9 years (<27–30 kg) 600,000 units, >27–30 kg 1,200,000 units single dose deep IM	As for penicillin G	

Contd...

Contd...

Name	*Formulations*	*Dosage and interval*	*Adverse effects*	*Drug interactions*
		Congenital syphilis—50,000 units/kg/dose (max 24 L units) once a week for 3 weeks. Early syphilis in adolescents—24 L units as single dose in 2 injection sites. If present for >1 year—24 L units as single dose in 2 injection sites once weekly for 3 doses		
Piperacillin *Generally used only in combination with tazobactam*	Inj: 1,000, 2,000, 4,000 mg	IV (by infusion or slow inj) P: <2 kg <7 days 75 mg/kg bd, N: 100 mg/kg tds; >28 days old: 50–75 mg/kg tds or qds M = 16,000	Anaphylactic and allergic reactions, drug fever, rash, leukopenia, convulsions with high doses	Probenecid delays excretion, inactivates aminoglycosides warfarin increase INR
B. Penicillinase resistant Cloxacillin	Inj: 250, 500 mg. Cap: 250, 500 mg. Syr: 125 mg/5 mL	Newborn IV/oral <7 days 25–50 mg/kg bd; 7–21 days 25–50 mg/tds, > 21 days 25–50 mg/kg qds. May be increased to 100 mg/kg/dose in severe infection (meningitis, cerebral abscess, staph osteitis). M = 12,000. Oral used only for minor infections. Oral <1 year 250 mg/day, 1–5 years 500 mg/day, 5–18 years 1 g in 4 divided doses	Anaphylactic and allergic reactions, drug fever, rash, urticaria, joint pains, serum sickness, GI upsets	Loss of potency when mixed with aminoglycoside-serythromycin, polymixin B, vitamin C. Sulpha, aspirin inhibit protein binding, increasing free cloxacillin level
C. Penicillins with beta-lactamase inhibitors Amoxicillin-clavulanate	Inj: *(Amoxy + Clavulanate)* 1,000 + 200, 500 + 100, 250 + 50	*Dosed on the amoxicillin component* Oral: N; 10–15 mg/kg bd.	Anaphylactic and allergic reactions, drug fever, rash, urticaria, perioral edema.	Probenecid increases amoxicillin levels

Contd...

Contd...

Name	*Formulations*	*Dosage and interval*	*Adverse effects*	*Drug interactions*
	Tab: 500 + 125, 400 + 57, 250 + 125, 200 + 28.5, Syr: 400+57, 200 + 28.5, 125 + 31.25	Children > 1 week 15–20 mg/kg bd. Higher doses of 40–45 mg/kg bd for infection due to intermediate resistance pneumococci. Oral: Give at the start of a meal. IV: 25–30 mg/kg of amoxicillin component tds	Nausea, epigastric distress, diarrhea more common	
Ampicillin-sulbactam	Inj: Ampicillin 1,000, 500 + sulbactam 500, 250. Tab: Ampicillin 220 + sulbactam 147	*Calculated on ampicillin* IV N: 50 mg/kg bd. 1–4 weeks 37.5–50 mg/kg qds. >4 weeks 50–100 mg/kg qds. M = 12,000 mg	Gastritis, diarrhea, anaphylactic and allergic reactions, drug fever, rash, urticaria	Probenecid increases ampicillin levels. Prolongation of prothrombin time with warfarin
Piperacillin-tazobactam	Inj: Vials 2,000 mg piperacillin + 250 mg tazobactam; 4,000 mg piperacillin + 500 mg tazobactam	Dosed on piperacillin component By IV infusion N: 90 mg/kg tds. Child: 75–100 mg/kg tds. M = 16,000	Anaphylactic and allergic reactions, drug fever, rash, leukopenia, convulsions with high doses	Probenecid delays excretion, inactivates aminoglycosides warfarin increase INR
Cephalosporins *First-generation* Cephalexin	Cap/Tab/DT: 125, 250, 500 mg. Syp: 125, 250 mg/5 mL Drp: 100 mg/mL	10–25 mg/kg qds Adolescent 250–500 mg 4 times daily. M = 4000 mg.	Diarrhea, dyspepsia, rarely nausea, vomiting. Allergic reactions (rash, urticaria and angioedema) uncommon. Rarely headache, dizziness and fatigue	Probenecid increases levels
Cefadroxil	Cap/Tab/DT: 125, 250, 500 1,000 mg. Syp: 125, 250 mg/5 mL Drp: 100 mg/mL	10–20 mg/kg bd Adolescent and adults 500–1,000 mg bd M = 2000 mg	Rash, pruritis, urticaria, angioedema rare. Rarely diarrhea, dyspepsia, nausea, vomiting, fatigue, headache, dizziness	Probenecid increases blood levels which may cause nephrotoxicity

Contd...

Contd...

Name	*Formulations*	*Dosage and interval*	*Adverse effects*	*Drug interactions*
			Reversible neutropenia, mild elevation in transaminases and Stevens–Johnson syndrome	
Cefazolin	Inj: Vials 125, 250, 500, 1,000	15–50 mg/kg tds M = 6,000	Skin rash, eosinophilia, convulsions, bone marrow supression	Probenecid increases levels of cefazolin. Prolongation of prothrombin time with warfarin. Nephrotoxicity with aminoglycosides
Second-generation Cefaclor	Tab/DT/Cap 250, 375, 500 Syp 125, 187.5, 250 mg/5 mL. Drp: 50 mg/mL	7–15 mg/kg tds. Orally < 1 year 62.5 mg, 1–5 years 125 mg, 6–18 years 250 mg/dose tds. Dose doubled in severe infection. M = 1,000	Diarrhea, vomiting, skin rash, urticaria, pruritus, eosinophilia, may cause serum sickness like reactions	Probenecid increases levels. Prolongation of prothrombin time with warfarin. Nephrotoxicity with aminoglycosides
Cefuroxime Oral formulation available as cefuroxime axetil	Inj: Vials 500, 750, 1,500 mg Tab: 125, 250, 500, 750 mg Syr: 125 mg/5 mL	Inj IV N: 25 mg/kg bd 1–4 weeks. 25 mg/kg tds (up to 50 mg/kg in severe infection) >4 weeks 25–mg/kg tds or qds (50–100 mg/kg in severe infection) M = 6,000 mg. Oral: 10–20 mg/kg bd or tds Adolescents and adults 500 mg bd Double the dose for severe LRTI	Hypersensitivity reactions including rashes and fever. Gastrointestinal disturbances like nausea, diarrhea and vomiting. Rarely transient rises in liver function tests	Increased chances of nephrotoxicity when using high doses along frusemide and/or aminoglycosides
Third-generation Cefotaxime	Inj: Vial 125, 250, 500, 1,000, 1,500	P: <2 kg <7 day 50–100 mg/kg bd, >7 day tds. N: (severe infections like meningitis)	Nausea, vomiting, skin rash, drug fever, anaphylaxis, leukopenia, thrombocytopenia, local pain	Probenecid delays excretion, increase risk of bleeding with warfarin

Contd...

Contd...

Name	*Formulations*	*Dosage and interval*	*Adverse effects*	*Drug interactions*
		50 mg/kg/dose <7 day bd, 7–21 days tds, 21–30 days 3–4 times. Child: 12.5 –50 mg/kg qds M = 12,000		
Ceftriaxone	Inj: Vial 100, 125, 200, 250, 500, 750, 1,000, 2,000	IM or IV 50–100 mg/kg od or 25–50 mg/kg bd. M = 4,000 mg	Pain at inj site. Hypersensitivity: skin rashes, drug fever and very rarely anaphylaxis. Transient rise in liver enzymes, biliary sludge formation. Diarrhea and pseudomembranous colitis rarely. Nephrotoxicity with high doses, neutropenia, thrombocytopenia, hemolytic anemia may occur. Competition with bilirubin binding to albumin may cause kernicterus at loewer bilirubin levels	Increased chances of nephrotoxicity with concomitant use of frusemide, aminoglycosides. Antagonism of bacterial killing by chloramphenicol
Ceftizoxime	Inj: Vials 200, 1,000	Child 30–50 mg/kg tds M = 12,000	Pain at inj site, rash, neutropenia, thrombocytopenia, eosinophilia	Probenecid slows excretion, increase risk of bleeding with warfarin, increase chances of nephrotoxicity with aminoglycosides
Ceftazidime	Inj: Vials 250, 500, 1,000	IV, IM N: <7 days and >7 days <1,200 g 30–50 mg/kg bd >7 days >1,200 g 30–50 mg/kg tds Child: 25–50 mg/kg tds M = 6,000	Pain at inj site, rash, neutropenia, thrombocytopenia, eosinophilia, positive Coomb's test	Possible antagonism of effect with chloramphenicol. Increase risk with other nephrotoxic drugs. Chemical inactivation if mixed with aminoglycosides

Contd...

Contd...

Name	*Formulations*	*Dosage and interval*	*Adverse effects*	*Drug interactions*
Cefoperazone	Inj: Vials: 250, 500, 1,000, 2,000	50–100 mg/kg bd M = 4000	Skin rash, urticaria, increase liver enzymes, reversible neutropenia, GI upset, hypoprothrombinemia	Probenecid increases levels. Increase chances of nephrotoxicity with frusemide, aminoglycosides. Antagonism of bacterial killing by chloramphenicol
Cefixime	Tab/DT 100, 200, 400. Syp: 50 mg/5 mL, 100 mg/5 mL	4 mg/kg bd or 8 mg/kg od 10 mg/kg bd for enteric fever M = 1,200	Mild changes in liver and renal function tests. Diarrhea, abdominal pain, nausea, vomiting, rash and headache. Thrombocytopenia, leukopenia, eosinophilia, pseudomembranous colitis (rare) and hypersensitivity reactions	False-positive reaction with benedicts test in urine
Cefpodoxime	Tab/DT: 50, 100, 200 mg Syr: 50, 100 mg/5 mL	Oral: 4.5 mg/kg bd or 9 mg/kg od M = 400 mg	Diarrhea, nausea, vomiting, abdominal pain. Occasionally headache, allergic reactions	Absorption decreased by antacids or histamine H_2 antagonists
Cefdinir	Cap/Tab: 300 Syp: 125 mg/5 mL.	7 mg/kg bd or 14 mg/kg od M = 600 mg	Abdominal pain, diarrhea, nausea, vomiting, constipation. Headache, dizziness, insomnia, somnolence, confusion, rash, pruritus. Hypotension, palpitation, anaphylaxis, angioedema	Therapeutic iron and antacids reduce absorption. Frusemide increase nephrotoxicity. Probenecid delays excretion
Fourth-generation Cefepime	Inj: 250, 500, 1,000, 2,000	N: <14 days 30 mg/kg bd IV/IM. >14 days 50 mg/kg bd IV/IM. Children IV 50 mg/kg every 8 h (maximum 2 g/dose). M = 6,000	Pain, inflammation at inj site, rash, pruritus, fever, GI upset, CNS symptoms, hemolytic anemia	Probencid delays excretion. Increase nephrotoxicity with frusemide, aminoglycosides

Contd...

Contd...

Name	*Formulations*	*Dosage and interval*	*Adverse effects*	*Drug interactions*
Cephalosporins with betalactam inhibitors				
Cefoperazone-sulbactam	Inj cefoperazone 1,000 + sulbactam 500; cefoperazone 1,000 + sulbactam 1,000	Dosed on the cefaperazone component	As for cefoperazone	As for cefoperazone
Monobactams				
Aztreonam	Inj: Vial 250, 500, 1,000, 2,000	IV dose (over 3–5 min or as infusion) 30 mg/kg P: <7 d <2 kg bd, >7 d <2 kg and <7 d >2 kg tds, >7 d >2 kg qds. In severe infection and cystic fibrosis in >2–12 years increase up to 50 mg/kg tds or qds 12–18 years 1 g tds or 2 g bd M = 8,000	Local reaction at injection site, altered taste, jaundice, rash. Thrombocytopenia, neutropenia may occur	Incompatible in solutions with metronidazole or vancomycin. Increase effect of warfarin
Glycopeptides, lipopeptides				
Vancomycin	Vials 500, 1,000	By IV infusion, 15 mg/kg od in P <28 weeks gestation; 18 hourly in P >28 weeks gestation and age <7 d; bd in P >7 d and N <7 d; tds in term N >7 d. Infants and child: 10 mg/kg qds. For meningitis 15 mg/kg qds. For critically sick patients loading dose of 30 mg/kg. For *C. difficile* colitis PO 125 mg or 10 mg/kg qds M = 2,000 mg Intrathecal doses. N: 2.5–5 mg od 1 month to 4 years 5 mg, 4–15 years 10 mg and > 15 years 20 mg od	Flushing soon after infusion, drug fever, neutropenia, nephrotoxicity, ototoxicity, anaphylactic reactions Should be given as infusion over 1–2 years to avoid redman reaction. Maintain trough levels >15–20 µg/mL	Additive effect with other drugs causing nephrotoxicity or ototoxicity. Increased neuromuscular blockade with other depolarizing agents

Contd...

Contd...

Name	*Formulations*	*Dosage and interval*	*Adverse effects*	*Drug interactions*
		Children with enlarged ventricles need higher doses. Adjust dose according to CSF levels aiming for a trough level of <10 mg/L		
Teicoplanin (teichomycin A)	Vials 200, 400	Age 0–2 months 16 mg/kg 1 dose and then 8 mg/kg IV od. Children 6–10 mg/kg od. For severe infections higher dose and bd for 1st 3 doses. Adults 6–12 mg/kg od. For severe infections higher dose bd for 1st three doses	Local reactions, fever, allergic reactions, anaphylaxis, nausea, diarrhea, thrombocytopenia, elevated SGPT, SGOT, Alk. PO4ase, urea, amylase	Chances of auditory and vestibular changes with concomitant other ototoxic drugs
Daptomycin	Vials 350 mg	For skin and soft tissue 4 mg/kg IV od. For endocarditis and bacteremia 6–8 mg/kg (up to 12 mg/kg)	Increase in CPK levels	Coadministration of statins increases myotoxicity
Sulphonamides Cotrimoxazole	Tab: *(Trimethoprim content)* 20 mg, 40 mg, 80 mg, 160 mg. Syr: 40 mg/5 mL. *(With sulfamethoxazole in ratio of 1:5)*	*Dosed on trimethoprim* not recommender <2 weeks. 2–4 weeks: 3 mg/kg loading, 2 mg/kg bd. >4 weeks: 4–6 mg/kg bd M = 320 mg For PCP pneumonia Treatment 5 mg/kg qds. For PCP prophylaxis 5 mg/kg/day od or thrice a week	Headache, sore tongue, rash (including SJ syndrome), nausea, vomiting, diarrhea, leukopenia, thrombocytopenia, megaloblastic anemia, jaundice, hemolysis in G6PD deficiency, pseudomembranous colitis. Can precipitate kernicterus in jaundiced neonates	Potentiates the anticoagulant activity of warfarin. Prolongs half-life of phenytoin. Increased toxicity of concomitant use of other antifolate drugs

Contd...

Contd...

Name	*Formulations*	*Dosage and interval*	*Adverse effects*	*Drug interactions*
Silver sulfadiazine	Skin cream 1%, eye drops 1%	Apply tds or qds to affected areas to adepth of 3 to 5 mm. Frequency of reapplication based on washing off due to patient activity or volume of exudates. Instil eye drops 4 hourly. Discard 50 g tubes 7 days after opening. Discard 250 g and 500 g pots 24 hours after opening	Hypersensitivity reactions, local itching, burning	Decrease metabolism of phenytoin, tolbutamide
Quinolones Nalidixic acid	Tab/DT: 125, 250, 500, 1,000. Syr: 300 mg/5 mL	18 mg/kg tds. For prolonged therapy reduce to 11 mg/kg tds Adolescents: 500–1,000 mg qds. UTI prophylaxis >2 months to 2 years: 15–30 mg/kg/day in od or bd doses. M: 4,000 mg in adolescents Children and infants ≥3 months: 55 mg/kg/day Infants <3 months: Not recommended	Diarrhea, nausea, vomiting, rash, photosensitivity headache, increase ICT, dizziness, vertigo, seizures psychosis, joint pains, diplopia, cholestasis, metabolic acidosis, hemolysis in G6PD deficiency	Increase bleeding with warfarin, probenecid increases plasma concentration of nalidixic acid. Antagonises effect of nitrofurantoin alcohol increase sedative effect
Norfloxacin	Tab/DT: 100, 200, 400, 800 mg. Syr: 100 mg/5 mL. Drp: 10 mg/mL eye drops 0.3%	6–10 mg/kg bd M = 800	Gastritis, anorexia, skin rash, SJ syndrome, sleep disturbances, irritability, depression, tinnitus, transient rise in liver enzymes, hemolysis in G6PD deficiency	Increase levels of theophylline and cyclosporine. Antacids interfere with absorption. Probenecid delays excretion. Increase bleeding with warfarin

Contd...

Contd...

Name	*Formulations*	*Dosage and interval*	*Adverse effects*	*Drug interactions*
Ciprofloxacin	Tab: 200, 250, 400, 500, 750 mg. Inj: 2 mg/mL 100 mL bottle eye drops 0.3%	Oral. N: 10 mg/kg bd. Children: 10–15 mg/kg bd M = 1,500 IV 7.5–12.5 mg/kg bd or tds (cystic fibrosis 30–40 mg/kg/day) M = 1,200. Max single dose IV 400 mg and oral 750 mg. Corneal ulcers: Apply throughout the day and night. First day: 2 drops every 15 min for 6 hours followed by 2 drops every 30 min for the rest of the day. 2nd day: 2 drops every hour and from 3rd to 14th day: 2 drops 4th hourly. Superficial infections of eye: 1–2 drops 4 times daily till 48 hours after the eye is clinically normal (use for max of 21 days)	Nausea, vomiting, diarrhea, anorexia, skin rash, SJ syndrome, insomnia, hallucinations, depression, seizures, tinnitus, deafness, transient rise in liver enzymes, arthropathy, hemolysis in G6PD deficiency	Antacids, milk and oral iron decrease absorption. Probenecid delays excretion. Increase bleeding with warfarin. Inreased levels of theophylline, increased risk of seizures with NSAIDs. Increased risk of QT prolongation with antiarrythmics, antimicrobials (azoles, macrolids), psychoactive drugs
Ofloxacin	Tab/DT: 50, 100, 200, 400. Syr: 50 mg/5 mL Inj: 2 mg/mL 100 mL bottle. Eye drops: 0.3%	Oral 7.5 mg/kg bd M = 800. IV 5–7.5 mg/kg bd M = 600	As for ciprofloxacin. Also leukopenia, eosinophilia	As for ciprofloxacin
Levofloxacin is an S-isomer of ofloxacin and has less side effects	Tab: 250, 500, 750 mg. Inj: 5 mg/mL 100 mL bottles	Pediatric dose not established 10 mg/kg od has been used M = 1,000	Nausea, vomiting, diarrhea, anorexia, skin rash, SJ syndrome, insomnia, hallucinations, depression, seizures, tinnitus, deafness, arthropathy, hemolysis in G6PD deficiency	As for ciprofloxacin

Contd...

Contd...

Name	*Formulations*	*Dosage and interval*	*Adverse effects*	*Drug interactions*
Moxifloxacin	Tab: 200, 400 mg. Inj: 2 mg/mL 200 mL bottle. Eye drp: 0.5%	Pediatric dose not established used as 10 mg/kg od. Adults 400 mg od	GI disturbances, CNS effects (as above), reversible arthralgia, hepatitis, tachycardia, pain at inj site	As for ciprofloxacin. Increased Q-T interval effect of other drugs
Nadifloxacin	Skin cream 0.1%	Apply bd	Pruritus, redness, flushes, contact dermatitis	None on local application
Aminoglycosides Streptomycin Many dose regimens exist for aminoglycosides depending on target concentration aimed for and patient groups treated. The doses shown here are generally accepted initial doses and dose adjustments should be made in the light of serum concentrations	750, 1,000 mg vials	IM 15–20 mg/kg od M = 1,000 For TB: Intermittent regimen: 15–20 mg/kg	Ototoxicity (vestibular and auditory), nephrotoxicity, neuromuscular blockade, pain at inj site	Increase nephrotoxicity with NSAIDs, cyclosporin, vancomycin, amphotericin B, cephalosporins. Increase ototoxicity with frusemide. Increase neuromuscular blockade, apnea with muscle relaxants
Kanamycin	500, 1,000 mg vials	IM 15 mg/kg od M = 1,000	Nephrotoxicity, ototoxicity, neuromuscular block	As above
Gentamicin	Inj: Vials 40 mg/mL and 10 mg/mL; Amp: 20, 40, 60, 80 mg Eye drops: 0.3%	5–7.5 mg/kg/day IM or IV infusion od, bd, tds M = 240 N: < 7 days 1,200–2,000 g 2.5 mg/kg once in 12–18 hours and >2,000 g 2.5 mg/kg bd; >7 days 1,200–2,000 g 2.5 mg/kg bd/tds; >2,000 g 2.5 mg/kg tds. Extended interval dose regimen by slow IV inj or infusion 32 weeks of	Nephrotoxicity with hematuria, renal failure; ototoxicity with tinnitus, hearing loss; vestibular toxicity with nausea, vomiting, dizziness, vertigo; hypomagnesemia	Increased nephrotoxicity with NSAIDs, cyclosporin, vancomycin, amphotericin B, cephalosporins. Increased ototoxicity with frusemide. Increase neuromuscular blockade, apnea with muscle relaxants

Contd...

Contd...

Name	*Formulations*	*Dosage and interval*	*Adverse effects*	*Drug interactions*
		gestation 4–5 mg/kg every 36 hours; >32 weeks of gestation 4–5 mg/kg every 24 hours. Children: <12 years 2.5 mg/kg tds; 12–18 years 2 mg/kg tds. Alternatively 5–7.5 mg/kg/24 hours IV or by infusion od. Intrathecal/ventricular: preservative free preparation: newborn 1 mg/24 hours; children 1–2 mg/24 hours; 16–18 years. Pseudomonal lung infection in cystic fibrosis. By nebulization Child 1 month to 2 years 40 mg bd; Child 2–8 years 80 mg bd; Child 8–18 years 160 mg bd.		
Netilmycin	Amp: 50 mg/mL; 100 mg/mL 2, 3 mL ampoules	N: IV 3 mg/dose bd. Increase to tds after 1 week age. Children: IV/IM <12 years 7.5 mg/kg/day and >12 years 6 mg/kg/day in 3 divided doses or 1 month 18 years 7.5 mg/kg as single dose daily. Intraperitoneal 7.5–10 mg/L in peritoneal dialysis fluid	Nephrotoxicity, ototoxicity	As above
Amikacin	Inj: 50 mg/mL, 125 mg/mL, 250 mg/mL	<35 weeks up to 14 days 10 mg/kg once daily and >14 days 10 mg/kg loading dose	As above; skin rash, tremors	As for gentamicin

Contd...

Contd...

Name	*Formulations*	*Dosage and interval*	*Adverse effects*	*Drug interactions*
		followed by 7.5 mg/kg/dose 2 times daily; >35 weeks <14 days 15 mg/kg as single dose daily and >14 days 10 mg/kg loading dose followed by 7.5 mg/kg/dose 2 times daily. Children (1 month to 18 years): IV/IM 7.5 mg/kg/dose bd or 15–22.5 mg/kg od M = 1,500		
Neomycin	Cap: 350 mg. Oint: 2%	Children: 3g/m^2/day q 6 hours. oral in hepatic coma. Adolescents: 0.25–1 g qds	Nephrotoxicity and ototoxicity (even with oral use)	As for fentamicin. Decrease absorption of digoxin, bile acids
Tobramycin	Vials 2 mL each; 10, 30, 40 mg/mL, Eye oint: 0.3%, Drp: 0.3%	Newborn: IV (over 3–5 min or infusion) < 32 weeks 4–5 mg/kg 36 hourly and >32 weeks 4–5 mg/kg od Child: IV/IM 2.5 mg/kg/dose tds or 7 mg/kg od. Pseudomonal lung infection in cystic fibrosis: Child 1 month to 18 years—initially 10 mg/kg (max 660 mg), chronic pulmonary *Pseudomonas aeruginosa* infection in patients with cystic fibrosis by nebulization Child 6–18 years: 300 mg bd	Nephrotoxicity, ototoxicity	As above. With concommittant indomethacin use, increase dosing intervals

Contd...

Contd...

Name	*Formulations*	*Dosage and interval*	*Adverse effects*	*Drug interactions*
		Intraventricular: newborn 1 mg/day, child 1–2 mg/day, adolescent 2–4 mg/day		
Sisomycin	Inj: 40 mg. Eye drops: 1%	Inj IM/IV 1–2 mg/kg tds. Eye Drp instil 1–2 Drp 4 hourly	Tinnitus, vertigo, deafness, CNS disturbances, nephrotoxicity. Transient eye irritation, hypersensitivity reactions	As for gentamicin. None on local application
Framycetin	Eye drops: 1% Ointment: 5%	Instil 1–2 drops tds or qds	Irritation, hypersensitivity reactions	None on local application
Macrolides Erythromycin	Cap/Tab/DT: 125, 250, 333, 500 mg. Syp: 100, 125, 250 mg/5 mL Drp: 100 mg/mL Eye oint: 0.1% Oint, lotion, gel, 2%, 3%, 4%	Oral: N: 10 mg/kg bd <7 d; tds if >7 d but <2 kg; 15 mg/kg tds if >2 kg, >7 d Child: 7.5–12.5 mg/kg qds. M = 1,000 Adolescents: 250–500 mg qds. max 2,000. Secondary prevention of rheumatic fever: oral 20 mg/kg/day max 500 mg bd. Uncomplicated gonorrhea, postexposure pertussis prophylaxis: 40–50 mg/kg/day (maximum 2 g/day) in four divided doses for 14 days. (For neonates: azithromycin is preferred). Pneumococcal prophylaxis: 1 month to 2 years 250 mg/day, 2–8 years	Gastritis, vomiting, abdominal pain, rash, false increase in SGOT levels. Reversible hearing loss with high doses. Contraindicated in liver disorder. If given to neonates, monitor for infantile hypertrophic pyloric stenosis	Increased digoxin, theophylline, warfarin, carbamezapine levels. Increased cardiac toxicity with cisapride, terfenadine and astemizole

Contd...

Contd...

Name	*Formulations*	*Dosage and interval*	*Adverse effects*	*Drug interactions*
		500 mg/day, >9 years 1 g/day in 2 divided doses. Gastric stasis: Oral/IV 1 month to 18 years—3 mg/kg 4 times daily		
Roxithromycin	Tab/DT: 50, 75 150, 300 Syr: 50, 100 mg/5 mL.	3–4 mg/kg bd	Nausea, vomiting, diarrhea, skin rash, transient increase in liver enzymes	Digoxin, terbinafin increase roxithromycin absorption
Clarithromycin	Tab: 125, 250, 500 mg Syr: 125 mg/5 mL	7.5 mg/kg bd M = 1,000 For *Helicobacter pylori:* 1–2 years 125 mg, 2–6 years 250 mg, 6–9 years 375 mg, 9–12 years 500 mg and 12–18 years 1 g/day in 2 divided doses along with amoxycillin/metronidazole and PPI. Bacterial endocarditis prophylaxis: 15 mg/kg (single dose max 500 mg) 30–60 minutes before procedure in those allergic to penicillin. Treatment and postexposure pertussis prophylaxis: infants > 6 months and children: 15 mg/kg/day max 1000 for 7 days. Not used in neonates	Nausea, vomiting, diarrhea, abdominal pain, blood dyscrasias, stomatitis, cholestatic jaundice, pseudomembranous colitis	Increased digoxin, theophylline, warfarin, carbamezapine levels. Cardiac arrythmias with terfenadine, astemizole, cisapride. Reduced dosage required with concommitant ritonavir treatment
Azithromycin	Inj: Vials: 30 mL (20 mg/mL) Tab: 1,000, 500, 250, 100 mg Syr: 200, 100 mg/5 mL	10 mg/kg od or 10 mg/kg on day 1 and then 5 mg/kg od >6 months <2 years M = 200 mg > 2 years < 7 yrs	Nausea, vomiting, diarrhea, flatulence, vertigo, headache, urticaria rash, cholestatic jaundice	Antacids reduce absorption. Increases absorption of digoxin and cyclosporin

Contd...

Contd...

Name	*Formulations*	*Dosage and interval*	*Adverse effects*	*Drug interactions*
		M = 300 mg 8–11 years M = 400 >12 M = 500 Group A beta-hemolytic streptococcal (GAS) pharyngitis and tonsillitis (primary prophylaxis of rheumatic fever): 12 mg/kg/day single dose for 5 days. Chlamydial infection in adolescents: single dose of 1 g orally. Bacterial endocarditis prophylaxis: 15 mg/kg (single dose max 500 mg) 30–60 minutes before procedure in children and adolescents allergic to penicillin. Enteric fever: 10–20 mg/kg od M = 1,000		
Spiramycin	Tab: 1.5 million units (MU) Syr: 0.375 MU/5 mL	< 1 year 0.375 MU, 1–2 years. 75 MU, 3–5 years 1.125 MU, 6–9 years 1.5 MU, 10–12 years 2.25 MU, > 12 years 3 MU. All doses bd For toxoplasmosis in pregnant women 1.5 g (4.5 MU bd orally	Nausea, vomiting, diarrhea, skin rash	Increases theophyline and carbamezapene levels if given concomitantly
Lincosamides Lincomycin	Inj: 300 mg/mL Cap: 250, 500 mg. Inj: 300, 600. Syr: 125 mg/5 mL	Inj. 10 mg/kg od or bd. Oral: 10–20 mg/kg bd	Diarrhea, severe pseudomembranous enterocolitis	Potentiates action of neuromuscular blocking agents

Contd...

Contd...

Name	*Formulations*	*Dosage and interval*	*Adverse effects*	*Drug interactions*
Clindamycin	Cap: 150 mg Gel/Oint: 5%	Oral 10 mg/kg tds or qds M = 1,800 mg N: <7 days, <2,000 g 5 mg/kg bd IV/IM; <7 days >2,000 g 5 mg/kg tds IV/IM; >7 days <1,200 g 5 mg/kg bd IV/IM; 1,200–2,000 g 5 mg/kg tds >2,000 g 20 mg/kg/day divided 8 hrly IV/IM. Children 10–15 mg/kg tds Falciparum malaria (alternate therapy) 20 mg/kg/day for 5 days. Acne: topical application as thin film bd with lotion and od with gel	Metallic taste in mouth. Stomach pain, nausea, vomiting, diarrhea. Pseudomembranous enterocolitis may occur. Steven–Johnson type of reactions may be seen	Erythromycin clindamycin antagonism. Increase neuromuscular blocking with similar drugs
Chloramphenicol	Inj: Vial 1,000 mg Tab/Cap: 250, 500 mg. Syr: 125 mg/5 mL Lotion: 100 mg/mL Eye drops: 0.5%, 1% Ear Drp: 1%, 5%	Oral, IV N: 1–4 weeks <2 kg: 12.5–25 mg/kg od. 1–4 weeks >2 kg 12.5–25 mg/kg bd. Monitor blood levels. Child >4 weeks 12.5–25 mg/kg qds. The higher dose for septicemia and meningitis. M = 1,000 mg (2,000 for severe infections)	Rash itching, peripheral and/or optic neuritis, sore throat, fever, weakness, bone marrow depression, grey baby syndrome	Levels increased by phenytoin and phenobarbitone Antagonizes bactericidal effect of penicillins
Oxazolidinones Linezolid	Tab: 600 Inj: 2 mg/mL 100 mL and 300 mL	Oral/IV (by infusion) doses: P: <7 d, gestational age <34 weeks 10 mg/kg bd >7 days 10 mg/kg tds	Headache, nausea, constipation, insomnia, liver dysfunction, thrombocytopenia, bone marrow suppression	Reversible inhibitor of MAO. Increase BP with dopamine, epinephrine, psuedoephedrine phenylpropanolamine, and with diet

Contd...

Contd...

Name	*Formulations*	*Dosage and interval*	*Adverse effects*	*Drug interactions*
		N, Child: 10 mg/kg tds ≥12 years: 600 mg bd M = 1200 For MDR/XDR TB or NTM 10 mg/kg once daily M = 600		high in tyramine and selective serotonin reuptake inhibitors
Tetracyclines Tetracycline	Cap/Tab: 250, 500 mg	>8 years age 5–10 mg/kg qds M = 2,000 Acne: topical application bd	Gastritis, diarrhea, pancreatitis, benign increase in intracranial tension, teeth discolouration, enamel hypoplasia	Iron, antacids decrease absorption, antagonistic to penicillins, decrease serum level with antiepileptics, warfarin effect potentiated
Oxytetracycline	Inj: 50 mg/mL Cap 250, 500 mg Eye oint: 10 mg/g	Age >8 years Inj IM/oral 10–20 mg/kg tds M = 2,000 Eye Oint: 5—10 mm ribbon bd or tds Acne: Oral 12–18 years 250–500 mg/dose bd Infections: 250–500 mg/dose qds	Pain at inj site, skin rash, nausea, gastritis, teeth discolouration, enamel hypoplasia	As for tetracycline
Demeclocycline	Tab/Cap: 150, 300 mg	Age > 8 yrs 3–6 mg/kg bd M = 450	As for oxytetracycline	As for tetracycline
Doxycycline	Cap/Tab/DT: 50, 100, 200 Syr: 5 mg/mL, 10 mg/mL	Oral: 3–4 mg/kg/day od or bd M = 200 IV 3–4 mg/kg loading and then once daily given bd Adults 200 loading and 100 bd Acne: Initial dose: 100 mg orally bd for 3–6 weeks or until improvement occurs	Can be used for children less than 8 years unlike other tetracyclines Skin rash, itching, nausea, vomiting, diarrhea	As for tetracycline

Contd...

Contd...

Name	*Formulations*	*Dosage and interval*	*Adverse effects*	*Drug interactions*
		Maintenance dose: 50–150 mg orally od. Cholera: single dose of 4 mg/kg (max 200 mg) Multidrug-resistant *P. falciparum* along with quinine at 3.5 mg/kg once a day for 7 days. Malaria chemoprophylaxis: Child (>8 years) 1.5 mg/kg od. M = 100 mg Uncomplicated urethral, endocervical, or rectal infections due to *Chlamydia trachomatis* or gonorrhoea: 100 mg bd orally Periodontitis: 20 mg orally twice a day for up to 9 months		
Minocycline	Tab: 100 mg	1.5 mg/kg bd. M = 200 Paucibacillary leprosy: 50 mg single dose, given as a combination with rifampicin and ofloxacin	Vestibular symptoms, reversible hypersensitivity pneumonitis	As for tetracycline
Tigecycline	Injection: 50 mg	1.5 mg/kg loading and then 1 mg/kg bd M = 200 mg	Nausea, vomiting Hepatic dysfunction	
Carbapenems Impenem-cilastatin	Inj: 500 mg	N: 20 mg/kg <7 d bd, 7–21 d tds, 21 days to 3 months qds. 3 months to 12 years 15–25 mg/kg qds, >12 years 500 mg qds. May be given as 1 g tds M = 3000	Hypersensitivity, GI intolerance, hepatic impairment, convulsions. Positive Coombs test	Increased risk of CNS side effects with gancyclovir and cyclosporin. Delayed excretion with probenecid

Contd...

Contd...

Name	*Formulations*	*Dosage and interval*	*Adverse effects*	*Drug interactions*
Meropenem	Inj: 500 mg	N: 20–40 mg/kg bd < 7 d; tds > 7 d Children: 20–40 mg/kg tds (max 500–1,000 mg/dose) Severe infections/meningitis 40 mg/kg tds M = 6,000/day or 2,000 mg/dose for serious infections	Allergy, GI intolerance, bone marrow suppression, elevated liver enzymes and rarely, seizures	Probenecid delays excretion
Ertapenem	Injection: 1 g	15 mg/kg bd M = 1,000	As for other carbapenems, seizures	
Miscellaneous Colistimethate	Inj: 1 million units/80 mg of salt. 2.6 mg of salt = 1 mg of Colistin base = 30,000 IU	Loading of 10–12 mg/kg or 150,000 units/kg and then 12 hours later as 5–6 mg/kg or 75,000 units/kg bd M 9 million units Nebulization 1–2 million units tds Intrathecal/intraventricular 10–20 mg	Nephrotoxicity, neurotoxicity	Increased nephrotoxicity when used in combination with diuretics
Polymyxin B	Vial: 5,00,000 U/50 mg (1 mg = 10,000 units)	Loading dose of 15,000–25,000 units/kg and then 12 hours later 7,500–12,500 units/kg bd M = 15,00,000	Pain, flushing, paraesthesia, nephrotoxicity, ototoxicity and neurological disturbances	Synergistic with cephalosporins. Increase nephrotoxicity with aminoglycosides
Fosfomycin	Oral satchet: 3,1 g IV: 4 g	Preterms 50 mg/kg bd Neonates 60–70 mg/kg tds Children 100 mg/kg tds M = 16,000	Hypernatremia	
Furazolidone	Tab: 100 mg Syr: 35 mg/5 mL	1.25 mg/kg qds. Adolescents 100 mg qds	Nausea, headache, dizziness, hemolysis in G6PD deficiency	Hypertensive crises with MAO inhibiters and nasal degcongestants, increase orthostatic hypotension with sedatives, narcotics

Contd...

Contd...

Name	*Formulations*	*Dosage and interval*	*Adverse effects*	*Drug interactions*
Nitrofurantoin	Tab 50, 100 mg	1.25–1.75 mg/kg qds. Adolescents 50–100 mg qds. Contraindicated in infants < 3 month age. UTI prophylaxis: 1–2.5 mg/kg/day at bedtime or in 2 divided doses (max 100 mg/24 hours)	Rash, tingling of face, vomiting, loss of appetite, drug fever, jaundice, peripheral neuropathy, hemolysis in G6PDD, benign increase ICT, pulmonary fibrosis	Probenecid delays excretion. Antagonizes effect of nalidixic acid, increase bactericidal activity by agents acidifying urine
Nitrofurazone	Oint, cream, powder 2%	Apply as per requirement	Local irritation, sensitivity reactions	None on local application
Fusidic acid	Oint 2%	Apply bd or tds	Hypersensitivity reactions (rare)	Increases risk of jaundice with rifampicin
Mupirocin	Oint, cream 2%	Apply to affected area tds Nasal application: to the inner surface of each nostril 2–3 times a day for 5–7 days	Stinging and dryness at application site	Mixing with other agents may reduce bactericidal effect

TABLE 2: Antimycobacterial agents.

Name	*Formulations*	*Dosage and route*	*Adverse effects*	*Drug interactions*
Isoniazid	Tab: 100, 300	10 mg/kg od for treatment and prophylaxis M = 300	Peripheral neuropathy, liver dysfunction, fever, CNS	Rifampicin, ethionamide (increase liver injury), Al salts (decrease INH absorption), CBZ, phenytoin (increase interacting drug levels), warfarin (increase INR), itraconazole (decrease itraconazole levels)
Ethambutol (EMB)	Tab: 200, 400,600,800	20–25 mg/kg od M = 1,600	Ocular toxicity (scotoma, decrease visual acuity, color blindness), drug fever, rash, mental confusion	Al salts, didanosine (decrease EMB and interacting drug absorption)

Contd...

Contd...

Name	*Formulations*	*Dosage and route*	*Adverse effects*	*Drug interactions*
Pyrazinamide (PZA)	Tab: 250, 300, 500, 750, 1,000 Susp: 250	30–35 mg/kg od M = 2,000 (1,500 if weight < 50 kg) (can be given in two divided doses also)	Vomiting, liver toxicity, rash, arthralgia, gout	INH, RMP (increase risk of hepatotoxicity)
Cycloserine	Tab/Cap: 250	10–20 mg/kg/day in 2 divided doses. M = 1,000 mg/day. Adolescent: 250–500 mg twice daily for 2 weeks and then increased to 500 mg to 1 g in divided doses	Peripheral neuropathy, seizures, delirium, psychosis	EMB, ethionamide (increase drowsiness), phenytion (increase phenytoin levels)
Ethionamide	Tab: 250	15 (10–20) mg/kg/day od or bd M = 1,000	Hepatic dysfunction, headache, nausea, vomiting, tremor, alopecia, gynecomastia	Cycloserine (increase neurotoxicity) INH, PZA, rifampicin (increase hepatotoxicity), INH (increase peripheral neuritis)
Para-aminosalicylic acid (PAS)	Granules	150–200 mg/kg/day given bd or tds M = 12,000	Hepatitis, fever, rash, goitrous hypothyroidism, leucopenia, hypokalemia	
Rifampicin (RMP),	Tab: 100, 150, 200, 300, 450, 600 Syp: 100	10–15 mg/kg od to be given on empty stomach. M = 600 Meningococcal infection prophylaxis: Oral <5 years 5 mg/kg/dose and >1 year 10 mg/kg/dose (max 600 mg/dose) bd for 2 days for meningococcal infection prophylaxis *Haemophilus influenzae* prophylaxis: Oral <3 months 10 mg/kg and >3 months	Hepatitis, fever, flu-like symptoms	Indanvir, nelfinavir, TMP-SMX, clarithromycin, fluconazole, ketoconazole (increase RMP levels), beta-blockers, cyclosporin, warfarin, corticosteroids, phenytoin, theophylline, digoxin, nifedepine (decreased interacting drug effect), nevirapine

Contd...

Contd...

Name	*Formulations*	*Dosage and route*	*Adverse effects*	*Drug interactions*
		20 mg/kg/dose (max 600 mg/ dose) once daily for 4 days. Staphylococcal infections (MRSA): 10–15 mg/kg od M 900 mg		(decreased nevirapine levels), INH and PZA (increased hepatotoxicity)
Dapsone	Tab: 100 mg	1–2 mg/kg od M = 100 For blistering skin conditions: Start at 0.5 mg/kg/ day and increase or decrease as necessary in 12.5 mg increments. Prophylaxis of *Pneumocystis jiroveci* in HIV: > 1 month: 2 mg/kg/ day (up to 100 mg) orally od	Fever, rash, nausea, anorexia, jaundice, headache, hemolysis (G6PDD), methemoglobin	Rifampicin, didanosine (decrease dapsone levels), pyrimethamine, azathioprine (increase marrow suppression)
Clofazimine	Cap: 50, 100 mg	For TB 2–3 mg/ kg od M = 200 In leprosy, 6 mg/ kg once a month. In multibacillary leprosy (in combination with dapsone and rifampicin) Adolescent, 50 mg od and 300 mg once a month Child 10–14 years, 50 mg on alternate days and 150 mg once a month Children <10 years: 1 mg/kg PO once daily plus an additional 6 mg/kg PO once per month in combination type 2 lepra reaction (erythema nodosum leprosum), adolescent, and child, 200–300 mg daily in 2 or 3 divided doses	Anorexia, nausea, diarrhea, photosensitivity with darkening of skin, itching	Increased ototoxicity and nephrotoxicity with other drugs with similar toxicity

TABLE 3: Antifungal agents.

Name	*Formulations*	*Dosage, route and interval*	*Adverse effects*	*Drug interactions*
Polyenes Amphotericin B dexocycholate	Vials: 50 mg.	Test dose of 1 mg in 10–50 mL of 5% dextrose over 20–30 minutes 0.6–1.3 mg/kg/day given in 5% dextrose over 4 hours (concentration is 1 mg/10 mL) Reduce nephrotoxicity by saline loading before the infusion Severe rigors respond to pethidine 25–50 mg Premedication with paracetamol, diphenhydramine, hydrocortisone has no effect on rigors and fever	Acute infusion reactions (40–80%): pain at site, fever, chills, nausea, vomiting, headache, dyspnea, muscle and joint pains, especialy with initial doses. Renal toxicity very common. (30–50%) hypokalemia, hypomagnesemia, azotemia, renal tubular acidosis, nephrocalcinosis. Less common anuria, hematuria, acute renal failure. Abnormal LFT, convulsions, diplopia, peripheral neuropathy. Infusion related and nephrotoxic	Increase renal toxicity with other nephrotoxic drugs. Steroids may worsen hypokalemia. Amphotericin-induced hypokalemia causes increase toxicity of digitalis and skeletal muscle relaxants. Flucytosine toxicity may be enchanced. AZT: Effects on bone marrow and renal function may be enhanced. Increase cyclosporin levels
Amphotericin B lipid complex (ABLC)	Vials: 50 mg	Test dose of 1 mg over 20–30 minutes 5 mg/kg/day single dose Infusion rate 2.5 mg/kg/hour Prepare in 5% dextrose Not to use inline filter	Infusion reactions faily common like AMB-D Lesser nephrotoxicity (25%) than AMB-D Fatal case of fat embolism reported	Same as amphotericin B deoxycholate
Amphotericin B colloidal dispersion (ABCD)	50 mg	Test dose of 1 mg over 20–30 minutes 3–5 mg/kg/day as infusion in 5% dextrose over 2–4 hours	Same as ABLC	Same as amphotericin B deoxycholate
Liposomal amphotericin B (L AMB)	50 mg	3–5 mg/kg/day as infusion in 5% dextrose over 2 hours	Infusion related side effects lower than AMB-D and ABLC and ABCD	Same as other amphotericin B deoxycholate

Contd...

Contd...

Name	*Formulations*	*Dosage, route and interval*	*Adverse effects*	*Drug interactions*
		Increase dose to 10 mg/kg/day in mucormycosis	(20–40%) Most occur within 5 minutes of infusion and respond to diphenhydramine and interruption of infusion Nephrotoxicity also lower than the others (20%)	
Nystatin	Tab: 5 lakh units (Can be chewed or applied after crushing for oral thrush). Liquid 100,000 u/mL	N: 1 lakh U qds, infants 2 lakh U qds, child 4–6 lakh U qds N and child (for oral candidiasis): 1 mL tds/qds, Oral candida in immunocompromised 1 mL 4–6 times a day, esophageal/ intestinal candida 5 mL or 1 tab 4–6 times daily	Rash, diarrhea, vomiting, rarely Steven–Johnson Syndrome	None known
Pyrimidine analogue 5-fluorocytosine		25 mg/kg qds M = 6,000 mg Drug level monitoring desirable	Nausea, vomiting, diarrhea, skin rash myelosuppression, hypocalcemia, hypokalemia, muscle weakness, cardiac arrest. Rarely, convulsions, headache	Cytarabine may reduce plasma concentrations of 5-fluorocytosine. Antacids delay absorption
Azoles Fluconazole	Inj: 400 mg Tab/DT: 50, 100, 150. Eye drop: 0.3%	Invasive infections Neonates 25 mg/ kg loading and 12 mg/kg od Children 12 mg/kg loading and 6 mg/ kg od M 800 loading and 400 daily Mucosal candidiasis 3 mg/ kg daily	Nausea, vomiting, abdominal pain, diarrhea, skin rash, elevated liver enzymes	Cycloserine, warfarin, phenytoin levels are increased

Contd...

Contd...

Name	*Formulations*	*Dosage, route and interval*	*Adverse effects*	*Drug interactions*
		Prophylaxis of candidiasis in neonates 3–6 mg/kg twice or thrice weekly		
Clotrimazole	Cream: 1%, 2% Mouth paint: 1% Dusting powder: 1% Ear drp: 1% Gel: 2% Vaginal pessaires: 100 mg	Topical and mouth application for oral thrush: 10–20 drops gently apply to buccal mucosa (covering all lesions) qds. Vaginal candidiasis: Apply 5 g gel or pessary deep into vagina at bedtime for 6 consecutive nights (not to be used during menstruation). Or 200 mg for 3 days or 500 mg single dose at bedtime. Scalp seborrhea: Apply liquid with selenium to scalp, massage gently, leave for 5 minutes and then rinse well with water 2–3 times/week. Otomycosis: Instill 4–5 drops in ear tds/qds	Side effects minimal. Skin irritation	None
Ketoconazole	Tab: 200 mg Lotion: 2% Shampoo: 2%	5–10 mg/kg od for pityriasis versicolor. Seborrheic dermatitis and dandruff: twice weekly for 2–4 weeks For tinea adolescent: 200 mg od. Serious infection may require 400 mg od. Children ≥2 years of age: 3.3–6.6 mg/kg od	Jaundice, itching, rash, headache, gynecomastia, GI upset, skin discoloration	Antacids, H2 blockers, rifampicin, cycloserine reduces drug levels

Contd...

Contd...

Name	*Formulations*	*Dosage, route and interval*	*Adverse effects*	*Drug interactions*
Itraconazole	Cap: 100 mg	<12 years 3–5 mg/kg and 12–18 years 100 mg od in tinea corporis, tinea cruris and oropharyngeal candidiasis. Aspergellosis: Allergic bronchopulmonary 3–5 mg/kg/day in 2 divided doses (M = 200)	Nausea and vomiting common, headache, hypertension, rash, hepatitis	Food increases bioavailablility. Carbamezapine, phenytoin phenobarbital INH, rifampicin, cyclosporine, antacids, H2 blockers decrease bioavailability
Voriconazole	Tablets: 200 mg IV preparation 200 mg	2–12 years 12–14 years (weight <50 kg) IV 9 mg/kg/dose twice daily day 1 and then 8 mg/kg/ dose twice daily Oral 9 mg/kg twice daily 12–14 years >50 kg ≥15 years 6 mg/kg twice daily on day 1 And then 4 mg/kg twice daily or 200 mg twice daily TDM needed, level is 1–6	Nausea, headache hepatic dysfunction, reversible dose-dependant visual disturbances	To be taken empty stomach Plenty of interactions due to inhibition of CYP 450 enzymes (see chapter on antifungals)
Posaconazole	Syrup: 40 mg/mL Inj: 300 mg	For children aged 18 years or older For treatment 400 mg bd or 200 mg qds and prophylaxis 200 mg tds IV 300 mg 12 hourly loading and then 300 mg once daily	Nausea, vomiting, diarrhea, fever and increased bilirubin	Same for other azoles
Miscellaneous Terbinafine	Tab: 250 mg Cream: 1%	3–6 mg/kg or >12 kg < 20 kg 62.5, >20 <40 kg 125, >40 kg 250 mg od. Topical 1–2 times daily	Oral: Mild GI disturbances, malaise, lethargy, rash. Local: Erythema, irritation, dryness	Cimetidine, rifampicin decrease metabolism

Contd...

Contd...

Name	*Formulations*	*Dosage, route and interval*	*Adverse effects*	*Drug interactions*
Griseofulvin	Tab: 125, 250, 375, 500 mg	2.5–5 mg/kg qds M = 500	Rash, nausea, vomiting, dizziness, drowsiness, headache, photosensitivity	Decreases effect of oral anticoagulants, barbiturates decrease effect of griseofulvin
Tolnaftate	Cream: 10 mg/mL Lotion: 10 mg/mL	Apply evenly to affected area and rub gently bd/tds	Stinging sensation	None on local application
Echinocandins Caspofungin	Injection: 70 mg and 50 mg	Neonatal 25 mg/m^2 or 2 mg/kg od Pediatric dose 50 mg/m^2 od Adult dose 70 mg/m^2 loading and then 50 mg od	Liver function abnormalities Fever, infusion reactions	Cyclosporine increases caspofungin levels Rifampicin, dexa, phenytoin, nevirapine and efavirenz reduce caspofungin levels Caspofungin reduces tac levels
Micafungin	Injection: 100 mg	Neonates 10 mg/kg od Children: 2–4 mg/kg od Adults 100 mg od M = 100	Liver tumors in rats	Micafungin increases cyclosporin and nifedipine levels
Anidulafungin	Injection: 200 mg and 100 mg	Not approved for children but doses of 3 mg/kg loading and 1.5 mg/kg have been used In adults loading dose of 200 mg and then 100 mg od	Same as echinocandins	Cyclosporine increases anidulafungin levels

TABLE 4: Antiviral agents.

Drug	*Formulations*	*Dose*	*Adverse effects*	*Drug interactions*
Acyclovir	Tab: 200,400,600 mg Syp: 400 mg/5 mL Inj: 250 mg Cre: 5% Oint: 2%, Eye Oint: 0.5%	Herpes simplex encephalitis IV <12 years: 20 mg/kg tds, >12 years 10 mg/kg tds for 14–21 days Chickenpox/herpes zoster Oral 20 mg/kg qds for 5 days Adults 800 mg 5 times daily	Local phlebitis at inj site reversible neurological reactions	ZDV: Extreme lethargy. Probenecid and cimetidine: Increase toxicity. Other nephrotoxic drugs: Increased renal damage

Contd...

Contd...

Drug	*Formulations*	*Dose*	*Adverse effects*	*Drug interactions*
		Complicated chickenpox/hereps zoster 10 mg/kg tds or 500 mg/m^2 tds For other indications see chapter on antivirals		
Gancyclovir	Pow Inj: 500 mg Cap: 250, 500 mg	5 mg/kg/dose BD IV (induction) × 21, then 5 mg/kg/dose orally	GI upsets, change of taste, bone marrow depression, renal toxicity, mental changes, cramps	Probenecid delays excretion. Dapsone, flucytosine, AZT, cotrimoxazole increase bone marrow toxicity. With imipenem increase seizures
Valganciclovir	Tab: 450 mg	Adults 900 mg bd (for treatment) and od for prophylaxis Pediatric dose 7X BSA X creat clearance	Same as ganciclovir	Same as ganciclovir
Famciclovir	Tab: 250, 500 mg	10 mg/kg tds	Headache, paraesthesiae rash, nausea, vomiting, diarrhea, fatigue	None significant clinically
Valacyclovir	Tablets: 500 mg	Chickenpox and herpes zoster 1 g thrice daily in adults		
Idoxuridine	Eye drops 0.1% Eye oint: 0.5%	1 drop	Burning sensation	None of clinical significance
Interferon alfa	Vials 0.45, 3 and 5 million units	3–6 million units/m^2 subcut. or IM od >12 yrs 3–10 million units/m^2. Usually 3 times/week (daily for hemangioma)		
Ribavarin	Cap: 100, 200 mg Syr: 50 mg/5 mL	3–5 mg/kg tds	Hypertension, respiratory effects, leukopenia, hemolytic anemia	

Contd...

Contd...

Drug	*Formulations*	*Dose*	*Adverse effects*	*Drug interactions*
Lamivudine	Tab: 100, 150, 300 Syr: 50 mg/5 mL	3–4 mg/kg. M = 300. Adolescents (weight ≥40 kg): 300 mg/day	Nausea, vomiting, diarrhea, abdominal pain, pancreatitis, peripheral neuropathy, optic neuritis, lactic acidosis and severe hepatomegaly with steatosis	Drug levels and effectivity increase by AZT, Cotrimoxazole increases blood levels of lamivudine
Amantadine	Cap: 100 mg	For influenza Limited role now in view of resistance 5–9 mg/kg od, M = 150 Influenza A virus infection: Oral-Children ≥10 years: 5 mg/kg/day in two divided doses, Max 200. < 10 years: 5 mg/kg/day in 2 divided doses. Max 150. Influenza A Px: adolescents: 200 mg/day od or 2 divided doses and continue for at least 10 days after exposure	Acute episodes of gout, anorexia, nausea, dysuria, agitation, dizziness, blurred vision	Increase anticholinergic effects with other atropine like agents. Increase drug levels of triamterene and hydrochlorthiazide
Oseltamivir	Tab: 75 mg Syrup: 30 mg/5 mL	<15 kg: 30 mg 15–24 kg: 45 mg 25–34 kg: 60 mg 35 kg and more 75 mg Given twice daily for treatment and once daily for prophylaxis Can consider doubling dose in the immunocompromised	GI side effects like nausea, vomiting and diarrhea and neurologic side effects like drowsiness	None significant
Zanamavir	Inhalation solution: 5 mg	For treatment and prophylaxis of influenza	Diarrhea, nausea, vomiting.	None reported

Contd...

Contd...

Drug	*Formulations*	*Dose*	*Adverse effects*	*Drug interactions*
		2 inhalations (5 mg each, 10 mg total) twice daily for treatment and once daily for prophlylaxis	Allergic reactions and neuropsychiatric events	
Foscarnet sodium	Inj: 24 mg/mL	90 mg/kg by slow infusion over 1–1/2–2 hours 40 mg/kg by slow infusion over 1–1/2–2 hours	Renal toxicity (33%) rash, mood disturbances, diarrhea, anorexia, vomiting, seizures, hypokalemia, dizziness, anemia, paresthesia, genital irritation and ulceration	Additive toxicity like hypokalemia and renal damage with IV pentamidine. Increase renal toxicity with other nephrotoxic drugs especialy amphotericin B
Cidofovir	Injection	For resistant CMV, HSV, VZV infections JC and BK virus Children 5 mg/kg once weekly for induction and then suppressive 3 mg/kg once weekly Adults induction 5 mg/kg once weekly and then every other week for suppressive therapy Prehydration with saline needed Proben acid mandatory prior to administration and then 2 and 8 hours after adminsitration	Severe nephrotoxicity (fanconi like syndrome) can occur with <2 doses Contraindicated if creatinine more than 1.5	Nephrotoxicity with other nephrotoxic drugs

TABLE 5: Antiparasitic agents.

Name	*Formulations*	*Dosage, interval and route*	*Adverse effects*	*Drug interactions*
Antimalarials Chloroquine	*Amount of Chloroquine base* Inj: 40 mg/mL Tab: 150, 300 mg Syr: 50 mg/5 mL	*Dosed on the base* 10 mg/kg loading M = 600, then 10 mg/kg after 24 hours and then at 48 hours M = 1,500	Nausea, vomiting, abdominal pain, rash, blurred vision, rarely neuropsychiatric disturbances	Antacids, kaolin decrease absorption of chloroquine. Increase blood digoxin levels.

Contd...

Contd...

Name	*Formulations*	*Dosage, interval and route*	*Adverse effects*	*Drug interactions*
		For prophylaxis: 1 month to 12 years 5 mg/kg, 12–18 years 300 mg once weekly. Start 1 week before entering and 4 weeks after leaving endemic area		Other antimalarials decrease antimalarial effect
Mefloquine	Tab: 250 mg	15 mg/kg loading, then 10 mg/kg 12 hours later M = 1,500 Prophylaxis: Start 1 week before entering malarious area and give weekly, continue for 4 weeks after return from malarious area. 5 mg/kg weekly M = 250	Nausea, vomiting, somnolence, dizziness, rash, neuropsychiatric disturbances including hallucinations disorientation, neuropathy and convulsions	With chloroquine, increase risk of convulsions. Ketoconazole, ampicillin, tetracycline and metclopramide increase levels of mefloquine. Increase cardiotoxicity with quinine, quinidine, digitalis, calcium channel blockers. Decreases blood levels of valproate and efficacy of typhoid vaccine
Quinine	Inj: 300 mg/mL Tab: 100, 300 mg Syr: 100, 150 mg/5 mL	Dosed on salt IV 20 mg/kg (M = 1,400) loading over 4 hours, then 10 mg/kg (M = 700) tds. IV infusion over 4 hours. As soon as possible change to oral. Oral 10 mg/kg tds M = 1,800	Distrubed vision, tinnitus, hearing loss, rash, gastritis, headache. Hypoglycemia and hypotension with IV use. Hemolysis in G6PD deficiency	Antacids and cimetidine reduce absorption of quinine. Reduces serum levels of digoxin
Artesunate	Inj: Vial 60, 150 mg/mL Tab: 50 mg	IV (or IM) 2.4 mg/kg loading and then 2.4 mg/kg 12 hours later and then on day 1, later 2.4 od (children below 20 kg 3 mg/kg) oral 4 mg/kg od	Mild GI disturbances, rarely hemolysis. Ist degree heart block	Drug levels increase by tetracycline, chloroquin, mefloquin and primaquin
Artemether	Inj: 80 mg/mL Tab: 40 mg	IM 3.2 on day 1, later 3.2 od; Oral 1.7 mg/kg twice daily	1st degree heart block, leukopenia, raised liver enzymes,	Increase cardiac toxicity with terfenadine, astemizole,

Contd...

Contd...

Name	*Formulations*	*Dosage, interval and route*	*Adverse effects*	*Drug interactions*
			nausea, vomiting, abdominal cramps, neurotoxicity	quinidine, procainamide, erythromycin, and tricyclic antidepressants. Tetracycline, mefloquine and pyrimethamine interfere with action of drug
Arteether	Inj: 75 mg/mL 1 mL and 2 mL ampoules	Inj IM only. 3 mg/kg od	Nausea, dizziness, vomiting, eosinophilia	As for artemether
Pyrimethamine-sulfadoxine	Tab: Pyrimethamine 25 mg, sulfadoxine 500 mg. Syr: Pyrimethamine 12.5 mg, 25 mg with sulfadoxine 250, 500 mg/5 mL respectively	1.25 mg/kg of the pyrimethamine component M = 75 of pyrimethamine	Unusual bleeding, rash bruising, sore throat, fever, leukopenia, thrombocytopenia, megaloblastic anemia	Antimetabolites, antirheumatics, cotrimoxazole increase bone marrow toxicity
Other parasitic agents Pyrimethamine (PYM) sulfadiazine (SDZ)	Pyrimethamine 25 mg Sulfadiazine 500 mg	Congenital toxoplasmosis Neonates: PYM 1 mg/kg od and SDZ 50 mg/kg bd Infants: PYM 1 mg/kg bd for 3 days and then 1 mg/kg od (M = 25 mg) and SDZ 30–50 mg/kg qds Folinic acid 10–20 mg thrice weekly Children with AIDS related toxoplasmosis PYM 3 mg/kg on day 1 and then 1.25 mg/kg and sulfadizine and SDZ 25 mg/kg qds	PYM: Bone marrow suppression SDZ: Rash, SJS, leukopenia, crystalluria	
Primaquine	Tab: 2.5, 7.5, 15 mg of the base	Dosed on the base 0.25–0.75 mg/kg od. M = 45 mg For G6PD patients: 1–12 yrs 0.5–0.75 mg/kg and 12–18 years 30 mg once in a week for 8 weeks	Nausea, vomiting, weakness, leukopenia, methemoglobinemia	May inhibit chloroquine metabolism. With other bone marrow depressants, increase toxicity

Contd...

Contd...

Name	*Formulations*	*Dosage, interval and route*	*Adverse effects*	*Drug interactions*
Other antiparasitic agents				
Metronidazole	Inj: 5 mg/mL, 100 mL bottles Tab: 200, 400 mg Syr: 100, 200 mg/5 mL Oral gel: 0.5%	Inj: N: 15 mg/kg loading followed 24 hrs later by 7.5 mg/kg/dose bd. Children Anaerobic infections: 7.5 mg/kg tds, amoebiasis 10–15 mg/kg tds M = 1,500 Oral: amoebiasis 10 mg/kg tds Giardiasis and Trichomoniasis: 5 mg/kg tds (for giardiasis also 40 mg/kg od for 3 days) M = 2,000 For *H. pylori* oral 1–6 years 100 mg, 6–12 years 200 mg and 12–18 years 400 mg/dose tds for 14 days with either amoxicillin/omeprazole or clarithromycin/omeprazole	Nausea, tingling, numbness, metallic taste, dark urine, headache, drowsiness, blood dyscrasias, gynecomastia	Increases levels and toxicity of warfarin, phenytoin, lithium. Cimetidine, rifampicin, phenobarbitone increase metronidazole metabolism
Tinidazole	Tab: 300, 500, 600, 1,000 Syr: 75, 150 mg/5 mL	10–15 mg/kg tds, 50 mg/kg stat for giardiasis M = 2,000	Nausea, tingling, numbness, metallic taste, neuropathy, leukopenia, seizures	Synergy with ampicillin, doxycycline and cotrimoxazole.
Secnidazole	Tab: 500, 1,000, 2,000 Syr: 500 mg/5 mL	15 mg/kg bd M = 2,000	Nausea, vomiting, glossitis, metallic taste, skin rash, leukopenia, headache	Increases levels and toxicity of warfarin, phenytoin, lithium. Cimetidine increase secnidazole metabolism
Ornidazole	Inj: 5 mg/mL Tab: 500 mg	40 mg/kg od	As for secnidazole	Increases levels and toxicity of warfarin, increases clearance of 5 fluorouracil

Contd...

Contd...

Name	*Formulations*	*Dosage, interval and route*	*Adverse effects*	*Drug interactions*
Hydroxyquinolones (quinidochlor, diiodohydroxyquinolin, broxyquinolin)	Tab: 250 Oint: 3%	10–15 mg/kg tds M = 2,000	Nausea, headache, dermatitis, diarrhea, goitre	With alcohol, antabuse like effect
Diloxanide furoate	Tab: 500 mg	6–7 mg/kg tds M = 1,500	Nausea, flatulence, itching, urticaria	Synergistic effect with metronidazole and tinidazole
Nitazoxanide	Tab: 200, 500 mg. Syr: 100 mg/5 mL	>1 <5 years 100 mg bd, >5 <10 years 200–250 mg bd, >11 years 500 mg bd	Pain abdomen and hyperhidrosis are most frequent. Nausea, vomiting, Diarrhea, weakness, myalgia, hypotension	Decreases the effect of warfarin.
Dehydroemetine	Inj: 30 mg/mL vials 1, 2 mL	1 mg/kg tds deep IM	Pain at inj site, vomiting, nausea, myalgia, hypotension, cardiac arrythmias	None reported
Piperazine citrate	Tab: 500 mg	50–75 mg/kg od Round worm: Children: 750 mg/year of age, max 4,000. Enterobiasis; 50 mg/kg od for 7 days 75 mg/kg single dose	Diarrhea, rash, incoordination, drowsiness, confusion, vomiting	Increase risk of abnormal movements with phenothiazine antipsychotics
Albendazole	Tab: 200, 400 Syr: 200 mg/5 mL	For intestinal worms: <2 years 200 mg, >2 years 400 mg stat. For giardiasis: 7.5–10 mg/kg bd M = 800 In neurocysticercosis: 15 mg/kg for 2–4 weeks. Take with food. Hydatid disease, echinococcosis: 15 mg/kg daily for 4 weeks. Repeat the dose after 14 days, if required for next such 3 doses.	Gastritis, dizziness, dry mouth, pruritus. Agranulocytosis or leukopenia (rare)	H_2 antagonists increase blood levels of albendazole. Increase action of oral antidiabetic agents. Serum concentrations are reduced by barbiturates, carbamazepine, phenytoin and rifampin

Contd...

Contd...

Name	*Formulations*	*Dosage, interval and route*	*Adverse effects*	*Drug interactions*
		Cutaneous larva migrans: <2 years 10 mg/kg bd for 5 days; 2–12 years 400 mg od for 5 days. Toxocariasis: 2–12 years 10 mg/kg up to maximum of 400 mg; 12–18 years 400 mg twice daily for 5 days		
Mebendazole	Tab: 100 mg Syr: 100 mg/5 mL	Enterobiasis 100 mg stat; other nematodes 100 mg bd. Or 500 mg single dose Cestodes: 200 mg bd for 3 consecutive days. May be repeated after 2 weeks	GI upset, skin rash, hair loss, agranulocytosis, hypospermia	As for albendazole
Pyrantel pamoate	Tab: 250 mg Syr: 250 mg/5 mL	11 mg/kg od M = 1,000 Repeat after 2 weeks. In heavy hookworm infestation, give for 2 successive days	Nausea, vomiting, headache, tenesmus, skin rash, headache, increase in SGOT can cause insomnia	Antagonizes piperazine
Niclosamide	Tab: 500 mg	<2 years 500 mg. 2–6 years 1 g, >7 years 2 g od. Give the dose in 2 divided doses one before breakfast and the rest 1 hour later. *Hymenolepis nana* (dwarf tapeworm): Oral single dose on first day and then od for the next 6 days. Initial day dose for <2, 2–6 and 7–18 years are 500 mg, 1 g and 2 g, respectively. No purgative is needed	Gastritis, diarrhea, skin rash, itching, dizziness, headache	No drug interactions reported

Contd...

Contd...

Name	*Formulations*	*Dosage, interval and route*	*Adverse effects*	*Drug interactions*
Tetramisole	Tab: 150 mg	3 mg/kg od	Gastritis, insomnia, dizziness, agranulocytosis	None clinically significant. Alcohol may cause flushing
Levamisole	Tab: 50, 150 mg Syr: 50 mg/5 mL	3–5 mg/kg od	As for tetramisole	Increase blood conc. of phenytoin and warfarin. Antabuse like reaction with alcohol
Sodium antimony gluconate	Cap: 250 mg	Dosed on the antimony 20 mg/kg IM/IV od	Joint pains, abdominal pain, nausea, anaphylaxis, renal failure, hemolysis with G6PD deficiency	With other nephrotoxic drugs, increase renal toxicity
Praziquantel	Tab: 600 mg	Intestinal cestodes: 10–15 mg/kg od. Neurocysticercosis 15 mg/kg tds	Nausea, abdominal pain, fever, dizziness, sedation, sweating, eosinophilia	Cimetidine increase and carbamezapene and phenytoin reduce blood levels of praziquantel
Pentamidine	Inj: 300 mg	2–4 mg/kg od IM/IV M = 300	Fatigue, metallic taste, hypotension, itching, vomiting, hypoglycaemia, leukopenia, thrombocytopenia	Increase chances of bleeding with anticoagulants, increase marrow suppression with other bone marrow toxicant drugs
Diethyl carbamazine	Tab: 50, 100 mg. Syr: 50, 120 mg/5 mL	1–2 mg/kg tds. For filariasis and visceral larva migrans, start with low dose of 0.3 mg/kg on day 1 and increase over 3 days. M = 300	Nausea, anorexia, skin rash, urticaria, fatigue, headache, dizziness	No known interactions
Ivermectin	Tab: 3, 6 mg	0.15–0.2 mg/kg single dose M = 1,200 Filariasis 150 μg/kg once a year for 10 years. If symptoms recur, then dose is given every 3 months instead of	Nausea, vomiting, constipation, abdominal pain, fatigue	Increases the effect of warfarin (increased INR)

Contd...

Contd...

Name	*Formulations*	*Dosage, interval and route*	*Adverse effects*	*Drug interactions*
		once a year. For mass treatments single dose of albendazole 400 mg + ivermectin 200 μg/kg every year. Scabies and pediculosis 200 μg/kg stat		
Benzyl benzoate	Emulsion: 25%	Apply over entire body except head and face once daily after bath for 3 days. Allow to remain on the body for 24 hours. Pediculosis shampoo, rinse, and dry hair and scalp well before applying benzyl benzoate. Rinse thoroughly and dry. After rinsing and drying, use a fine-toothed comb (less than 0.3 mm between the teeth) to remove any remaining nits	Irritation of eyes and mucous membrane, hypersensitivity	None reported
Permethrin	Lotion: 1%, 5%	For scabies apply all over body Single topical application of up to: 1 tube for children >12 years. Half a tube for children aged 6–12 years. A quarter of a tube for children aged 1–5 years. An eighth of a tube for children aged 2 months to 1 year. If necessary a second application may be given not less than 7 days after the initial application	Transient burning and stinging sensation, pruritus, tingling, mild erythema	None reported

Contd...

Contd...

Name	*Formulations*	*Dosage, interval and route*	*Adverse effects*	*Drug interactions*
		Apply to whole body excluding head. Wash off after 8–12 hours. Pediculosis capitis (head lice) (cream rinse) Apply to clean damp hair, leave on for 10 minutes, rinse and dry		
Crotamiton	Lotion, cream: 10%	After patient has a warm bath and dried, rub well into the entire body surface excluding face and scalp. Repeat od preferably in the evening for 3–5 days	Skin irritation allergic reactions	None reported

Note: *Abbreviations for Tables 1 to 5:*

[bd: twice a day; BP: blood pressure; Cap: capsule (amount per Capsule); CNS: central nervous system; CPK: creatine phosphokinase; Cre: cream (amount % w/w); CSF: cerebrospinal fluid; d: day(s) dosage is in mg/kg/dose unless otherwise stated; Drp: drops (amount per mL); DT: dispersible tablet (amount per tablet); GI: gastrointestinal; G6PD: glucose-6-phosphate dehydrogenase; G6PDD: glucose-6-phosphate dehydrogenase deficiency; IM: intramuscular; IV: intravenous; Inj: injection (amount per vial or per mL as stated); Lot: lotion (amount % w/w); LRTI: lower respiratory tract infection; M: maximum (ceiling) dose (per day); MAO: monoamine oxidase; MDR: multidrug-resistant; N: newborn; od: once in a day; NSAIDs: nonsteroidal anti-inflammatory drugs; Oint: ointment/cream (amount % w/w); P: premature baby; qds: four times a day; PCP: *Pneumocystis carinii pneumonia*; PPI: proton-pump inhibitor; SGOT: serum glutamic-oxaloacetic transaminase; SGPT: serum glutamic pyruvic transaminase; Syp: syrup/suspension (amount per 5 mL); Tab: tablet (amount per tablet); TB: tuberculosis; tds: thrice in a day; UTI: urinary tract infection; XDR: extensively drug-resistant]

RECOMMENDED READING

1. Davies EG, Elliman DAC, Hart CA, et al. Manual of Childhood Infections, 2nd edition. Philipadia: WB Saunders; 2002.
2. Gilbert DN. Sanford Guide for Antimicrobial Therapy 2018, 48th edition. Sperryville, VA: Sanford Guide; 2018.
3. IAP. (2018). IAP Drug Formulary 2019. [online] Available from http://iapdrugformulary.com/ [Accessed January, 2019].
4. Moon TD, Oberelman RA. Antiparasitic Therapy in Children. Peditar Clin N Am. 2005;52:917-48.
5. Passi Publication. (2006). Drug Index. [online] Available from http://www.passi.org/indexes.html [Accessed January, 2019].

Index

B

C

D

E

F

G

H

I

J

K

L

M

O

P

T

U

V

W

Y

Z